Handbook of
PULMONARY AND CRITICAL CARE MEDICINE

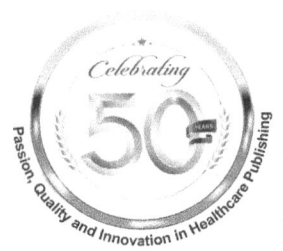

Handbook of
PULMONARY AND CRITICAL CARE MEDICINE

Second Edition

Editor-in-Chief
SK Jindal MD FAMS FNCCP FICS FCCP
Emeritus Professor (Pulmonary Medicine)
Postgraduate Institute of Medical Education and Research
Chandigarh, India
Medical Director
Jindal Clinics, Chandigarh

Foreword
Randeep Guleria

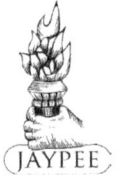

JAYPEE BROTHERS MEDICAL PUBLISHERS
The Health Sciences Publisher
New Delhi | London | Panama

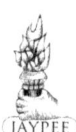 **Jaypee Brothers Medical Publishers (P) Ltd**

Headquarters
Jaypee Brothers Medical Publishers (P) Ltd
4838/24, Ansari Road, Daryaganj
New Delhi 110 002, India
Phone: +91-11-43574357
Fax: +91-11-43574314
Email: jaypee@jaypeebrothers.com

Overseas Offices

J.P. Medical Ltd
83 Victoria Street, London
SW1H 0HW (UK)
Phone: +44 20 3170 8910
Fax: +44 (0)20 3008 6180
Email: info@jpmedpub.com

Jaypee-Highlights Medical Publishers Inc
City of Knowledge, Bld. 235, 2nd Floor
Clayton, Panama City, Panama
Phone: +1 507-301-0496
Fax: +1 507-301-0499
Email: cservice@jphmedical.com

Jaypee Brothers Medical Publishers (P) Ltd
Bhotahity, Kathmandu, Nepal
Phone: +977-9741283608
Email: kathmandu@jaypeebrothers.com

Website: www.jaypeebrothers.com
Website: www.jaypeedigital.com

© 2019, Jaypee Brothers Medical Publishers

The views and opinions expressed in this book are solely those of the original contributor(s)/author(s) and do not necessarily represent those of editor(s) of the book.

All rights reserved. No part of this publication may be reproduced, stored or transmitted in any form or by any means, electronic, mechanical, photocopying, recording or otherwise, without the prior permission in writing of the publishers.

All brand names and product names used in this book are trade names, service marks, trademarks or registered trademarks of their respective owners. The publisher is not associated with any product or vendor mentioned in this book.

Medical knowledge and practice change constantly. This book is designed to provide accurate, authoritative information about the subject matter in question. However, readers are advised to check the most current information available on procedures included and check information from the manufacturer of each product to be administered, to verify the recommended dose, formula, method and duration of administration, adverse effects and contraindications. It is the responsibility of the practitioner to take all appropriate safety precautions. Neither the publisher nor the author(s)/editor(s) assume any liability for any injury and/or damage to persons or property arising from or related to use of material in this book.

This book is sold on the understanding that the publisher is not engaged in providing professional medical services. If such advice or services are required, the services of a competent medical professional should be sought.

Every effort has been made where necessary to contact holders of copyright to obtain permission to reproduce copyright material. If any have been inadvertently overlooked, the publisher will be pleased to make the necessary arrangements at the first opportunity. The **CD/DVD-ROM** (if any) provided in the sealed envelope with this book is complimentary and free of cost. **Not meant for sale.**

Inquiries for bulk sales may be solicited at: jaypee@jaypeebrothers.com

Handbook of Pulmonary and Critical Care Medicine

First Edition: 2012

Second Edition: **2019**

ISBN 978-93-5270-615-0

Dedicated to
The memories of my parents who made a doctor out of me, Dr SK Malik who handed over the reins to me and Dr Dheeraj Gupta, a trusted colleague and friend who tirelessly helped in shaping this specialty.

Contributors

AG Ghoshal MD DNB FCCP
Director
National Allergy Asthma Bronchitis Institute
Kolkata, West Bengal, India

AK Janmeja MD
Former Professor and Head
Department of Pulmonary Medicine
Government Medical College
Chandigarh, India

AN Aggarwal MD DM
Professor and Head
Department of Pulmonary Medicine
Postgraduate Institute of Medical
Education and Research
Chandigarh, India

Abha Chandra MD
Professor and Head
Department of Cardiothoracic and
Vascular Surgery
Sri Venkateswara Institute of Medical
Sciences
Tirupati, Andhra Pradesh, India

Abinash Singh Paul MD DM
Consultant Pulmonologist
Life Line Hospital
Dubai, UAE

Aditya Jindal DNB DM FCCP
Consultant Interventional Pulmonology
and Intensivist
Jindal Clinics, Chandigarh, India

Ajay Handa MD DNB DM FCCP FAPS
Senior Advisor (Medicine and Pulmonary
Medicine)
Professor of Internal Medicine
Rajiv Gandhi University of Health
Sciences (RGUHS), Bengaluru
Command Hospital Air Force
Bengaluru, Karnataka, India

Ajmal Khan MD DM
Assistant Professor
Department of Pulmonary Medicine
Sanjay Gandhi Postgraduate Institute
of Medical Education and Research
Lucknow, Uttar Pradesh, India

Alladi Mohan MD
Chief
Division of Pulmonary, Critical Care and
Sleep Medicine
Professor and Head
Department of Medicine
Sri Venkateswara Institute of Medical
Sciences
Tirupati, Andhra Pradesh, India

Amanjit Bal MD DNB MAMS
Additional Professor
Department of Histopathology
Postgraduate Institute of Medical
Education and Research
Chandigarh, India

Arjun Srinivasan MD DM
Pulomonary and Critical Care Medicine
Kovai Medical Center and Hospital (KMCH)
Specialty Hospital
Chennai, Tamil Nadu, India

Arun S Shet MD
Department of Medical Oncology
St John's National Academy of Health
Sciences
Bengaluru, Karnataka, India

Arunabh Talwar MD FCCP
Department of Pulmonary
Critical Care and Sleep Medicine
North Shore University Hospital
Manhasset, New York
Professor of Medicine
Hofstra North Shore- LIJ School of Medicine
New Hyde Park, New York, USA

Arunaloke Chakrabarti MD
Professor and Head
Department of Medical Microbiology
Postgraduate Institute of Medical
Educationand and Research
Chandigarh, India

Arvind H Kate MD
Institute of Pulmonology
Medical Research and Development
Mumbai, Maharashtra, India

Ashim Das MD
Professor
Department of Histopathology
Postgraduate Institute of Medical
Education and Research
Chandigarh, India

Ashok Shah MD
Former Director Professor
Department of Pulmonary Medicine,
Vallabhbhai Patel Chest Institute
New Delhi, India

Atul C Mehta MBBS FACP FCCP
Department of Pulmonary Medicine
Cleveland Clinic
Cleveland, Ohio, USA

B Vijayalakshmi Devi MD
Additional Professor
Department of Radiodiagnosis
Sri Venkateswara Institute of Medical
Sciences
Tirupati, Andhra Pradesh, India

Baishakhi Ghosh MD
Research Student
Chest Research Foundation, Pune
Research Scholar
Symbiosis International University
Pune, Maharashtra, India

Balamugesh T MD DM FCCP
Professor
Department of Pulmonary Medicine
Christian Medical College
Vellore, Tamil Nadu, India

Basil Varkey MD FRCP FCCP
Professor Emeritus of Medicine
Medical College of Wisconsin
Milwaukee, Wisconsin, USA

Bharat Bhushan Sharma MD
Assistant Professor
Pulmonary and Allergy Division
Sawai Man Singh (SMS) Medical College
Jaipur, Rajasthan, India

Bill Brashier DTCD
Former Head
Academic Clinical and Molecular Research
Chest Research Foundation
Pune, Maharashtra, India

C Ravindran MD DTCD MBA
Professor and Head
Pulmonary Medicine
DM Wayanad Institute of Medical Sciences
Calicut, Kerala, India

Carmen Luraschi-Monjagatta MD
University of Southern California
Keck School of Medicine of USC
Los Angeles, California, USA

Chandramani Panjabi MD
Head, Respiratory Medicine
Mata Chanan Devi Hospital
New Delhi, India

Charles Feldman MB BCh PhD DSc
Department of Internal Medicine
University of the Witwatersrand Medical
School
Parktown, Johannesburg, South Africa

Charles Peng MD
Pulmonary, Critical Care and Sleep
Medicine Fellow
Pulmonary Hypertension Center
Icahn School of Medicine at Mount Sinai
Mount Sinai Beth Israel
New York City, New York, USA

D Behera MD FCCP
Professor
Department of Pulmonary Medicine
Postgraduate Institute of Medical
Education and Research
Chandigarh, India

D Robert McCaffree
MD MSHA Master FCCP
Regents' Professor of Medicine Pulmonary
Disease and Critical Care Section
University of Oklahoma
Health Science Center
Oklahoma City, Oklahoma, USA

Contributors

Daniel E Banks MD MS
Professor
Department of Medicine
Uniformed Services University of Health Sciences
Bethesda, Maryland, USA

David Honeybourne MD
Consultant Physician and Clinical Director
Honorary Clinical Reader in Respiratory Medicine and Biological Sciences
Department of Respiratory Medicine
Birmingham Heartlands Hospital
Birmingham, UK

Deepak Aggarwal MD
Assistant Professor
Department of Pulmonary Medicine
Government Medical College
Chandigarh, India

Devasahayam J Christopher MD FCCP FRCP
Professor and Head
Department of Respiratory Medicine
Christian Medical College
Vellore, Tamil Nadu, India

Dheeraj Gupta MD DM
Former Professor
Department of Pulmonary Medicine
Postgraduate Institute of Medical Education and Research
Chandigarh, India

Dhruva Chaudhry MD DM
Professor and Head
Department of Pulmonary and Critical Care Medicine
Pt Bhagwat Dayal Sharma Postgraduate Institute of Medical Sciences
Rohtak, Haryana, India

Dilip V Maydeo MD
Professor of TB and Respiratory Diseases
KJ Somaiya Medical College
Mumbai, Maharashtra, India

Dinkar Bhasin MD
Deaprtment of Medicine
All India Institute of Medical Sciences
New Delhi, India

G Gaude MD
Professor and Head
Department of Pulmonary Medicine
Jawaharlal Nehru Medical College
Belgaum, Karnataka, India

GA D'Souza MD
Professor and Head
Department of Pulmonary Medicine
St John's Medical College
Bengaluru, Karnataka, India

GC Khilnani MD
Professor
Department of Pulmonary, Critical care and Sleep Medicine
All India Institute of Medical Sciences
New Delhi, India

Gaurav Prakash MD DM
Associate Professor
Bone Marrow Transplantation
Department of Internal Medicine
Postgraduate Institute of Medical Education and Research
Chandigarh, India

Gautam Ahluwalia MD FAPS FICP FIACM
Professor
Department of Medicine
Dayanand Medical College and Hospital
Ludhiana, Punjab, India

Girish Raju MD
Department of Medical Oncology
St John's National Academy of Health Sciences
Bengaluru, Karnataka, India

Gwen Skloot MD
Associate Professor of Medicine
Ichan School of Medicine at Mount Sinai
New York City, New York, USA

Gyanendra Agrawal MD DM
Consultant Pulmonologist
Jaypee Group of Hospitals
Noida, Uttar Pradesh, India

H Shigemitsu MD FCCP
Professor of Medicine
Chief, Division of Pulmonary and Critical Care Medicine
Fellowship Program Director
University of Nevada, School of Medicine
Las Vegas, Nevada, USA

Harakh V Dedhia MBBS
Former Professor of Medicine
Section of Pulmonary and Critical Care Medicine
West Virginia University School of Medicine
Morgantown, West Virginia, USA

Inderpaul Singh Sehgal MD DM
Assistant Professor
Department of Pulmonary Medicine
Postgraduate Institute of Medical Education and Research
Chandigarh, India

Indu Verma PhD
Professor
Department of Biochemistry
Postgraduate Institute of Medical Education and Research
Chandigarh, India

Javid Ahmad Malik MD DM FCCP
Additional Professor and Head
Department of Pulmonary Medicine
SKIMS Medical College
Srinagar, Jammu and Kashmir, India

Jaydeep Odhwani
BJ Medical College
Ahmedabad, Gujarat, India

Jean I Keddissi MD
Professor of Medicine
Pulmonary Disease and Critical Care Section
University of Oklahoma Health Science Center
Oklahoma City, Oklahoma, USA

Jeba S Jenifer MD Dip Pal Med
Associate Professor
Palliative Care Unit
Christian Medical College
Vellore, Tamil Nadu, India

Jyothi E MD DTCD
Assistant Professor
Department of Pulmonary Medicine
Government Medical College
Kozhikode, Kerala, India

Kalpalatha K Guntupalli
MD FCCP FCCM MACP
Professor of Medicine
Chief, Pulmonary, Critical Care and Sleep Medicine
Baylor College of Medicine
Houston, Texas, USA

Karakontaki F MD
Sismanoglio General Hospital
Athens, Greece

Karan Madan MD DM
Assistant Professor
Department of Pulmonary, Critical Care and Sleep Medicine
All India Institute of Medical Sciences
New Delhi, India

Kripesh Ranjan Sarmah MD MNAMS
Assistant Professor
Department of Pulmonary Medicine
Guwahati Medical College
Guwahati, Assam, India

Krishna K Singh PhD
Senior Technical Team Lead
Siemens Healthcare Diagnostics
Tarrytown, New York, USA

Kumar Utsav MD
BJ Medical College
Ahmedabad, Gujarat, India

Lakhbir K Dhaliwal MD
Former Professor and Head
Department of Obstetrics and Gynecology
Postgraduate Institute of Medical Education and Research
Chandigarh

Lakshmi Mudambi MD
Pulmonary-Critical Care Medicine
Baylor College of Medicine
Houston, Texas, USA

Liesel D'silva MD DETRD
Senior Medical Advisor
Specialist in Respiratory Medicine
Mumbai, Maharashtra, India

Contributors

Liziamma George MD FCCP
Associate Professor of Clinical Medicine
Weill Medical College
Director, Medical Intensive Care Unit
New York Methodist Hospital
Brooklyn, New York, USA

Madhur Kalyan MSc
Senior Research Fellow
Department of Biochemistry
Postgraduate Institute of Medical
Education and Research
Chandigarh, India

Malay Sarkar MD
Professor
Department of Pulmonary Medicine
Indira Gandhi Medical College
Shimla, Himachal Pradesh, India

Mamta Kalra PhD
Senior Scientist Immatics US Inc
Houston, Texas, USA

Manabu Nonaka MD
Nippon Medical School
Tokyo, Japan

Mark Astiz MD
Weil Medical College, New York
Methodist Hospital
Brooklyn, New York, USA

Miyuki Hayashi MD
Nippon Medical School
Tokyo, Japan

Monica Barne MBBS
Chest Research Foundation
Pune, Maharashtra, India

N Goel MD
Assistant Professor
Department of Pulmonary Medicine
Vallabhbhai Patel Chest Institute
University of Delhi
New Delhi, India

Nagarjuna V Maturu MD DM
Pulmonologist and Somnologist
Yashoda Hospitals
Hyderabad, Telangana, India

Navneet Singh MD DM FACP FCCP FICS
Additional Professor
Department of Pulmonary Medicine
Postgraduate Institute of Medical
Education and Research
Chandigarh, India

Ngozi Orjioke MD
University of Southern California
School of Medicine
Los Angeles, California, USA

Nikhil C Sarangdhar MBBS
Assistant Professor
Department of TB and Respiratory Diseases
KJ Somaiya Medical College
Mumbai, Maharashtra, India

Nikhil Gupta MD
Assistant Professor
Department of Medicine
Era's Lucknow Medical College
Lucknow, Uttar Pradesh, India

Nusrat Shafiq MD DM
Additional Professor
Department of Pharmacology
Postgraduate Institute of Medical
Education and Research
Chandigarh, India

Om P Sharma MD
Former Professor of Medicine
Keck School of Medicine
Division of Pulmonary and Critical Care
Medicine
University of Southern California
Los Angeles, California, USA

P Baruwa MD
Senior Consultant
Tuberculosis and Respiratory Medicine
Gauhati, Assam, India

PR Mohapatra MD
Professor and Head
Department of Pulmonary Medicine
All India Institute of Medical Sciences
Bhubaneswar, Odisha, India

PS Shankar MD FRCP FAMS DSc DLitt
Emeritus Professor of Medicine
Rajiv Gandhi University of Health
Sciences, Bengaluru
SMV Medical College, Puducherry
KBN Institute of Medical Sciences
Kalaburagi, Karnataka, India

PS Tampi MD DM
Consultant
Bombay Hospital and Medical Research
Centre
Mumbai, Maharashtra, India

Pankaj Malhotra MD MAMS
Professor
Department of Internal Medicine
Postgraduate Institute of Medical
Education and Research
Chandigarh, India

Parameswaran Nair MD PhD
Professor of Medicine
Division of Respirology
McMaster University
Hamilton, Ontario, Canada

Peter J Barnes FRS FMedSci
Margaret Turner-Warwick Professor of
Medicine
Head of Respiratory Medicine
Imperial College London
Airway Disease Section
National Heart and Lung Institute
London, UK

Polychronopoulos V MD PhD FCCP
Director
3rd Chest Department
Sismanoglio General Hospital
Athens, Greece

Prahlad Rai Gupta MD DM
Former Professor
Department of Pulmonary Medicine
Sawai Man Singh (SMS) Medical College
Jaipur, Rajasthan, India
(Consultant, Shalby Hospital, Jaipur)

Pralay Sarkar MD DM
Assistant Professor
Department of Pulmonary and Critical
Care Medicine
Baylor College of Medicine
Houston, Texas, USA

Prashant Chhajed MD DNB
Director of Pulmonology and Center for
Sleep Disorders
Fortis Hiranandani Hospital
Mumbai, Maharashtra, India

Preyas Vaidya MD
Institute of Pulmonolgy
Medical Research and Development
Mumbai, Maharashtra, India

Preeti Verma MD
Department of Obstetrics and Gynecology
Chandigarh, India

R Caroli MD
Consultant Pulmonologist
Fortis Hospital
Noida, Uttar Pradesh, India

Rachael A Evans MB ChB MRCP (UK) PhD
Division of Respiratory Medicine
West Park Healthcare Centre
University of Toronto
Toronto, Ontario, Canada

Raja Dhar MD MRCP MSc
Consultant Pulmonary and Critical Care
Medicine
Fortis Hospital
Kolkata, West Bengal, India

Rajendra Prasad
MD DTCD FAMS FCCP FNCCP
Head
Department of Pulmonary Medicine
Era's Lucknow Medical College
Lucknow, Uttar Pradesh, India

Rajesh N Solanki MD FNCCP
Professor, Head, Unit II
Department of Pulmonary Medicine
BJ Medical College
Ahmedabad, Gujarat, India

Contributors

Rama Murthy Sakamuri PhD
Post-Doctoral Fellow
Department of Pathology
New York University Langone Medical Centre
New York City, New York, USA

Richa Gupta MD
Assistant Professor
Department of Pulmonary Medicine
Christian Medical College and Hospital
Vellore, Tamil Nadu, India

Ritesh Agarwal MD DM
Professor
Department of Pulmonary Medicine
Postgraduate Institute of Medical Education and Research
Chandigarh, India

Roger S Goldstein
MB ChB FRCP FCRP FCCP
Department of Respiratory Medicine
West Park Healthcare Centre
Toronto, Ontario, Canada

Romica Latawa PhD
Department of Biochemistry
Postgraduate Institute of Medical Education and Research
Chandigarh, India

Ronald Anderson PhD
Division of Pulmonology
Department of Internal Medicine
University of the Witwatersrand
Johannesburg, South Africa

Roxana Sulica MD
Director
Pulmonary Hypertension Program
Assistant Professor of Medicine
Icahn School of Medicine at Mount Sinai
Mount Sinai Beth Israel
New York City, New York, USA

Rubal Patel MD
Tift Regional Medical Center
Tifton, Georgia, USA

Ruby Pawankar MD PhD
Professor of Rhinology and Allergy
Department of Otolaryngology
Nippon Medical School
Tokyo, Japan

Ruchi Bansal MD
Department of Medicine
Divison of Pulmonary, Critical Care and Sleep Medicine
New York Methodist Hospital
Brooklyn, New York, USA

S Kashyap MD
Professor and Head
Department of Pulmonary Medicine
Director
Kalpana Chawla Government Medical College
Karnal, Haryana, India

SK Jindal
MD FAMS FNCCP FICS FCCP
Emeritus Professor (Pulmonary Medicine)
Postgraduate Institute of Medical Education and Research
Chandigarh
Medical Director
Jindal Clinics, Chandigarh, India

Sahajal Dhooria MD DM
Assistant Professor
Department of Pulmonary Medicine
Postgraduate Institute of Medical Education and Research
Chandigarh, India

Samir Malhotra MD
Professor
Department of Pharmacology
Postgraduate Institute of Medical Education and Research
Chandigarh, India

Sanjay Jain MD
Professor
Department of Internal Medicine
Postgraduate Institute of Medical Education and Research
Chandigarh, India

Sanjeev Mehta MD
Consultant
Lilavati Hospital, Bhartiya Arogya Nidhi
Hospital Bandra (West)
Mumbai, Maharashtra, India

Sean E Hesselbacher MD
Baylor College of Medicine
Ben Taub General Hospital
Houston, Texas, USA

Shingo Yamanishi
Nippon Medical School
Tokyo, Japan

Shu Hashimoto MD PhD
Nihon University
Tokyo, Japan

Sidney S Braman MD FCCP
Professor of Medicine
Ichan School of Medicine at Mount Sinai
New York City, New York, USA

Sneha Limaye MBBS
Research Fellow
Chest Research Foundation
Pune, Maharashtra, India

Srinivas Rajagopala MD DM
Assistant Professor of Chest Diseases
Department of Medicine
St John's Medical College and Hospital
Bengaluru, Karnataka, India

Stagaki E MD
Consultant
3rd Chest Department
Sismanoglio General Hospital
Athens, Greece

Stuti Agarwal PhD
Senior Research Fellow
Department of Biochemistry
Postgraduate Institute of Medical
Education and Research
Chandigarh, India

Subhash Varma MD
Professor and Head
Department of Internal Medicine
Postgraduate Institute of Medical
Education and Research
Chandigarh, India

Suman Laal PhD
Associate Professor
Department of Pathology
New York University
Langone Medical Centre
Veterans Affairs New York Harbor
Healthcare System
New York City, New York, USA

Sundeep Salvi MD DNB PhD FCCP
Director
Chest Research Foundation
Pune, Maharashtra, India

Surendra K Sharma MD PhD
Ex-Professor and Head
Department of Medicine
All India Institute of Medical Sciences
New Delhi, India

Uma Devraj MD
Associate Professor
Department of Pulmonary Medicine
St John's Medical College
Bengaluru, Karnataka, India

Umesh Jindal MD
Senior Consultant and Director
Jindal IVF and Sant Memorial Nursing Home
Chandigarh, India

VK Jindal PhD
Honorary Professor of Physics
Advanced Centre for Physics
Panjab University
Chandigarh, India

VK Vijayan MD PhD DSc FAMS
Advisor to Director-General
Indian Council of Medical Research (ICMR)
Bhopal Memorial Hospital and Research
Centre and National Institute for Research
in Environmental Health
Bhopal, Madhya Pradesh, India

VR Pattabhi Raman MD
Consultant Pulmonologist
Kovai Medical Center and Hospital
Coimbatore, Tamil Nadu, India

Vijay Hadda MD
Assistant Professor
Department of Pulmonary, Critical Care
and Sleep Medicine
All India Institute of Medical Sciences
New Delhi, India

Vikram Jaggi MD DNB
Medical Director
Asthma Chest Allergy Centres
New Delhi, India

Virendra Singh MD
Consultant Pulmonary Physician
Asthma Bhawan
Jaipur, Rajasthan, India

Vishwanath Gella MD DM
Senior Consultant Pulmonologist
Continental Hospitals
Hyderabad, Telangana, India

Walter G Shakespeare MD
Division of Pulmonary and Critical Care Medicine
Baylor College of Medicine
Houston, Texas, USA

William J Martin Jr MD
Associate Director
National Institute for Environmental Health Sciences
Director
Office of Translational Research
National Institutes of Health
North Carolina, USA

Zeenat Safdar MD FACP FCCP
Associate Professor of Medicine
Director
Baylor Pulmonary Hypertension Center
Pulmonary and Critical Care Medicine
Baylor College of Medicine
Houston, Texas, USA

Foreword

It is indeed a pleasure to write a foreword to this very useful *Handbook of Pulmonary and Critical Care Medicine* (2nd edition) by Professor SK Jindal. In my mind, this is something that is needed not only for students but also for internists and specialists as well. Pulmonary and critical care medicine is a rapidly changing field of medicine and one of the fastest growing specialties. For everyone, this handbook is a ready reckoner and something which we all should have on our desks. Often a clinical or a busy student needs to have a readily available source to clarify problems or to help in being sure about the diagnosis or management strategy. This handbook is ideally suited for such a need. It has a wealth of up-to-date knowledge which is easy to access. It is concise and very user friendly. It covers multiple areas including pathophysiology, radiology and clinical management in an integrated manner and is therefore easy to read and refer to.

Being a teacher for now more than 30 years, I have seen how rapidly and radically pulmonary and critical care medicine has evolved. From being a tuberculosis driven specialty, it has become a specialty which has so much of internal medicine and has evolved with new areas like sleep medicine and interventional pulmonology, now considered an integral part of "pulmonary medicine". Recognizing this, we now have a very active DM program in "pulmonary medicine" which is one of the most sought after program by postgraduates. Also, there has been an exponential increase in medical knowledge over the last 20 years. Some feel that this has led to an enormous accumulation of knowledge and multiple options being available, without a clarity as to what is ideal and what is best for the patient. It is important for both internists and specialists to stay in touch with the changing times. This book is therefore essential in today's time.

I would like to take this opportunity to congratulate the authors and Professor SK Jindal for coming out with this excellent handbook and greatly appreciate the hard work that has been put in writing this book.

Randeep Guleria
MD DM FAMS
Padma Shree and B C Roy Awardee (Eminent Medical Person)
Director and CEO
All India Institute of Medical Sciences
New Delhi, India

Preface to the Second Edition

'No bubble is so iridescent or floats longer than that blown by the successful teacher'
William Osler, 1911

There have been rapid advances in the field of medicine in the last few years but the three most significant developments in India and several other countries relate to the fast expansion of drugs and devices for diagnosis and treatment of diseases as well in the numbers of medical manpower. This has been particularly so in case of the specialties such as Pulmonary and Critical Care Medicine. In India for example, there have been introduction of post-doctoral DM courses in the subject at the super-specialty level at several new centers. These developments have created, at least temporarily, a relative shortage of resources and lack of standardization. There also exists an imbalance between the demand for and availability of good teaching and learning resources. It is true that there is an enormous amount of knowledge available on the internet and various publications which have increased in an exponential fashion. Caught with contradictory and sometimes antagonistic information, a student finds it often confusing and sometimes misguiding. It is therefore important to maintain the credibility of the source of information.

In medicine, a textbook is usually the most credible source since it contains the distilled and critical information which has stood the test of time as well as the standards of practice. Moreover, a good textbook contains chapters contributed by eminent and experienced teachers of different subjects. Our *Textbook of Pulmonary and Critical Care Medicine* adequately fulfils those criteria. But it requires time and focussed attention to absorb the contents of the textbook which is not often feasible in a busy clinical practice when quick decisions are needed. *Handbook of Pulmonary and Critical Care Medicine* which contains the concise information on important subjects serves the purpose. It is a summarized version of the Textbook published last year. Some of the important chapters of the textbook had to be excluded from this abbreviated edition because of the limitation of total page requirement. I am sure that the students and medical practitioners including the pulmonary physicians will find it easy to carry as a *'vade mecum'*—it should serve as a pocket-reference in their day-to-day practice.

SK Jindal

Preface to the First Edition

"The physician ought to know literature.... To be able to understand or to explain what he reads".
Isidore of Seville (570–636)

The specialty of Pulmonary and Critical Care Medicine has quickly grown in size and expanded in scope in a short span of time. So also has increased the need of a wider availability of reliable, authoritative and multidimensional educational resources in the subject. Today's pulmonologists are required to know a lot more about systemic illnesses and sister-specialties, besides the primary diseases of the lungs. Pulmonary critical care and invasive interventions have also become essential in pulmonary practice.

It is less than a year when the *Textbook of Pulmonary and Critical Care Medicine* edited by ourselves was first published. Since then, there has been a growing demand to come with an abridged version for convenience and easy readability. This handbook is an effort in that direction to enable the busy and ever on-the-run students and practitioners to quickly go through the contents. Needless to say that the postgraduates as well as the students need to consult the textbook for a more comprehensive and in-depth knowledge of the subject.

For purposes of brevity, it was not possible to include all the chapters in the handbook. For the same reason, the bibliography as well as a large number of figures and tables of the original chapters were excluded from the handbook. The handbook, however, not just serves the purpose of quick browsing of the contents but also provides an opportunity to read the carefully dissected factual information of the subjects. I do hope that the readers will find it useful and informative.

SK Jindal

Acknowledgments

I am thankful to Drs Suhail Raoof and PS Shankar as well as my departmental colleagues Drs D Behera, AN Aggarwal, Ritesh Agarwal, Navneet Singh, Sahajal Dhooria and Inderpaul Singh Sehgal who had contributed and edited the 2nd edition of *Textbook of Pulmonary and Critical Care Medicine*—the main source of this Handbook even though myself and my son, Dr Aditya Jindal take the onus of abridging. I am also obliged to a large number of friends and eminent authors from across the globe to spare their time with valuable contributions.

I greatly appreciate the help rendered my erstwhile secretary, Ms Manju Aggarwal in the preparation of the manuscript and M/s Jaypee Brothers Medical Publishers (P) Ltd, New Delhi, India in taking the challenge of publication.

Contents

1. **Introduction**   1
   SK Jindal
   - History   1
   - Respiratory System Function   2
   - Ventilation-Perfusion (V/Q) Relationships   2
   - Respiratory Defenses   3

2. **Applied Respiratory Physics**   4
   SK Jindal, VK Jindal
   - Atom, Element, Molecule, and Compound   4
   - Molecular Movement   5
   - Atomic and Molecular Weights   5
   - Physical Properties of Gases   5
   - Gas Laws   8
   - Gas Solution and Tension   10
   - Vapor   10
   - Expression of Gas Volumes and Pressures   11
   - Flow of Gases   11
   - Deposition   13
   - Diffusion   13

3. **History and Physical Examination**   15
   Prahlad Rai Gupta
   - History Taking   15
   - History of Treatment   17
   - Physical Examination   18

4. **Pulmonary Function Tests**   22
   AN Aggarwal
   - Spirometry   22
   - Peak Expiratory Flow   25
   - Static Lung Volumes   26
   - Diffusing Capacity of Lungs   27
   - Exercise Testing   28
   - Other Tests   30

5. **Interpretation of Arterial Blood Gases and Acid–Base Abnormalities**   32
   Aditya Jindal
   - Basic Concepts   33
   - Overview of Acid–Base Pathophysiology in the Body   33
   - Types of Acid–Base Disorders   34
   - Anion Gap   36
   - Acid–Base Disorders   37

6. **Tuberculosis: Overview** — 40
   Stuti Agarwal, Romica Latawa, Indu Verma
   - Route and Spread of Infection   40
   - Mycobacterial Groups   41
   - Mycobacterial Identification   42
   - Mycobacterial Drug Resistance   43

7. **Immunology and Pathogenesis** — 44
   Madhur Kalyan, Krishna K Singh, Indu Verma
   - Mycobacterium Tuberculosis Infection and Overview of Immunopathogenesis   44
   - Immune Responses to Tuberculosis   46

8. **Pulmonary Tuberculosis: Clinical Features and Diagnosis** — 50
   S Kashyap, Malay Sarkar
   - Postprimary Pulmonary Tuberculosis   50
   - Symptoms and Signs   51
   - Tuberculosis in the Elderly   52
   - Miliary Tuberculosis   52
   - HIV and Tuberculosis   53
   - Pleural Effusion   53
   - Paradoxical Response   53
   - Physical Examination   53
   - Diagnosis of Tuberculosis   54
   - Extrapulmonary Tuberculosis   57

9. **Molecular Diagnosis of Tuberculosis** — 58
   Rama Murthy Sakamuri, Mamta Kalra, Indu Verma, Suman Laal
   - Diagnosis of Tuberculosis: Beyond the Microscopy   58

10. **Management of Tuberculosis** — 63
    D Behera
    - Prevention of Drug Resistance   63
    - Early Bactericidal Activity   64
    - Sterilizing Action   64
    - New Patients   65
    - Previously Treated Cases   67

11. **Prevention of Tuberculosis** — 68
    Rajesh N Solanki, Jaydeep Odhwani, Kumar Utsav
    - Primordial Prevention   68
    - Primary Prevention   68
    - Secondary Prevention   70
    - Tertiary Prevention   73

12. **Extrapulmonary Tuberculosis** — 74
    AK Janmeja, PR Mohapatra, Deepak Aggarwal
    - Diagnosis   74
    - Treatment of Extrapulmonary Tuberculosis   75
    - Lymph Node Tuberculosis   75
    - Pleural Effusion   76
    - Bone and Joint Tuberculosis   76
    - Central Nervous System Tuberculosis   79

- Abdominal Tuberculosis *81*
- Genitourinary Tuberculosis *82*
- Skin Tuberculosis *83*
- Pericardial Tuberculosis *83*
- Hepatic Tuberculosis *84*

13. Multidrug Resistant Tuberculosis — 86
Surendra K Sharma, Dinkar Bhasin
- Definitions *86*
- Diagnosis *87*
- Management *87*

14. Treatment of Tuberculosis in Special Situations — 91
Rajendra Prasad, Nikhil Gupta
- Treatment of Tuberculosis in Pregnancy and Lactation *91*
- Treatment of Tuberculosis in Renal Insufficiency *92*
- Treatment of Tuberculosis in Liver Disease *93*

15. Tuberculosis and Human Immunodeficiency Virus Infection — 95
Aditya Jindal, SK Jindal
- Epidemiology *95*
- Pathogenesis *95*
- Clinical Features *97*
- Diagnosis *98*
- Management *98*

16. Nontuberculous Mycobacterial Diseases — 102
PS Shankar, SK Jindal
- Classification *102*
- Human Disease *103*
- Summary *105*

17. Community-acquired Pneumonia — 106
Charles Feldman, Ronald Anderson
- Microbial Etiology *106*
- Risk Factors *107*
- Pathogenesis with Particular Reference to the *Pneumococcus* *107*
- Diagnostic Testing *108*
- Prognosis *109*
- Treatment *110*

18. Pulmonary Fungal Infections — 112
Arunaloke Chakrabarti
- Types of Infections *112*

19. Nosocomial Pneumonia — 118
Vishwanath Gella, SK Jindal
- Definitions *118*
- Pathogenesis *119*
- Prevention of Hospital-acquired Pneumonia and Ventilator-associated Pneumonia *119*
- Diagnosis *121*
- Treatment *123*

20. **Lung Abscess** 125
    C Ravindran, Jyothi E
    - Epidemiology *125*
    - Classification *125*
    - Etiology *126*
    - Pathogenesis *126*
    - Pathology *126*
    - Clinical Features *127*
    - Laboratory Diagnosis *127*
    - Complications *128*
    - Treatment *129*
    - Prognosis *130*

21. **Bronchiectasis and Cystic Fibrosis** 131
    David Honeybourne *131*
    Bronchiectasis *131*
    - Pathology *131*
    - Physiology *132*
    - Etiology *132*
    - Symptoms and Signs *132*
    - Diagnosis *133*
    - Microbiology *134*
    - Treatment *134*
    - Complications *136*
    - Prognosis *136*

    Cystic Fibrosis *136*
    - Diagnosis *137*
    - Clinical Features *138*
    - Infections and Treatment *138*

22. **Anaerobic Bacterial Infections of the Lungs and the Pleura** 141
    Ashok Shah, Chandramani Panjabi
    - Pathophysiology *141*
    - Other Predisposing Factors *141*
    - Natural History and Clinical Classification *142*
    - Anaerobes and Upper Respiratory Syndromes *143*
    - Clinical Features *144*
    - Laboratory Diagnosis *145*
    - Treatment *145*

23. **Bronchial Asthma Epidemiology** 147
    SK Jindal
    - Epidemiology *148*
    - Disease Burden *149*
    - Risk Factors of Asthma *149*

24. **Airway Inflammation and Remodeling** 153
    Ruby Pawankar, Shu Hashimoto, Miyuki Hayashi, Shingo Yamanishi, Manabu Nonaka
    - Chronic Inflammation in Allergic Rhinitis and Asthma *154*
    - Remodeling in Asthma *156*

25. Asthma Diagnosis *Liesel D'silva, Parameswaran Nair* • Clinical Diagnosis 158 • Tests for Diagnosis and Monitoring 159 • Diagnostic Challenges 162	158
26. Control and Management of Stable Asthma *Sidney S Braman, Gwen Skloot* • Goals of Asthma Treatment 165 • Essential Components of Asthma Care 166	165
27. Acute Asthma Exacerbations *Aditya Jindal* • Triggers Causing Exacerbations 171 • Diagnosis and Evaluation of Severity 172 • Management 173	171
28. Allergen Desensitization *Vikram Jaggi* • Definition 177 • Mechanisms of Allergen Immunotherapy 177	177
29. Patient Education in Asthma *Bharat Bhushan Sharma, Virendra Singh* • Goals of Asthma Education Programs 184 • Benefits of Asthma Education Programs 185 • Methods and Settings 185 • Asthma Education Program Components 185 • Problems in Patient Education 186	184
30. Pharmacotherapy of Bronchial Asthma *Nusrat Shafiq, Samir Malhotra* **Controllers: Anti-inflammatory Agents 187** • Corticosteroids 187 • Leukotriene Receptor Antagonists 189 • Mast Cell Stabilizers 191 **Relievers—Bronchodilators 192** • Beta-2 Adrenergic Agonists 192 • Methylxanthines (Xanthines) 196 • Anticholinergic Agents 198	187
31. Allergic Bronchopulmonary Aspergillosis *Ritesh Agarwal* • Epidemiology 200 • Pathogenesis 201 • Pathology 201 • Clinical Features 202 • Laboratory Findings 202 • Diagnosis and Diagnostic Criteria 205 • Management 205 • Allergic Bronchopulmonary Mycosis 207	200

32. **Burden of Chronic Obstructive Pulmonary Disease** — 208
    Monica Barne, Sundeep Salvi
    - Mortality due to Chronic Obstructive Pulmonary Disease *208*
    - Prevalence of Chronic Obstructive Pulmonary Disease *209*
    - Disability Adjusted Life Years (DALYS) due to Chronic Obstructive Pulmonary Disease *211*

33. **Risk Factors for Chronic Obstructive Pulmonary Disease** — 213
    Sneha Limaye, Sundeep Salvi 213
    - Tobacco Smoking *213*
    - Environmental Tobacco Smoke *214*
    - Household Air Pollution *214*
    - Mosquito Coil Smoke *215*
    - Outdoor Air Pollution *215*
    - Chronic Obstructive Pulmonary Disease Associated with Occupational Exposures *215*
    - Chronic Obstructive Pulmonary Disease Associated with Pulmonary Tuberculosis *216*
    - Chronic Asthma *216*
    - Genetic Factors *216*
    - Socioeconomic Status *217*

34. **Pathophysiology of Chronic Obstructive Pulmonary Disease** — 218
    Bill Brashier, Sundeep Salvi, Baishakhi Ghosh
    - Inflammatory Changes *218*
    - New Insights into Small Airway Obstruction *221*
    - Chronic Obstructive Pulmonary Disease as a Disease of Systemic Inflammation *221*

35. **Systemic Manifestations and Comorbidities of Chronic Obstructive Pulmonary Disease** — 223
    SK Jindal, PS Shankar
    - Pathogenesis *223*
    - Systemic Manifestations *224*
    - Therapeutic Considerations *228*

36. **Treatment of Chronic Obstructive Pulmonary Disease** — 229
    Peter J Barnes
    - Risk Factors and their Prevention *229*
    - Pharmacotherapy *230*
    - Supplementary Oxygen *235*
    - Antibiotics *236*
    - Other Drug Therapies *236*
    - Nonpharmacological Treatments *238*

37. **Acute Exacerbations of Chronic Obstructive Pulmonary Disease** — 239
    Raja Dhar, AG Ghoshal
    - Copd Exacerbation *239*

38. **Pulmonary Rehabilitation** — 245
    Rachael A Evans, Roger S Goldstein
    - Role and Definition of Pulmonary Rehabilitation *245*
    - Changing Pulmonary Rehabilitation Population—Whom to Refer? *246*

- Outcome Measures *247*
- Core Components of a Pulmonary Rehabilitation Program *248*
- Maintenance *249*
- Mobility Aids *250*
- Rehabilitation Team *250*
- Setting *250*
- Exacerbations *250*
- Performance Enhancement *250*

39. Bullous Lung Diseases   252
Aditya Jindal, Gyanendra Agrawal
- Pathogenesis *252*
- Etiology *253*
- Clinical Presentation *254*
- Radiologic Features *254*
- Pulmonary Function Tests *254*
- Natural History *255*
- Complications *255*
- Treatment *255*

40. Upper and Central Airways Obstruction   257
VR Pattabhi Raman
- Physiological Considerations *257*
- Clinical Features *258*
- Diagnosis *258*
- Acute Upper Airway Obstruction *259*
- Chronic Upper Airway Obstruction *261*
- Therapeutic Considerations *264*

41. Interstitial Lung Diseases   266
Nagarjuna V Maturu, Dheeraj Gupta
- Etiology and Classification *266*
- Epidemiology *268*
- Pathology *268*
- Pathogenesis *268*
- Diagnostic Approach *269*
- Treatment *271*
- Acute Exacerbation of ILD *273*
- Prognosis *274*

42. Idiopathic Interstitial Pneumonias   275
H Shigemitsu, Ngozi Orjioke, Carmen Luraschi-Monjagatta
- Diagnosis *275*
- Histological Features *276*
- Idiopathic Pulmonary Fibrosis *276*
- Nonspecific Interstitial Pneumonia *278*
- Desquamative Interstitial Pneumonia *279*
- Respiratory Bronchiolitis-associated Interstitial Lung Disease *280*
- Cryptogenic Organizing Pneumonia *281*
- Acute Interstitial Pneumonia *282*
- Lymphoid Interstitial Pneumonia *282*
- Idiopathic Pleuroparenchymal Fibroelastosis *283*
- Unclassifiable Idiopathic Interstitial Pneumonia *284*

43. **Sarcoidosis** 285
    Dheeraj Gupta, Sahajal Dhooria, Om P Sharma
    - Etiology and Risk Factors 285
    - Pathogenesis and Immunology 286
    - Pathology 286
    - Clinical Features 287
    - Diagnosis 289
    - Treatment 291
    - Prognosis and Mortality 293

44. **Pulmonary Eosinophilic Disorders** 294
    Subhash Varma, Aditya Jindal
    - Eosinophils 294
    - Pulmonary Eosinophilic Disorders 296
    - Approach to Diagnosis and Conclusion 304

45. **Infiltrative and Deposition Diseases** 305
    Pralay Sarkar, Arunabh Talwar
    - Pulmonary Amyloidosis 305
    - Lysosomal Storage Disorders 307

46. **Bronchiolitis** 312
    Gyanendra Agrawal, Dheeraj Gupta
    - General Features of Bronchiolar Disorders 312
    - Clinical Presentations 312
    - Practical Approach for Diagnosis of Bronchiolar Disorders 315

47. **High-altitude Problems** 317
    Ajay Handa
    - Physical Changes with Altitude 317
    - Physiological Adaptation to High Altitude 317
    - Specific Altitude-related Illnesses 318
    - Effects of High Altitude on Existing Lung Diseases 320

48. **Aviation and Space Travel** 322
    Ajay Handa
    - Respiratory Physiology with Altitude 322
    - Preflight Assessment 323
    - Prescribing In-flight oxygen 324
    - Space Travel 325
    - Microgravity and Weightlessness 325

49. **Lung Disease in Coal Workers** 327
    Harakh V Dedhia, Daniel E Banks
    - Clinical Features of Coal Dust Exposure 327
    - Pathology of Coal Worker Pneumoconiosis 329
    - Management of CMDLD 330

50. **Silicosis** 333
    PS Shankar, SK Jindal
    - Occupational Exposure 333
    - Pathogenesis 334
    - Forms of Silicosis 334
    - Clinical Features 336

- Diagnosis *336*
- Prognosis *339*
- Treatment *339*

51. Berylliosis 340
PS Shankar
- Acute Beryllium Disease *340*
- Chronic Beryllium Disease *340*
- Pathogenesis *341*
- Clinical and Radiological Features *341*
- Diagnosis *342*
- Treatment *342*

52. Metal-induced Lung Disease 344
Dilip V Maydeo, Nikhil C Sarangdhar
- Types *344*
- Epidemiology *344*
- Pathogenesis *345*
- Types of Immune Responses in Metal-induced Lung Disease *345*
- Clinical Presentation and Diagnosis *345*
- Approach *346*
- Treatment *347*

53. Health Risks of Asbestos Fiber Inhalation 348
Daniel E Banks, Harakh V Dedhia
- Asbestosis *349*
- Asbestos Fibers and the Pleural Space *350*
- Diffuse Pleural Thickening: Fibrosis of the Visceral Pleura *350*
- Pleural Plaques: Fibrosis of the Parietal Pleura *351*
- Malignant Mesothelioma *352*
- Lung Cancer *353*

54. Occupational Asthma 354
PS Shankar, G Gaude
- Agents Causing Occupational Asthma *355*
- Pathogenetic Mechanisms of Occupational Asthma *357*
- Diagnosis *357*
- Management *359*
- Prognosis *360*

55. Hypersensitivity Pneumonitis 361
PS Shankar
- Etiology *361*
- Pathogenesis *362*
- Pathology *363*
- Clinical Presentation *363*
- Diagnosis *364*
- Management and Prevention *365*
- Prognosis *366*

56. Toxic Inhalations and Thermal Lung Injuries 367
VK Vijayan, N Goel, R Caroli
- Determinants of Inhalational Lung Injury *367*
- Clinical Presentations of Inhalational Injury *368*

- Systemic Illnesses from Inhaled Toxins 371
- Smoke Inhalation Lung Injury 372
- Management 372

57. Drug-induced Respiratory Disease 373
William J Martin Jr
- Drugs Associated with Respiratory Toxicity 373
- Diagnosis and Management of Drug-induced Respiratory Disease 376

58. Epidemiology and Etiopathogenesis of Lung Cancer 378
Nagarjuna V Maturu, Navneet Singh
- Lung Cancer in India 378
- Histological Patterns 378
- Risk Factors 379
- Molecular Biology of Lung Cancer 383

59. Pathology of Lung Tumors 385
Amanjit Bal, Ashim Das
- Preinvasive Lesions 385
- Classification of Lung Cancer 386
- Epithelial Tumors 386
- Neuroendocrine Lesions of the Lung 388
- Staging of Lung Tumors 389

60. Lung Cancer: Clinical Manifestations 391
Javid Ahmad Malik
- Local Manifestations 391
- Metastatic Manifestations 393
- Endocrine Syndromes 396
- Neurological Syndromes 397
- Hematological Syndromes 399
- Skeletal 399
- Miscellaneous Syndromes 400

61. Diagnosis and Staging of Lung Cancer 401
Nagarjuna V Maturu, Ajmal Khan, Navneet Singh
- Diagnosis of Lung Cancer 401
- Staging of Nonsmall-cell Lung Cancer 403
- Staging of Small-cell Lung Cancer 405

62. Approach to Management of Lung Cancer in India 407
Navneet Singh, Nagarjuna V Maturu, Digambar Behera
- Treatment of Lung Cancer 407
- Palliation 413

63. Targeted Agents for Nonsmall Cell Lung Cancer 415
Nagarjuna V Maturu, Navneet Singh
- Epidermal Growth Factor Receptor–Tyrosine Kinase Inhibitors 415
- Anaplastic Lymphoma Kinase Inhibitors 418
- Vascular Endothelial Growth Factor Inhibitors 419

64. Hematopoietic and Lymphoid Neoplasm of Lungs 420
Gaurav Prakash, Pankaj Malhotra
- Lymphomas 420
- Lymphomatoid Granulomatosis 425

- Secondary Involvement of Lung by Other Systemic Hematopoietic and Lymphoid Disorders *426*

65. Solitary Pulmonary Nodule — 428
Alladi Mohan, B Vijayalakshmi Devi, Abha Chandra
- Terminology *428*
- Etiology *429*
- Clinical Evaluation *430*
- Imaging Studies *430*
- Management *435*

66. Mediastinal Disorders — 436
Arjun Srinivasan, SK Jindal
- Imaging of Mediastinum *437*
- Diseases of Mediastinum *438*
- Tumors and Cysts of Mediastinum *441*

67. Diseases of the Chest Wall — 447
Balamugesh T
- Kyphoscoliosis *447*
- Thoracoplasty *449*
- Pectus Excavatum *450*
- Pectus Carinatum *450*
- Ankylosing Spondylosis *450*
- Obesity *451*
- Flail Chest *452*
- Miscellaneous Conditions *452*

68. Diffuse Alveolar Hemorrhage — 454
Stagaki E, Karakontaki F, Polychronopoulos V
- Diffuse Alveolar Hemorrhage Syndromes *454*
- Causes *457*
- Other Causes of Diffuse Alveolar Hemorrhage *464*

69. Pulmonary Hypertension: A Third World Perspective — 466
Lakshmi Mudambi, Zeenat Safdar
- Clinical Features *467*
- Physical Examination *468*
- Diagnostic Evaluation *468*
- Pathophysiology *470*
- Management *471*

70. Pulmonary Thromboembolism — 473
Devasahayam J Christopher, Richa Gupta
- Pathophysiology *473*
- Risk Factors *475*
- Clinical Features *475*
- Diagnosis *476*
- Management *478*

71. Pulmonary Vascular Malformations — 482
Gautam Ahluwalia
- Hereditary Hemorrhagic Telangiectasias or Rendu–Osler–Weber Syndrome *483*

- Pathogenesis 483
- Clinical Features 484
- Investigations 484
- Management 485
- Other Pulmonary Vascular Malformations 485

72. **Approach to Respiratory Sleep Disorders** 488
    Ruchi Bansal
    - Sleep History 488
    - Physical Examination 489
    - Nocturnal Polysomnography 490
    - Out-of-center Sleep Testing 490
    - Sleep Questionnaires 491
    - Respiratory Disorders During Sleep 491

73. **Respiratory Sleep Disorders** 493
    Aditya Jindal
    - Classification 493

74. **Respiratory Failure** 499
    Abinash Singh Paul, Ritesh Agarwal
    - Classification 499
    - Mechanisms 500
    - Clinical Manifestations 502
    - Diagnosis 502
    - Treatment 503

75. **Acute Respiratory Distress Syndrome** 507
    Jean I Keddissi, D Robert McCaffree
    - Etiology 507
    - Clinical Picture 508
    - Pathophysiology 508
    - Management 509
    - Prognosis and Outcome 513

76. **Sepsis** 514
    Sean E Hesselbacher, Walter G Shakespeare, Kalpalatha K Guntupalli
    - Pathogenesis 514
    - Clinical Features and Evaluation 515
    - Prognosis 516
    - Management 517
    - Goals of Care 520
    - Special Considerations 521

77. **Nonpulmonary Critical Care** 522
    Liziamma George, Mark Astiz
    - Gastrointestinal Disease in Critical Care 522
    - Hematology in Critical Care 526
    - Renal Disease in Critical Care 528
    - Endocrine Emergencies in Critical Care 529
    - Neurological Disorders in Critical Care 531

78. **Critical Care in Nonpulmonary Conditions: Poisoning, Envenomation, and Environmental Injuries** — 535
Dhruva Chaudhry, Inderpaul Singh Sehgal
- Poisoning *535*
- Envenomation *541*
- Environmental Injuries *544*

79. **Pulmonary Hypertension in the Intensive Care Unit** — 548
Charles Peng, Roxana Sulica
- Right Heart in Health and Disease *548*
- Pulmonary Hypertension in the Critically Ill Patient *549*
- Right Ventricular Failure in Patients with Preexisting Pulmonary Arterial Hypertension *551*
- Management of the Pulmonary Arterial Hypertension Patient with Decompensated Right Heart Failure *552*
- Perioperative Management of the Patient with Pulmonary Arterial Hypertension *554*

80. **Mechanical Ventilation: General Principles and Modes** — 555
GC Khilnani, Vijay Hadda
- Indications of Mechanical Ventilation *555*
- Basic Aspects of Mechanical Ventilation *556*
- Modes of Mechanical Ventilation *557*
- Newer Modes of Mechanical Ventilation *565*
- Initiating Mechanical Ventilation *567*
- Complications of Mechanical Ventilation *568*

81. **Noninvasive Ventilation** — 570
GC Khilnani, Vijay Hadda
- Technical Aspect of Noninvasive Ventilation *570*
- Steps to Successful Provision of Noninvasive Positive Pressure Ventilation *573*
- Clinical Uses of Noninvasive Positive Pressure Ventilation: Evidence and Recommendations *575*

82. **Blood Gas Monitoring** — 579
Inderpaul Singh Sehgal, Ritesh Agarwal
- Arterial Sampling *579*
- Arterial Cannulation *580*
- Noninvasive Blood Gas Monitoring *581*

83. **Cutaneous Capnography** — 585
Preyas Vaidya, Arvind H Kate, Prashant Chhajed
- Site for Measurement *585*
- Factors Influencing $PcCO_2$ Monitoring *586*
- Medical Applications of $PcCO_2$ Monitoring *586*
- Clinical Settings for the Use of Cutaneous Capnography *587*

84. **Nutritional Management and General Care in the Intensive Care Unit** — 591
Inderpaul Singh Sehgal, Navneet Singh
- Malnutrition in Critical Illness *591*
- Refeeding Syndrome *593*

- Assessment of Nutritional Status in Critically Ill Patients 593
- Goals and Principles of Nutritional Support 593
- Timing of Initiation of Nutritional Support 594
- Route of Administration of Nutritional Support 594
- Quantity and Volume of Nutrition Support 595
- Delivery of Enteral Nutrition and Its Determinants 596
- General Care in ICU 598

85. **Management of Complex Airways Diseases** 601
   Rubal Patel, Atul C Mehta
   - Difficult Airway Situations 601
   - Indications for Artificial Airway 602
   - Techniques 605
   - Alternative Airway Techniques 607

86. **Analgesia and Sedation in the ICU** 609
   Karan Madan, Ritesh Agarwal
   - Teamwork (Multidisciplinary Management) and Patient-focused Care 609
   - Initial Evaluation and Medication Reconciliation 610
   - Consequences of Off-target Sedation and Analgesia 610
   - Assessment of Pain, Sedation, and Agitation in the ICU 610
   - Objective Measurement of the Cerebral Activity in the ICU 612
   - Management of Analgesia and Sedation in the ICU 612
   - Recent Developments and Novel Approaches 618

87. **Weaning from Mechanical Ventilation** 621
   Ajmal Khan, Ritesh Agarwal
   - Pathophysiology of Weaning 622
   - Outcome of Weaning 623
   - Assessment for Weaning 623
   - Techniques of Weaning 624

88. **Hyperbaric Oxygen Therapy** 628
   PS Tampi, SK Jindal
   - Rationale of Hyperbaric Oxygen 628
   - Other Physiological Effects of Hyperbaric Oxygenation 629
   - Beneficial Effects of HBO_2 629
   - Mechanism of Action of HBO_2 629
   - Indications 630
   - HBO_2 in Pediatric Age Group 633
   - Potential New Indications 633
   - Contraindications 633
   - Complications 634

89. **Pleura: Anatomy and Physiology** 635
   Srinivas Rajagopala
   - Anatomy of the Pleura 635
   - Development of the Pleural Membranes 636
   - Histology of the Pleura 636
   - Pleural Fluid: Normal Volume and Cellular Contents 636
   - Physiology and Pathophysiology of Pleural Fluid Turnover 637
   - Physiological Changes with a Pleural Effusion 638
   - Physiological Changes with Pneumothorax 638

- Pleural Manometry *638*
- Pleural Ultrasound *639*

90. Tubercular Pleural Effusion **640**
Pranab Baruwa, Kripesh Ranjan Sarmah
- Pathology and Pathogenesis *640*
- Clinical Features *641*
- Diagnosis *641*
- Management *645*
- Complication of TB Pleural Effusion *646*

91. Parapneumonic Effusion and Empyema **648**
Devasahayam J Christopher
- Definitions *648*
- Pathogenesis *649*
- Epidemiology *649*
- Bacteriology *650*
- Clinical Features and Diagnosis *650*
- Treatment *652*

92. Malignant Pleural Effusions and Pleurodesis **655**
Srinivas Rajagopala
- Etiology of Malignant Effusions *655*
- Pathogenesis of Metastasis and Effusions *656*
- Clinical Presentation *656*
- Radiological Findings *657*
- Diagnosis *657*
- Management *659*
- Prognosis *663*

93. Pneumothorax **664**
Uma Devraj, GA D'Souza
- Definitions *664*
- Pathophysiology *665*
- Resolution of Pneumothorax *665*
- Etiology *665*
- Laboratory Investigations and Diagnosis *667*
- Recurrence Rates *668*
- Treatment *668*

94. Malignant Pleural Mesothelioma **674**
Arun S Shet, Girish Raju, GA D'Souza
- Epidemiology *674*
- Pathogenesis *675*
- Pathology *675*
- Clinical Presentation *676*
- Diagnostic Approach *676*
- Treatment *676*

95. Pulmonary Involvement in Connective Tissue Diseases **680**
Om P Sharma, Aditya Jindal
- Rheumatoid Arthritis *680*
- Systemic Sclerosis *684*
- Sjögren's Syndrome *686*

- Systemic Lupus Erythematosus *687*
- Dermatomyositis and Polymyositis *691*
- Ankylosing Spondylitis *692*
- Mixed Connective Tissue Disease *693*

96. **Pulmonary Manifestations of Other System Diseases** 695
    Ajmal Khan, SK Jindal
    - Cardiovascular Diseases *695*
    - Neuromuscular Diseases *697*
    - Endocrine Disorders *703*
    - Gastrointestinal Diseases *706*
    - Hepatic Disorders *709*
    - Renal Diseases *712*

97. **Pulmonary Involvement in Tropical Diseases** 714
    Sanjay Jain, SK Jindal
    - Malaria *714*
    - Typhoid *716*
    - Leptospirosis *717*
    - Dengue *718*
    - Amebiasis *719*

98. **Pulmonary Diseases in Pregnancy** 721
    Lakhbir K Dhaliwal, Preeti Verma, Umesh Jindal
    - Dyspnea During Pregnancy *722*
    - Asthma in Pregnancy *722*
    - Pneumonia in Pregnancy *726*
    - Tuberculosis and Pregnancy *730*
    - Pulmonary Thromboembolism *732*
    - Pregnancy-specific Problems *734*

99. **Rare Lung Diseases** 737
    Sanjeev Mehta, PS Shankar
    - Pulmonary Alveolar Phospholipoproteinosis *737*
    - Pulmonary Calcification and Ossification Syndromes *740*
    - Pulmonary Alveolar Microlithiasis *742*

100. **Ethics in Respiratory Care** 744
     Basil Varkey
     - Ethics Education *744*
     - Ethics in End-of-life Care *749*
     - A Conceptual Model for Patient Care *751*

101. **End-of-Life Care** 753
     Jeba S Jenifer, SK Jindal
     - Components *754*
     - Common Symptoms *754*
     - Diagnosing Dying and Providing Terminal Care *757*
     - End-of-life Care in the Intensive Care Unit *758*

Index *761*

CHAPTER

1

Introduction

SK Jindal

HISTORY

Breathing was perhaps the most vital physiological sign of life noticed by the ancient man. The number of total breaths was supposed to be fixed during life of an individual. Though there is little mention on the role of the lungs in the archaic Medicine, the anatomy of lungs was perhaps known in those periods. The oldest and best known image of the respiratory tract which dates back to 30th century BC comes from an Egyptian hieroglyph that depicts a wind pipe with a pair of lungs. Ancient Egyptians also believed that breathing was the most vital to life. Ebers Papyrus (c. 1550 BC), a detailed document on medicine of that time, written on papyri was accidently unearthed in Thebes in 1862. The papyrus, more than 20 meters long, was purchased and translated into German in 1873 by Georg Ebers. Considered to be knowledge imparted by Thoth the Egyptian God of learning and medicine, it mentioned about remedies for a number of diseases, including asthma.

The presence of lung diseases such as tuberculosis and asthma was variously described in the ancient Egyptian, Greek, Indian (Vedic) and Chinese civilizations of the prebiblical periods. The concept of gas exchange and the role of the lungs to maintain life, however, were not known until the 12th century of the medieval era. The saga of both tuberculosis and asthma independently runs back by 3000 years. The two are also amongst the few diseases which continue to exist in a manner that was recognized in the past.

The earliest mention of respiration can perhaps be traced to Erasistratus of Alexandria in Egypt who in 300 BC had postulated that it was the interplay between the air and the blood which produced the "pneuma" or the spirit essential for life.

RESPIRATORY SYSTEM FUNCTION

The thoracic cavity bound externally by the thoracic-cage contains the lungs and the mediastinal structures between the two lungs. The thoracic cage is formed by the ribs and intercostal muscles, lined internally by the parietal pleurae. The lungs are lined on the surface by the visceral pleurae.

The respiratory systems essentially comprise of three different structural and functional units:
1. Respiratory tract (from the nose and the mouth to the alveoli), meant for air conduction.
2. Lung parenchyma (the alveoli and the surrounding interstitium, which includes the blood capillaries, lymphatics and interstitial matrix with several different kinds of cells).
3. Respiratory regulatory system.

The chest wall, respiratory muscles and the respiratory center constitute the ventilatory apparatus or the pump responsible for movement of air in and out of the lungs. On the other hand, gas exchange happens in the lungs at the alveolar level.

Gas exchange by human lungs is achieved with the help of four processes, which are also variably interdependent:
1. *Ventilation:* To and fro movement between the atmosphere and the gas exchanging units of lung
2. *Circulation:* Supply and distribution of blood through the pulmonary capillaries
3. *Diffusion:* The movement of O_2 and carbon dioxide across the air-blood barrier between alveoli and pulmonary capillaries
4. Ventilation-perfusion relationships

VENTILATION-PERFUSION (V/Q) RELATIONSHIPS

The ratio of pulmonary ventilation to pulmonary blood flow for the whole lung at rest is about 0.8–1 (4–6 L/min ventilation divided by 5–6 L/min blood flow), and this matching of distribution of ventilation and perfusion is the most important determinant of gas exchange. The ventilation-perfusion mismatch is the final common pathway to cause hypoxemia in most pulmonary diseases. An area of lung that is well perfused, but under ventilated acts as a right to left shunt (physiological shunt) whereas an area that is well ventilated, but under perfused acts like a dead space (physiological dead space). The spectrum of V/Q ratios in a healthy lung would vary between zero (perfused, but not ventilated) to infinity (ventilated, but not perfused).

The ideal V/Q ratio of one indicates perfectly matched ventilation and perfusion. Although V/Q mismatch includes both physiologic shunt and physiologic dead space, but in clinical parlance, the term generally denotes physiologic shunt as physiologic dead space, is rarely, if ever the cause of hypoxemia.

The alveolar PO_2 appears to be the most important factor involved in regulating the distribution of ventilation-perfusion within the lung. In this respect, hypoxic pulmonary vasoconstriction can be considered as part of a negative feedback loop. For example, in lung units with low V/Q ratios, there is a fall in local alveolar PO_2, and constriction of associated microcirculation reduces the local pulmonary blood flow. This tends to restore the local V/Q ratio toward its normal value. This effect can be appreciated in the residents of high altitudes, who are exposed constantly to lower ambient O_2 concentrations. Residents of high altitudes have better V/Q matching than sea level residents, as reflected by a smaller alveolar-arterial PO_2 difference.

The intensity of hypoxic pulmonary vasoconstriction varies among different lung regions, and probably depends on the smooth muscle tone in different vessels. The nitric oxide-mediated mechanism may also be important in patients with inflammatory lung diseases, in whom the production of nitric oxide is increased. The loss of local hypoxic vasoconstriction would worsen ventilation-perfusion mismatch.

RESPIRATORY DEFENSES

The respiratory tract is exposed to environmental toxic substances, such as the smoke, soot, dust and chemicals in the atmosphere, and also to a wide range of organisms such as viruses, bacteria, fungi and parasites. It has been calculated that the average individual inhales about 8 microorganisms per minute or about 10,000 per day. The magnitude of this atmospheric insult on the respiratory tract is much greater in the developing countries.

The defense against foreign material within the lungs is a critical physiological function. This is accomplished by passive mechanisms, such as the branching nature of the respiratory tract and the regulation of airway lining fluid composition. The first line of respiratory defense consists of mechanisms, such as the physical barrier; reflexes, including sneezing and coughing; production of mucus; mucociliary clearance; transport of IgA and antimicrobial mediators (defensins, lysozyme, lactoferrin, lectins).

These defenses can be overcome by a large number of organisms and inhibitory factors of pathogens, by compromised effectiveness resulting from air pollutants (e.g. cigarette smoke, ozone) or interference with protective mechanisms (e.g. endotracheal intubation or tracheostomy) or genetic defects (e.g. cystic fibrosis). Following exposure to airborne microorganisms (bio-aerosols) in air, the defense mechanisms are able to eliminate most of the larger microorganisms; however, smaller particles and spores may be trapped within the lung tissue, which pose health risks. The impact on health depends on the interaction between genetic differences in the host, agent and environments (duration and exposure dose).

The vulnerability of individuals to the inhaled substances varies widely depending on age, atopic status, nutrition and coexisting conditions. It is, therefore, vital for respiratory clinicians to have a clear understanding of the normal defenses of the respiratory tract.

CHAPTER 2

Applied Respiratory Physics

SK Jindal, VK Jindal

Matter can exist in three different forms in nature—solid, liquid, or gas; although plasma, a fourth state of matter has also been identified under the extremes of temperature and pressure. In nature, matter is either an element made from similar atoms, e.g. iron or a compound made from two or more types of atoms, e.g. water (H_2O).

ATOM, ELEMENT, MOLECULE, AND COMPOUND

An atom is the smallest part of an element, which acts like a "building block". On the further subdivision of an atom, the elemental properties are lost and therefore, subatomic constituents of all atoms are identical. Atoms of certain elements (e.g. hydrogen and helium) can exist in free state (H, He) and there is no difference between the atoms and molecules of these elements. Atoms of many other elements (such as oxygen) do not exist free, but combine with other atoms of the same element to form molecules (e.g. O_2, i.e. O + O). Atoms of different elements may form molecules or compounds. Hydrogen can exist in atomic or molecular form; whereas, nitrogen and oxygen occur in molecular form (N_2 and O_2).

All substances consist of exceedingly small particles called molecules. There are about 10^{19} molecules in 1 mL of air under the normal conditions of temperature (T) and pressure (P). A molecule possesses the distinctive properties of the parent element or compound. A molecule is found to consist of two or more atoms of same kind or of different kinds. The number of molecules comprising a macroscopic quantity of a gas is enormous typically around 10^{23} molecules. The number of molecules and their velocity determine many properties of gases.

A compound is composed of two or more elements united chemically to form a substance different from the individual elements forming that compound. For example, carbon dioxide is a compound of carbon and oxygen. On subdivisions, the compound loses its properties and may resume those of the constituent elements. Both elements and compounds exist as molecules as the smallest component.

MOLECULAR MOVEMENT

All the molecules of matter are in a state of incessant motion. This is known as Brownian movement and forms the basis of the kinetic theory of matter. This motion results from temperature—the higher the temperature, the larger the velocity of the molecules. At absolute zero temperature, the velocity of a classical molecule goes to zero. Molecules of a gas have great mobility and travel longer distances before colliding with other molecules. It is because of this mobility that a gas has no fixed shape and mixes readily with other gases.

ATOMIC AND MOLECULAR WEIGHTS

The mass of an atom is concentrated at its nucleus, which contains a definite number of neutrons and protons of identical masses. The neutrons or protons are also called *nucleons*. The mass of a nucleon is $\approx 1.6 \times 10^{-24}$ g (sometimes also called *atomic mass unit*—amu). Therefore, total number of nucleons of an atom determines the mass of an atom and is usually called *atomic weight*. This H´ atom has atomic weight equaling 1; whereas, O´ atom has atomic weight equaling 16, though their actual masses are around $1 \times 1.6 \times 10^{-24}$ g and $16 \times 1.6 \times 10^{-24}$ g, respectively. Similarly, *molecular weight* is determined by summing up atomic weights of the constituent atoms forming that molecule.

Volume at NTP (normal temperature 0°C, and pressure 760 mm Hg) is 22.4 liters for any gas. Quantity of any substance equaling molecular weight as g has 6.02×10^{23} molecules and as a gas, occupies 22.4 liters at NTP. Equal volume of gases at the same temperature and pressure contains equal number of molecules *(Avogadro's hypothesis)*.

PHYSICAL PROPERTIES OF GASES

The air we normally breathe is a mixture of gases of which oxygen and nitrogen constitute the main bulk. Breathing of additional or supplemental gases is required in abnormal situations. The physical properties of these gases influence the mechanics of normal breathing, as well as the therapeutic strategies.

Volume

Volume is the space occupied by a gas. The volume of a cuboid-shaped vessel is determined by the multiplication of internal length, width, and height of the vessel. It is expressed in cubic centimeters (cc), cubic feet or liters (L), etc. (1 L ≡ 1,000 cc or mL).

$$Volume = Length \times Width \times Height$$

A 10 cm cube has the volume equaling 1 L. Volume (V) of a container of uniform cross-sectional area (A) and height (h) is determined by V = A × h. The gas shall occupy the available volume irrespective of the amount (mass) of gas. For example, if a small vessel containing oxygen is emptied in a larger vessel, the entire volume of the larger vessel will be occupied by the same amount of gas.

Mass and Weight

Mass

Mass is the bulk or the total mass of number of molecules of the gas. In the above mentioned example, the mass of the gas in two cylinders shall remain the same, although the volume has changed. The number of molecules per unit of volume in the two vessels has changed, i.e. lesser number of molecules per unit volume in the larger vessel.

Weight

Weight is often used synonymously with mass. Weight is determined by the pull of gravity on mass (i.e. m × g). Since the force of gravity on the earth is nearly constant, mass is equivalent to weight on the surface of the earth. In fact, weight is scaled to indicate mass and therefore both represent the same thing.

Density

Density is expressed as the weight in grams of 1 liter of a gas. Since the weight of 22.4 liters of a gas is that of a gram molecule of that gas, 1 liter of gas shall weigh molecular weight/22.4 gm. Relative density is just a number without units and shows how much a particular gas is heavier or lighter with respect to air. It is also measured in g/cc, which will equal 1/1,000 in value to that in g/L.

$$\text{Molecular weight of oxygen} = 32$$
$$\text{Density} = 32/22.4$$
$$= 1.43 \text{ g/L}$$

The density of a gas is also expressed as relative to the density of air. Density of air shall vary depending upon its composition. For all practical purposes, it comprises of one volume of oxygen (about 20%) and four volumes of nitrogen (about 80%). At NTP, the density of air is (32 × 1/5 + 28 × 4/5)/22.4 = 1.3 g/L. Therefore, the density of oxygen relative to that of air is 1.1. Relative density is just a number without units and shows how much a particular gas is heavier or lighter with respect to air.

Pressure (P)

The gas molecules are always in a state of motion and constantly bombard the walls of the container. The force (F) applied to (or acting upon) a unit area (A) of the wall is called the gas pressure (P = F/A). The closer the molecules, the greater the number, which strikes each unit area; and therefore, the greater the pressure applied. Also, larger the velocity (or temperature), larger is the impact on the walls, leading to greater pressure.

Gas pressure is generally considered as that of a stationary gas when the pressure exerted is the same at any point in a gas container. The pressure is usually expressed in the millimeters of mercury (mm Hg) or centimeters of water (cm H_2O) or pounds per square inch (psi). 1 millimeter of mercury means force on a unit area (1 cm²) on which 1 mm of height of Hg is placed. Pressure is also measured in bars. 1 bar of pressure is 10^6 dynes/cm² or 10^5 Pa and is nearly 1 atm (1 atm = 1.0197 bar).

Atmospheric Pressure

Atmospheric air is pulled to the earth by gravity and generates a force upon the surface of the earth, resulting in atmospheric pressure. Atmospheric pressure is the sum of pressures of all gases (e.g. N_2, O_2, and CO_2 present in air). It is measured with the help of a glass tube filled with either mercury or water (manometer). The height of the column of mercury (or water) multiplied by its density is a measure of the atmospheric pressure. Standard pressure is measured at sea level and expressed in mm Hg (torr) or cm H_2O.

Partial Pressure

In a mixture of gases in a container, each gas exerts the same pressure, which it would if it alone occupied the container. There is no interference from the presence of other gas(es). The pressure exerted by each individual gas is called the partial pressure. The total pressure exerted by the mixture of gases is equal to the sum of the partial pressures of all the gases contained in the mixture (*Dalton's law*). The partial pressure is determined by the fraction of the concentration of the gas in the mixture.

The atmospheric air has a total pressure of 760 mm Hg when dry at sea level. The partial pressures of N_2 (79%) and O_2 (21%), therefore, are as follows:

$$P_{N2} = 79\% \text{ of } P = 600.4 \text{ mm Hg}$$
$$P_{O2} = 21\% \text{ of } P = 159.6 \text{ mm Hg}$$

Other Body Pressures

The presence of air or fluid in other body cavities exerts different pressures in similar fashion as in the lungs (Table 2.1). The interval pressures in the body are also influenced by outside environmental pressures. The total pressure is therefore the sum of the external plus the internal pressure (*gauge pressure*). For example, the internal pressures will rise in hyperbaric conditions and decrease in hypobaric conditions as at high altitudes.

Temperature and Heat

Temperature is the thermal state of a substance, which determines whether the substance will give or receive heat from another substance in contact. It is

TABLE 2.1: Some important pressures (mm Hg) in normal human body.

Pressure	Expressed in mmHg
• Alveolar	760
• Arterial blood	
– Systolic	100–195
– Diastolic	60–85
• Venous blood	3–7
• Capillaries	
– Arterial end	30
– Venous end	10

an indication of the level of molecular activity. Heat is the thermal energy of a substance, which can be given to or abstracted from it. Temperature is the measurement of heat.

Calorie is the unit of heat. It is defined as the quantity of heat required to raise the temperature of 1 g of water by 1°C. As an example, if 1 calorie is required to raise the temperature of 1 g of water by 1°C, 1,000 calories will be required for 1,000 g of water. The caloric value of food is expressed by a larger heat unit, i.e. the kilocalorie (cal or kcal), which is equivalent to 1,000 cal.

GAS LAWS

There is a definite and simple relationship which connects pressure, temperature and volume of any gas of a given concentration. These laws are valid for ideal gases only, where the assumption that the gas particles are very small and do not interact with each other is valid.

Boyle's Law

Pressure (P) of a gas is inversely proportional to its volume (V) provided the absolute temperature (T) of the mass of gas is kept constant. In other words, the product of pressure and volume remains constant. It follows immediately from the ideal gas equation:

$$P \propto 1/V \text{ or } P \times V = \text{Constant, if } T \text{ is constant. Or } P_1 V_1 = P_2 V_2$$

The application of this law in respiratory physiology is best exemplified in the use of body plethysmography to measure total lung capacity. It is also employed in many mechanical ventilators whereby the gas is driven into patient's lungs or into the cylinder of the ventilator by the upstroke and downstroke movements of the piston.

Charles' Law

When pressure and mass of a gas are kept constant, the volume of the gas will vary directly with its absolute temperature. Again from gas equation:

$$V/T = \text{Constant } (K), \text{ if } P \text{ is constant}$$

It is because of this reason that volumes measured with the help of lung function equipment (at room temperature) are a little lower than those at body temperature (37°C) and need to be corrected for the same. If the temperature of a container of a gas is lowered, the volume shrinks. Therefore, more gas can be stored in the same cylinder at a lower temperature.

Gay-Lussac's Law

Temperature and pressure of a gas are directly proportional when the volume and mass are kept constant.

$$P \propto T \text{ or } P/T = K \text{ at constant } V$$

It implies an increase in pressure if the temperature is increased. For this reason, safety valves are provided with devices using high pressure gases to vent high pressures in case there is an accidental heating.

General Gas Law

Assume N ideal noninteracting molecules of a gas each of mass m are contained in a cube of volume V. They are in motion if the temperature is above 0°K (0°K = –273°C). If the temperature is T in Kelvin, the kinetic energy from each molecule is of the order of kT, where k is called Boltzmann constant [K = 1.38 × 10^{-16} centimeter–gram–second (CGS) units]. Because of this kinetic motion, the molecules of the gas keep bombarding the walls of the cube and exert pressure. The pressure increase results in extra energy (obtainable from force × distance or p × volume relation).

It may be stated here that under the conditions of lower temperature and high pressure, the gas changes its state to liquid. This is because the gas molecules get attracted to each other (van der Waals forces) rather than being repelled. The higher pressure condenses the molecules and the lower temperature reduces their activity. The temperature at which the gas turns into liquid is the "critical temperature" of that gas. For oxygen, it is –116°C. A pressure of 50 atmospheres is required to liquefy oxygen at –116°C. To keep the oxygen in a liquid form at 1 atmosphere in a flask open to the atmosphere, the temperature is lowered to below –183°C. This principle forms the basis of the availability of oxygen in the liquid form for storage and ambulatory use.

Henry's Law

The amount of gas that enters into physical solution in a liquid is directly proportional to the partial pressure of the gas. For example, the greater the partial pressure of oxygen in the alveoli, the greater the solubility in plasma.

Graham's Law

The rate of diffusion (D) of a gas is inversely proportional to the square root of its density (d).

$$D_1 d_2 = D_2 d_1$$

Therefore, a light gas (such as helium) will diffuse at a faster rate than a heavier gas (such as oxygen).

Bernoulli's Principle

Flow of a gas through a partially obstructed tube can be described by Bernoulli's principle, i.e. the pressure required to produce flow is the difference in velocity at two points and the density of the gas.

GAS SOLUTION AND TENSION

The amount of gas dissolved in a liquid is directly proportional to the pressure of the gas (*Henry's law*). It also varies with the temperature—lesser amount is dissolved at the same pressure, if temperature is increased. A state of equilibrium is reached when no further gas dissolves in the liquid. This is a state of full saturation with the gas at a given temperature and pressure. The gas in solution is said to exert the same "tension" as the partial pressure of the gas over the liquid in equilibrium with it. For example, when the partial pressure of oxygen in alveoli is 100 mm Hg, the tension of O_2 in alveolar capillaries is 100 mm Hg. At this pressure, 0.3 cc of oxygen at NTP dissolves in 100 cc of water. The weight of oxygen dissolved in 100 cc of water is $1.3 \times 0.3/1,000 = 0.0004$ g (1.3 g/L is the density of oxygen).

The amount of oxygen dissolved in plasma or water is the same (0.004 g/100 mL). This is quite sufficient to supply all the oxygen necessary for the metabolism of the body.

VAPOR

Vapor is defined as the gaseous state of a substance, which, at room temperature and pressure, is a liquid. On the other hand, a gas at room temperature exists only in the gaseous state. Like any other gas, the molecules of a vapor are continuously in violent motion and bombard the walls of the container. The force exerted on each unit area is called the pressure of the vapor (*vapor pressure*).

A vapor in a mixture of gases obeys the same laws as the gases. The partial pressure of the vapor in a mixture bears the same proportion to the total pressure as the volume, i.e. it depends on the percent (or fractional) concentration in the mixture. For example, the concentration of about 16% of water vapors in air at NTP, which is sufficient to saturate air with water vapors, exerts a pressure of 16% of 760 mm Hg (47 mm Hg).

The presence of water vapors in air or oxygen is referred to as *humidity*. It is largely through the process of evaporation that the molecules of water (or any other liquid) evaporate into the overlying air (or any other gas in a container).

The molecules leave the liquid substance when their kinetic energy exceeds the surface tension of the liquid. If a liquid is kept in a closed container for long, a state of equilibrium is reached when the number of molecules returning to the liquid (*condensation*) is exactly equal to the number leaving it (*evaporation*).

This is called the saturation point. This is further dependent upon temperature; if the temperature increases, the number of molecules leaving the liquid also increase and the saturation point is raised, i.e. there is a greater amount of vapors in the same amount of gas. Reverse happens with a fall in temperature.

The air we breathe is normally humid due to the presence of water vapor. The actual amount of water vapor present in air is expressed as "relative humidity", which is defined as the ratio of the amount of water vapor present in a given volume with the amount of water vapor, which the air (or the gas) is capable of holding at the given temperature, in the same volume. The humidity of air varies with the atmospheric conditions. Once inhaled in the lungs, air gets fully saturated. The amount of water vapor required to saturate the alveolar air at body temperature and pressure is the body humidity.

The presence of water vapor in the inhaled air exerts its own partial pressure, and lowers the pressures of constituent gases of air—oxygen and nitrogen. Therefore, PN_2 or PO_2 is calculated as a proportion of the atmospheric pressure minus water vapor pressure, i.e. $P - PH_2O$. When fully saturated, PH_2O of atmospheric air is equal to 47 mm Hg. Therefore, $PO_2 = (P - PH_2O) \times 21\% = (760 - 47) \times 0.21 = 150$ mm Hg. The rest, i.e. $760 - (150 + 47)$ would be approximately the PN_2.

EXPRESSION OF GAS VOLUMES AND PRESSURES

In view of the effects of temperature, pressure, and humidity on all gases, these are expressed with reference to those conditions. Some of the common expressions are:
- Standard (or normal) temperature and pressure (STP) or NTP temperature 0°C; pressure 760 mm Hg
- STPD—D indicates "dry" = complete absence of water vapor
- Ambient temperature and pressure—dry or saturated (ATPD or ATPS). Ambient implies the room conditions.
- Body temperature and pressure saturated (BTPS)—body temperature (usually 37°C), ambient pressure, and water vapor pressure (47 mm Hg).

Normally, gas volume measurements are made in the ambient conditions. Conversion is required to express the volume at BTPS or STPD. STPD is used for the uniformity of expression. This is done by multiplying with conversion factors. Tables of conversion factors from ATPS to STPD, STPD to BTPS, or BTPS to ATPS are available in most laboratories. Such corrections are also required to express volume of a gas (such as O_2) produced in the laboratory. The volume is expressed at STPD, which is different than that produced at ATPS.

FLOW OF GASES

Flow is the movement of particles of a liquid or a gas from higher to lower pressure. It is expressed in the terms of volume per unit time, e.g. liters per minute or per second (L/min or L/sec). The movement of air into the lungs during inspiration and out into the atmosphere during expiration is accomplished by the flow of air through tracheobronchial tree. Similarly, oxygen flows from a container cylinder to the lungs or a ventilator through connecting tubes as long as there is a pressure difference.

The flow is described as laminar, if it is smooth and gas particles move along lines parallel to the walls of the tube. But it is turbulent, if the lines of flow are irregular, broken up, and disorderly. Whether the flow is laminar or turbulent, it has to meet a certain resistance while moving from one to the other end of the tube. The laminar flow is described by the *Hagen–Poiseuille equation*, i.e. $V = \Pi \gamma^4 \Delta P/(8 \eta l)$.

Resistance

Resistance is defined by the pressure difference under given conditions—between the entry and the exit points of a tube. The resistance is dependent on the tube length (l) and diameter. It is also directly proportional to the velocity of flow (V) or rate in case of laminar flow. The flow is also viscosity (η) dependent and density independent. When the flow is turbulent, the resistance rises for steeply.

Laminar flow through a straight tube of uniform size is inversely proportional to the length (l) of the tube and directly to the fourth power of radius (r).

When the flow exceeds a *"critical flow rate"*, the laminar flow is replaced by the turbulent flow throughout the length of the tube. Turbulent flow is less efficient since the ∇P varies directly with V^2. Turbulent flow is density dependent and viscosity independent. The critical flow varies directly with the internal diameter of the tube—the larger the diameter, the greater the flow. At a flow below the critical rate, local turbulence may occur as a result of irregularities in the pathways of the gas. During oxygen administration, this may occur due to the constriction of kinking of the tubes.

Turbulence

Turbulence in a flowing system can also be predicted by Reynolds number. It is the ratio between inertial (density dependent, viscosity independent) and viscous (viscosity dependent, density independent) forces—a dimensionless number.

Flow is "laminar" when the number is less than 2,000 and "turbulent" when it is more than 3,000. Turbulent flow is dominated by inertial forces producing random eddies and flow fluctuations. Between 2,000 and 3,000, the flow is transitional, i.e. neither fully laminar nor fully turbulent.

Flow through Orifices

An orifice is a narrow opening of a tube. Unlike a tube, the diameter of the fluid pathway of the orifice exceeds the length. The greater the diameter compared to the length, the more does the opening approach the "ideal" orifice. The flow through an orifice depends on the diameter (or the cross-section area) of the orifice and the difference in pressures on either side of the orifice.

The intrinsic property of a liquid that influences its flow, which we earlier termed as resistance, is called viscosity. It is attributed to the internal friction between different layers, which move at different speeds. While the laminar flow largely depends on viscosity, it is the density, which determines the flow when turbulent. The coefficient of viscosity is equal to the force per unit area necessary to maintain the unit difference of velocity between two parallel planes.

The flow through an orifice is at least partially turbulent. The lower the density, i.e. the lighter the gas, the greater is its volume flow for any given pressure difference on the either side of the orifice.

Heliox

Heliox is a mixture of oxygen with helium (He) in varying concentrations, commonly as 20% oxygen and 80% helium. It has a lower density than that of air, i.e. oxygen (21%) with nitrogen (79%). Resistance offered to the flow of heliox is lower than that of air and of oxygen and depends on the fractional concentrations. It diffuses 1.8 times faster than oxygen. This fact is exploited in clinical practice for the treatment of acute respiratory distress of obstructive airway diseases, such as asthma when the flow is highly turbulent. Heliox diffuses faster than oxygen through partially obstructed airways. In view of the lower resistance offered to heliox, the breathing effort is considerably reduced and the crisis tide over.

DEPOSITION

The particular matter inhaled in the lungs gets deposited in the tracheobronchial tree and the alveoli. The alveolar deposits have the potential to penetrate the alveolar walls and migrate to the bloodstream. The deposition is influenced by multiple factors such as the particle size, the acinus morphometry, the type of airflow, breathing patterns, and lung heterogeneities.

DIFFUSION

The molecules in a fluid (liquid or gas), unlike in a solid, move freely in all directions. The time taken by a molecule to travel a given distance depends upon its closeness to other molecules, and the intermolecular spaces. The gas molecules do not necessarily collide with the neighboring molecules when they move around or across a membrane.

Diffusion across a membrane is determined by the difference in concentrations between the two neighboring layers of the solution. The rate of diffusion is proportional to the gradient of concentration, i.e. the change of concentration per unit length in the direction of diffusion (*Fick's law*). Diffusion also depends on molecular movement. The rates of diffusion of gases at similar partial pressures through a porous membrane are inversely proportional to the square roots of their molecular weights (*Graham's law*).

Solubility

Another factor, which determines diffusion across a wet film, is the solubility of the gas. The rate of diffusion is directly proportional to the solubility of the gas in the fluid.

Permeability

A membrane is permeable, if it allows the particular molecules to pass through, i.e. across the membrane. Permeability of different membranes to the molecules of different substances (solid, liquid, or gases) is variable.

Osmosis

Osmosis is the migration of molecules of a solvent across a membrane. The pressure, which stops the transfer of molecules, is called the osmotic pressure of the solution. The osmotic pressure of a solution depends only on the number of dissolved particles per liter and not on the nature of the substances, which is dissolved.

The diffusion mechanisms also depend upon the pressures, volume, and filtration. In respiratory system, the diffusion of gases and fluids across the alveolar membrane are critically important for normal gas-exchange functions of the lung and in the maintenance of a fluid balance.

CHAPTER 3

History and Physical Examination

Prahlad Rai Gupta

INTRODUCTION

Clinical history and physical examination continue to play an important role in the assessment of medical illness in a given patient. Quick decisions regarding treatment are often made on the basis of clinical evaluation alone. Such subjective, context dependent reasoning is integral to clinical judgment and is especially useful to diagnose rare diseases.

HISTORY TAKING

The guiding principle to history taking is: "listen to the patient as if he is revealing the diagnosis". Allow him to speak about his illness in his own words. Avoid unnecessary interruptions except when it becomes essential to seek details on certain issues.

Cough

Cough is a reflexive or deliberate explosive expiratory act. It is normally physiological and meant to clear the airways, but may become troublesome at times. History should cover the duration and characteristics of cough, whether it is dry or productive of sputum or blood, the provocative factors, i.e. cold, smoke, change of posture or eating and what are the accompanying symptoms to find out its likely cause.

Sputum

A patient having productive cough should be asked about the time course, amount, character, viscosity, taste, and color of the sputum. Early morning sputum in smokers suggests chronic bronchitis but if it occurs while lying down/going to bed, it points to underlying bronchiectasis or lung abscess. Most children and adult females usually do not spit but swallow their sputum; the presence of sputum should be assessed by the sound of their cough. It is usually not possible to measure the exact amount of sputum, but its quantum can be accessed from the number of spits, spoonfuls or cupfuls. Sputum may be very foul smelling in lung abscess or bronchiectasis. It is better to inspect the sample of sputum as the patient may not be able to describe its exact character, viscosity, and color.

Hemoptysis

Hemoptysis is coughing out blood from respiratory tract, mainly the lungs. Mild hemoptysis, often seen as blood streaking, is a common symptom with severe sough. Efforts should be made to differentiate true hemoptysis from hematemesis, epistaxis or bleeding from oral cavity by asking the patient about the temporal pattern of blood spitting. Hematemesis generally follows nausea, vomiting or retching; in epistaxis, the patient feels sensation of postnasal drip or bleeding from nares without coughing but hemoptysis follows coughing. The type of blood in the expectorate can also help to detect the source (bright red often mixed with frothy sputum in hemoptysis versus the dark black, often in clumps and mixed with food, in hematemesis).

Chest Pain

Chest pain is a common complaint, but the patient's perception about its gravity may vary. To some, it is a warning of potential life-threatening illness and they may seek repeated consultations even when the symptom is trivial. Others, including those with serious illnesses, may tend to ignore. However, a physician should never discard the symptom without exploring its etiology. Chest pain may have its origin from disorders of chest wall, pleura, lungs, heart/great vessels, esophagus and subdiaphragmatic structures. History of chest pain should include its duration, location, radiation to other areas and character, i.e. heaviness, tearing, burning, stabbing, sharp needle like, urge to eructate or merely a discomfort (dull ache or boring).

Dyspnea

Dyspnea is an unpleasant or uncomfortable awareness of breathing. A host of pulmonary, cardiac or other disorders may lead to dyspnea. History should cover its duration, onset (sudden or insidious), severity, and exacerbating or relieving factors, i.e. exertion or rest, supine or sitting position or exposure to cold, dust, smoke, and allergens. Associated symptoms may provide useful clue to the cause of dyspnea. A patient with psychogenic dyspnea is symptomatic more often during rest than on exertion.

Upper Respiratory Tract Symptoms

A brief history of upper respiratory tract symptoms, more particularly running of nose, itching, sneezing, congestion, discharge of blood or blood mixed secretions or blocked nose, should always be obtained while assessing a patient for respiratory illness.

General Symptoms

Once the assessment of the respiratory symptoms is over, the patient should be asked for the presence of general symptoms and those pertaining to other systems. Presence of fever, loss of appetite, weight loss or anemia signifies serious illness. History of associated urinary symptoms, dysphasia, joint pain, and skin lesions may point to an important systemic illness. Symptoms pertaining to cardiac and neuromuscular diseases may unravel the cause of respiratory illness, particularly of dyspnea.

Past Medical History

Past medical history of the patient may give an important clue to the etiology of the current illness. Ask about childhood illnesses like fever, cough and cold; if recurrent, as these may end up with diagnoses of asthma, chronic obstructive pulmonary disease (COPD) or bronchiectasis during adult life. Chest injuries in past (particularly those with hemothorax) may indicate frozen chest. History of loss of consciousness in the past may point to lung abscess. Surgery or pregnancy in recent past suggests pulmonary thromboembolism. Indeed, history of infections, trauma, surgery, malignancies or prolonged bed rest in the past, all may provide important clue to the diagnosis of the current illness. Important lifestyle diseases that may have impact on respiratory system include diabetes mellitus and obesity. History of allergy to food, drugs and/or dust may give an important clue to the diagnosis of rhinitis/asthma. History of wheezy bronchitis in childhood is also helpful in diagnosis of asthma in adults.

HISTORY OF TREATMENT

Most patients visit a pulmonologist only after consulting their family physician. It is therefore, always worthwhile to ask the patient about the details of such consultations, investigations already done, diagnosis made, treatment offered, and the outcome thereof. A correct diagnosis may have been missed for want of time and skill and even if a diagnosis was correctly made, the treatment may be wanting in the terms of drugs, dosages, and compliance. Past history of incorrect or irregular treatment of tuberculosis (TB) may point to drug failure (and drug resistance), relapse or sequelae such as bronchiectasis, aspergilloma or chronic necrotizing pulmonary aspergillosis. Drugs taken for other illnesses may sometimes be responsible for the current illness.

Personal History

Patient's lifestyle and personal habits like smoking or alcohol consumption, along with the details of the quantity, frequency and its duration, are integral parts of a good history-taking. Exposure to pets and animals may be responsible for a serious or recurrent respiratory illness. Present or past occupational exposure to organic dust like bagasse or hay or inorganic dust like silica, coal or asbestos may at times help to unravel the diagnosis in most difficult clinical situations.

PHYSICAL EXAMINATION

After the history-taking, the clinician already has some idea regarding the likely diagnosis and what to expect of the physical examination. Yet a systematic approach to the latter is always rewarding and may obviate the need for unnecessary investigations at a later stage.

General Physical Examination

Always begin with assessment of the general appearance, mental faculty, and breathing pattern of the patient. Note down the presence of wheeze, stridor or voice abnormality, if any. An anxious look indicates acute illness while the presence of fatigue and cachexia point to a chronic disease or malignancy. A plethoric appearance may be seen in polycythemia, most commonly as a result of chronic lung disease or superior vena cava (SVC) obstruction. Look at the tongue, soft palate and the nail beds for cyanosis, anemia or polycythemia, at fingers for clubbing, at face, neck, hands, and feet for edema (generalized, localized or differential); and neck for any lymphadenopathy or abnormal pulsations/fullness of veins. Record vital signs, i.e. pulse (rate, rhythm, and character), respiration (type, rate and regularity), blood pressure, and temperature. Also look for any nicotine stains on the intertriginous surfaces of the second and third fingers which may point to the smoking habit (in cigarette or *bidi* smokers). Similar stains may be present on the palm in *chillum* or *hookah* smokers.

Breathing Pattern

Breathing pattern should be observed throughout the clinical examination. Normal breathing is quiet without any sound. The usual respiratory rate is between 12 and 18 per minute. An increased respiratory rate (tachypnea) is seen in the presence of a respiratory disease such as asthma, chronic obstructive lung disease, restrictive lung diseases, pulmonary artery hypertension or hypoxia of any etiology. Tachypnea may be also present in nonrespiratory conditions such as congestive heart failure, severe anemia or tension and anxiety. A slow respiratory rate (bradypnea) may be caused by depressed respiratory drive due to drug overdose (e.g. sedative or narcotics) or the presence of central nervous system lesions. Use of the accessory muscles of respiration or pursed lip breathing, which indicate severe illness, should be recorded.

Cyanosis

Cyanosis is the bluish discoloration of the tongue and the soft palate (central, when it mostly reflects arterial hypoxemia) or of nail beds and lips (peripheral, when it may also reflect arterial hypoxemia due to low blood flow). Central cyanosis mostly occurs due to severe chronic hypoxemia of pulmonary or cardiac origin and is often associated with polycythemia. Peripheral cyanosis (often with edema) affecting face, neck (and sometimes the upper limbs) may indicate SVC obstruction, and that of lower limbs, the inferior vena cava obstruction.

Clubbing

Clubbing is defined by the presence of diffuse bulbous enlargement of the terminal phalanges. Early clubbing is characterized by thickening of the fibroelastic tissue of the nail bed. These changes are best seen by the loss of the normally present angle between the nail-base and the adjacent dorsal surface of the finger. This finding can be appreciated when the finger is viewed from the side. Finger clubbing can occur in various pulmonary, cardiac, and abdominal diseases. Rarely clubbing may be congenital (familial) in origin.

Lymphadenopathy

Lymphadenopathy is abnormal enlargement of lymph glands (mostly > 0.5 cm in size) at neck, axilla, groin, and other external or internal sites. Note down the number, size, consistency, and fixity of the lymph nodes to each other, the underlying tissues or to the overlying skin. Large fixed masses indicate metastasis, while firm and matted nodes point to TB. Lymph nodes in Hodgkin's lymphoma are classically described as large, soft, and rubbery in character.

Miscellaneous Physical Findings

All components of the upper respiratory tract (nasal cavity, nasopharynx, nasal sinuses, oropharynx, and the larynx) need to be examined sequentially as this may help clinch the diagnosis, e.g. discharging nasal lesion in GPA (Wegener's granulomatosis). Thyroid gland should also be examined to detect abnormality in its shape, size, and consistency. Other lesions that may provide clue to the underlying respiratory pathology include skin lesions such as erythema nodosum in sarcoidosis and TB; malar rash in systemic lupus erythematosus and dermatomyositis; subcutaneous nodules in metastatic carcinoma and eye lesions such as phlyctenular conjunctivitis in TB; Horner's syndrome in lung cancer; iridocyclitis in TB and sarcoidosis; chemosis in SVC obstruction and flapping tremors in type II respiratory failure (hypercapnea).

Examination of the Chest

Traditionally, the scheme of chest examination includes inspection, palpation, percussion, and auscultation in that order, but some physicians combine inspection with palpation. It is best done in good day light with the patient in the sitting posture and arms at the side.

Percussion is important to compare the degree of resonance over the equivalent areas on the two sides of chest and then focus on the area of interest to detect a generalized or localized abnormality. Note for an area of tenderness, if any. The character of percussion note may point to the underlying pathology. A stony dull percussion note indicates pleural effusion, more so, if the breath sounds and vocal resonance are decreased. A dull note with increased bronchial breath sounds and bronchophony indicates consolidation but with shrunken chest and decreased breath sounds, it indicates atelectasis. Hyper resonant note indicates pneumothorax, more so when the chest appears fuller and the breath sounds and/or vocal resonance are decreased or absent.

Listen to lung sounds for its character and quality over all the parts of the chest wall, on both the sides, using the diaphragm of stethoscope. Breath sounds are vesicular in character (low frequency rustling sound with longer inspiration than expiration and without a pause in between) over the healthy lungs and are best heard at the lung bases. When the breath sound is blowing in character and loud in mid-expiration, it is called as broncho-vesicular. In a normal person, such a breath sound may be heard over the lung apices. Bronchial breathing consists of a high-pitched blowing sound of hollow character. It is heard during both inspiration and expiration and separated by a brief pause. Bronchial breathing is normally heard over trachea or larynx. When heard over a part of the chest wall, it is abnormal and indicates consolidation of the underlying lung. It is produced due to the increased transmission of high-pitched breath sounds to the chest wall through the solid lung which now acts as a bridge between the airways and the chest wall. Breath sounds are decreased in intensity when there is fluid (effusion) or air (pneumothorax) in the pleural cavity. Presence of atelectasis due to airway obstruction also decreases the breath sounds due to diminished transmission of sounds from airways to the chest wall.

Extra sounds such as wheezes, crackles and/or pleural rub may be heard in disease states. Wheezes are continuous, high-pitched sounds, often musical in character, which arise from air moving in the narrowed airways, e.g. in asthma. They are more marked during expiration, usually associated with prolonged expiratory time. Low-pitched sound (rhonchus) may be heard at a localized area such as obstruction of a large airway by a tumor. Crackles are discontinuous, "popping" or bubbling sounds. Presence of secretions in the larger airways may cause coarser, gurgling sounds which may be heard during inspiration as well as expiration. Finer crackles, usually during early inspiration, are commonly heard in the presence of restrictive lung disorders such as the pulmonary edema and pulmonary fibrosis. They are produced due to snap-opening of the small airways. Rub is a localized cracking or rubbing sound, often associated with chest pain and is heard during inspiration as well as expiration (to and fro character).

Systemic Examination

Examination of other systems may provide vital clues in the assessment of a patient with respiratory illness. Certain skin lesions are an essential part of the pulmonary disease, i.e. erythema nodosum in TB and sarcoidosis; Kaposi's sarcoma in AIDS; larva migrans in Loeffler's syndrome; metastatic nodule in lung carcinoma; and "Mat" telangiectasia in Osler–Weber–Rendu disease. Skin lesions may also manifest as the complication of drugs, i.e. Stevens–Johnson syndrome in a patient of TB on antitubercular treatment or be a part of a systemic disease having pulmonary manifestations, i.e. lupus pernio, flashy papules and erythema nodosum in sarcoidosis, malar rash and discoid lesions (often accompanied by telangiectasia, atrophy and scarring) in systemic lupus erythematosus. Besides, certain primary skin diseases like erythema multiforme may have pulmonary complications.

Examination of the joints may show symmetrical arthritis of small joints (rheumatoid arthritis) or large joints (Behçet disease). Examination of cardiovascular system may unravel cor pulmonale complicating the hypoxemia of pulmonary diseases or unravel the underlying pericardial, myocardial, endocardial or valvular lesions of the heart or aneurysmal lesions of vessels that complicate the respiratory diseases. Similarly, examination of abdomen may reveal advanced cirrhosis that leads to hepatopulmonary syndrome, while neurological examination may reveal the signs of metastatic brain lesion in an otherwise occult lung cancer.

Bedside Measurement of Lung Functions

Measurement of forced expiratory time has been used to detect the presence of airway obstruction in a patient at bedside. The length of time taken to walk 6 meter distance (6MWD) is a simple test of lung function. Peak expiratory flow measurements and oxymetry can also be considered as essential components of the initial clinical and physical assessment.

Examination of Chest Skiagrams

Many chest physicians now consider examination of the respiratory system as incomplete without perusal of the recent and past skiagrams of the chest. It provides a visual appreciation of the respiratory illness and helps planning of further investigations. Occasionally, situation may arise where the clinical findings may not correlate with the X-ray findings and the latter will prevail over the former in making clinical judgment.

In summary, the importance of history-taking and physical examination should never be underestimated, in spite of the ever expanding diagnostic armamentarium. Patients expect and appreciate some degree of physical examination by the doctor. Besides being a powerful diagnostic tool, it helps as healing-ritual and promotes physician-patient relationship. While over-reliance on physical findings and stress on mandatory demonstration of individual physical signs is unnecessary, the importance of history-taking remains critical for diagnosis as well as for comprehensive management.

CHAPTER 4

Pulmonary Function Tests

AN Aggarwal

INTRODUCTION

There is as yet no single test that can provide sufficiently detailed information on all aspects of lung function. Instead, depending on the clinical scenario, one must do one or more procedures to answer a particular question. Further, the available options vary greatly in terms of ease of conducting the test, equipment and technician requirements, test performance characteristics, and procedure cost.

SPIROMETRY

Spirometry is the most common and most widely used lung function test, although its true potential still needs to be realized. One needs to pay careful attention to follow the standard procedures while performing and interpreting the test. Because the residual volume in lungs cannot be exhaled, spirometric measurements are limited to the vital capacity and its subdivisions (Fig. 4.1).

Indications and Contraindications

The most common indication for doing the test is a functional evaluation of patients with lung disease. The presence of spirometric abnormalities, as well as the degree of impairment, provides useful information about the disease severity and pulmonary reserve of the patient. Serial measurements can provide information about disease progression, as well as response to prescribed treatment. The test also has an important role in clinical trials. Spirometry is also used as a screening tool for studies in epidemiologic surveys, and to screen at-risk populations for subclinical disease (for example,

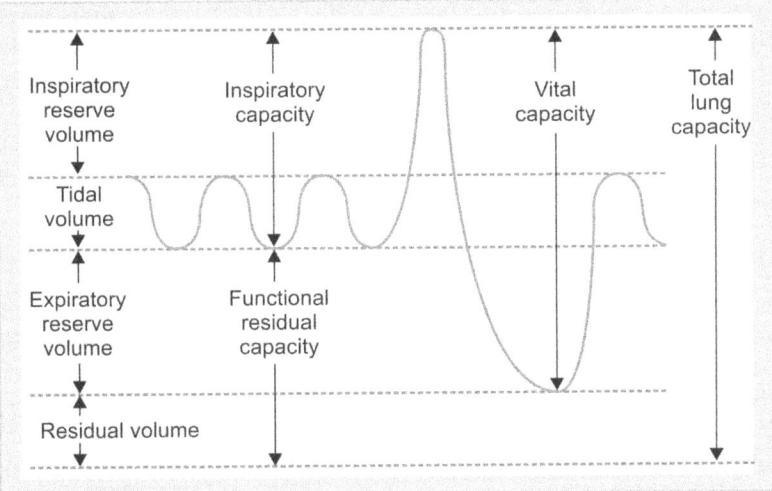

Fig. 4.1: Various lung volumes and capacities in relation to the spirometry tracing. Note that residual volume cannot be determined through conventional spirometry.

preoperative assessment, or detecting chronic obstructive pulmonary disease (COPD) among asymptomatic smokers). The test is also utilized in occupational setting, both for detecting work-related respiratory disorders, and for disability assessment in symptomatic people (for example, as part of compensation procedures). Finally, spirometry is an important research tool for understanding pathophysiology and temporal course of several diseases.

Any benefit from the information obtained through this test should be carefully weighed against patient discomfort and risk. The test is better avoided in pregnant and severely dyspneic patients. It should also not be carried out in patients where pressure swings due to a forced expiratory maneuver can worsen existing conditions (such as ruptured tympanic membrane, bronchopleural fistula, ongoing hemoptysis, etc.). Uncooperative patients, and those on life support systems, should also not undergo the test.

Equipment

A wide range of apparatus, ranging from handheld portable devices to large equipment, and from predominantly manual to completely automated systems, is available to perform spirometry. Although many factors such as cost, patient load, clinical requirements, etc. determine the choice of machine, it is important to use one that confirms to some minimum technical specifications necessary to obtain valid results.

Most commercially available spirometers nowadays are computerized systems that employ a transducer to convert a mechanical signal to an electrical one, and display the output in a fashion understood by the operator. These equipment can be divided into two broad categories: (1) volume displacement spirometers and (2) flow-sensing spirometers. The former work with volume as the primary output, and flow is a derived parameter. Such machines can have a water seal, a dry-rolling seal, or a bellows type design. Flow sensing devices can either be electronic turbines, or use electronic pneumotachometers (sensors that estimate airflow from the change in pressure occurring across a suitable resistance), which in turn can have a flow-resistive, a heated wire, or an ultrasonic design. As opposed to volume displacement spirometers, these machines measure flow as the primary signal, which is time-integrated to yield volume estimates.

Reference Values

The basic purpose of pulmonary function testing is to identify persons with abnormal lung function. To know what is abnormal, we must first define what is normal. Predicted normal values can be obtained from studies carried out in healthy subjects. They are usually in the form of a regression equation describing the predicted value as a function of gender and anthropometric data (e.g. height, weight, etc.), and differ greatly with ethnicity. Any value below the predicted normal is not necessarily reduced, since the normal value is a range rather than a fixed point. This introduces the concept of "lower limit of normal" or LLN, which can be defined in several ways. The simplest (and most widely used) method is to use a fixed percentage of predicted value. For example, a value less than 80% of predicted FEV1 can be considered abnormal. However, there is very little statistical or physiological basis for such an approach. A more valid approach is to use lower 95% confidence limits of the regression equation, or subtract 1.645 times the standard error of estimate of the regression equation from the predicted value, to define the LLN. Any value below the corresponding LLN is considered abnormal. It is very important to use norms derived from individuals largely similar to the patients being generally tested at any pulmonary function laboratory. Therefore standard Caucasian norms, often incorporated into spirometer softwares, should be avoided, and locally appropriate reference equations preferred wherever available.

Interpretation and Patterns in Common Disorders

Interpreting lung function data is not just about looking at numbers generated by the spirometer. Both the volume-time curve and the flow-volume loop must also be evaluated with regard to their technical quality, size and shape, and various components, before making a final interpretation. Often such graphical analysis provides additional important information not obtainable from the numerical data. If available, the postbronchodilator graphs should also be similarly evaluated and compared to baseline curves. The clinical data provided in the requisition form is equally important in helping to reach any conclusion, especially in borderline situations.

Broadly, the interpretation of spirometric data involves only three numerical variables: FEV1, VC and FEV1/VC. The largest observed values of FEV1 and VC available from among at least three acceptable and reproducible tests should be used as the key parameters for interpretation, even if these individual observations are derived from different test maneuvers. If both forced and relaxed VC maneuvers have been performed, the larger value of VC amongst the FVC and SVC measurements should be used for interpretation. The large numbers of other variables, often available from computerized spirometer outputs, usually provide no additional information, and are best excluded from a standard interpretative algorithm.

Any spirometry record with normal FEV1, VC and FEV1/VC (i.e. all values more than their corresponding LLN values) should be interpreted as normal. Any spirometry record with FEV1/VC value below its predicted LLN should be interpreted as having an obstructive abnormality. This approach is superior to the use of fixed cut-offs in correctly identifying patients with airflow limitation, especially among the elderly.

Any spirometry record with a normal FEV1/VC (i.e. value above corresponding LLN), coupled with a reduced VC (i.e. value below corresponding LLN), is suggestive of a restrictive abnormality. In situations where statistically valid LLN figures are not available (or not practical to use, as in field settings), observed VC ratio less than 80% of predicted value is often used to define reduction in VC. Restrictive defects are common in conditions with loss of functioning lung parenchyma (e.g. diffuse parenchymal lung diseases, lung collapse/atelectasis, pneumonia, after lung resection). Such defects are also observed in neuromuscular diseases (due to reduction in generation of force needed for a FVC maneuver) as well as disorders of chest wall and pleura (e.g. massive pleural effusion, pleural fibrosis, obesity, and kyphoscoliosis). True restriction is defined as reduction in total lung capacity. A mixed (obstructive plus restrictive) defect also cannot be diagnosed solely based on spirometry. A disproportionately low VC in face of a reduced FEV1/VC can either represent air trapping (with consequent increase in RV at the expense of VC, as in severe emphysema), or a true reduction in TLC (as in COPD with pneumonia). There is no universally accepted scheme of severity categorization.

The flow-volume loop may also provide a clue to underlying pathology. A small and concave or scooped curve suggests obstructive disorder. A small curve with steep slope suggests restriction. A small and flat curve suggests central airway obstruction. In disorders with variable intrathoracic obstruction, only the expiratory component of the loop is flat, whereas in disorders with variable extrathoracic obstruction, only the inspiratory component is flat. Both components are flat in lesions causing fixed airway obstruction.

Bronchodilator responsiveness (BDR) is considered to be present if the increase in FEV1 and/or VC (15-30 minutes after inhalation of 400 µg salbutamol) in the postbronchodilator study is both more than 12% and more than 200 mL over baseline values. Although an oversimplification, patients with asthma tend to have BDR much more frequently than those with COPD. It must be noted that lack of BDR does not necessarily imply poor clinical response to bronchodilators in either condition.

PEAK EXPIRATORY FLOW

Peak expiratory flow (PEF) is defined as highest flow achieved from a maximum forced expiratory maneuver started without hesitation from a position of maximal lung inflation. It can be measured either as a part of the spirometry procedure on the same instrument (with values derived from the flow volume curve), or separately using peak flow meters. The first meter specifically designed to measure this index of lung function was developed more than 50 years ago (Wright meter). Subsequently, a more portable, lower cost version (the "Mini-Wright" peak flow meter) was developed, and other designs and copies have since then become available across the world.

Although PEF is fairly well reproducible for an individual, the normal range of PEF in healthy individuals is rather wide. As a result, predicted values of PEF cannot be used to detect lung disease, since there is substantial overlap between values in patients with lung diseases and normal persons. Further, since PEF recordings are both flow and volume dependent, they tend to get reduced in both obstructive and restrictive disorders. Hence in general notion that diminished PEF is a marker of airway obstruction is also not correct. While a normal PEF can reliably rule out airway obstruction, a low PEF does not necessarily indicate the same. The degree of reduction in PEF does not correlate well with the severity of obstruction described by the degree of reduction in FEV1. PEF measurements generally underestimate the degree of airway obstruction, as determined from FEV1 measurements.

STATIC LUNG VOLUMES

Since spirometry cannot measure RV, it is not possible to determine FRC and TLC from this test. Other techniques are needed for the purpose. These methods are generally based on principles in which airflow velocity plays no role (in contrast to spirometry), and hence the term "static lung volumes" is often used for these measurements. Three techniques may be used: (a) open circuit nitrogen washout, (b) closed circuit inert gas dilution, and (c) whole body plethysmography. Determination of static lung volumes is helpful in ascertaining true restrictive physiology, and differentiating between obstructive and restrictive disorders. Comparison between TLC estimated through gas dilution and plethysmographic methods can also quantify the extent of air trapping within the lungs.

Whole Body Plethysmography

In contrast to gas dilution techniques, plethysmography measures the total volume of air in the thoracic cavity, including gas trapped in bullae and other noncommunicating spaces (e.g. air within pleura or esophagus). Plethysmographically determined FRC is therefore often referred to as thoracic gas volume (TGV). Although several different types of body plethysmographs are available, the "volume constant" type is the most widely used.

Interpretation

A decrease in TLC is diagnostic of a restrictive defect. In parenchymal restriction (e.g. lung fibrosis), RV and TLC are reduced proportionately, resulting in a normal RV/TLC ratio. In extrapulmonary restriction (e.g. chest wall or neuromuscular disorders), RV is usually normal (or sometimes even increased), resulting in an increased RV/TLC ratio. On the other hand, TLC might be increased in acromegaly, or in conditions like emphysema, as a result of air trapping. An increase in RV/TLC ratio, with an obstructive defect on spirometry, is a good indicator of air trapping. In conditions characterized by non-communicating air in the lungs (e.g. emphysema, bullae, etc.), whole body plethysmography provides a better estimate of the lung volume, since gas dilution techniques measure only the volume of air that is freely exchanged during breathing. In fact, the difference in volumes calculated by the two techniques may provide some indication to the volume of noncommunicating air present in the lungs. Estimation of static lung volumes is also necessary to diagnose mixed obstructive-restrictive defects, with a combination of reduced FEV1/VC ratio and reduced TLC.

DIFFUSING CAPACITY OF LUNGS

Measurement of pulmonary diffusing capacity allows us to assess the ability of lungs to transport gas from inspired air to the red blood cells in pulmonary capillary network. It is, however, a misnomer, since gas transfer does not depend solely on diffusion across the alveocapillary membrane, and it is not a "capacity" in that there is no theoretical maximal limit. Many laboratories therefore employ the term "transfer factor" instead.

The diffusing capacity for carbon monoxide (DLCO) is the generally measured index. This is because carbon monoxide uptake is easily measurable, and the gas essentially follows the same pathway as oxygen during transport from alveolar air to red blood cells, and ultimate binding to hemoglobin. DLCO is the uptake of carbon monoxide from lungs per unit time per unit of carbon monoxide driving pressure. The test is usually performed for screening for diffuse lung diseases and pulmonary vascular disorders, precise characterization of airflow limitation, differential diagnosis and severity assessment of restrictive ventilatory defects, disability evaluation, and preoperative assessment. There are no absolute contraindications. However, for technical reasons, most machines cannot measure DLCO in individuals with an extremely low VC (usually <1.5 L) or severely dyspneic patients unable to hold breath for a sufficient time. The test cannot be performed on many patients receiving supplemental oxygen, as this needs to be discontinued before and throughout the test procedure.

Methodology

Diffusing capacity for carbon monoxide can be measured using a single breath method, an intrabreath method, or a rebreathing technique. The first is most commonly used, as it is simpler and better standardized. DLCO is calculated from the total lung volume, breath-hold time, and the initial and final alveolar carbon monoxide concentrations. It is a product of the subject's total lung capacity and rate of carbon monoxide uptake during the breath-hold time. An estimate of the total lung capacity and the initial alveolar carbon monoxide concentration is obtained from the tracer gas concentration in exhaled gas.

The test can be repeated after an interval of at least 5 minutes. Generally, a mean value is reported from two acceptable tests whose results agree within 2 mL/min/mm Hg.

Interpretation

In contrast to other pulmonary function tests, observed DLCO values must be normalized to key nonrespiratory variables. Hemoglobin concentration is important as it removes the carbon monoxide from the blood, thus providing a nearly constant gradient for gas transfer. Anemic patients may thus have a lower DLCO, and the measurement should therefore be corrected for this factor in such patients. Smokers tend to have a small baseline level of blood carbon monoxide, and thus the transfer gradient may be less than for nonsmokers. If available, blood carboxyhemoglobin levels may be used to compensate for this anomaly.

As with other lung function tests, the patient's result is interpreted by comparing it with a corresponding reference value. It must be noted that the degree of variability of DLCO (both for a given subject and for the population) is much higher than the results of other lung function tests. In case serial tests are performed, a DLCO result can also be compared to previous values to detect any sizeable change. Normalizing the DLCO to patient's alveolar volume may provide additional information about the reason for an abnormal result. When alveolar volume is reduced (either because of true restriction or due to noncommunicating air spaces), the ratio of DLCO to alveolar volume is relatively preserved. The ratio is however decreased if alveolar volume is increased (as in emphysema) or normal (as in anemia, or nonperfusion of ventilated alveoli).

EXERCISE TESTING

Exercise testing is generally indicated for (a) evaluation of exercise intolerance, (b) evaluation of unexplained breathlessness, (c) preoperative assessment, and (d) formulation of exercise prescriptions. Detailed evaluation can give some clue about whether the underlying disorder is predominantly cardiovascular or respiratory in origin. Exercise testing can range from gross and crude assessments to highly detailed and standardized evaluation using computerized equipment. The two most regularly employed types of exercise testing for evaluating pulmonary diseases are the 6-minute walk test (6MWT) and a formal complete cardiopulmonary exercise testing (CPET).

Basic Modalities

Stair climbing remains the most basic exercise test that asks patients to climb stairs till they get limited by symptoms. There is, however, no consensus on how to standardize the procedure, and several variations (such as climbing at own pace or at brisk pace, climbing with or without holding handrails) are used. Results are generally reported as number of stairs or number of flights of stairs.

Step tests ask the subject to walk up and down on a stool or bench at a specified rate. Several variations exist with regard to height of steps, number of steps, and the frequency of step-ups. The most popular is the Master two-step test. The test is well-suited to field use, and subjects can achieve close to their maximal exercise capacity.

The 6MWT is a simple procedure that assesses the maximum distance that a subject can walk on flat surface at his/her own pace in 6 minutes. The test provides a global estimate functional capacity, but does not provide any specific information on individual systems (cardiac, pulmonary, hematologic, and musculoskeletal) involved in exercise. The test is also sensitive to patient effort. The 6MWT is the most popular among the basic exercise tests as it is simple, practical and well standardized, and involves an activity familiar to almost everyone. A measured corridor, usually about 30 meters, is used, and the subject walks to and fro in this space at a self-determined pace. If a long corridor is not available, the test can be performed on a treadmill, although pacing and control are not as optimal and the distance walked is usually less. The test has good reproducibility and good correlation with other measures of functional status. For this reason, the 6MWT is the preferred investigation when a complete CPET is not available. Norms for healthy Indian men have recently become available.

The shuttle walk test uses an audio signal from a metronome to dictate the walking pace. Walking speed is incrementally increased every minute while the subject walks to and fro on a 10-meter straight path. The test is terminated when the subject can no longer maintain the required speed. Hence, the test correlates better with maximal symptom limited tests such as the CPET, rather than the submaximal tests like 6MWT. However, the test is more complicated than 6MWT, and may result in more frequent cardiac complications in the absence of electrocardiographic monitoring.

Exercise testing may sometimes be used to diagnose airway hyperreactivity due to exercise in patients with unexplained dyspnea. Exercise induced bronchospasm (EIB) is described as a self-limiting bronchospastic event occurring immediately after strong exercise. Typically, greater than 10–15% reduction in FEV1 and/or FVC is observed. EIB is caused by loss of heat, water, or both, from the airways during exercise.

Cardiopulmonary Exercise Testing

The CPET is a more complex investigation that involves exercise at incrementally increasing intensity. The test is terminated when symptoms limit further exercise, or the maximal exercise capacity is achieved. A computerized protocol provides breath-by-breath information on respiratory gas exchange, airflow, oxygen consumption, carbon dioxide production, and cardiac variables (such as heart rate, blood pressure, etc.). The subject exercises on either a treadmill or on a bicycle ergometer; the latter may however be preferable as work rate can be directly measured.

Electrocardiographic and noninvasive blood pressure monitoring accompanies the test. In addition, oxygen saturation is continuously monitored through pulse oximetry. Real-time data on ventilatory and gas exchange parameters is obtained by asking the subject to breathe through a mouthpiece connected to a spirometer and metabolic cart. Flow, volume, and exhaled oxygen and carbon dioxide concentrations are measured. Either incremental or constant work protocol can be used. The test is terminated when the subject (a) gets exhausted, fatigued or distressed, (b) develops signs of cardiovascular instability (ischemia, arrhythmia, substantial blood pressure elevation, etc.), or (c) develops significant hypoxemia.

Although data for a large number of monitored and calculated variables is generated, interpretation and clinical correlation depends on judicious integration of all available information. No single parameter is diagnostic of a cause for exercise limitation. Four basic measurements are critical in describing the response to exercise: oxygen consumption, carbon dioxide production, heart rate, and minute ventilation. Under steady state conditions, measured oxygen uptake (VO_2) equals metabolic oxygen consumption, and measured carbon dioxide output (VCO_2) is the same as its metabolic production. Both VO_2 and VCO_2 can be mathematically computed from expired gas concentrations.

The test is highly sensitive in identification of subclinical disease than other lung function tests conducted at rest. Therefore, CPET can be performed for preoperative assessment, disability evaluation, and selection of candidates for heart and/or lung transplantation. The test is also useful in determining whether breathlessness results from cardiac or pulmonary component among patients who have disorders of both organ systems.

OTHER TESTS

Airway Hyperresponsiveness

Airway hyperresponsiveness (AHR), a characteristic feature of bronchial asthma, is an increased sensitivity of airways to a variety of inhaled agents. AHR is classically measured using inhalation challenges with airway constrictor agonists, such as histamine or methacholine, which result in direct bronchoconstriction. Recently, inhaled mannitol solution has also become available for this purpose and acts by inducing osmotic changes in the airway. Exercise can also be used to test for AHR.

Airway Resistance

Airway resistance can be clinically estimated using several approaches such as interrupter technique, forced oscillation technique, and whole body plethysmography. The interrupter technique is the simplest, and requires monitoring airway pressure and airflow. Airway resistance is not normally determined for clinical purposes, but may provide additional information in the evaluation of patients suspected to have obstructive disorders. The range of normal airway resistance is not well defined, and generally values higher than 2.8 cm H_2O/L/s are considered abnormal.

Pulmonary Mechanics

The elastic properties of the lungs are determined by relating alterations in volume of air in the lungs to the corresponding changes in the lung's recoil. A body plethysmograph is usually used to determine the static pulmonary mechanics. Lung recoil force is measured as the transpulmonary pressure. This is the difference between the alveolar and pleural pressures; the former is measured at mouth under static conditions with shutter at mouth closed and glottis open, and the latter is quantified through pressure measurement from a thin balloon placed in the lower third of esophagus and connected to a pressure transducer.

Respiratory Muscle Function

Estimation of maximal respiratory pressures is a simple technique to assess global respiratory muscle function. A manometer is used to record highest pressures during maximal inhalation and exhalation, which can be sustained for at least 1 second. Maximal expiratory pressure (MEP) is roughly twice as much as maximal inspiratory pressures (MIP). The test is commonly used during evaluation of respiratory muscle weakness in patients with neuromuscular disorders. It is also used as one of the several parameters to assess weaning potential in patients receiving mechanical ventilation. Abnormal muscle strength is identified by comparing observed values to reference data; such data is also available for the Indian population. Values are generally higher among men, and decline with age. A reduction in both MIP and MEP indicates generalized skeletal muscle weakness. A low MIP with normal MEP suggests isolated inspiratory muscle weakness (usually diaphragmatic). Isolated expiratory muscle weakness (normal MIP and low MEP) is rare.

The sniff nasal inspiratory pressure (SNIP) is a noninvasive test of inspiratory strength. The test is performed by wedging a catheter into one nostril and asking the subject to sniff through the other nostril. Pressure measured in the obstructed nostril. The SNIP correlates strongly with transdiaphragmatic pressure and the MIP, but provides no information on expiratory muscle function.

Transdiaphragmatic pressure can be measured after insertion of esophageal and gastric balloon catheters. This allows functional assessment during inspiration, expiration, a sniff, a cough, or phrenic nerve stimulation. Although the technique is highly complex and invasive, it is the best measure of respiratory muscle strength. However, a wide normal range limits its clinical utility.

CHAPTER 5

Interpretation of Arterial Blood Gases and Acid–Base Abnormalities

Aditya Jindal

Acid–base and oxygenation abnormalities are among the most common clinical problems faced, both in routine medical clinics and in the intensive care unit. Proper interpretation and analysis of the blood gas report following a step-wise approach can lead to major changes in the treatment protocols and be lifesaving for the patient (Flowchart 5.1). Unfortunately, this is one area where most medical personnel face problems.

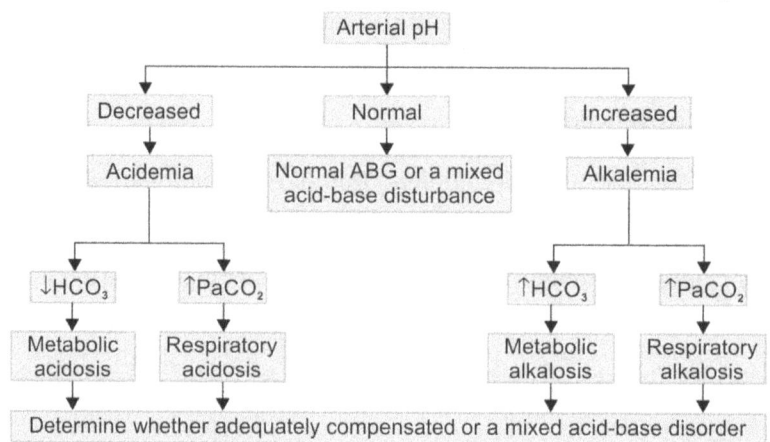

Flowchart 5.1: Stepwise approach to interpretation of arterial blood gases.

(pH: potential of hydrogen; ABG: arterial blood gas; PaCO$_2$: arterial partial pressure of carbon dioxide; HCO$_3$: bicarbonate)

BASIC CONCEPTS

Definitions

Acids and Bases

Acids and bases have been defined variably over the centuries. An acid has been defined based on its sourness quotient, bitter taste, and ability to neutralize alkaline solutions. Modern definitions include those of Arrhenius, i.e. ability to produce hydrogen ions when dissolved in water; the Van–Slyke definition based on electrolytes; the Bronsted-Lowry definition (an acid is a substance that can donate protons); and finally, the Lewis definition (an acid is a substance that can accept a pair of electrons to form a covalent bond). Conversely, a base is defined as a substance that produces hydroxyl ions when dissolved in water (Arrhenius) or that which can accept protons (Bronsted-Lowry) or that which can donate electrons to form a covalent bond (Lewis).

Buffer

A buffer is defined as a substance, which reacts with acids and bases and minimizes changes in the pH of a solution.

pH

The pH is the negative logarithm of the hydrogen ion concentration in a solution and is used to represent the acid-base status of a solution. The pH of body fluids is maintained in a specific range depending on the anatomical compartment. The accepted normal range for blood is 7.36–7.44.

Henderson-Hasselbalch Equation

This equation describes the correlation between the respiratory and metabolic compartments involved in acid-base balance in a mathematical way. Essentially, it relates the hydrogen ion concentration to the balance between carbon dioxide (CO_2) and bicarbonate (HCO_3^-) ions. For the purpose of comprehension, it can be expressed simply as:

$$H^+ \mu\ CO_2/HCO_3^-$$

This means that the H^+ concentration and the pH are dependent upon these two factors. Any increase in CO_2 would lead to an increase in the H^+ or decrease in pH or acidosis, while a decrease would decrease the H^+ or increase the pH or alkalosis. Conversely, decrease in HCO_3^- concentration would decrease the pH leading to acidosis, while increase in HCO_3^- would lead to alkalosis. If the pH change is primarily due to change in the CO_2, it is termed respiratory; while if it is due to change in the HCO_3^-, it is termed metabolic.

OVERVIEW OF ACID–BASE PATHOPHYSIOLOGY IN THE BODY

The body is not a static system but a dynamic one with continuous changes in the internal and external milieu. From the perspective of acid-base balance, the following changes are important:

- *Respiration*: The addition of oxygen to and removal of CO_2 from the system
- *Nutrition*: The addition of nutrients like fats, carbohydrates, proteins, etc. to the system, which acts as acid or alkali loads
- *Excretion*: Both renal and gastrointestinal; removal of acid or base from the body
- *Disease*: Leads to excess or lack of acid or base in the body.

The body has various autoregulatory mechanisms to maintain the acid–base homeostasis. Change in the pH would lead to disruption in organ functioning. Additionally, pH variations would lead to changes in ionization of proteins and other molecules, which would further disrupt functioning. The potential impact is huge and widespread—almost all body systems would be involved. The acid–base status (and by default, the pH) needs to be maintained in a stable range, which is appropriate for life.

TYPES OF ACID–BASE DISORDERS

Interpretation of the Henderson-Hasselbalch equation leads to categorization of acid–base disorders as either metabolic or respiratory. Metabolic disorders are due to primary changes in HCO_3^-, while respiratory disorders are due to primary changes in CO_2. These may be further categorized as metabolic acidosis and alkalosis and respiratory acidosis and alkalosis. The normal ranges of the pH, partial pressure of CO_2 (pCO_2), and HCO_3^- are given in Table 5.1.

The pH is normally tightly regulated within the mentioned range; pCO_2: HCO_3^- ratio should not change significantly, i.e. for a primary change in the CO_2 the HCO_3^- would change in the opposite direction and vice-versa. This is also known as a secondary or compensatory response. For example, if the HCO_3^- decreases and leads to a primary metabolic acidosis, the CO_2 will also decrease in order to maintain a relatively constant pCO_2/HCO_3^- ratio and thus the pH (Table 5.2). However, it must be remembered that in disease conditions, the compensatory responses are never strong enough to completely correct the

TABLE 5.1: The normal ranges of the potential of hydrogen (pH), partial pressure of CO_2 (pCO_2), and bicarbonate (HCO_3^-).

Parameter	Normal range
pH	7.36–7.44
pCO_2	36–44 mm Hg
HCO_3^-	22–26 mEq/L

TABLE 5.2: Acid–base abnormalities and compensatory changes based on the Henderson-Hasselbalch equation.

Disorder	Primary change	Compensatory response
Metabolic acidosis	↓ HCO_3^-	↑ CO_2
Metabolic alkalosis	↑ HCO_3^-	↓ CO_2
Respiratory acidosis	↑ CO_2	↑ HCO_3^-
Respiratory alkalosis	↓ CO_2	↓ HCO_3^-

(HCO_3^-: bicarbonate; CO_2: carbon dioxide; ↓: decrease; ↑: increase)

acid–base abnormality but serve only to limit the change in the pH. The amount of compensation expected in response to any pH change can be calculated and compared with the actual change to have occurred. One must also remember that respiratory compensation for primary metabolic acid–base abnormalities occurs faster (minutes to hours) as compared to metabolic compensation for primary respiratory disorders (hours to days).

It is pertinent to add here that it is entirely possible for two or more separate acid–base disorders to exist simultaneously. These can be detected based on calculation of the compensation. As an example, a patient of chronic obstructive pulmonary disease may have both metabolic acidosis due to sepsis and a respiratory acidosis due to the underlying disease.

Respiratory Compensation

Compensation by the respiratory system for metabolic acid–base abnormalities, as mentioned before, is prompt. It is mediated through the peripheral chemoreceptors, which are present in the carotid bodies.

Primary Metabolic Acidosis

A primary metabolic acidosis will lead to a fall in the HCO_3^- levels and a fall in the pH. In compensation, the respiratory system will increase ventilation and blow off CO_2, so as to limit this fall, i.e. respiratory compensation.

Primary Metabolic Alkalosis

A primary metabolic alkalosis will be associated with elevated HCO_3^- levels. In compensation, the CO_2 levels will increase.

The calculations for metabolic alkalosis are not as accurate as in metabolic acidosis; however, they do give a general idea of the expected responses. If the expected pCO_2 is equivalent to the measured pCO_2, the response is known as a compensated metabolic alkalosis. If the measures pCO_2 is less than the expected pCO_2, it means that there is additional respiratory alkalosis and this is known as primary metabolic alkalosis with superadded respiratory alkalosis. Similarly, if the measured pCO_2 is more than the expected, there is an additional respiratory acidosis and the condition is known as primary metabolic alkalosis with superadded respiratory acidosis.

Metabolic Compensation

Metabolic compensation to primary respiratory abnormalities is mediated by the kidneys. As mentioned earlier, the time course is somewhat delayed. However, this is also dependent upon the chronicity of the disease. For acute conditions, renal buffering may start as early as 5–10 minutes; while in chronic conditions, buffering may take from 2–3 days and indeed may be continuous as the primary disease continues to worsen.

Clinically, metabolic responses may be divided into acute and chronic—acute before the onset of compensation and chronic after the compensatory response is well established. The kidney generates this compensatory response by varying the reabsorption of HCO_3^-. The kidney responds more effectively over a period of time; therefore, the magnitude of the chronic compensatory response is always greater than that of the acute response.

Primary Respiratory Acidosis

The metabolic response to a primary respiratory acidosis will be an increase in the HCO_3^- levels. As mentioned in the previous sections, the expected response can be calculated and compared with the expected to determine the adequacy of compensation and also the coexistence of secondary disorders.

Primary Respiratory Alkalosis

As expected, the metabolic response will be a decrease in the HCO_3^- levels. Also, this can acute or chronic and can be interpreted as mentioned under the other acid–base disorders.

ANION GAP

The anion gap is a theoretical concept; it is a value, which is calculated from the concentration of electrolytes in serum. It has been used in the differential diagnosis of acid–base disorders, especially metabolic acidosis. The anion gap reflects the value of the unmeasured anions in serum.

The total negative charge in human plasma must be balanced by the total positive charge to maintain electroneutrality. The total positive charge in the serum is the sum total of the positively charged ions and other particles in the serum. These include cations such as sodium, potassium, calcium, and magnesium and also cationic proteins. As the contribution of the sodium ion to the net positive charge is significantly out of proportion to the other cations, only sodium is considered in the calculation of the anion gap. Similarly, the negatively charged particles include chloride, HCO_3^-, anionic proteins, inorganic phosphate, sulfate, and organic anions, only the concentrations of chloride and HCO_3^- are considered in the calculation of the net negative charge.

So, the anion gap, while calculated from the concentrations of sodium, chloride, and HCO_3^- ions, represents the difference between the unmeasured anions and cations in serum. Traditionally, the normal anion gap value ranges from 8–16 mEq/L. However, use of ion-specific electrodes has led to a decrease in the normal anion gap; it is essential for clinicians to know the normal range from their respective clinical laboratory.

It is obvious from the above equation that the anion gap will change with either decrease or increase in the levels of the unmeasured anions and/or cations.

The anion gap needs to be corrected for hypoalbuminemia before using it to interpret acid–base abnormalities. Albumin is the major unmeasured anion in serum and hypoalbuminemia will therefore lead to the determination of a falsely low anion gap. This is especially important in critically ill patients in the intensive care unit because of the high prevalence of hypoalbuminemia.

The most common cause of elevated anion gap is metabolic acidosis. The anion gap can be used for the classification of metabolic acidosis and can also help in the differential diagnosis. Metabolic acidosis involves an increase in the acid load in serum. Addition or underexcretion of organic anions to serum leads to an increase in the unmeasured anion fraction in serum and further on to an elevated anion gap. However, some causes of metabolic acidosis are also associated with a normal anion gap. The underlying mechanisms are not entirely clear; however, it is postulated that the retention of chloride by the kidneys to maintain electroneutrality may be responsible.

ACID-BASE DISORDERS

The clinical features of acid-base disorders are more dependent on the underlying clinical conditions rather than due the presence of acidosis or alkalosis per se. However, severe pH changes will lead to clinical features that are independent and superimposed over that of the underlying disease.

Acidosis

Severe acidosis is considered to exist when the pH falls below 7.20. This can affect multiple systems including the cardiovascular, respiratory, and others. The cardiovascular complications include decrease in the blood pressure and cardiac output, reduction in the arrhythmia threshold, decrease in the renal and hepatic blood flow, and shift of blood from the peripheral to the central circulation. These effects, compounded by a decrease in myocardial contractility, predispose to pulmonary edema with even minor fluid shifts. Acidosis also promotes hyperventilation and dyspnea (known as Kussmaul respiration) and also the weakening and early exhaustion of respiratory muscles. The metabolic effects of acidosis include development of insulin resistance, inhibition of anaerobic glycolysis, increase in metabolic demands, depletion of adenosine triphosphate (ATP), and protein denaturation. Ultimately, severe acidosis may lead to mental obtundation and coma.

Metabolic Acidosis

Metabolic acidosis may be classified into high and normal anion gap metabolic acidosis for purposes of differential diagnosis. The treatment of metabolic acidosis is mainly dependent on the underlying cause. However, in severe acidosis, alkali therapy may be given in order to temporarily increase the pH and prevent the development of the adverse effects of acidosis.

Acidotic conditions where the acidosis is due to the accumulation of metabolizable anions (lactic acidosis and ketoacidosis) need not be given alkali therapy till the acidosis is severe (pH < 7.2). This is because the accumulated anions will be converted to HCO_3^- ions in a few hours, if proper treatment is instituted and the kidneys are functioning normally. However, in conditions such as hyperchloremic acidosis, renal failure and acidosis due to accumulation of nonmetabolizable ions (renal failure and toxin ingestion), where the conversion to HCO_3^- is not possible and regeneration by the kidneys is either limited or slow in onset, alkali therapy is indicated earlier.

The most common compound used is intravenous sodium bicarbonate. The use of HCO_3^- therapy has been associated with several complications such as fluid overload and pulmonary edema and paradoxical worsening of the acidosis due to conversion of the HCO_3^- ion to CO_2. Although, CO_2-consuming compounds such as Carbicarb and tromethamine (THAM) have been used to prevent the latter complication, they have not shown significant benefit in clinical trials.

Respiratory Acidosis

The division into acute and chronic is purely for the purposes of diagnostic simplification—it should be remembered that any cause of chronic respiratory acidosis may present acutely due to worsening of the underlying disease and other precipitating factors like infections.

The treatment is mainly dependent upon the acuteness of presentation and the underlying disease. Patients with rapid onset of respiratory acidosis may require admission in an intensive care unit with intubation and mechanical ventilation. Chronically acidotic patients need to be treated holistically with realistic treatment end-goals and priority given to relief of symptoms. These patients may require long-term noninvasive ventilation, which dramatically increases the quality of life in some cases.

Alkalosis

Both respiratory and metabolic alkalosis may present with similar clinical features. Mild alkalosis is usually asymptomatic; symptoms start to appear as the severity increases (severe alkalosis is defined as a pH > 7.6). At this pH, arteriolar constriction occurs, which leads to restriction of cerebral and cardiac circulation. Cardiac effects include reduction in the anginal threshold and predisposition to refractory supraventricular and ventricular arrhythmias. These are more prominent in patients with underlying heart disease. Alkalosis is associated with electrolyte abnormalities like hypocalcemia, hypomagnesemia, hypophosphatemia, and hypokalemia. Additionally, there may be stimulation of anaerobic glycolysis with anion production, leading to an increase in the anion gap. Alkalosis also leads to hypoventilation, which though a compensatory response, can after be life-threatening in patients with inadequate respiratory reserve. Finally, the neurological compilations include tingling, numbness, paresthesias, tetany, lethargy, seizures, and mental obtundation progressing on to coma. These may be worsened by the associated electrolyte abnormalities.

Metabolic Alkalosis

The most common causes of metabolic acidosis include vomiting and nasogastric aspiration.

Treatment: The treatment is directed to the underlying cause. Use of antiemetics in vomiting and proton pump inhibitors in cases of pronged gastric aspiration may be sufficient. Likewise, reduction in diuretic dose or addition of potassium-sparing diuretics may ameliorate the clinical condition. In severe cases, exogenous acid administration, in the form of 0.1 N hydrochloric acid may be required.

Respiratory Alkalosis

Respiratory alkalosis is the most commonly encountered acid–base abnormality in humans, primary because of its presence in normal pregnancy and at high altitudes, situations in which it is physiological rather than pathological.

The treatment of respiratory alkalosis is primarily directed towards the cause. However, in cases of anxiety hyperventilation, distressing symptoms can be temporarily ameliorated by rebreathing into a closed bag, in order to increase the CO_2 levels.

CHAPTER

6

Tuberculosis: Overview

Stuti Agarwal, Romica Latawa, Indu Verma

INTRODUCTION

Tuberculosis, known since antiquity, has been a major killer of men and animals throughout the world. The disease was known to consume the whole body, hence called as "phthisis" which was the Greek equivalent of "consumption". Tuberculosis is an infectious illness caused by *Mycobacterium tuberculosis* or tubercle bacillus (TB). The bacillus is also referred to the acid fast bacillus (AFB) because of the characteristics on Ziehl–Neelsen (ZN) staining. But a few other mycobacteria may also show acid-fastness on staining.

ROUTE AND SPREAD OF INFECTION

Mycobacterium tuberculosis commonly transmits through aerosols, enters the host via mucosal surface of the respiratory tract and harbors the lung rich in oxygen supply, which provides a suitable environment for this slow replicating pathogen. The complex immune responses mounted against *M. tuberculosis* are well defined at cellular level and involve both innate and adaptive immune responses. The phagocytic cells engulf the bacteria, rapid inflammatory response is induced followed by adaptive immune response leading to accumulation of a variety of immune cells followed by the formation of granulomas, characterized by a relatively small number of infected phagocytes surrounded by activated monocytes/macrophages and activated lymphocytes. One of the most remarkable features of nonsporulating *M. tuberculosis* is its ability to remain dormant within an individual for decades before reactivating into active tuberculosis.

Latent TB is a kind of subclinical infection caused by exposure to *M. tuberculosis*. Following the exposure, there is activation of host's immune response to control bacillary growth and arrest further progression of infection in a quiescent state. It is a state of mycobacteria surviving in closed necrotic lesions. *M. tuberculosis* can surpass the immune response and breach the protective barrier and can disseminate into various organs of the body through blood and lymph. Mycobacterium can also establish itself within tissues other than lung, such as, lymph nodes, eye, bone, meninges, etc. causing extrapulmonary tuberculosis. Newer sites of mycobacterial infection have also been elucidated showing presence of viable mycobacterium in kidney, liver, and spleen. Further, viable mycobacteria have been recovered from bone marrow mesenchymal stem cells suggesting that stem cells in bone marrow can act as favorable and protective niche for survival and persistence of mycobacteria.

MYCOBACTERIAL GROUPS

The most important of mycobacterial group is *M. tuberculosis* complex (MTC), which includes *M. tuberculosis, Mycobacterium leprae, Mycobacterium bovis,* and *Mycobacterium africanum*. *M. tuberculosis* and *M. leprae* cause tuberculosis and leprosy, respectively in humans. *M. bovis* causes tuberculosis in cattle and humans. Some mycobacteria are saprophytes (living on decaying organic matter), while others are obligate parasites. Most are found as free-living forms in soil, water or diseased tissues of animals. The other group "atypical mycobacteria" that is different from typical *M. tuberculosis complex*, depending upon in vitro characteristics is the Nontuberculous mycobacteria (NTM). In 1950s, it was divided into four categories on the basis of Runyon classification: photochromogens (pigment producing on light exposure), e.g. *Mycobacterium kansasii, Mycobacterium marinum*; Scotochromogens (pigment producing), e.g. *Mycobacterium scrofulaceum, Mycobacterium xenopi*; Nonchromogens (no pigment production), e.g. *Mycobacterium avium* complex (MAC), *Mycobacterium terrae* complex; and rapidly growing mycobacteria, e.g. *Mycobacterium chelonae*, and *Mycobacterium fortuitum*.

Mycobacterium avium and *Mycobacterium intracellulare* are closely related species commonly grouped to form *M. avium* complex that is implicated as a potential pathogen for both animals and humans. Atypical mycobacteria like *M. avium* complex, *M. kansasii, M. fortuitum,* and *M. chelonae* cause opportunistic infections in patients with human immunodeficiency virus (HIV)/acquired immunodeficiency syndrome (AIDS) or systemic immunosuppression of which *M. avium* complex is the most common; *M. avium* being highly significant clinically. In patients with HIV infection and/or AIDS, opportunistic infections are commonly caused by atypical mycobacteria such as *M. avium* complex, *M. kansasii, M. fortuitum,* and *M. chelonae* which are otherwise essentially saprophytic in healthy individuals. *M. avium,* is the most clinically significant of the environmental mycobacteria that opportunistically infects susceptible humans having systemic immunosuppression. *Mycobacterium abscessus, Mycobacterium massiliense,* and *Mycobacterium bolletii* together comprise *M. abscessus* complex, has been implicated as most common NTM in developed countries after *M. avium* complex.

Mycobacterium pathogenicity is attributed to various genes and cellular components they encode, which are known as virulence factors. The most important of these are the transcription regulators that constitute approximately 0.6% of the total mycobacterial genome and other are genes that encode for various cell surface components particularly unique to pathogenic mycobacteria. Another important functional genomic region of *M. tuberculosis* is dormancy regulon that encodes for dormancy and stress-related genes.

MYCOBACTERIAL IDENTIFICATION

The most common laboratory identification of *M. tuberculosis* complex species includes smear microscopy based on ZN staining and culture on solid egg-based LJ medium coupled with phenotypic characterization such as the growth rate, colony morphology, pigmentation and antibiotic susceptibility testing (AST). Several highly sensitive broth-based fully automated culture system (BACTEC460 and MGIT960) are now routinely being used in many mycobacteriology laboratories to complement microscopy as well as to increase the speed and accuracy of TB diagnosis. It is also possible to distinguish *M. tuberculosis* and *M. avium* using culture and a battery of biochemical tests, but these are complicated and time consuming. The biochemical tests, which are specific for *M. tuberculosis* are niacin reduction test, nitrate test and urease test. On the other hand, tellurite reduction and catalase tests are positive specifically for *M. avium* complex species. There has been a marked increase in different novel assays not only for the identification of *M. tuberculosis* complex but also for detection of drug resistance. A more sensitive alternative to ZN stain is a fluorochrome auramine stain that has been introduced in many TB diagnostic laboratories throughout the world.

For the identification of isoniazid (INH) and rifampin (RIF) drug-resistant isolates, microscopic observation drug susceptibility (MODS) assay is an inexpensive and simple broth-microtiter method. However, the assay requires training and technical expertise along with infrastructure (BSL3 laboratory) and equipment. A number of molecular assays have been developed to detect the presence of *M. tuberculosis* as well as resistance to INH/RIF. Line probe assay (LPA) involves the extraction of DNA from mycobacterial isolates followed by PCR and hybridization of labeled PCR products with oligonucleotide probes immobilized on strip that are visualized colorimetrically. The assay has been recommended by WHO in 2008 for detection of drug resistance in mycobacteria. Loop-mediated isothermal amplification assay (Eiken Chemical Company) is another molecular method for detection of *M. tuberculosis* in clinical samples. The GeneXpert *M. tuberculosis*/RIF (Cepheid), which is considered as most efficient mycobacterial identification technique and being endorsed by WHO is a self-enclosed rapid PCR device that can detect *M. tuberculosis* complex and rifampin resistant mycobacterial species but is unable to detect isoniazid resistance. Lack of technical expertise and infrastructure required for these advanced molecular methods for mycobacterial identification impedes their successful implementation in developing countries.

MYCOBACTERIAL DRUG RESISTANCE

Comparative genomic analysis has revealed that *M. tuberculosis* complex has evolved by extensive horizontal gene transfer and recombination events creating several genomic and molecular changes in the *M. tuberculosis* complex. This has led to the emergence of more host-adapted pathogenic and virulent *M. tuberculosis*. Many gene gain/loss events, mutation, and conversion have arisen leading to *M. tuberculosis*-specific genetic elements that contribute to its virulence. The gene content evolution in *M. tuberculosis* is mostly driven by uneven gene gain/loss in gene families, e.g. transposable elements and fatty acid metabolism-related gene families, large number of insertions and deletions (Indels) in drug-resistance associated loci and PE-PGRS-related genes (contribute to antigenic variability), lineage-specific changes within the amino-acid sequences of transcription regulators and nucleotide sequences of promoter sites, overexpression of genes related to drug efflux pumps as well as chromosomal mutations like single nucleotide polymorphism.

The adaptation of mycobacteria within the host leads to selection of mutations within species making it more pathogenic and virulent. Whole-genome based approaches have elucidated that multi/extremely drug resistant (MDR/XDR) strains and more virulent strains of *M. tuberculosis* with enhanced resistance and fitness like Beijing are consequence of gene expansion. This suggests that the development of drug-resistance within clinical isolates is a highly diversified and complex process involving variations in the selection intensity of mutations. It also depends on distribution of SNPs and Indels within the genome contributing to nucleotide diversity. As a result of these mutations, there is altered expression of various genes as well as encoding of novel functional proteins which further leads to phenotypic diversity within clinical isolates and different levels of drug resistance.

To sum up, considerable information is now available regarding the chemical structure of *M. tuberculosis* unique cell envelope and *M. tuberculosis* genome which has provided a wealth of information that can be important for the understanding of the molecular basis of *M. tuberculosis* pathogenicity. This in turn can be translated into the development of new drugs, diagnostic tests and vaccines to combat tuberculosis.

CHAPTER 7

Immunology and Pathogenesis

Madhur Kalyan, Krishna K Singh, Indu Verma

INTRODUCTION

In approximately 5-10% of individuals who get infected with *Mycobacterium tuberculosis (M. tuberculosis)*, the bacteria continue to replicate, resulting into clinical TB. In the remaining 90-95% of infected individuals, effective immune responses are elicited, which contain the bacteria in granulomas where they persist latently for several years.

MYCOBACTERIUM TUBERCULOSIS INFECTION AND OVERVIEW OF IMMUNOPATHOGENESIS

The current view of TB pathogenesis in humans can still be pictured as a multiple-stage process, which was described over a decade ago using the rabbit model of TB. Overall, it is a kind of tug of war between host immune system and tubercle bacillus (Flowchart 7.1).

The first stage starts with the inhalation of small airborne droplet (1-5 μm) which can remain in the environment for several hours. The infectious droplets pass through the upper parts of the airways where the majority of bacilli are trapped in mucus and removed by cilia. The remaining droplets containing bacteria settle in the alveoli of distal airways where they are engulfed nonspecifically by activated alveolar macrophages, Dendritic Cells (DCs) and probably by alveolar epithelial cells also.

Second stage begins with the replication of bacilli in alveolar macrophages, to some extent in DCs and possibly in alveolar epithelial cells. The bacilli multiply in these cells until they burst; the released bacilli are ingested by other alveolar macrophages. It is followed by a localized proinflammatory response

Immunology and Pathogenesis

Flowchart 7.1: Various stages in the pathogenesis of tuberculosis

1st Stage
- Inhalation of airborne droplets containing *M.tb*
- ↓
- Travel through the respiratory tract to the alveoli/distal airways
- ↓
- Engulfment by activated alveolar macrophages, dendritic cells (and ? alv. epithelial cells)
- ↓

2nd Stage
- Replication of *M.tb*
- ↓
- Bursting of cells, release of bacilli—entrance into other cells
- ↓
- Local proinflammatory response Recruitment of mononuclear and DCs
- ↓
- Infected macrophages, DCs spread to lymph nodes (LNs)
- ↓

3rd Stage
- T-cell activation in LNs—initiation of cell-mediated immunity (CMI)
- ↓
- Migration of activated T cells
- ↓
- Formation of granulomas

Branches:
- Liquefaction of granulomas
- Neutrophil influx
 → **Primary TB**

- Containment of *M.tb* (Dormant bacilli)
 → **Latent TB**

leading to recruitment of mononuclear and DCs from neighboring blood vessels thus providing new host cells for the expansion of bacterial population and also inducing the alveolar macrophages to invade the lung epithelium. The accumulation of these cells at the site of infection initiates the early lesion formation in the lung. Simultaneously, the bacilli ingested macrophages and DCs disseminate to lymph nodes via the lymphatic system or probably by the direct breaching of alveolar wall.

The arrival of the bacilli-containing macrophages and DCs to the lymph nodes initiates the cell-mediated immunity (CMI), which is the beginning of the third stage of pathogenesis. T-cell activation starts in lymph nodes draining the lung and the development of CMI occurs between 2 weeks and 8 weeks postinfection in the majority of individuals. The activation of T-cells leads to their expansion followed by migration to the infection site in the lung where they activate macrophages and induce the formation of granulomas. In humans, the granuloma is the hallmark of pulmonary TB, characterized by a central acellular eosinophilic region of caseous necrosis surrounded by concentric layers of macrophages, large epitheloid cells, multinucleated giant Langhan's cells and lymphocytes. The central necrotic core of the granuloma with sparse mycobacterial is surrounded by two layers of cells. Foamy macrophages (macrophages filled with lipid containing bodies) infected with mycobacteria have been demonstrated in the interface region flanking the necrotic core in the granulomas of TB patients.

During the early phase of granuloma formation, the structure is highly vascularized, however at the "late" stages, the caseous portion of the granuloma becomes hypoxic; bacilli stop replicating and enter into a dormant phase. The infected individuals at this stage show no overt sign of disease and categorized as individuals with latent TB. Although it is well known that *M. tuberculosis* may remain in a nonreplicating dormant state for years together, exact niche for its survival and maintaining such a state is still not precisely known. A recent study suggested that *M. tuberculosis* may persist in a mesenchymal subpopulation of human bone marrow stem cells from patients previously treated for pulmonary TB and of mouse bone marrow stem cells from a mouse model of non-replicating *M. tuberculosis* infection.

In the majority of latently infected individuals, the bacilli remain dormant for their entire life and never cause TB. Unfortunately in some of these individuals, at the time when their immune system becomes weak, the tubercle bacilli out—smart the host immune response and start undergoing intracellular replication. This results into extensive macrophage death and necrosis and the granuloma starts liquefying to form cavity, which permits the spill of numerous viable bacilli into airways. In late-stage disease, neutrophil influx has also been implicated in the tissue damage and the dissemination of infectious bacteria into the airways in TB patients. This final stage of TB pathogenesis completes with development of productive cough, which promotes the spread of viable bacilli in the aerosol droplets to other individuals.

Although most cases of reactivation of dormant *M. tuberculosis* involve the pulmonary site, there might also be a possibility that it persists in and reactivates from other sites distinct from lungs which can subsequently cause extrapulmonary tuberculosis.

IMMUNE RESPONSES TO TUBERCULOSIS

Currently, the mechanism of immune defense against mycobacteria is not clearly known; both innate and adaptive immune systems are involved in providing immunity against *M. tuberculosis*.

Innate Immunity

In general, innate immune system recognizes microbes immediately after infection by using receptors and induces secretion of a range of chemokines and cytokines, which direct the recruitment of various immune cells, including the phagocytic cells to the site of infection to kill the microbes.

Role of Phagocytic and Other Cells

Macrophages and dendritic cells comprise the major phagocytic cells in immunity against tuberculosis. The uptake of *M. tuberculosis* by alveolar macrophages represents the first step in the innate host defense against TB. Following mycobacterial infection, macrophages can differentiate either into type 1 or type 2 macrophages producing IL-23 or IL-10 respectively, thus leading to either protection or suppression of immunity to tuberculosis. The type 2 macrophages that produce IL-10 can also promote adoption of T-regulatory (T_{reg}) phenotype by CD4+ T-cells.

In spite of the potent bactericidal activity of macrophages, *M. tuberculosis* is able to survive and replicate in these cells by avoiding the killing mechanisms. It has been shown that *M. tuberculosis* survive inside macrophage by avoiding the fusion of phagosomes with lysosomes.

Amongst the other cells that are involved in immunity against TB are the natural killer (NK) cells and neutrophils. NK cells are one of the major components of innate immune system and provide the first line of defense against infection.

Just like NK cells neutrophils also have been shown to have a protective role in against *M. tuberculosis,* at least in the early stages of TB infection, as these are attracted to the site of infection thereby restricting the growth of *M. tuberculosis* and secreting various chemokines and cytokines on interaction with *M. tuberculosis*. It is also observed that the ingestion of apoptotic neutrophils by macrophages enhances *M. tuberculosis* killing.

Antimicrobial peptides, known as naturally occurring antibiotics, are not only one of the important constituents of innate immunity but also serve as signaling molecules in regulation of both innate and adaptive immune system. Cathelicidin, defensin, and hepcidin are the AMPs that have antimycobacterial actions. In addition to direct killing cathlicidin has also been shown to act as an immunomodulator. The defensins are the most profuse type of peptides present in mammals. Majority of peptides produced by neutrophils are human neutrophil defensins or human neutrophil peptides. These peptides have been shown to co-localize with *M. tuberculosis* in the early endosomes, following engulfment of infected neutrophils by macrophages, as a result of which bacterial burden is reduced. In addition to the direct killing effects, defensins also trigger the Th1 response resulting in enhanced production of proinflammatory cytokines (TNF-α, IL-12, IFN-γ) and hence protection against TB.

Cytokines and Chemokines Bridging the Innate and Adaptive Immunity

An efficient control of mycobacterial infection requires an effective balance between innate and adaptive immune responses mediated by cytokines and chemokines that develop proper inflammatory responses. The control of *M. tuberculosis* infection depends on the appropriate development of inflammatory responses because improper responses can cause chronic infection and associated pathology. IL-12 secreted from infected macrophages and DCs induces IFN-g which ultimately leads to down modulation of IL-10 and IL-4 and hence results in differentiation of T cells to Th1 cells. Infected macrophages and dendritic cells produce Interleukin-12 (IL-12), the crucial cytokine in controlling early *M. tuberculosis* infection.

Role of IFN-γ in human TB has been demonstrated by studies which show that those individuals are more susceptible to infections with mycobacteria having defect in either IFN-γ or IFN-γ receptor genes. Besides IFN-γ, TNF-α, a proinflammatory cytokine secreted by macrophages, DCs and T-cells also enhance the killing of mycobacteria intracellularly as well as formation of granuloma by induction of reactive nitrogen intermediates and IFN-γ.

IL-4 is another anti-inflammatory cytokine that has been implicated in various intracellular infections including *M. tuberculosis* for its harmful effects by suppressing IFN-γ production and macrophage activation. Another anti-inflammatory cytokine that is implicated in suppressing protective immunity to *M. tuberculosis* is transforming growth factor (TGF)-β. Production of TGF-β by monocytes and DCs is induced by mycobacterial components specifically by ManLAM.

In addition to above-mentioned cytokines, several investigators have shown that *M. tuberculosis* or its components induce chemokines from monocytes, macrophages, multinucleated giant cells, DCs, granulocytes, etc.

Adaptive Immunity

Although, *M. tuberculosis* infection elicits both humoral and cell-mediated immune responses, due to intracellular residence of *M. tuberculosis*, it is well accepted that only cell-mediated immunity provides protection against TB. In recent years it has been shown that humoral immune responses also play important role in protection to TB.

Cell-mediated Immunity

The T-cells which comprise of CD4+ T-helper cells (Th), CD8+ cytotoxic T-cells (CTLs), γδT-cells, regulatory T-cells (T-regulatory cells), memory T-cells and unconventional CD1 restricted T-cells play main role in providing cell-mediated immunity.

Role of CD4+/CD8+ T-cells: In human, the protective role of CD4+ T-cells during *M. tuberculosis* infection has been suggested by enhanced occurrence of both primary and reactivated TB in HIV-infected individuals showing loss of these cells. Although, the mechanism of protection by CD4+ T-cells is not clear, so far studies suggest that during *M. tuberculosis* infection, CD4+ T-cells of Th1 type activate macrophages primarily through IFN-γ production. Other antimycobacterial mechanisms suggested for these cells include apoptosis of infected macrophages, release of ATP and lymphotoxin α3 (LTα3) or TNF-β for control of *M. tuberculosis* infection.

Role of regulatory T (T_{reg}) cells: T_{reg} cells express CD4, CD25 and Foxp3 and are found to suppress the proliferation and function of CD4+ CD25-cells and inhibit the production of IFN-γ by secreting IL-10 and TGF-β. Besides CD4+ CD25+ FoxP3+ T_{reg} cell subsets, CD8+ T_{reg} cells that inhibit the T-cell proliferation and production of cytokines are also described.

Role of γδ T-cells: During mycobacterial infection, γδT-cells are rapidly recruited to lung, secrete IFN-γ and kill *M. tuberculosis* infected cells. In humans, γδT-cells recognize mycobacterial nonpeptidic phosphoantigens without any requirement for MHC molecules leading to the secretion of Th1 cytokines primarily IFN-γ and killing of *M. tuberculosis* infected cells. The occurrence of increased size of granuloma and enhanced numbers of neutrophils in granuloma of *M. tuberculosis* infected γδTCR-KO mice suggested that γδT-cells are involved in the regulation of granuloma formation.

Role of memory T (T_M) cells: Although, role of T_M cells in providing protection against *M. tuberculosis* infection is poorly defined, persistence of latent *M. tuberculosis* infection in most of the infected individuals suggest the involvement of these cells in controlling *M. tuberculosis* infection during latency.

Humoral Immunity

Historically, it is accepted that B cells play no significant role in providing protection against *M. tuberculosis* infection. Although, studies of *M. tuberculosis* infection in B-cell deficient mice have yielded variable results, data from *M. tuberculosis* infected B-cell-deficient mice and polymeric Ig receptor knockout mice deficient in secretory IgA have convincingly demonstrated a role of B cells and antibodies in protection against *M. tuberculosis* infection.

CONCLUSION

In conclusion, a complex interaction of multiple cell types of host immune system is important for optimal immunity against mycobacteria. The cross talk between *M. tuberculosis* and the host immune system determines the infection outcome. Once *M. tuberculosis* is taken up by alveolar macrophages, possibly by other cells too, and if infection is established, activation of macrophages, DCs, NK cells and T-cells lead to production of various chemokines and cytokines that regulate a central nonspecific inflammatory immune response. Fate of infection is determined by this initial response which either leads to progressive growth of *M. tuberculosis* or the containment of infection.

CHAPTER

8

Pulmonary Tuberculosis: Clinical Features and Diagnosis

S Kashyap, Malay Sarkar

INTRODUCTION

The clinical features of tuberculosis (TB) depend upon the site and the type of involvement. They are rarely diagnostic. Primary infection consists of inhalation and implantation of mycobacteria in the lung parenchyma. The primary lung lesion is called as the Ranke or Ghon complex, which comprises the primary focus, draining lymphatics, and the lymph node. Often, the primary complex resolves or calcifies. These healed foci may frequently contain dormant mycobacteria producing a state of latent infection. In a minority of infected individuals (10%), the disease progresses during the initial weeks or months after infection, and the patient develops the typical symptoms of progressive primary TB. Disseminated or miliary TB may develop in people with immunosuppression or with an overwhelming infection.

POSTPRIMARY PULMONARY TUBERCULOSIS

Endogenous reactivation of the dormant mycobacteria is the most common cause of postprimary TB. Coinfection with HIV is the strongest known risk factor for progression from latent infection to active TB. Other known risk factors are malnutrition, drug, and alcohol abuse; coexistent medical conditions, such as diabetes, malignancy, silicosis, post-transplantation, corticosteroid, or other immunosuppressive and biological therapies. Tobacco smoking and biomass fuel exposure also predispose to TB.

Reactivation can occur at any site; however, lung is the most common site of reactivation. Postprimary disease differs from primary TB in its preferential apical localization, a strong immune response, marked presence of caseation necrosis and cavities. Traditionally, primary and postprimary TB are described in children and adults, respectively. Due to the presence of large number of immunocompromised patients and aging populations, atypical and "mixed" radioclinical patterns are frequently observed in adults with the consequent fading of the age-related distinction between primary and postprimary TB.

SYMPTOMS AND SIGNS

Pulmonary tuberculosis (PTB) is a disease with protean manifestations, often associated with nonspecific constitutional and specific respiratory signs and symptoms. Constitutional symptoms include tiredness, malaise, weight loss, fever, night sweats, anorexia, and headache. In miliary TB, fever can have morning spikes. They are generally attributed to the release of various cytokines in the systemic circulation. Symptoms are minimal or absent until the disease is in an advanced stage. Complete absence of symptoms has been reported in 4.9% of active adult PTB cases, majority of patients are from countries with endemic TB. Most patients develop symptoms insidiously; although acute manifestations have been also reported.

Cough is the most predominant symptom in TB. In the initial stages, cough is dry, but subsequently there occurs the production of mucoid or mucopurulent sputum, generally in small amounts. Sometimes, sputum may also be streaked with blood. At the onset, it is more in the early morning; with progression of disease, it becomes persistent throughout day and night. Cough is less frequent in tubercular pleural effusion.

Hemoptysis is usually mild in TB, but occasionally, it can be massive. When massive, it is mostly of bronchial artery or nonpulmonary systemic artery origin. Rarely, hemoptysis can also be the presenting symptom. Both active and inactive TB can produce hemoptysis. There are several mechanisms, which can cause hemoptysis in PTB (Box 8.1). Rasmussen's aneurysm is a rare complication of cavitary PTB caused by granulomatous weakening of a pulmonary arterial wall. It can present as the repeated episodes of minor hemoptysis or occasionally as major hemoptysis. Incidence of Rasmussen's aneurysm is 4% in patients with advanced cavitary disease.

Breathlessness, which is a late symptom in PTB, may result from extensive pulmonary involvement, bronchial obstruction, pneumothorax, and pleural effusion. Rarely, patients with miliary TB or TB bronchopneumonia may present with the symptoms of respiratory failure.

BOX 8.1: Mechanisms of hemoptysis in tuberculosis.

Necrosis of pulmonary venules and capillaries in early stages
Rupture of Rasmussen's aneurysm
Post-tubercular bronchiectasis
Mycetoma in tubercular cavity
Broncholiths
Scar carcinoma—very rarely

Involvement of pleural surface can cause pleuritic chest pain. Pain is referred to ipsilateral shoulder in diaphragmatic pleurisy and to upper abdomen in costal pleural involvement. Pneumothorax due to TB can also cause acute pleuritic chest pain. Sometimes, chest pain can be dull and poorly localized. Chest pain is an early and relatively frequent symptom and it disappears within 2 or 3 weeks after effective treatment is started.

The most common cause of hoarseness of voice in PTB is the associated laryngeal TB. Rarely, inflamed TB nodes or the retraction of left upper lobe bronchus by cicatrization atelectasis can cause recurrent laryngeal nerve palsy and hoarseness of voice.

TUBERCULOSIS IN THE ELDERLY

The elderly population is particularly susceptible to TB because of the age-induced decline in cell-mediated immunity. More specifically, impairment of helper T-lymphocyte functions and subsequently defects in secretion and response to different cytokines are particularly important in increasing the susceptibility of TB in elderly subjects. Elderly individual is also more likely to suffer from various immunosuppressive conditions. There are several characteristics features of TB in the elderly. After exposure, elderly subjects are more likely to become infected with *Mycobacterium tuberculosis* than younger subjects; they also develop tuberculous diseases more easily after contracting infection. Mortality from TB is also high in this population.

Delayed diagnosis is not uncommon as the clinicoradiological presentations of TB are often atypical in the elderly. Some patients may present with only nonpulmonary symptoms, such as unexplained weight loss, weakness, or change in cognitive status. Classical symptoms, such as night sweats, fever, and hemoptysis, are less frequently observed in the elderly. Fever is infrequent, because of age-associated decrease in pyrogenic response. Cavitation is less common in elderly age group, which can explain the lower frequency of hemoptysis. Lower lobe involvement is also common. Potential of adverse drug reactions is also high in elderly subjects.

MILIARY TUBERCULOSIS

Miliary TB consists of disseminated millet like lesions in the lungs and other solid organs. It is more commonly present in cases of extrapulmonary cases, especially in immunocompromised patients. It is present in about 2% of all types of TB patients. Clinical symptoms are generally nonspecific, which may include fever, malaise, general ill health, and weight loss. Respiratory symptoms, such as dry cough, may also be present in some cases. Diagnosis is often suspected on chest roentgenography. Classical miliary shadows on plain chest X-ray are present in only half the case. Associated meningeal TB is commonly seen in up to 30% of adult patients. Choroidal miliary lesions are characteristically seen on fundal examination as pale, graywhite nodules of less than one quarter the size of optic disk, usually located within 2 cm of the optic nerve.

Hematogenous dissemination of mycobacteria can occasionally lead to sepsis and septic shock. It was known as Landouzy septicemia or sepsis tuberculosa acutissima in the past. It is most commonly noted in immunocompromised patients, especially in patients with HIV, but may also occur in immunocompetent patients.

HIV AND TUBERCULOSIS

Presence of TB in HIV-infected patients usually depends on the CD4 lymphocyte count and degree of immunosuppression. TB is less common and less severe in patients with CD4 counts of greater than 200 cells/cm^3. Chest radiographic findings in these patients are often limited to upper lobe infiltrates with or without cavitation. On the other hand, patients with advanced HIV disease (CD4 T-lymphocyte count <200/cm^3) are more likely to have atypical presentation, such as the lower lobe predominance, adenopathy, and absence of cavities. Extrapulmonary and disseminated disease is common in advanced HIV infection, occurring in 63% of patients. Severely immunocompromised patients can have sepsis-like syndrome with high fevers.

PLEURAL EFFUSION

Pleural effusion is more commonly seen in primary TB, although it is not altogether uncommon in postprimary forms in adults. It frequently presents with chest pain or dullness, breathlessness, and cough. Sputum production, hemoptysis, and weight loss are less common features.

PARADOXICAL RESPONSE

Paradoxical reaction in TB is defined by the increase in clinical features and/or appearance of new symptoms and lesions in a patient after the initiation of antitubercular therapy. This is typically seen in tuberculous pleural effusion, lymphadenopathy, and sometimes with intracranial tuberculomas. It can be possibly attributed to the release of various proinflammatory cytokines following rapid killing of mycobacteria and stimulation of T-helper lymphocytes. Paradoxical reaction is particularly common in up to 30% patients with cervical lymphadenopathy; whereas, it is rare in those with intrathoracic lymphadenopathy.

PHYSICAL EXAMINATION

Wasting is a classic feature of TB caused by a combination of factors, e.g. lack of appetite, increased losses, and altered metabolism as part of the inflammatory and immune responses.

Wasting also carries poor prognosis by causing increased mortality in patients with TB. It is usually seen in advanced disease and indicates the loss of both fat and lean tissues.

Other general physical features may consist of lymph node enlargement and skin lesions, such as erythema nodosum or erythema induratum. Reactive arthritis and amyloidosis are other occasional manifestations. A major constraint of physical examination of respiratory system is its failure to detect mild or even moderate illness despite apparent radiographic abnormalities. Post-tussive crackles constitute an important sign, demonstrated on deep inhalation followed by full exhalation and coughing at the end of exhalation. Fine crackles are heard over the areas of TB infiltrations, particularly at the apices. In endobronchial TB, localized wheezing may be heard. In tubercular consolidation, high-pitched bronchial breathing may be audible; whereas in superficial large cavities, cavernous breathing may be audible. In tubercular pleurisy, pleural rub is often detected. Signs of volume contraction are often present in advanced disease with extensive fibrosis.

DIAGNOSIS OF TUBERCULOSIS

Laboratory testing for TB includes tests for latent TB infection as well as for TB disease. In latent TB infection, individuals are harboring live *M. tuberculosis*, but do not show any clinical evidence or signs and symptoms of active disease. TB, on the other hand, is the clinically manifested illness caused by *M. tuberculosis* complex. Tests for latent tuberculosis infection (LTBI) include tuberculin skin test (TST) and interferon-gamma release assays (IGRAs).

Tuberculin Skin Test

Tuberculin skin test is the oldest diagnostic test still in use in the modern medical practice. The material used for this purpose is purified protein derivative (PPD). It is injected intradermally, and indicates delayed type hypersensitivity response in exposed individuals. In tuberculin test, the area of induration (not erythema is measured after 48–72 hours of administration of PPD). In India, induration of more than 15 mm is taken as positive TST in immunocompetent person with no known risk factors for TB. PPD has low sensitivity particularly in immunocompromised individuals (elderly, malnourished, HIV infection, and other immunosuppressive conditions). In HIV infected patients, a cutoff of more than or equal to 5 mm of induration is considered as positive response. More than 50% of normal healthy individuals show positive TST in this country. Moreover, it is nonspecific since PPD contains more than 200 mycobacterial proteins shared by different mycobacteria.

Interferon Gamma Release Assays

Interferon gamma release assay is more specific than TST to look for tuberculous infection. Interferon gamma is released by sensitized lymphocytes whenever exposed to TB antigens, such as ESAT-6 and culture filtrate protein-10. These antigens are encoded by region of difference 1 (*RD1*) genes. These are present in *M. tuberculosis* but absent in most nontuberculous mycobacteria (NTMs) and bacillus Calmette-Guerin (BCG) vaccine strain, therefore, specific to *M.*

tuberculosis. Like TST, however, the use of IGRA tests cannot differentiate latent infection from active disease. This is particularly problematic in high-TB burden countries where the prevalence of latent infection is very high. Result of IGRA is not affected by prior BCG vaccination. The IGRA does not require a return visit, has no variability of skin test readings, and there is no induction of boosting phenomenon on repeat testing. High-diagnostic sensitivity has also been observed in young children for T-SPOT TB test and in immunosuppressed populations for both T-SPOT TB test and to a lesser extent to QuantiFERON TB Gold.

Chest Radiology

Chest radiography is an important tool in suspecting the diagnosis of PTB. Chest X-rays are mostly abnormal in immunocompetent patients, but may be normal in about 10–15% of HIV-infected patients. No radiological features are typical of TB and various other lung diseases can radiologically mimic TB. Radiological manifestations have been traditionally described in children and adults on the basis of primary and postprimary TB. Recently, these age-wise distinctions of radiological manifestations have been blurred due to several reasons.

Tuberculoma is a sharply marginated round or oval lesion of 0.5–4.0 cm in diameter, detected in approximately 5% of patients with postprimary TB. The location of tuberculoma has been variably reported in upper and lower lobes. About 20–30% of tuberculomas in adults may ultimately calcify. In up to 80% of cases, smaller satellite lesions were seen in the immediate vicinity of the main lesion.

Presence of infiltrates, tree-in-bud appearances, consolidation, fibrosis, and cavitation are some of the common findings seen on chest radiography. Miliary pattern on chest X-ray is seen in up to 2% cases. Hilar and mediastinal lymphadenopathy are more commonly seen in primary TB.

Another important radiological characteristic of PTB is sequelae of TB. It includes open-healed cavity, mycetoma within cavity, and tubercular destroyed lung (TDL).

Sputum Microscopy

Sputum microscopy is cheap, rapid, easy to perform, and widely available diagnostic procedure to detect mycobacteria in clinical specimens. However, there are certain limitations of sputum microscopy. Sputum microscopy is not a highly sensitive tool, and it requires a minimal of 5,000–10,000 bacilli per mL of sputum to reliably identify the bacilli. It cannot differentiate *M. tuberculosis* from other mycobacteria. Sputum microscopy may also fail to diagnose paucibacillary and extrapulmonary tuberculosis (EPTB), the incidence of which is disproportionately higher in high HIV-prevalent areas. The smear is more likely to be positive in patients who have cavitary disease and multilobar infiltrates. The result of smear microscopy is influenced by several variables like type of the specimen, thickness of the smear, technical preparation of the slide, and experience of the laboratory personnel examining the smear. Sensitivity of sputum microscopy is increased, if sputum is liquefied and concentrated by centrifugation or sedimentation prior to acid-fast staining.

Other microorganisms that may take up acid-fast stains, albeit weakly, are *Rhodococcus, Nocardia, Legionella micdadei*, and cysts of *Cryptosporidium, Isospora*, and *Cyclospora*. Fluorescence microscopy requires staining with the dye auramine–rhodamine. The mycobacteria appear bright yellow rods against inky black background. In comparison with Ziehl–Neelsen microscopy, fluorescence microscopy has shown a 10% increase in sensitivity.

Induced Sputum Examination

There are several advantages of sputum induction:
- Diagnostic yield of single induced sputum is at least equivalent to that of one bronchoscopy with bronchoalveolar lavage (BAL) in the terms of positivity on both smear and culture for mycobacteria. The diagnostic yield of induced sputum can be increased with significantly higher detection rates than with bronchoscopy alone when multiple (three or more) specimens are used.
- Smear microscopy and culture positivity rates of 91–98% and 99–100%, respectively, have been reported with multiple specimens.

Fiberoptic Bronchoscopy

The main role of fiberoptic bronchoscopy (FOB) in diagnosing PTB includes patients who are sputum smear negative for acid-fast bacilli (AFB) or who do not produce adequate sputum, particularly, if an immediate diagnosis is required or if alterative diagnoses are being entertained. It is also useful for follow-up studies in endobronchial TB to detect bronchostenosis. Different bronchoscopic modalities to obtain samples include the bronchial aspirate, BAL, brushings, transbronchial lung biopsy (TBLB), and transbronchial needle aspiration (TBNA). FOB is also useful in the diagnosis of tuberculous intrathoracic lymphadenopathy by using TBNA technique. Postbronchoscopy sputum is also helpful in increasing the diagnostic yield in TB. It can increase culture yield by 7%.

Mycobacterial Cultures

Mycobacterial culture is the gold standard for the diagnosis of TB. It is more sensitive than sputum microscopy, requires 10–100 bacilli/mL of sputum to detect *M. tuberculosis*. About 25–60% of patients with culture-positive PTB may show negative smears. Culture not only increases the sensitivity of diagnosis, but also helps in species identification, drug susceptibility testing, and genotyping.

EXTRAPULMONARY TUBERCULOSIS

Extrapulmonary tuberculosis is reported in about 15-20% cases in immunocompetent adults, though it accounts for as high as 50% in HIV-infected patients. The most common sites of involvement include the lymph nodes, pleura, bones, and joints. Central nervous, gastrointestinal, and genitourinary systems are also frequently involved. However, it can involve any organ. Lymph node TB is the most common form of EPTB in India and other developing countries. Diagnosis of EPTB can pose a challenge to the clinicians due to various reasons—(i) signs and symptoms are most often nonspecific, (ii) paucibacillary nature of samples decreases the sensitivity of diagnostic tests, and (iii) EPTB involves relatively inaccessible sites, so the retrieval of samples for diagnosis is a difficult job. The tests for diagnosis, however, are the same as for PTB.

CHAPTER 9

Molecular Diagnosis of Tuberculosis

Rama Murthy Sakamuri, Mamta Kalra, Indu Verma, Suman Laal

INTRODUCTION

There is no single diagnostic test that can detect tuberculosis (TB) at all the different stages or the different forms of TB; a combination of clinical suspicion, microscopic examination of smears made directly from sputum for presence of acid-fast bacilli (AFB) and radiological findings are used for diagnosis.

DIAGNOSIS OF TUBERCULOSIS: BEYOND THE MICROSCOPY

Direct sputum microscopy has been used for TB diagnosis since the 1880s; it remains the primary tool for TB diagnosis, even 120 years later. More sensitive and specific diagnostic tests have emerged in the last few decades, but are too expensive and technically challenging for implementation in the high burden, low-resource settings.

Nucleic Acid Amplification: Detection-based Diagnostic Test for Tuberculosis

The use of nucleic acid amplification (NAA)-based diagnosis has led to significant improvement in rapid diagnosis of TB in the resource-rich countries. According to the latest report by the UNITAID, WHO, on the TB diagnostics technologies, NAA-based diagnostic tests are currently the largest group of tests for TB. These tests use different methods to extract nucleic acids from the specimens, amplify specific regions in *Mycobacterium tuberculosis* (*MTB*) genome and to detect the amplified product. Most of the currently commercially available or under development TB-NAA diagnostics products are based on polymerase chain reaction (PCR) hybridization, real-time PCR or isothermal amplification.

Real-time PCR is a quantitative method that combines the two steps, i.e. amplification and detection into one step and is based on hybridization of the amplified segments (DNA) with different fluorescent probes. The main advantage of real-time PCR is its ability to yield the results in 1.5–2 hours after DNA extraction and its high sensitivity. In addition, problems with cross-contamination are reduced because the detection occurs in a closed system.

The CDC guidelines recommend that "NAA testing be performed on at least one respiratory specimen from each patient with signs and symptoms of pulmonary TB for whom a diagnosis of TB is considered but not established and for whom the test result would alter case management and TB control activities". Since all the current tests require trained personnel, specialized equipment and are expensive, they are rarely used in the TB-endemic countries and cannot be integrated into routine patient care.

Tests for Species Identification of Mycobacteria

Prompt identification of *Mycobacterium* species has become increasingly important with the increase in NTM infections, especially in HIV-infected individuals. NTMs require a different treatment regimen and a lack of response to standard antituberculous drugs can be confused with drug resistance. Thus, adequate disease management requires precise classification of mycobacteria. Conventional methods of *Mycobacterium* species identification include biochemical tests and phenotypic characteristics by culturing that are simple and do not require any sophisticated equipment; these tests are laborious and cumbersome, take several days for results, thus, delaying prompt and accurate identification of bacteria. Newly developed molecular methods are attractive alternatives for rapid identification of mycobacteria, especially *MTB* complex. Several molecular commercial tests are currently available for rapid identification of mycobacterial species from culture isolates.

Microarray-based TB diagnostic tests are in development stages. These tests are being developed to identify or quantify multiple targets in the same assay; the high throughput capability makes these tests important for high-burden settings. In all these products initially gene targets are amplified using PCR, the amplicons are fluorescently labeled, denatured, then hybridized to the complementary DNA oligonucleotides printed on the arrays and signal intensity is measured using a fluorescence reader. These products not only help to aid in the identification of *Mycobacterium* species but will also aid in drug-resistance screening.

Diagnostic Tests for Drug Resistance of *Mycobacterium tuberculosis*

Even as efforts to devise improved diagnostic tests for TB are ongoing, there has been an alarming increase in the incidence of multidrug-resistant TB

(MDR-TB) and extensively drug-resistant TB (XDR-TB) in several parts of the world. MDR-TB is defined as resistance to both INH and rifampicin (RIF) and XDR-TB is defined as MDR-TB with additional resistance to any fluoroquinolone and at least one of the three injectable second-line drugs (SLDs)—capreomycin, kanamycin, and amikacin. As per the WHO estimates, almost 25% of the 5 million cases of MDR-TB that emerged globally in 2012 were from India.

Conventional diagnosis of DR-TB by the proportion method, absolute concentration method or the resistance ratio method takes several weeks even with the rapid-culture (BACTEC 460, MB/BacT, MGIT)-based methods since the primary isolation and culture of *MTB* from the clinical specimens is followed by susceptibility testing in cultures. During this time, transmission of resistant bacteria continues and patients are treated with inappropriate regimens, potentially amplifying resistance.

Rifampicin is the key drug in the first-line chemotherapy of TB, it is estimated that over 90% of the RIF-resistant strains are also INH-resistant. The line probe assays (LPAs) were the first *MTB* molecular assays that were endorsed by WHO. Initially, two commercial assays for rapid detection of drug resistance in *MTB* were developed, the INNO-LiPA RIFTB assay (innogenetics NV, Belgium) for the detection of resistance to rifampicin and the GenoType MTBDRPlus (Hain Lifescience, Germany) for simultaneous detection of rifampicin and isoniazid resistance. The basis of both assays is reverse solid phase hybridization. Currently, there are several LPA-based products in development or field evaluation for rapid detection of both first and SLD resistance.

The second TB-NAA test approved by WHO is GeneXpert® MTB/RIF assay (Cepheid, Sunnyvale, CA) which simultaneously detects *MTB* and rifampicin resistance. The Cepheid GeneXpert system is an integrated diagnostic system that performs sample processing and real-time PCR analysis test in a single hands-free two-hour step. The assay is designed to perform a hemi-nested molecular beacon assay, which uses six molecular beacons to amplify a sequence of *rpoB* gene specific to the *MTB* complex organisms and probe for mutations in the RRDR (rifampicin-resistance determining region) of the *rpoB* gene.

The GeneXpert MTB/RIF assay is closed system format (cartridge based) and fully automated with nucleic acid extraction, amplification and detection process, hence reduces hands-on time and detection of undesirable nucleic acids. This fully automated approach is first of its kind in TB diagnosis. Since the sample processing is automated, this assay has fewer biosafety hazards compared to direct smear microscopy. Several studies have demonstrated the diagnostic accuracy of GeneXpert MTB/RIF assay in both the high-income and resource-limited settings. A recent meta-analysis, reported that the GeneXpert MTB/RIF test has 89% and 99% pooled sensitivity and specificity respectively for TB diagnosis; the pooled sensitivity and specificity for rifampicin resistance is 95% and 98% respectively. The sensitivity for TB diagnosis is lower in smear negative (67%), extra-pulmonary tuberculosis (EPTB) (80%), children

(65.1–75.9%) and HIV-positive individuals (79%). Despite these promising results, GeneXpert MTB/RIF assay has several limitations including the inability to differentiate live from dead bacteria, the difficulty in detection of mixed infections and operational limitations such as the high cost of the equipment and the cartridges, air-conditioned environment for the machines, requirement for uninterrupted power supply, maintenance and annual calibration of the machine, etc.

Microarray technology is also being evaluated for detection of drug resistance in *MTB*. The microarrays or DNA biochips allow simultaneous detection of multiple mutations. A low-density oligonucleotide chip has been reported to detect mutations associated with INH, RIF, SM, KM, and EMB with sensitivities of 69%, 93%, 86%, 80%, and 85%, respectively.

The usefulness of all molecular tests is limited by the fact that not all drug-resistant isolates have mutations in the hotspots of genes associated with drug resistance. These strains still require phenotype-based assays for detection. Secondly, the molecular tests are unable to detect minor populations of drug-resistant organisms in primary culture from clinical samples.

Sample Collection, Processing, and Extraction of Nucleic Acids for Nucleic Acid Amplification Tests

The purity and integrity of nucleic acids extracted from clinical sample greatly influence the results of NAA tests. The sample collection, type of specimen used, nucleic acid extraction method and inhibitors in the nucleic acid after nucleic acid extraction influences the NAA test results. Although most of the molecular assays are based on sputum sample from pulmonary TB patients, the clinical samples from EPTB patients are from other body fluids such as cerebrospinal fluid, bronchiolar alveolar lavage, pleural fluid, abscess, lymph, biopsy, fine-needle aspiration for TB diagnosis.

Acquisition of adequate and quality clinical sample is important for accurate diagnosis. Sputum collection is a challenge in paucibacillary, HIV+, pediatric, and EPTB patients. Sputum induction and concentration methods are used to get improved sample collection. Decontamination of the clinical sample is another critical component to remove the contaminants and inactivate *MTB* in the clinical sample. N-acetyl cysteine and NaOH decontamination method is commonly used for *MTB* culture from sputum sample.

Clinical Impact of the Sensitive Molecular Tests on Tuberculosis Patients

The high-burden TB-endemic countries urgently require simple, accurate point-of-care diagnostic tests that can replace and improve upon microscopy without requiring laboratory infrastructure and highly trained personnel. Although multiple new molecular tests for TB diagnosis are rapidly being developed; several match the sensitivity and specificity of GeneXpert but will be less expensive, their contribution to rapid diagnosis of TB and slow the

TB epidemic remains to be assessed. Most new molecular tests continue to be too expensive for routine use as point-of-care tests in peripheral facilities. No molecular test as yet matches the sensitivity of liquid culture, and even liquid cultures do not provide bacteriological confirmation in approximately 25–30% of the PTB patients, and approximately 50% of the patients with EPTB. Furthermore, NAA tests and cultures cannot be used for routine screening of high-risk populations. Rapid and simple point-of-care tests that are not based on detection of bacteria or bacterial antigen/nucleic acids are required for screening active TB, identify different forms of TB, paucibacillary pulmonary and EPTB.

Optimal Tuberculosis Test

It is important to appreciate the differences between the developed and developing countries in regard to TB. Unfortunately, the diagnostic tests that are used in the industrialized world as well as the resources required for monitoring treatment are too expensive and technically difficult for routine use in resource-limited countries. The patient burden is enormous; accuracy of microscopy is limited and facilities for culture-confirmation are rarely available.

The ideal diagnostic marker for TB would be a universal marker that can:
- Replace and improve upon sputum microscopy.
- Identify patients with EPTB (TB meningitis, skeletal TB, genitourinary TB, gastrointestinal TB, and TB lymphadenitis), many of which are not accessible to microscopy.
- Identify HIV-infected TB patients, in whom TB progresses rapidly and fatally, but the low bacterial burden in the sputum makes detection of bacteria or bacterial molecules difficult, and the immune dysfunction preclude use of cellular immune-based diagnostic assays.
- Diagnose pediatric TB patients who rarely produce sputum and are currently diagnosed based on epidemiologic, clinical and radiological suspicion rather than microbiological confirmation.
- Identify a potential TB patient during the window period from infection to clinical disease.
- Simultaneously detect drug resistance.

In conclusion, in view of the absence of a single universal marker, a set of new diagnostic tests may be able to fulfill these criteria. Not only must the new diagnostic tests detect the myriad forms and stages of TB with high sensitivity, but they must also be highly specific.

CHAPTER 10

Management of Tuberculosis

D Behera

INTRODUCTION

Chemotherapy is the mainstay of treatment of tuberculosis. Duration of chemotherapy got reduced from 18 months to 6 months following addition of rifampin (R) and pyrazinamide (Z) to isoniazid (H) and streptomycin (S) for management of tuberculosis. The short-course of 6 months has also achieved cures in 95% or more of patients, which is considered as the gold standard of the efficacy of any chemotherapy program. Short-course chemotherapy is now widely accepted as the treatment of choice for pulmonary tuberculosis.

The antituberculosis drugs vary in (i) their bactericidal action, defined as their ability to kill a large number of actively metabolizing bacilli rapidly; (ii) their sterilizing action, defined as their capacity to kill special populations of slowly or intermittently metabolizing semidormant bacilli, the so-called "persisters"; (iii) their ability to prevent the emergence of acquired resistance by suppressing drug-resistant mutants present in all large bacterial populations, and (iv) their suitability for intermittent use.

PREVENTION OF DRUG RESISTANCE

Drugs can be graded according to their activity in preventing the emergence of resistance to a second drug, usually isoniazid. Even populations of tubercle bacilli, which are not exposed to antitubercular drugs, contain small proportions of drug-resistant mutants. The proportion of such mutants in wild strains is 1 in 10^5–10^6 for streptomycin, isoniazid and ethambutol, and 1 in 10^7 for rifampicin. If inadequate drug combinations are used, these mutants are likely to replace the killed susceptible bacilli and give rise to drug-resistant disease. The effectiveness of drugs in preventing the emergence of acquired resistance depends upon the extent to which they can inhibit bacilli continuously, whatever their rate of metabolism, even if there is some irregularity in taking drugs.

Isoniazid and rifampicin are the most effective at preventing the emergence of resistance to other drugs, and streptomycin and ethambutol are only slightly less. Pyrazinamide (Z) is less effective; para-aminosalicylic acid (PAS) and thiacetazone are the least effective. Activity of a drug is assessed from the results of clinical studies of the treatment of smear positive pulmonary tuberculosis in which the drug concerned is given in a two-drug combination with isoniazid. Drug gradings are based on the proportion of patients who fail during treatment with the emergence of isoniazid resistance. This proportion is about 0.5% for rifampicin (high activity) and 13–15% for thiacetazone (low activity).

EARLY BACTERICIDAL ACTIVITY

Most of the antitubercular drugs (INH, rifampin, streptomycin, pyrazinamide) have bactericidal activity. Of them, isoniazid kills the largest number of bacilli early during the first 2 days of chemotherapy at a rate of $0.72 \log_{10}$ cfu/mL/day when given alone and the kill of other drugs is increased considerably by $0.36 \log_{10}$ cfu/mL/day when isoniazid is added to them in the treatment. Next in order of bactericidal activity are ethambutol and rifampin with rates of kill of $0.25 \log_{10}$ cfu/mL/day and $0.19 \log_{10}$ cfu/mL/day, respectively. They add little or nothing to the activity of second drugs. Streptomycin, thiacetazone, and pyrazinamide are just bactericidal with rates of kill of 0.09–$0.04 \log_{10}$ cfu/mL/day.

STERILIZING ACTION

Sterilizing activity is the ability to kill all or virtually all of the bacilli in the lesions as rapidly as possible. As the speed of killing gets progressively slower during chemotherapy, sterilizing activity measures the speed with which the last few viable bacilli are killed. This activity is assessed in man by (i) proportion of sputum cultures that are negative at 2 months, or round about that time, after the start of treatment, and (ii) the proportion of relapses that occur after chemotherapy has been stopped. The sterilizing activity of a drug indicates its suitability for incorporation in short-course regimens. The two drugs with the greatest sterilizing activity are rifampicin and pyrazinamide. Isoniazid is less active, taking longer time to sterilize lesions. Though less active than isoniazid, addition of streptomycin or thiacetazone to a regimen probably increases its sterilizing activity to a very small extent. Ethambutol virtually has no sterilizing activity.

Site of Tubercular Disease (Pulmonary or Extrapulmonary)

In general, recommended treatment regimens are similar for both pulmonary and extrapulmonary tuberculosis and are the same irrespective of the site of disease, although some authorities recommend a prolonged continuation phase for tubercular meningitis. Pulmonary tuberculosis refers to disease involving the pulmonary parenchyma and intrathoracic tuberculous lymphadenitis.

Suitability for Intermittent Use

Isoniazid, rifampicin, pyrazinamide, streptomycin and ethambutol are all effective when given twice or thrice a week. The relative activities of the main antitubercular drugs in each of the above three functions are summarized in Table 10.1.

NEW PATIENTS

New patients are defined as those who have no history of prior TB treatment or who received less than 1 month of anti-TB drugs (regardless of whether their smear or culture results are positive or not).

New patients are presumed to have drug-susceptible TB with two exceptions:
1. Where there is a high prevalence of isoniazid resistance in the new patients.
or
2. If they have developed active TB after known contact with a patient documented to have drug-resistant TB, they are likely to have a similar drug resistance pattern to the source case and DST should be carried out at the start of treatment. While DST results of the patient are awaited, a regimen based on the DST of the presumed source case should be started.

The 2-month rifampicin regimen (2HRZE/6HE) is associated with more relapses and deaths than the 6-month rifampicin regimen (2HRZE/4HR).

The WHO recommends the following treatment regimen for new patients presumed or known to have drug-susceptible TB. *New patients with pulmonary TB should receive a regimen containing 6 months of rifampicin: 2HRZE/4HR* (Strong/High grade of evidence). Patients of extrapulmonary TB require similar duration of treatment for 6 months. Longer therapy of 9–12 months is

TABLE 10.1: Grading of activities of antituberculosis drugs.

Extent of activity	Prevention of resistance	Early bactericidal	Sterilizing
High	Isoniazid	Isoniazid	Rifampicin
	Rifampicin		Pyrazinamide
		Ethambutol	
	Ethambutol	Rifampicin	Isoniazid
	Streptomycin		
		Streptomycin	Streptomycin
	Pyrazinamide	Pyrazinamide	Thiacetazone
Low	Thiacetazone	Thiacetazone	Ethambutol

recommended for patients of TB of central nervous system, bones or joints. WHO further recommends that the National TB Control Programs provide supervision and support for all TB patients in order to ensure completion of the full course of therapy.

The other important recommendation of WHO is that the 2HRZE/6HE treatment regimen should be phased out (Strong/High grade of evidence). In terms of dosing frequency for HIV-negative patients, the systematic review found little evidence of differences in failure or relapse rates with daily or three times weekly regimens. However, patients receiving three times weekly dosing throughout therapy had higher rates of acquired drug resistance than patients who received drugs daily throughout the treatment. In patients with pretreatment isoniazid resistance, three times weekly dosing during the intensive phase was associated with significantly higher risks of failure and acquired drug resistance than daily dosing during the intensive phase.

Other Important Recommendations

Wherever feasible, the optimal dosing frequency for new a patients with pulmonary TB is daily throughout the course of therapy (Strong/High grade of evidence).

In terms of dosing frequency for HIV-negative patients, the systematic review found little evidence of differences in failure or relapse rates with daily or three times weekly regimens. However, rates of acquired drug resistance were higher among patients receiving three times weekly dosing throughout therapy than among patients who received daily drug administration throughout treatment. Moreover, in patients with pretreatment isoniazid resistance, three times weekly dosing during the intensive phase was associated with significantly higher risks of failure and acquired drug resistance, particularly to rifampicin, than daily dosing during the intensive phase.

Mediastinal lymphadenitis and pleural effusions without radiographic parenchymal involvement are taken as extrapulmonary tuberculosis. A patient with both pulmonary and extrapulmonary tuberculosis is categorized as a case of pulmonary tuberculosis. The case definition of an extrapulmonary case with several sites affected depends upon the site representing the most severe form of the disease.

Severity of Disease

Bacillary load, extent of disease and anatomical site of involvement are taken into account in defining the severity of the disease. Involvement of an anatomical site results in classification as severe disease if there is either a significant acute threat to life as in pericardial tuberculosis, or a risk of subsequent severe sequel with handicap as in spinal tuberculosis, or both as in tuberculous meningitis. Thus, the following forms of extrapulmonary tuberculosis are classified as severe: Meningitis, miliary, pericarditis, peritonitis, and bilateral or extensive pleural effusion, spinal, intestinal and genitourinary. Other forms of extrapulmonary tuberculosis like lymphadenitis, unilateral pleural effusion, and bone (excluding spine), peripheral joint, and skin are classified as less severe.

PREVIOUSLY TREATED CASES

History of the Previous Treatment

By this information, a case is defined whether a patient had previous antitubercular treatment or not. By this case definition, patients who are at increased risk of acquired drug resistance are identified for the prescription of appropriate treatment; and for epidemiological monitoring. Although smear-negative and extrapulmonary cases may also be treatment failures, relapses, or chronic cases, this is rare. The importance of case definitions as above is important for registration, notification and to define treatment categories.

In populations where isoniazid resistance is known or suspected to be high, the new TB patients should receive HRE as therapy in the continuation phase as an acceptable alternative to HR. While there is a pressing need to prevent multidrug resistance (MDR), the most effective regimen for the treatment of isoniazid-resistant TB is not known. There is inadequate evidence to quantify the ability of ethambutol to "protect rifampicin" in patients with pretreatment isoniazid resistance. There is no sufficient evidence for ocular toxicity from ethambutol but the risk of permanent blindness exists. Thus, further research is urgently needed to define the level of isoniazid resistance that would warrant the addition of ethambutol (or other drugs) to the continuation phase of the standard new patient regimen in TB programs where isoniazid drug susceptibility testing is not done (or results are unavailable) before the continuation phase begins. Daily (rather than three times weekly) intensive-phase dosing may also help to prevent acquired drug resistance in TB patients starting treatment with isoniazid resistance. Patients with isoniazid resistance treated with a three times weekly intensive phase had significantly higher risks of failure and acquired drug resistance than those treated with daily dosing during the intensive phase.

CONCLUSION

In summary, tuberculosis is a completely curable disease provided the treatment is given according to the standard national guidelines whether in the programmatic conditions or outside the National Program. There is no place for liberty in TB treatment. Treatment should be instituted early to prevent the drug sequelae which may not be completely controllable with drugs. The battle is to be fought both to treat the condition and to prevent the emergence of drug resistance.

CHAPTER 11

Prevention of Tuberculosis

Rajesh N Solanki, Jaydeep Odhwani, Kumar Utsav

There are multiple levels of prevention that are crucial to decrease the mortality and morbidity of the disease, i.e. primordial, primary, secondary, and tertiary prevention. Community-based interventions were found to be most effective for prevention and control of tuberculosis (TB).

PRIMORDIAL PREVENTION

Adoption of proper lifestyle, especially in the early childhood, is the basis of primordial prevention. For TB, it will involve the following measures:
- Nutritional interventions
- Environmental modifications (especially healthy housing and proper sanitation, improved socioeconomic status)
- Appropriate health education and behavioral changes.

PRIMARY PREVENTION

Primary prevention efforts aim at reducing an individual's susceptibility to the disease, illness, or injury. Education, changes in lifestyle, and behavior modification are components of primary prevention. TB is infectious when it occurs in the lungs or larynx. TB that occurs elsewhere in the body in isolation is usually not infectious.

Administrative Measures

The aim of administrative interventions in any healthcare facility which manages patients with suspected TB is to reduce the total time period that such a patient stays in the healthcare facility, reduce airborne transmission to other patients and healthcare workers (HCWs) in this limited time period, all rooms require more than 6–12 air changes per hour. Administration should also ensure rapid diagnostic evaluation, rapid initiation of treatment, limit employee, and visitor exposure.

Outpatient Area
Reducing the overall stay of such patients in the healthcare facility is likely to prove the single most effective measure of reducing airborne disease transmission in these areas. This can be achieved by fast tracking these patients, which can be accomplished by several measures that are not mutually exclusive.
- *Screening*
- *Education on cough etiquette and respiratory hygiene*
- *Patient segregation.*

Inpatient Care Facilities
- *Need-based hospitalization of TB patients*
- *Establish separate rooms, wards, or areas within wards for patients with infectious respiratory diseases*
- *Cough hygiene and adequate sputum disposal*
- *Establish safe radiology procedures for patients with infectious respiratory disease, including smear-positive TB cases or TB suspects.*

Environmental Controls
Environmental control measures are the second-line of defense for preventing the spread of TB in healthcare settings. Environmental controls include ventilation (natural and mechanical), ultraviolet germicidal irradiation (UVGI), filtration, and other methods of air cleaning. Environmental controls work on the same basic principle—dilution of infectious particles through real or "effective" air exchange.

Ventilation
In the case of ventilation, the dilution occurs through the introduction of fresh, uninfected air, and removal of the infected air.

Natural ventilation: It refers to fresh air that enters and leaves a room or other area through openings such as windows or doors. Simple natural ventilation can be optimized by maximizing the size of the windows, opening up fixed window panes, by locating windows on opposing walls, and by the use of propeller "mixing fans".

Mechanical ventilation: It uses fans to drive the airflow through a building. Mechanical ventilation can be fully controlled and combined with air conditioning and filtration systems as is normally done in some office buildings. Mechanical ventilation also includes "mixed mode ventilation", in which exhaust and/or supply fans are used in combination with natural ventilation to obtain adequate dilution when sufficient ventilation rate cannot be achieved by natural ventilation alone.

The simplest form of mechanical ventilation is the use of "exhaust fans", placed for instance in windows to move air from inside a room to the outdoors.

Direction control of airflow: It is recommended in specific high-risk settings where infectious patients with drug-resistant TB are managed. Natural ventilation would allow potentially infected air to cross HCWs.

Ultraviolet Germicidal Irradiation (UVGI)

Mycobacterium tuberculosis (MTB) is sensitive to germicidal radiation of ultraviolet rays found in the UV-C portion of the ultraviolet spectrum. The use of UVGI lamps is reserved for high-risk areas (laboratory, sputum collection area, poorly ventilated spaces, etc.), where other environmental measures are not sufficient due to climatic or structural constraints.

Sputum collection area: This area must be designed outside in the open to allow the bacilli get naturally dispersed by air and killed by sun. In a closed room, the concentration of bacilli will be high.

Filtration (HEPA Filters)

Filtration is another option to remove infectious particles from the air. Situations where HEPA filter might be considered include the bronchoscopy suits, laboratories, and individual TB patient room.

Personal Protection

Health staff: TB is transmitted mainly via the respiratory route. Only anti-inhalation masks (high-filtration masks, N95 masks) are capable of preventing inhalation of the bacilli.

All members of the staff, whether caregiver or not must wear these masks under the following conditions, when:
- In contact with contagious patients
- Collecting sputum samples and preparing slides
- Collecting and disposing the sputum containers.

In addition to wearing a mask, which is a specific protective measure, standard precautions (hand hygiene, gown, etc.) apply in TB wards, just as they do in any other hospital department.

Vaccines

The only vaccination for TB in the market is the bacillus Calmette–Guérin (BCG) vaccine. It has poor efficacy ranging from 0% to 80%. The BCG vaccine is routinely given in India to the newborn after birth. It is not recommended in the United States because secondary prevention techniques are greatly hindered by the BCG vaccine, which can interfere with the management of persons who are possibly infected with MTB.

SECONDARY PREVENTION

Screening

Secondary prevention denotes the identification of people who have already developed a disease at an early stage in the natural history. This is achieved through screening and early intervention.

Screening tests and preventive therapy accomplish secondary prevention efforts. This is particularly important for high-risk population groups such as the HCW, prisoners, and inmates of common living facilities. Implementation of preventive therapy (treatment with anti-TB drugs) reduces the risk that TB infection will progress to TB disease. Early identification and successful treatment of persons with TB disease remain the most effective means of preventing disease transmission. Some of the screening methods applied for identification of high-risk group populations are as given below:

1. *Symptomatic screening*
2. *Radiographic screening*
3. *Detection of latent tuberculosis infection*

The US Centers for Disease Control and Prevention (CDC) recommends a strategy to identify those who have latent tuberculosis infection (LTBI) and, if indicated, the use of chemotherapy to prevent the latent infection from progressing to active TB disease. There are two tests that can be used to help detect LTBI:

1. *Tuberculin skin test*
2. *QuantiFERON-TB gold*: QFT-G is more sensitive than the TST. The test is highly specific and unaffected by BCG vaccination status, a major cause of false-positive TST response.

Chemoprophylaxis

Chemoprophylaxis is most often the treatment for primary infection in order to sterilize the lesions and prevent the development of active TB. In the literal sense of the term, it is more a treatment than chemoprophylaxis. It may reduce the risk of developing TB by up to 90% in a patient with primary infection. It usually consists of daily administration of isoniazid (INH) 5 mg/kg (maximum 300 mg/day) for 6 months in both children and adults. The effectiveness of INH prophylaxis depends on the sensitivity to INH. The use of INH must be avoided in patients with severe or chronic active hepatitis. It should be administered with caution to patients who regularly consume alcohol.

Chemoprophylaxis for Newborn Infant of Sputum Smear-positive Mother

In all the cases, where the mother is sputum smear-positive at birth of child, chemoprophylaxis is administered to the child for 6 months; BCG vaccination is done afterwards (BCG vaccine should not be given during administration of INH).

If a child develops signs of TB immediately or subsequently (in general, only evident after approximately 2–8 weeks), e.g. arrested growth, splenohepatomegaly, jaundice, sometimes, pneumonia, she/he should receive complete anti-TB treatment after exclusion of other possible medical causes.

If a tuberculin skin test is possible, the approach is to administer INH for 3 months, followed by a tuberculin skin test. If the tuberculin skin test is positive, INH is continued for 3 more months. If the tuberculin skin test is negative, stop INH and administer the BCG vaccine.

- The child should not be separated from her/his mother unless she/he is severely ill. Breastfeeding should be continued. INH is not effective in cases where there is primary resistance against the drug (which varies according to the area) as well as in cases where there is a problem of secondary resistance in the mother. The child must, therefore, be closely monitored in all cases.
- If a mother presents with TB during pregnancy or if the sputum becomes negative under the treatment, it is sufficient to vaccinate the child at birth and to monitor him/her thereafter.

Children under 5 years of Age in Contact with Mantoux-positive Patients

If suspicion of TB exists before administering chemoprophylaxis, it is imperative to rule out active TB. If TB is suspected, the child should undergo complete curative treatment. If not, prophylaxis should be administered for 6 months. Chemoprophylaxis is administered for 6 months regardless of the vaccination status, if the child is healthy. Vaccination and monitoring is recommended, if prophylaxis is not possible to administer.

The use of tuberculin skin test may help to better specify indications for prophylaxis. In practice, it is simpler and prudent to systematically administer prophylaxis, when indicated.

Chemoprophylaxis in HIV Patients

The use of antiretroviral therapy (ART) in HIV patients causes up to 80% of risk reduction, without the use of INH. This, in itself, is the best chemoprophylaxis. The target population for chemoprophylaxis among HIV-seropositive includes all Mantoux (PPD) positive individuals who do not have active TB and could include PPD negative individuals living in high-prevalence region for TB.

The optimal duration of preventive therapy with single drug INH, daily or twice weekly, should be greater than 6 months to provide the maximum degree of protection against TB. The effectiveness of preventive therapy should be evaluated at regular intervals by monitoring patients for drug adherence, drug toxicity, and for the development of TB.

Chemoprophylaxis in tuberculin negative HIV-infected persons: Tuberculin skin test negative, HIV-infected persons from high-risk groups or from areas with a high prevalence of *MTB* infection may be at increased risk of primary or reactivation TB.

Prerequisite to initiate preventive therapy: Prior to starting an individual on preventive treatment for TB, it is essential to ensure that he/she does not have active TB. At times, it is difficult to exclude TB even when the chest radiograph is normal and two sputum smears are negative for acid-fast bacilli (AFB). Where mycobacterial culture facilities are available, sputum culture can be used to definitively diagnose TB. In general, it is safe to presume that completely asymptomatic individuals are unlikely to have TB.

Duration of preventive therapy: There is the evidence to suggest that preventive therapy is efficacious in HIV-positive persons with tuberculin reactions greater than 5 mm and that optimal duration of INH preventive therapy (using a single drug) should be greater than 6 months to provide the maximum degree of protection against TB.

Current recommendations for preventive therapy against TB in HIV-infected persons:
- *WHO recommendation*: INH is recommended drug (5 mg/kg to maximum 300 mg) to be taken daily, as self-administered therapy for 6 months. Individuals should be seen monthly and given only 1 month's supply of medication at each visit.
- *CDC recommendation*: INH is chosen for prevention of TB in persons with HIV infection. It is recommended for 9 months rather than 6 months of rifampicin. Pyrazinamide may be offered daily for 2 months to contacts of patients with INH-resistant and rifampicin-susceptible TB.
- *American Thoracic Society*: INH is recommended for 12 months as prophylaxis in persons infected with HIV infection.

Chemoprophylaxis and Multidrug-resistant Tuberculosis

Among contacts of patients with multidrug-resistant tuberculosis (MDR-TB), the use of INH is questionable. Although alternative prophylaxis treatments have been suggested, there is no consensus regarding the choice of the drug(s) and the duration of treatment. Prompt treatment of MDR-TB is the most effective way of preventing the spread of infection to others. The following measures should be taken to prevent spread of MDR-TB disease:
- Early diagnosis and appropriate treatment of MDR-TB cases
- Screening of contacts as per the Revised National Tuberculosis Control Program (RNTCP) guidelines.

TERTIARY PREVENTION

The treatment of people who have already developed a disease is often described as tertiary prevention. The final strategy used for preventing and controlling TB is the identification and treatment of patients with active TB. An individual with active TB is infectious. Special precautions or isolation may be necessary to avoid transmission to others. Once the individual begins treatment and continues to follow the prescribed regimen, the individual becomes usually noninfectious within days or weeks.

CONCLUSION

Primary prevention of TB is most essential to prevent the spread of the disease in the community. It is however equally important to adopt secondary prevention in the exposed and high-risk populations. Treatment of patients to help contain communication to others is an important step in tertiary prevention strategies.

CHAPTER 12

Extrapulmonary Tuberculosis

AK Janmeja, PR Mohapatra, Deepak Aggarwal

INTRODUCTION

Extrapulmonary TB (EPTB) constitutes about 15–20% of all TB cases, which rises to nearly 50% among human immunodeficiency virus-tuberculosis (HIV-TB) coinfection. The proportion of EPTB has shown an upward trend in the recent years both in the developed and developing countries. In presence of HIV coinfection, lymph node or central nervous system tuberculosis (CNS-TB) is quite commonly seen. Almost any organ can be involved in tuberculosis but lymph node tuberculosis and pleural tuberculosis together contribute to around 75% of the total pool of EPTB cases, followed by bone and joint tuberculosis, genitourinary tuberculosis (GUTB), tuberculous meningitis (TBM), abdominal, and disseminated miliary tuberculosis.

DIAGNOSIS

Diagnosis of EPTB is generally more difficult than that of pulmonary tuberculosis. Most forms of EPTB are of paucibacillary nature, making it imperative to depend on investigations other than the gold standard for the diagnosis, i.e. demonstration of causative tubercle bacilli on microscopy. The classical constitutional clinical features like low-grade evening pyrexia, anorexia, weight loss, malaise, and fatigue are also not regular manifestations. Sometimes, the disease may even present as the pyrexia of unknown origin.

Extrapulmonary TB manifestations are nonspecific, not significantly different in the HIV-infected or the noninfected patients, however, extensive disease, inadequate or delayed treatment and HIV coinfection are the factors associated with increased mortality. For the diagnosis of EPTB, all efforts must be exhausted to isolate of tubercle bacilli from the body fluids or the biopsy specimens. Role of adenosine deaminase (ADA) estimation in tuberculous fluid collections in various types of EPTB has been found helpful in reaching the diagnosis. Application of molecular methods, such as polymerase chain reaction (PCR), assay targeting IS6110, multiplex PCR and RT-PCR have also been reported useful in the diagnosis of EPTB, particularly where there is strong clinical suspicion, and conventional techniques are not conclusive.

Neither tuberculin skin test (TST) nor interferon-gamma release assay (IGRA) is recommended for the diagnosis of tubercular disease as these tests depict the immune response against tubercular antigens and do not provide information on the presence of active tuberculosis disease. The serological assays have shown unsatisfying diagnostic accuracies (low specificity and sensitivity) and their use has been banned by WHO.

TREATMENT OF EXTRAPULMONARY TUBERCULOSIS

Antituberculosis drug therapy alone is quite adequate to achieve cure in the majority of cases caused by typical tubercle bacilli, including EPTB. The recommended treatment comprises of short-course chemotherapy regimens of 6 months duration, in which four drugs, i.e. isoniazid (H), rifampicin (R), pyrazinamide (Z), and ethambutol (E) are given in the initial intensive phase of two months duration followed by two drugs (HR) for the next four months in the continuation phase. The Revised National Tuberculosis Control Program (RNTCP) of the Government of India and several other similar national control programs elsewhere follow the WHO recommended directly observed therapy short course (DOTS) strategy under which drugs are administered intermittently thrice a week.

LYMPH NODE TUBERCULOSIS

Lymph node tuberculosis is more commonly seen in the Asian, Hispanic, and African-American populations. Cervical, axillary, inguinal or chest wall nodes are the common involved sites. About 10% cases may also have concomitant mediastinal lymph node disease, which may be due to the retrograde spread. Hilar or mediastinal lymph nodes are frequently involved in primary tuberculosis and in HIV-infected patients particularly.

Lymph node tuberculosis is often a localized manifestation of systemic spread of tuberculous infection. Initially, at the time of primary infection, tubercle bacilli get into the lungs through inhalation and form a primary complex. During this stage, there occurs hematogenous and lymphatic spread of infection to the rest of the body, where they remain dormant in the majority of infected subjects.

Often, the lymph nodes are small, discrete and grow very slowly, but occasionally they grow faster, become tender or painful. The absence of warmth and redness on overlying skin earns it a peculiar name, "cold abscess" which is almost synonymous with tuberculous etiology of the abscess. Sometimes, in an immune-compromised host or in HIV infection, the abscess grows very fast making the overlying skin warm, erythematous and painful, mimicking an acute pyogenic abscess. Such abscesses may burst and form chronic discharging sinuses or ulcers. Tuberculous sinuses characteristically have thin, bluish, undermined edges, while the discharge is usually watery.

Also, concomitant pulmonary tuberculosis and intrathoracic or intra-abdominal lymph node involvement is more common in HIV-infected cases. Apart from the classical symptoms of local visible swelling, the enlarged nodes may result in signs and symptoms due to obstruction or pressure on adjacent viscera, e.g. mediastinal lymphadenopathy can cause dysphagia, tracheoesophageal or esophagomediastinal fistula, etc. chylothorax, chyluria or chylous ascites may develop as a result of pressure on thoracic duct due to upper abdominal or mediastinal lymphadenopathy. Although rare, obstructive jaundice due to biliary duct compression by enlarged lymph nodes at porta hepatis has also been reported.

The gold standard for diagnosis of tuberculous lymphadenitis is the excision biopsy. Fine-needle aspiration cytology (FNAC) and/or pus from the involved glands are often helpful. Although, the tubercle bacilli positivity rate is not very impressive, larger biopsy sample may show positivity rate up to 50–70%. Infrequent demonstration of bacilli on direct smear examination is basically due to the paucibacillary nature of the disease. In selected cases, endoscopic ultrasound-guided FNAC can also be used for assessing mediastinal and abdominal lymphadenopathy. It is a safe, minimally invasive, accurate, outpatient diagnostic modality and can be used early in suspected EPTB.

While treating lymph node tuberculosis, a unique paradoxical phenomenon is encountered in some cases during the course drug therapy. There occurs further enlargement of already diseased nodes or even new lymph nodes might appear ipsilaterally or contralaterally in the same or different group of lymph nodes. These lymph nodes tend to regress spontaneously on continuation of the same drug regimens without any alteration. Hence, there is no need of changing the drug regimen in such situations. This phenomenon is mostly attributable to hypersensitivity toward tuberculous-proteins released due to the bactericidal action of drugs or the disrupted macrophages. The phenomenon of paradoxical response to tuberculosis chemotherapy is also termed as immune reconstitution inflammatory syndrome (IRIS).

PLEURAL EFFUSION

Tuberculous pleural effusion is the most common type of EPTB after lymph node disease. Nearly 20% of all EPTB cases both in HIV-infected and non-infected patients are pleural effusion cases (details discussed in the section on "Pleural Diseases").

BONE AND JOINT TUBERCULOSIS

Spinal Tuberculosis (Pott's Disease)

Spinal tuberculosis is the most common type of osseous tuberculosis and nearly half of the bone and joint cases are due to spinal involvement. Usually weightbearing joints are affected by tuberculosis. In spinal tuberculosis, lower thoracic and upper lumbar vertebrae are commonly affected, followed by middle thoracic and cervical region vertebrae. Usually, more than one adjacent vertebrae are involved and the body of the vertebra is predominantly affected rather than its other elements.

The tubercle bacilli reach skeletal tissue as a result of hematogenous spread during primary tuberculous infection. Paradiskal, anterior, and central vertebral lesions are commonly encountered. The disease originates in the cancellous area of bone close to the superior or the inferior end-plates and extends into intervertebral disk after penetrating the subchondral bone plate and thence to the body of adjacent vertebra. With further progression, there occurs the demineralization of end plates and softening of body leading to vertebral collapse or anterior wedging. This is responsible for typical angulation or gibbus deformity in the spine seen in Pott's disease patients. The spread of disease may also follow subanterior longitudinal ligament route. The subligamentous downward spread of tuberculous abscess away from the primarily involved vertebrae can cause the destruction of anterior surface of other vertebral bodies.

The exudate tends to spread following the path of least resistance along with fascial planes, vasculature and nerves, and may present as cold abscesses elsewhere. Commonly, such abscesses are seen as a paravertebral abscess, psoas abscess in lumbar region, or abscess in iliac fossa, and some even gravitate below the inguinal ligament on medial side of thigh. Sometimes, it spreads laterally from the iliac fossa over the iliac crest. Rarely, it tracks with gluteal or femoral vessels to form gluteal or Scarpa's triangle abscess. If the cervical spine is involved with tuberculosis, the exudates track down in prevertebral area as a retropharyngeal abscess, which may mechanically cause deglutition and respiratory difficulty or hoarseness of voice. Accumulation of pus in the mediastinum may present as posterior mediastinal mass from where it can spread to the pleural cavity, esophagus or trachea.

Usual constitutional symptoms may be seen well before the localizing signs become actually perceivable in spinal tuberculosis. Often, local signs at the involved site or at the site of extended disease are more prominent. The characteristic clinical features include local pain, local tenderness, stiffness, and spasm of the muscles progressing on to cold abscess and spinal deformity. The progression of disease is generally slow varying from few months to few years, average duration ranging from 4 months to 11 months. Neurological deficits are more common with the involvement of thoracic and cervical regions.

Paraplegia (Pott's paraplegia) develops in about 30% cases of Pott's disease. Generally, it has been described as paraplegia of active disease (early onset paraplegia) and paraplegia of healed disease (late onset paraplegia). Early onset paraplegia develops during active disease due to mechanical pressure caused by formation of debris, pus and granulation tissue. Sometimes, nonmechanical causes are responsible for such neurological complications. Late onset paraplegia develops after a variable period in a patient with healed tuberculosis possibly due to the formation of a ridge of bone anterior to cord, fibrosis of dura mater or gliosis of cord, etc.

Plain radiography reveals narrowing or disappearance of disk space, area of destruction in the body and wedging or collapse of the vertebral bodies. The bony changes become perceivable on plain radiograph only about 5–6 months after the onset of pathology. However, CT and MRI scans may pick up such lesions quite early; also, the extent of associated complications is demarcated better with these investigations.

The CT and MR imaging are particularly useful to study the status of the spinal cord or the canal and to pick up the involvement of posterior elements of vertebrae. Some of the complications, such as the prevertebral abscess in neck region and the typical fusiform abscess in the dorsal spine area, can also be appreciated better with such imaging techniques. Healed psoas abscess may show calcification too. Often, typical clinicoradiological or MR imagings are quite adequate to diagnose spinal tuberculosis. However, in atypical presentations, differentiation is necessary from conditions like pyogenic osteomyelitis, mycotic infection, syphilis, neoplasia, multiple myeloma, lymphoma, chondroma, metastasis, traumatic fracture or sarcoidosis, and others. In such situations, biopsy of the affected vertebra and culture of its contents would be necessary to clinch the diagnosis.

Tuberculous Arthritis

Tuberculous arthritis is typically a monoarticular disease, although multiple joint involvements have been described in literature. About 15% of all skeletal tuberculosis cases are attributed by hip joint and about 10% cases by knee joint TB but shoulder joint is uncommonly involved. Involvement of joint may occur as a result of direct extension from adjacent tuberculous osteomyelitis or through hematogenous spread occurred during primary tuberculosis. Clinicopathological staging of joint tuberculosis usually decides the clinical features for that stage. Pain and circumferential limitation of joint movements are typical clinical features in such cases. Osteolytic areas, tuberculous sequestration along with the loss of the definition of articular margins are encountered in joint tuberculosis. In advanced stages, periarticular osteoporosis, peripheral bony erosions and gradual reduction in joint space constitute a radiological triad suggestive of joint tuberculosis. Often, pyogenic, fungal, and rheumatoid arthritis may also need differentiation from joint tuberculosis.

Poncet's Disease

This is defined as parainfective polyarthritis in which active tuberculosis is located anywhere in the body, not necessarily in the affected joints and tubercle bacilli are never isolated from the involved joints. Commonly, the lymph node is the extra-articular site of active tuberculous disease. This is basically a tuberculous hypersensitivity phenomenon, commonly accompanied by strongly positive TST or erythema nodosum. In addition to pain, swelling and tenderness of the involved joints, other constitutional features, fever, etc. are generally present. The joint synovial fluid is exudative type, sterile, negative for TB bacilli and even PCR is negative for *Mycobacterium* DNA. The condition responds very well to the standard drug treatment of primary tuberculous disease.

Tuberculosis Osteomyelitis

Osteomyelitis is usually seen in the bones of extremities involving small bones of hands and feet like phalanges, metacarpals, and metatarsals. Although tuberculosis can involve any bone, the long bone disease is rare. The disease commonly presents with clinical features, such as, pain, swelling with raised temperature, tenderness, and boggy soft tissue at the involved site. An abscess or sinus may also be encountered over the involved bone. The condition often needs differentiation from chronic pyogenic osteomyelitis and neoplasia. The typical radiographic picture reveals honey combing, sequestration of diaphysis and subperiosteal new bone formation.

Treatment of Bone and Joint Tuberculosis

Overall consensus is that spinal tuberculosis without neurological involvement and without unsightly deformity is a medical condition. Combined management is the modality of choice, which comprises of orthopedic intervention by an orthopedician if necessary and tuberculosis drug therapy under supervision of a physician. The basic principles of tuberculosis drug therapy regimens essentially remain the same as for pulmonary tuberculosis. Short-course chemotherapy of 9 months duration is quite adequate.

CENTRAL NERVOUS SYSTEM TUBERCULOSIS

Although only about 5% of all EPTB cases are contributed by CNS-TB, the latter has relatively high morbidity and mortality in comparison to other EPTB types. Human immunodeficiency virus has further compounded the risk for the development of CNS-TB.

Tubercle bacilli reach the brain parenchyma and the meninges during the stage of hematogenous spread of primary complex formation. Thereupon, these bacilli form tiny lesions prior to the development of delayed hypersensitivity or cell-mediated immunity. Consequent upon development of cell-mediated immunity, these lesions get resolved by natural healing in more than 95% cases. Later in life, such lesions may get reactivated and present with variety of different clinical forms of CNS-TB. Once reactivated, the foci may rupture into the subarachnoid space leading to arachnoiditis or grow intracranially as tuberculomas. Nearly, 20% of such patients have concomitant miliary tuberculosis. Occasionally, direct extension from tuberculosis of contiguous parts would lead to CNS-TB, like from skull bone tuberculosis, tuberculous otitis or spondylitis, etc. Rarely, extradural tuberculous abscess may occur with vault tuberculosis.

Tuberculous meningitis usually develops as a complication of primary tuberculosis, hence commonly seen in early childhood, but may occur at any age. The initial symptoms of disease are nonspecific in the form of loss of appetite, irritability, malaise, vomiting, headache, changed behavior, drowsiness or even convulsions. These features usually mark the prodromal stage of the disease, which may last for 2–8 weeks. Neck retraction or rigidity may be accompanied at this stage due to meningeal inflammation. In infants, fontanel may be found bulging on physical examination. Around 50% cases have papilledema, but usually without the loss of vision. Increasing hydrocephalus is responsible for decreasing consciousness and brain damage. Choroid tubercles may also be seen in some cases.

Cerebrospinal fluid findings play a vital role in the diagnosis of CNS-TB. Usually, CSF is clear and its glucose level is less than 40% of the corresponding blood glucose level. Proteins in CSF are in the range of 100–200 mg/dL usually, although it may exceed 1 g/dL in the presence of spinal block due to coexisting spinal meningitis. If allowed to stand, one can see the cobweb formation in CSF.

In the presence of HIV infection, CSF remains unremarkable and is not helpful in making of the diagnosis. Nevertheless, CSF must be sent in HIV-infected patients for acid-fast bacilli (AFB) culture, as it may come out to be positive in up to 50% cases. Sterile CSF culture for bacteria, fungi, and negative Gram's staining are supportive of TBM diagnosis. WHO has endorsed automated, hemi-nested real-time PCR Xpert MTB/RIF over other conventional tests for diagnosis of TB meningitis.

Tuberculous meningitis is a serious form of tuberculosis in the terms of morbidity and mortality, hence a better prognosis can only be anticipated if the disease is detected at an early stage and right treatment is initiated without wasting time. Isoniazid, pyrazinamide and ethionamide penetrate the blood-brain barrier (BBB) adequately; rifampicin enters poorly while streptomycin and ethambutol cross BBB adequately only when meninges are inflamed. Four drugs (HRZS/E) should be included in the intensive phase. Ethambutol is avoided in comatose patients because vision cannot be monitored. Therefore, streptomycin should be substituted for ethambutol accordingly. Intrathecal streptomycin is no longer used. The optimum duration of TB drug therapy in TBM is still debatable. Meta-analysis of available literature suggests that 6-month regimens are as affective as longer duration regimens provided the bacteria are fully susceptible to first-line drugs. However, chemotherapy for 9–12 months of treatment is recommended for TBM, because of the serious risk of mortality and morbidity.

Use of corticosteroids is somewhat controversial. Although its use does not benefit stage I, but it improves prognosis in stage II and III disease. Therefore, if nothing is suggestive of drug resistance and fungal etiology is ruled out, corticosteroid should be used as adjuvant to tuberculosis drug therapy in stage II and III TBM. In adults, dexamethasone 0.4 mg/kg/24 hours can be given, with a tapering course over 6–8 weeks. Surgery is sometimes necessary for the management of hydrocephalus, as an early drainage improves the outcome. Surgical drainage of intracranial or extradural abscess will also be necessary.

Tuberculomas usually regress with chemotherapy; therefore, a trial of at least 2 months drug therapy must be given before surgery.

ABDOMINAL TUBERCULOSIS

Abdominal tuberculosis encompasses tuberculosis of gastrointestinal tract (GIT) anywhere from esophagus to anus, peritoneum, mesentery, omentum, mesenteric lymph nodes, hepatobiliary system, spleen, and pancreas. The entity accounts for 3% of all EPTB cases. In abdominal tuberculosis concomitant pulmonary lesions are also found in about 25% of cases.

The tuberculous infection can reach the abdominal organs through hematogenous spread during its primary infection stage, due to swallowing of tubercle bacilli loaded sputum in pulmonary tuberculosis patients, through direct extension from adjacent organ harboring tuberculosis and occasionally by lymphatics spread. Transmission through milk from cattle suffering with bovine TB is not common these days due to the universal practice of pasteurization or boiling of milk before consumption.

The most common site for abdominal TB is the ileocecal region possibly because of the abundance of lymphoid tissue in the Peyer's patches, physiological stasis and minimal digestive work undertaken in this part of intestine allowing more stagnation time to bacilli for invasion. The disease spreading from lymph nodes, intestine or from fallopian tubes usually leads to peritoneal tuberculosis. In about 30% cases, lymph node and peritoneal tuberculosis may be seen even without the intestinal disease.

Grossly, intestinal tuberculosis is classified as ulcerative, ulcero-hyperplastic and hyperplastic type. While ulcerative and hyperplastic forms (stricture form) are seen in small intestine, ulcerohyperplastic form is found in colon and ileocecal region. Tuberculous peritonitis occurs in different forms: ascitic, encysted, and fibrinous. It sometimes gives a feel as an abdominal mass comprising of a mesentery and thickened omentum. Granulomas are commonly found in the lymph nodes.

Clinical presentation of abdominal tuberculosis is quite protean, may mimic many acute or chronic intestinal ailments. Nearly two-thirds cases of abdominal tuberculosis are young adults of 20–40 years of age with slight preponderance for female gender. The onset of symptoms may be acute, chronic or acute on chronic. Often, about one-third present as acute abdomen with pain in right iliac fossa mimicking acute appendicitis or as acute intestinal obstruction, while the remaining two-thirds have insidious onset with symptoms like pain in abdomen. Constitutional symptoms such as low-grade fever, malaise, anorexia, and weight loss are often present. Pain in abdomen is seen in around 80–95% cases, while alternate constipation and diarrhea are seen in about 9–20% cases. Other features like a moving ball of wind in abdomen, nausea, vomiting, and melena may also be found. Features of malabsorption are also encountered in some cases.

No characteristic physical signs are described for abdominal tuberculosis, the popular classical "doughy" feel of the abdomen has only been observed in 6–11% cases in Indian series, however, not reported in some large series. Right iliac tenderness like that in acute appendicitis or lump in this region mimicking carcinoma or appendicular abscess may be felt in these cases. The signs of acute or subacute small intestinal obstruction like abdominal distension, vomiting, and absolute constipation with or without a palpable mass may be encountered as per the pathological stage of the disease. Many other clinical features ensue depending upon the involved organ or the site and type of involvement.

Treatment is essentially the same as for pulmonary tuberculosis. All patients of abdominal tuberculosis should be treated with short-course chemotherapy for 6 months duration. The routine use of adjuvant corticosteroid is not advisable in such cases. Surgery in the form of intestinal resection and end-to-end anastomosis, is occasionally required, only if there is mechanical obstruction. It is particularly indicated for strictures of longer than 12 cm with involvement at multiple sites.

GENITOURINARY TUBERCULOSIS

Genitourinary tuberculosis is a significant problem in the developing world and around 9% of all EPTB cases in India are estimated to be suffering from GUTB. Often, the disease continues to progress late because of the delayed diagnosis. Most GUTB patients present with renal failure, bladder and ureteric strictures, which could have been easily averted, had there been timely diagnosis and treatment there upon 3–4% cases of pulmonary TB also have concomitant GUTB commonly involving kidneys, bladder, urethra, and genital tract.

The most common clinical presentation of urological tuberculosis is sterile pyuria and painless hematuria. Patient may present incidentally or with the symptoms of dysuria, hematuria, frank pyuria, fever and renal mass. These features are quite suggestive of urinary tract infection but for any isolation of common bacterial growth on culture.

Infertility, either primary or secondary is a common presentation of female genital tuberculosis. In India, one-third cases of tubal disease infertility are attributed to tuberculosis. Alterations in menstrual pattern (menorrhagia, amenorrhea or postmenopausal bleeding, etc.) are common features in such patients. Female genital tuberculosis may sometimes be mistaken for ovarian malignancy. The differentiation is further complicated by the presence of high levels of CA-125, which are also described in gynecological tuberculosis. Primary female genital tuberculosis is rare, usually seen when the male partner suffers from active GUTB. Mostly, genital TB is almost always secondary to tuberculosis elsewhere in the body. Commonly, the infection spreads directly from active abdominal tuberculous pathology.

Standard 6-month tuberculosis chemotherapy is advised; however, controlled clinical trials are lacking for short-course chemotherapy in GUTB. Adjuvant corticosteroids are recommended to avert ureteric stricture formation. Steroids have also been found helpful in the treatment of tuberculous interstitial nephritis. Sometimes, surgery, such as nephrectomy is necessary for destroyed nonfunctioning kidney. Partial nephrectomy, ureteric stricture dilatation and bladder reconstruction may be required as per the indication in some cases.

SKIN TUBERCULOSIS

Skin tuberculosis contributes 1–2.5% share of all skin disease cases and the ailment is more commonly found in poor socioeconomic strata of the society. There are three main types of skin tuberculosis determined by the presence of previous sensitization to tubercle bacilli, immune response of the host and route of inoculation by tubercle bacilli. In order of frequency, these are lupus vulgaris, tuberculosis verrucosa cutis and scrofuloderma. These three types are seen in persons who had previously been infected with tubercle bacilli and have delayed hypersensitivity to the tubercle bacilli. In absence of previous sensitization, the disease may occur in the form of tuberculous chancres and miliary tuberculosis of skin. Tuberculids are the hypersensitivity lesions of skin, which occur as a result of tuberculosis elsewhere in the body.

PERICARDIAL TUBERCULOSIS

Tuberculous involvement of pericardium is usually secondary to tuberculosis elsewhere in the body. Nearly 1–8% of pulmonary tuberculosis patients have concomitant pericardial tuberculosis. Out of all acute pericarditis cases, about 4% in developed countries and 60–80% cases in the developing countries are due to tuberculous pathology.

Direct extension from tuberculous mediastinal lymphadenitis is the most common route for the involvement of pericardium. The infection may also reach pericardium through lymphatic and hematogenous routes from tuberculous lesions of lungs, kidneys, bones or other organs. The pericardium is infrequently involved by breakdown and contiguous spread from a tuberculous lesion in the lung. Pericardial tuberculosis has following four pathological stages: (i) dry pericarditis, (ii) effusive pericarditis, (iii) absorptive, and (iv) constrictive pericarditis stage. Patient may present during any stage of the pathological progress. Invariably, the pericardial fluid is straw colored and exudative type; very rarely there could be frank pus in the pericardium due to intense inflammation.

The pericardium may contain somewhere between 15 mL and 3,500 mL of fluid. When the fluid collection occurs at very rapid rate, the patient may develop cardiac tamponade. Within a few weeks of development of pericardial effusion, there occurs thickening especially of the visceral pericardium resulting into effusive constrictive pericarditis. In the absence of effective antituberculosis therapy, progressive fibrosis may lead to chronic constrictive pericarditis. Complete obliteration of pericardium due to fibrosis interferes with the proper cardiac functioning. Sometimes, the disease may involve the myocardium, ultimately leading to its myonecrosis and muscle atrophy. Around 15% of patients show pericardial calcification, but it is reported in around 75% in some studies.

The disease is usually seen during third to fifth decades of life. Gradual onset tuberculous toxemia with anorexia, weight loss, malaise, low-grade evening temperature, and early fatigability are usual presentations of pericardial tuberculosis. In around 20% cases, pericardial effusion may present as acute cardiac tamponade with tachycardia, high jugular venous pressure and feeling of retrosternal compression.

Effusive-constrictive pericarditis patients usually show cardiomegaly, edema feet and elevated jugular venous pressure. In chronic constrictive pericarditis, there occurs the impediment of venous return due to tough encasement of the heart; however, heart shape and size remain normal. This causes pulmonary and systemic congestion leading ultimately to shortness of breath, orthopnea with edema, ascites, and pulsus paradoxus. Long-standing elevation of venous pressure may cause protein-losing enteropathy and resultant hypoproteinemia. Ascites is more prominent, called ascites praecox.

Pericardiocentesis is performed for diagnostic tests of the fluid as well as for therapeutic purpose in cardiac tamponade. Pericardiocentesis should preferably be done under echocardiography employing apical approach. Pericardial fluid characteristics are exactly the same as encountered in tuberculous pleural effusion as far as its physical, cellular, TB bacilli isolation, or ADA level, etc. are concerned, and the same diagnostic standards are applicable for both the conditions. Pericardial tissue taken by open biopsy may reveal typical granulomas with caseation necrosis in around 60% cases.

If not treated, the disease is almost always fatal and even with specific treatment the mortality is 3–14%. Medical treatment using standard 6-month short-course tuberculosis chemotherapy is successful in achieving the cure. Addition of corticosteroids has been found associated with reduction in the frequency of pericardiocentesis and mortality.

HEPATIC TUBERCULOSIS

Hepatic tuberculosis is relatively uncommon form of extrapulmonary tuberculosis. It is secondary to pulmonary or gastrointestinal tuberculosis. Hepatic involvement has been reported in 10–15% of patients with pulmonary tuberculosis, and commonly found in patients with disseminated tuberculosis. Hepatic tuberculosis generally occurs due to the reactivation of an old tuberculous focus, or on rare occasions as a result of a primary hepatic infection.

The clinical diagnosis of hepatic tuberculosis is difficult. Usually, symptoms and signs in this condition are nonspecific. Other than the constitutional symptoms, abdominal pain is present in 65–87% and jaundice in 20–35% patients. Jaundice may be caused by extra- or intrahepatic biliary obstruction. Hepatomegaly is frequently encountered. The laboratory investigations frequently reveal increase in alkaline phosphatase with normal transaminases. The definitive diagnosis of tuberculous liver abscess needs microbiological and pathological examination of the specimen from the abscess. Aspiration of the liver lesion under the guidance of USG or CT can provide a precise specimen for confirmation.

Hepatic tuberculosis is treated with similar standard 6-month regimen (2HRZE/S, 4HR) as for other forms of tuberculosis. Drainage is occasionally required, especially for large abscess.

CONCLUSION

In conclusion, clinical manifestations of extrapulmonary TB are varied depending upon the organ of involvement. Diagnosis is generally difficult because of the relative rarity as well as because of the problems associated with obtaining samples to look for mycobacterial demonstration. Mantoux test for skin sensitivity and IGRA test are too non-specific for a high-burden country. But for a few exception such as for meningeal, spinal or cardiac TB, management of extrapulmonary TB is done on the same lines as for pulmonary TB.

CHAPTER 13

Multidrug Resistant Tuberculosis

Surendra K Sharma, Dinkar Bhasin

INTRODUCTION

Globally, around 3.5% of new and 20.5% of previously treated tuberculosis (TB) patients are estimated to suffer from multidrug resistant TB (MDR-TB) and about 9% of them have extensively drug-resistant TB (XDR-TB). An estimated of 13% of the total number of people who developed TB were human immunodeficiency virus (HIV) positive.

Drug-resistant TB has emerged due to selection of mutant strains of the bacteria. The major cause can be attributed to improper treatment regimens and failure to adherence to the treatment regimen.

DEFINITIONS

Multidrug-resistant TB is defined when the bacilli isolated from a clinical specimen are resistant to rifampicin and isoniazid with or without resistance to any other first-line antitubercular drug. Rifampicin resistance is taken as a surrogate marker for MDR-TB and if the clinical specimen is resistant to rifampicin, the patient is put on MDR-TB treatment.

Microbiological isolates depicting resistance to isoniazid, rifampicin, one fluoroquinolone (ofloxacin, levofloxacin, or moxifloxacin) and a second-line injectable anti-tubercular drug (kanamycin, amikacin, or capreomycin) are labeled extensively drug-resistant TB (XDR-TB).

Recently, TB bacilli have been isolated that have shown resistance to all known anti-tubercular drugs. These strains have been characterized as totally drug-resistant tuberculosis (TDR-TB) or extremely drug resistant (XXDR-TB), and have also been isolated from India.

Drug resistance can be classified as primary or acquired. Primary drug resistance refers to the cases, which have previously never received anti-TB treatment. Acquired drug resistance cases are those, which have previously been given anti-TB drugs in the past.

DIAGNOSIS

Detection of MDR and XDR-TB are purely based on laboratory diagnosis. The diagnosis of drug-resistant TB requires isolation and culture of the tubercle bacilli followed by DST in a quality-assured, accredited laboratory. Limited resources and high burden of MDR-TB burden result in serious diagnostic challenges.

Diagnostic Modalities

Rapid detection is essential to control the growing problem of TB. Molecular methods which can help to detect genetic mutations associated with phenotypic resistance include cartridge-based nucleic acid amplification (CBNAAT) and line probe assay (LPA). CBNAAT or Xpert MTB/RIF is a rapid molecular test of high sensitivity and specificity for detection of mycobacteria and rifampicin resistance. Though, Xpert MTB/RIF only gives data on rifampicin resistance, this is considered equivalent to MDR-TB, sufficient evidence to initiate treatment for the MDR-TB while awaiting conventional drug-susceptibility test results.

MANAGEMENT

Counseling of patients is often an under-recognized aspect of disease management. Various issues need to be discussed, such as the nature of the disease, the nature of treatment he/she is about to undergo, the duration of treatment, the possibility of adverse drug reactions (ADR), the need for strict adherence to treatment, the need for daily injections for at least 6 months–9 months and need for initial/subsequent hospitalization, if needed.

Pretreatment Evaluation

To ensure a good treatment outcome, a pretreatment evaluation (PTE) is mandatory. The rationale behind PTE is to identify the patients who are at high risk of developing adverse drug reactions when put on MDR-TB treatment. It includes measurement of height, weight (to decide the drug dose according to appropriate weight band), total blood count, blood sugar levels (to rule out diabetes), renal function tests, liver function tests, thyroid stimulation hormone, chest X-ray, pregnancy test for all women of reproductive age-group, electrocardiogram (to check the QT interval) and psychiatric evaluation.

Treatment

Three different strategies can be used in management of drug-resistant TB, viz.: (a) standardized treatment, (b) empirical treatment, or (c) individualized treatment.

Standardized treatment refers to the use of a fixed combination of drugs for treating all patients. The regimen is usually based on the DST profile of population at large. Empirical treatment, on the other hand, uses those drugs to which the individual has not been previously exposed for less than 1 month and hence, presumed to be effective. Individualized treatment is based on individual DST results and uses only those drugs with proven in-vitro susceptibility. Initiation of an empirical regimen till DST results are available and then switching over to an individualized regimen is probably the best strategy to achieve the highest cure rates.

The greatest advantage of a standardized treatment, when provided on a programmatic basis, is the easy availability, low cost and directly observed treatment ensuring regular and complete therapy. This is the most appropriate approach for a resource-limited setting like India. Standardized treatment regimen used for treatment of MDR-TB under the Revised National Tuberculosis Control Program (RNTCP) consists of 18-month duration. Six drugs (kanamycin, ofloxacin, ethionamide, pyrazinamide, ethambutol and cycloserine) are used for the first 6–9 months of the intensive phase followed by 18 months of continuation phase with the use of ofloxacin, ethionamide, ethambutol and cycloserine.

Patients in whom subsequent cultures show resistance to other drugs as well, moxifloxacin can be replaced for isolates resistant to ofloxacin, and capreomycin for isolates resistant to kanamycin in addition to H and R. Isolates resistant to both ofloxacin and kanamycin in addition to H and R should be treated with XDR regimen. PAS is reserved as a substitute to patients not tolerating cycloserine or ethionamide. The recommended schedule for follow-up, sputum examination in the intensive phase is at 3rd, 4th, 5th, 6th and 7th month and in the continuation phase at 9th, 12th, 15th and 18th, 21st and 24th month. Duration of intensive phase is decided by prior culture results (smear conversion is not considered). Patient is shifted into continuation phase after at least 6 months of therapy and at least three consecutive negative culture results of sputum or other clinical specimen. If cultures remain positive, intensive phase can be extended for up to 9 months beyond which continuation phase is initiated irrespective of culture results. While all positive samples should be subjected to second-line DST, a high suspicion should be kept for patients who remain persistently culture positive.

Extensively drug-resistant TB is treated aggressively with seven drugs (capreomycin, para-aminosalicylic acid, moxifloxacin, high-dose isoniazid, clofazimine, linezolid and amoxicillin/clavulanate) for 6–12 months. Treatment is continued for another 18 months with para-aminosalicylic acid, moxifloxacin, high-dose isoniazid, clofazimine, linezolid, amoxicillin/clavulanate. Bedaquiline, which inhibits mycobacterial ATP synthase, is a promising new anti-TB drug reserved for drug-resistant TB.

New Drug Delivery System

Newer drug delivery systems have been developed over the last few years, which include liposomes, microparticles and nanoparticles. These drug delivery systems are more advantageous over the conventional drugs as they help in improving adherence of patients to anti-TB treatment, reduce the drug burden and also shorten the duration of anti-TB treatment. Nanoparticles help in a targeted drug delivery system, which can help in combating the TB bacillus in the body.

Adverse Drug Reactions

Adverse effects are common with drugs used for drug-resistant TB and responsible for poor compliance. Hepatitis, skin reactions, dyspepsia and arthralgias are common and frequently responsible for discontinuation of therapy. The other side effects may include anemia, thrombocytopenia, peripheral neuropathy, QT interval prolongation, and nausea. The side effects are more common in the presence of concurrent HIV infection and prior history of hepatitis.

Follow-Up of Patients

Close follow-up and monitoring are mandatory for patients with MDR and XDR-TB to ensure strict compliance to the regime, prompt identification, management of adverse drug reactions, early detection and treatment of treatment failure. Directly observed treatment (DOT) is integral for close follow-up and monitoring. Monitoring of patients on MDR- and XDR-TB treatment requires not only careful clinical examination, but also appropriate laboratory investigations like chest radiographs, renal and liver function tests, serum electrolytes and thyroid profile at appropriate time intervals for prompt identification of adverse reactions. Frequent sputum examination is required during treatment as per laid down criteria in the RNTCP.

Regimen Reinforcement

One must never add a single drug to a failing regimen. Resistance develops rapidly to the new drug in such a situation. In patients who have persistent positive sputum microscopy after several months of treatment (e.g. 3 months), there is a need to incorporate additional agents in their treatment regimen, a concept called "regimen reinforcement". In this circumstance, there are no other viable four- or five-drug combination regimens that can be given. Thus, any remaining effective agents may be added, or current agents switched, based on the latest drug-resistance testing pattern.

Surgical Management of Drug-resistant Tuberculosis

Cavities in a destroyed lung of TB patients act as reservoirs for large bacillary load. These cavities actively replicate bacteria even in patients, which are sputum culture negative. The rationale behind surgery is to help in a significant decrease in the bacillary load.

A number of surgical procedures have been recommended depending upon the site and extent of lesions. Common indications for surgical treatment include the following: (i) persistence of culture positivity despite the extended treatment; (ii) treatment failure and extensive patterns of drug resistance; (iii) local cavitary disease that is amenable to resection. Pre- and postoperative care, specialized surgical facilities, safe blood transfusion services, and stringent infection control measures are additional considerations during surgical management.

Treatment Outcomes

According to the RNTCP guidelines, treatment outcome was categorized as cured, defaulted, failure and death. A patient can be declared cured after complete treatment for at least 24 months with the last five cultures negative. However, patient having two or more of the last five cultures positive is considered as treatment failure. A patient who interrupts treatment for two or more consecutive months can be considered as a defaulter.

CONCLUSION

In conclusion, drug resistance is a man-made phenomenon. Every effort should be made to diagnose and treat drug-sensitive TB effectively at the grassroot level and prevent the development of drug resistance. MDR-TB or XDR-TB is a laboratory diagnosis and, therefore, requires quality laboratory support for timely and accurate results.

CHAPTER 14

Treatment of Tuberculosis in Special Situations

Rajendra Prasad, Nikhil Gupta

INTRODUCTION

Treatment of tuberculosis poses a difficult clinical problem in special situations such as pregnancy, renal insufficiency, and liver diseases. There are various concerns regarding dosage, toxicity, and the method of administration of drugs. Some antituberculosis drugs are metabolized in liver; while others are excreted either unchanged or in metabolized form, by the renal route. Their secretion in milk and ability to cross placenta is important in the situations of lactation and pregnancy, where there is concern of safety of the baby.

TREATMENT OF TUBERCULOSIS IN PREGNANCY AND LACTATION

Isoniazid is considered safe in pregnancy, except for some chance of postpartum hepatitis. The American Thoracic Society (ATS) recommends supplementation with pyridoxine during pregnancy (25 mg/day). Use of rifampicin and ethambutol is also safe. Data regarding other rifamycins (rifabutin and rifapentine) is insufficient and, thus, they should be cautiously used. Safety regarding pyrazinamide cannot be assured, but when used for 6-month regimen, the benefits may outweigh the possible risk.

Streptomycin may cause congenital deafness, as this drug interferes with the development of ear. Other injectables, like amikacin, kanamycin, and capreomycin having pharmacokinetics similar to streptomycin, may also cause fetal nephrotoxicity and ototoxicity. Ethionamide and prothionamide are contraindicated in pregnancy, as they are found teratogenic in animal studies. Cycloserine crosses placenta, its safety in pregnancy is not established;

it should be avoided and used only if no other suitable alternatives are available. Para-aminosalicylic acid (PAS) has been frequently used in pregnancy without any major toxicity in the past. Since no well-designed study has been done to ascertain its safety in pregnancy, it should be used only in the absence of any other alternative.

Fluoroquinolones being toxic and inhibitor of growing cartilage in animals should be avoided in pregnancy. Similarly, clarithromycin is not safe in pregnancy, as higher dose has been associated with embryotoxicity. There are no data on its use in pregnancy; may be considered when other treatment options are limited.

Treatment of tuberculosis in a pregnant woman is far less hazardous than leaving the disease untreated, both with regard to the baby and the mother. Untreated disease leads to increased risks of low birth-weight infant, congenital tuberculosis, miscarriages, and other complications. Treatment regimen consists of the standard four primary drugs, i.e. isoniazid, rifampicin, ethambutol, and pyrazinamide. If pyrazinamide is not given, the duration is prolonged to 9 months. Streptomycin is avoided during pregnancy. Most of the first-line drugs are reported to cross the placenta. But no teratogenic effect has been reported with their use.

Termination of pregnancy is not recommended in women who are on first-line antituberculosis drugs. But those on second- or third-line reserve drugs should be counseled for possible adverse effects. Breastfeeding should not be discouraged, as the amount of drugs secreted in milk is insufficient to cause any toxic or therapeutic effect. It is important to administer supplemental pyridoxine for the nursing mother. The newborn should also be given pyridoxine even if no isoniazid is being used for the infant. All antituberculosis drugs can be used during lactation, except fluoroquinolones. Baby of a woman who has taken rifampicin during pregnancy should receive vitamin K at birth to avoid the risk of postnatal hemorrhage. Rifampicin may induce metabolism of vitamin K and hamper hepatic synthesis of vitamin K-dependent coagulation factors.

Women taking oral hormonal contraceptives should be counseled for possible contraceptive failure and occurrence of pregnancy. This is especially so in women on rifampicin-containing antitubercular treatment regimen, because of the induction of metabolism of contraceptive drug by rifampicin.

TREATMENT OF TUBERCULOSIS IN RENAL INSUFFICIENCY

The basic treatment regimen remains the same as for any other patient of tuberculosis. The dose and duration of drugs, which are excreted by kidneys (ethambutol and pyrazinamide) need alterations usually based on creatinine clearance. If creatinine clearance is below 70 mL/min, ethambutol should be given in the lowest recommended dosage. Frequency of ethambutol (15–20 mg/kg) should be reduced to alternate days (three times a week), if the creatinine clearance is below 30 mL/min. Pyrazinamide, fluoroquinolones, streptomycin, and other aminoglycosides are also given three times a week in such a situation.

Hemodialysis, which removes the drugs from the body, will devoid of their beneficial effects. Administration of drug after hemodialysis will avoid the premature removal of the drug. Premature removal of second-line drugs, by hemodialysis, may further aggravate the problem of drug resistance by exposing the tubercle bacillus to subtherapeutic drug concentrations. Rifampicin, isoniazid, and ethambutol are removed to a much less extent by hemodialysis, but pyrazinamide is removed to a significant extent. Thus, there is no need to use supplemental dosages of isoniazid, rifampicin, and ethambutol for patients of end-stage renal disease undergoing hemodialysis. Usually, hemodialysis does not pose significant problem, if drugs are given after the procedure.

Some of the antituberculosis drugs, e.g. rifampicin are sometimes reported to induce acute kidney failure and hemolysis of immunological nature. There is also an increased risk of tuberculosis in patients with chronic renal failure.

TREATMENT OF TUBERCULOSIS IN LIVER DISEASE

Treatment of tuberculosis with deranged liver functions presents with two major clinical scenes. First is the issue of antitubercular drug-induced hepatotoxicity and second is the use of antitubercular drugs in persons with pre-existing liver disease. Various antitubercular drugs are potentially hepatotoxic and administration of these drugs may aggravate liver disease in a patient with compromised liver function. Drugs like ethambutol, streptomycin, kanamycin, amikacin, and capreomycin are safe in liver disease, as they are neither significantly metabolized nor toxic to liver.

Drug-induced Hepatotoxicity

The period of latency between the start of drug regimen and the occurrence of drug-induced hepatitis is usually 4–9 days. About 10–30% of patients receiving antituberculosis therapy may normally have the transient rise of bilirubin and liver enzymes to about one to three times the normal, during the first 2 months of therapy.

The incidence of isoniazid-induced clinical hepatitis is not as high as was previously thought. Hepatitis occurs in 0.6% patients, if isoniazid is given alone; but it is 1.6%, if given with drugs other than rifampicin. With rifampicin, the incidence of hepatitis is 2.7%. Risk of drug-induced hepatitis increases with age. It is reported to be about 2% in persons aged 50-64 years. Fatal hepatitis is reported in a rare case (0.023%). If it is given to patient with preexisting liver disease, it may accumulate in the body and further increase the risk of drug-induced hepatitis. In such a situation, frequent monitoring of hepatic transaminases is indicated. There is increased risk of peripheral neuropathy in alcoholic liver disease. Therefore, pyridoxine (10 mg/day) should be given to these patients.

All the three primary drugs (isoniazid, rifampicin, and pyrazinamide) can cause hepatotoxicity. Pyrazinamide is most hepatotoxic. Rifampicin is least likely to cause liver damage but can cause cholestatic jaundice. The second-line drugs such as ethionamide, prothionamide, and PAS may also cause hepatotoxicity but less often than the first-line drugs. Hepatitis is rare with fluoroquinolones.

Ethionamide, similar in structure to that of isoniazid, can cause liver toxicity in about 2% patients, and should be cautiously used in the presence of pre-existing liver disease. PAS may cause clinical hepatitis in 0.3% cases. Since pharmacokinetics of PAS is not significantly altered in liver disease, it could be used in usual doses and usual regimen. Cycloserine can be safely used in liver disease, except in the case of alcohol-related hepatitis, where it increases the risk of seizures. Thioacetazone is hepatotoxic and it should be avoided. Fluoroquinolones, except ciprofloxacin, are safe for use in liver disease.

Advanced age, female sex, poor nutritional status, preexisting liver disease, chronic alcoholism, hepatitis B carrier state, and slow acetylator status are considered risk factors for antitubercular drug-induced hepatitis.

It is often difficult to find the culprit drug in a multidrug regimen causing drug-induced hepatitis. The rise in serum transaminase activity within 15 days of starting regimen is usually attributed to rifampicin, but if it occurs after 1 month, it is usually attributed to pyrazinamide.

If a patient on antituberculosis therapy develops mild and transient elevation of serum bilirubin or liver enzymes, treatment need not be stopped. They usually come down during the course of the treatment. If a patient develops hepatitis-related symptoms with the significant elevation of bilirubin and liver enzymes, treatment should be stopped and viral hepatitis should be ruled out by serology. Drugs should be gradually reintroduced one by one starting from less hepatotoxic drug first, after liver functions come down to normal, and with close monitoring for deterioration.

Antituberculosis Treatment with Preexisting Liver Disease

All antitubercular drugs can be used in patients with stable liver disease. But it is better to use drugs without any known or at least with lesser hepatotoxicity. In case of advanced or unstable liver disease, it is advisable to avoid. Pyrazinamide is avoided in patients of chronic liver disease, such as cirrhosis or chronic active hepatitis. Ethambutol can be safely used, while rifampicin and isoniazid are used depending upon the urgency of indication with greater care and close monitoring of liver function.

In conclusion, different options are used for treatment of tuberculosis with deranged liver functions; mild derangements in liver enzymes require merely a close watch on the liver function without modifying the regimen while the progressively declining hepatic reserves prohibit the use of any potential hepatotoxic drug requiring a substantial revision of the antitubercular regimen.

CHAPTER
15

Tuberculosis and Human Immunodeficiency Virus Infection

Aditya Jindal, SK Jindal

INTRODUCTION

Both tuberculosis (TB) and human immunodeficiency virus (HIV) infections are deadlier together; TB causing one quarter of acquired immunodeficiency syndrome (AIDS)-related deaths and HIV infecting at least 15% of patients with TB worldwide. TB is the most common opportunistic infection in HIV-infected persons in several countries, including India.

EPIDEMIOLOGY

There are an estimated 33.2 million persons infected with HIV; of whom, about one-third are also infected with *Mycobacterium tuberculosis*. The TB incidence in HIV-infected persons is about 100-fold in the general population. According to the WHO/UNAIDS estimates, up to half of the patients with HIV or AIDS develop TB.

Although the HIV–TB scene in several countries is dismal, there is some evidence of a declining trend in India. The estimated number of people living with HIV/AIDS (PLWHA) in India has been revised to 2.5 million people from the earlier reported figure of 5.7 million. The revised figures are also likely to reflect the reduced HIV–TB burden.

PATHOGENESIS

Both TB and HIV suppress the host's immune responses even though the mechanisms are not fully understood. There is the evidence to suggest that the susceptibility to dual infection is also influenced by inborn errors of immunity, and genetic polymorphisms.

There are several immunological defects in HIV infection, which predispose to TB and encourage HIV–TB coinfection (Box 15.1). HIV infection is primarily responsible for impaired cell-mediated immunity (CMI) by causing a decline in the number and function of CD4++ subset of T-cells. *Mycobacterium tuberculosis* infection may induce nuclear factor binding to the NF-KB sequences in the HIV replication. The increased HIV replication by *M. tuberculosis* sets a vicious cycle in both promoting growth of each other and, therefore, the continuing damage to the host cells. Tuberculosis can occur in patients with HIV infection at all levels, but the type, severity and manifestations depend on the CD4+ T-lymphocyte counts. The greater the degree of immunosuppression and the lower the CD4+ counts, more likely the atypical presentation.

As the immunosuppression progresses, there occurs increased likelihood of infection by atypical and opportunistic mycobacteria and decreased tuberculin reactivity. Granuloma formation is impaired while the lesions show high content of intracellular organisms. The absence of an inflammatory cellular response in the presence of a large number of organisms and "naked necrosis" is sometimes referred to as "nonreactive" form of TB.

Human immunodeficiency virus-infected patients with TB may be less infectious than those without HIV infection. TB in HIV-infected patients is generally extrapulmonary or, if pulmonary, paucibacillary, with fewer bacilli in the sputum. This, however, is not always true. There are other studies, which report the opposite findings. In HIV-infected communities with HIV–TB coinfection, the number of persons with communicable TB keeps on multiplying with increased transmission to other people regardless of their HIV status.

Human immunodeficiency virus infection increases the rate of TB reactivation in a previously infected patient (latent TB). The annual risk of

BOX 15.1: Immune alterations/defects in human immunodeficiency virus (HIV) infection, which predispose to tuberculosis (TB).

- *CD4++ T cells*: Decline in number
  - Depletion
  - Functional impairment
  - Diminished recruitment and activation
- Impairment of macrophages and peripheral blood monocytes
- Increased secretion of Th-2 cytokines [interleukin 4 (IL-4) and IL-10] by the mononuclear cells.
- Failure of macrophage differentiation (to epithelioid cells)
- Lack of formation of Langhans giant cells
- *Enhanced HIV replication by*:
  - Increased production of tumor necrosis factor alpha (TNF-α) by *Mycobacterium tuberculosis*
  - *Mycobacterium tuberculosis* and its cell wall components
  - Beta chemokine monocyte chemotactic protein
  - Downregulation of chemokines.

developing TB in a PLWHA, coinfected with *M. tuberculosis,* is 5-15%. Both reactivation of previous infection and exogenous reinfection are reported to occur in these patients. Possibly, reactivation is the more likely mechanism in low prevalence Western countries with a lower level of exposure to patients with active disease, although the occurrence of new infection has been also shown with the help of restriction fragment length polymorphism (RFLP) analysis. New infections from different strains are, however, common in the high TB-burden countries.

CLINICAL FEATURES

The clinical features of TB in HIV-infected patients depend upon the severity of immunosuppression. The presentation in early HIV disease is almost similar to that observed in otherwise healthy individuals, in whom pulmonary disease with focal infiltration and cavities is more common, while extrapulmonary manifestations and other atypical features are common when the CD4+ counts are less than 200/mm.

"Typical" pulmonary disease presenting with fever and other constitutional symptoms, cough, expectoration and hemoptysis is not uncommon. Several of these patients are diagnosed to have HIV coinfection only on serological tests. On the other hand, several series have emphasized the frequent presence of disseminated disease with extrapulmonary organ involvement. Night sweats, fatigue, diarrhea and hepatosplenomegaly are other common features in these patients.

Both pleural and parenchymal pulmonary involvements are common in HIV-TB coinfection. Pleural fluid in the presence of HIV infection may more often show the presence of acid-fast bacilli (AFB), on both smear and culture examinations. These mycobacteria may also show the presence of drug resistance, similar to that seen in parenchymal TB.

Occurrence of TB in an HIV-infected patient in the previous 2 years is also used for HIV/AIDS staging. It is categorized as clinical stage 3 disease in case of pulmonary and stage 4 in case of extrapulmonary TB. Systemic manifestations include the presence of associated/complicating illnesses attributed to HIV immunosuppression. Recurrent pneumonias, diarrhea, herpes zoster infection, and mucosal (oral/genital/ gastrointestinal) ulcerations are common. Weight loss of more than 10 kg or more than 20% of original weight loss is an important AIDS-defining criterion.

The clinical and radiological manifestations of multidrug-resistant tuberculosis (MDR-TB) in HIV-infected individuals are generally similar to those of MDR-TB in non-HIV infected patients, but pose greater problems of symptom and severity control due to poor treatment with pulmonary cavitary and/or disseminated disease. Higher mortality rates are reported in MDR-TB patients with than in those without HIV infection. Transmission rate of MDR-TB in HIV infection is also high.

DIAGNOSIS

Diagnosis of TB in HIV-infected patients is established on the same lines and methods as in non-HIV-infected patients. However, diagnosis in the presence of HIV infection is somewhat difficult in view of the difficulties of AFB demonstration in cases of extrapulmonary and noncavitary pulmonary TB. There is lesser likelihood of sputum smear and culture positivity in the presence of HIV infection. Radiological diagnosis of TB is nonspecific. This is especially so in the presence of HIV coinfection when the chest X-ray findings are generally atypical. Moreover, the chest radiology is frequently negative in extrapulmonary manifestations of TB. There is some recent evidence to suggest the use of FDG-PET and PET/CT for early diagnosis, identification of extrapulmonary TB, staging of TB and assessment of response to therapy. More importantly, one relies on cytological and/or histopathological examination for the demonstration of caseation, granuloma formation (which are ill-formed and rare) and AFB. Investigational procedures, such as fine-needle aspiration biopsy, pleural fluid aspiration, lumbar puncture, forceps biopsy, bronchoscopic or transbronchial biopsy, and other methods are used to obtain the appropriate specimens for these examinations.

Interpretation of the tuberculin skin test (TST) in the presence of HIV infection for the diagnosis of TB is somewhat difficult, especially in the high TB prevalence countries. A positive TST is considered as suggestive of TB-infection or latent TB in any individual, more so in the presence of HIV infection in whom the test sensitivity is further reduced. In countries such as India, where there is presence of TB infection diagnosed by a positive TST in up to 40–50% of the normal healthy population, the positive test cannot be considered as an indication for treatment in non-HIV individuals.

The interferon-gamma release assays (IGRA) like TST, are unable to differentiate between TB infection and active TB disease. We do not have figures on positive IGRA in otherwise healthy people, but the interpretation is somewhat similar to that of TST. The updated guidelines for using IGRA in the United States suggest their use as aids in diagnosing TB infection in different populations. It is not possible to make such a recommendation of their use to guide the treatment in India.

MANAGEMENT

The greatest challenge in managing HIV-TB coinfection lies in the simultaneous treatment of both the infections and, frequently, of other concomitant opportunistic infections. The basic principles of treatment are similar as for TB treatment in non-HIV patients. One needs to consider the HIV-related problems, such as the compliance with the therapy, presence of drug resistance, the level of immunosuppression and presence of complicating or other coinfections. The outcomes of treatment in the presence of HIV infection are similar, if the basic principles are adequately taken care of:

The four primary drugs, rifampicin (R), isoniazid (H), pyrazinamide (Z), and ethambutol (E) constitute the mainstay of treatment in drug-susceptible TB, administered as the standard two-phase regimen: initial intensive phase of 2 months of all the four drugs, followed by the maintenance phase of H and R for four months (2HRZE, 4HR).

Treatment of HIV–TB with directly observed therapy has been shown to prolong life, prevent drug resistance and quickly render a TB patient noninfectious. It is the most effective method of promoting adherence to TB treatment, particularly in the presence of HIV coinfection.

The issues related to intermittent versus daily regime and the optimum duration of therapy have remained somewhat debatable. Most of the studies of standard 6 months regimen (2 HRZE, 4 HR) have shown similar rates of treatment failure and relapse among HIV-infected and non-HIV-infected patients. The current recommendation is to use standard 6 months regimen for all cases and to extend to 9 months for patients with delayed clinical (continued symptoms) or microbiological response (sputum culture positivity) at 2 months.

Management of MDR-TB and extensively drug-resistant TB (XDR-TB) in the HIV-infected patients poses the biggest challenge. The choice of drugs and the duration of therapy for MDR-TB are variably recommended. Generally, the treatment duration is guided by AFB smear and culture reports. Most regimens contain 4–6 drugs, administered for at least 18 months after culture conversion, but extended to 24 months in patients with extensive pulmonary damage. As per the Revised National Tuberculosis Control Program (RNTCP) recommendations, the regimen for MDR-TB comprises six drugs (kanamycin, ofloxacin, ethionamide, pyrazinamide, ethambutol, and cycloserine) during the 6–9 months of the intensive phase followed by four drugs (ofloxacin, ethionamide, cycloserine, and ethambutol) for the 18 months of the continuation phase.

Management of XDR-TB involves the use of toxic but less potent drugs with poorer outcomes than in MDR-TB cases. The medication adherence is reported to be poorer for anti-TB drugs than the anti-HIV drugs in a prospective cohort of XDR-TB/HIV coinfected patients.

A number of new drugs are in various phases of development with the aim of reduction in the number of drugs, as well duration of therapy. No drug as yet has proven to achieve the goals. Linezolid, delamanid, and bedaquiline are some of new anti-TB drugs for XDR-TB. There is a growing evidence to suggest the concurrent use of host-directed adjunctive therapies to enhance the role of pathogen-directed therapy. Immunotherapy, including the vaccines and vitamin D, has also been used as adjunctive treatments.

Concurrent treatment of both TB and HIV infections has significantly improved the outcome of patients. HIV treatment with highly active antiretroviral therapy (HAART) comprises a combination of at least three antiretroviral (ARV) drugs. There are four major groups of antiviral drugs, which are currently available; that include:

- Protease inhibitors

- Reverse transcriptase inhibitors
- Viral integrase enzyme inhibitors
- Viral entry inhibitors.

Antiretroviral treatment does not completely cure the disease, but effectively suppresses the viral replication. Antiretroviral therapy is costly and required to be continued lifelong. The ARV drugs also have a high-toxicity profile.

The short-term risk of HIV disease progression in HIV-related TB is related to the degree of immunosuppression (measured by CD4+ cell count or CD4+ cell percentage). Patients with advanced immunosuppression (CD4+ T cell counts <100/μL) are likely to develop treatment failure, relapses, and development of MDR-TB.

Combination of antiretroviral therapy (ART) along with antitubercular therapy (ATT) has the potential of overlapping adverse effects of both the therapies. Moreover, the presence of other opportunistic infections adds further to the complication list. HIV-related complications (e.g. thrombocytopenia) cause additional problems. Drug–drug interaction is an important problem, especially seen with the use of rifamycins, which increase the synthesis of a number of hepatic enzyme system. Rifampicin use results in a marked decrease in the concentrations of ARV agents, such as the protease inhibitors, which are metabolized by *CYP3A*. Rifabutin, with which the *CYP3A* expression is much less marked, is generally considered as an alternate drug. The dosages of these drugs, when used in combinations, are therefore altered to maintain effective concentrations. Thiacetazone should not be used in HIV–TB coinfection.

In view of the drug–drug interactions, the ART was withheld during the ATT administration in the past. The WHO recommends that irrespective of the CD4+ count, all HIV-TB patients should be given ART. It is now believed that an early institution of ART helps in an early control of immunosuppression and improves mortality in patients with CD4+ T-cell count of less than 200 cells/mm^3. In such patients, ART is started as soon as ATT is tolerated within the first 2 weeks to 2 months. If the CD4+ T-cell count is between 200 cells/mm^3 and 350 cells/mm^3, ART can start after the first 2 months of ATT. ART in patients with CD4+ counts of more than 350/mm^3 can be deferred until ATT is completed.

In India, the integrated activities of the national programs (RNTCP and National AIDS Control Programme), facilitate the treatment of HIV-TB coinfection. The ARV treatment is provided through the Integrated Testing and Counseling Centres and ATT through the Directly Observed Treatment, Short-course (DOTS) centers. The fewer number of ART centers, however, is a limiting factor. The choice of regimens for ATT under RNTCP is made on the basis of standard categorization for different forms of TB irrespective of the HIV status.

Improvement in immunity following ARV therapy results in an increase in inflammatory response to mycobacteria in TB lesions. The worsening of clinical symptoms following institution of both ATT and ARV is termed as the immune reconstitution inflammatory syndrome (IRIS). This paradoxical reaction is often noticed particularly with lymph node and pleural TB.

The common features of IRIS comprise fever, increase in lymphadenopathy, effusion, and pulmonary infiltrates. Occasionally, there is worsening of meningeal, central nervous system, hepatopulmonary, soft tissue or other forms of TB when it can even be life-threatening. The tuberculin skin reaction may become positive in a few cases.

Bacillus Calmette-Guérin (BCG) vaccination in an HIV-positive child is a cause of concern in view of the reports of local complications and disseminated BCG disease. The risk is not substantiated by the results of prospective studies in HIV-infected and non-HIV-infected infants. As per current recommendations, routine BCG vaccination in infants in the high HIV prevalence areas is not withheld, but it should not be given to known HIV-infected individuals.

CHAPTER 16

Nontuberculous Mycobacterial Diseases

PS Shankar, SK Jindal

INTRODUCTION

The nontuberculous mycobacteria (NTM) are also known as atypical mycobacteria, anonymous mycobacteria, or mycobacteria other than tubercle bacilli (MOTT). They are weak pathogens distinct from *Mycobacterium tuberculosis* in their characteristics. NTM are ubiquitously distributed in the environment, hence also called as environmental mycobacteria. Often, these organisms inhabit the respiratory passages as commensals. Pulmonary infection from NTM though rare, can cause disease similar to tuberculosis. They more commonly infect the skin, soft tissue, lymph nodes, implant devices, wounds, bones and joints. Occasionally, the infection is disseminated systemically in patients who are immunosuppressed or who suffer from acquired immunodeficiency syndrome (AIDS).

CLASSIFICATION

Earnest Runyon classified small, rod-shaped, atypical mycobacteria into four groups based primarily on colony morphology, pigmentation and growth characteristics: group I or photochromogens, such as *Mycobacterium* (M.) *kansasii*; group II or scotochromogen e.g. *M. scrofulaceum*; group III or nonchromogens, such as *Mycobacterium avium* and *Mycobacterium intracellulare* (*Mycobacterium avium* complex or *M. avium* and *M. intracellulare*, MAI). The organisms which belong to Group IV grow within 3 to 5 days on culture, hence referred as *rapid growers*. They do not change color on exposure to light, hence nonchromogens. *M. fortuitum, M. chelonae* and *M. smegmatis* are examples of this group. They often produce subcutaneous abscesses.

Recently, the mycobacterial species are classified on the basis of genetic differences, such as the sequence differences in the 16S ribosomal RNA. The

NTM species are divided into the rapid (Group IV) and slow growers (group I, II, and III). There is also an intermediate growing group that includes *M. marinum* and *M. gordonae*. They also vary in their nutritional requirements and grow on either the simple media or on the media supplemented with nutrients.

HUMAN DISEASE

Chronic pulmonary infection generally occurs in elderly persons by *M. avium* complex and *M. kansasii*. Cervical lymphadenopathy occurs in children from *M. scrofulaceum* while skin and soft-tissue infections may develop from *M. fortuitum*, *M. chelonae*, *M. xenopi* and *M. ulcerans*. Exposure of humans to NTM through bathing, swimming and drinking especially through cuts and abrasions is common. But risk of infection is generally less. Disseminated lesions are found in immunocompromised patients with infection from *M. avium* complex. Sometimes, *M. chelonae* may cause very indolent pulmonary infection.

Clinical Features

Infection in a healthy person from NTM (commonly *M. kansasii* and *M. avium* complex) presents a picture of chronic pulmonary disease resembling tuberculosis. The lung infiltrates are more diffuse and nodular in appearance. Cavitary disease is common. Mediastinal lymph node involvement and pleural effusion are uncommon. The lymph nodes, skin, soft tissues, bones and joints are other important sites of NTM infection.

Pulmonary Disease

The condition may present in one of three different forms: a tuberculosis-like pattern; nodular bronchiectasis and hypersensitivity pneumonitis. The classical TB-like presentation commonly occurs in older male smokers frequently with underlying chronic obstructive pulmonary disease. It is more indolent than typical tuberculosis and presents with cough and expectoration. Though there can be fever, night sweats, weight loss, and hemoptysis occasionally, these constitutional symptoms are less severe. The progress of the disease is slow. These patients may have preexistent pulmonary diseases, such as chronic obstructive pulmonary disease (COPD), bronchiectasis, cystic fibrosis, primary ciliary dyskinesia, silicosis and even prior pulmonary tuberculosis. The disease is more common in persons with diabetes and a history of smoking.

A *nonclassical* form of illness has been described. It is noted in postmenopausal, nonsmoker women. Though the condition has an insidious onset with chronic cough, it is not associated with any existing lung disease seen in *classical* form. The constitutional symptoms are rare. Hypersensitivity pneumonitis may present a typical episodic picture on exposure, such as to *M. avium* complex. This type of presentation commonly occurs in workers exposed to metal-working fluids and on exposure to aerosolizer MAC in association with indoor hot tub use MAC infection can present with any of the three different forms.

There are variable clinical patterns of NTM infection in patients with immune suppression, malignancies, solid organ transplantation and cystic fibrosis. The disseminated infection may occur in patients with immunosuppression due to hematological malignancy or immunosuppressive agents. Its incidence has shown an increase in patients with advanced stages of AIDS especially from *M. avium* complex. The condition presents with persistent fever, weight loss, anorexia and weakness. The pulmonary symptoms are infrequent and exhibit cough or dyspnea. There can be vomiting, diarrhea and abdominal pain. There is generalized lymphadenopathy, hepatomegaly, splenomegaly and nodular skin lesions. The condition is noted in children and young adults.

Diagnosis

Diagnosis of NTM pulmonary disease is made on the basis of the presence of a variety of clinical, radiological and microbiological criteria, several of which may only suggest them confirm the etiology.

The radiographic appearance in *classic* form of NTM disease resembles chronic indolent tuberculosis. The most common radiological pattern is fibronodular infiltrates involving the upper lobes especially apical and posterior segments. Unlike tuberculosis, the cavities are thin-walled with little surrounding infiltrate. The *nonclassical* form of disease is characterized by multiple bilateral opacities, similar to those in bronchiectasis.

The pleural involvement, especially effusion, is rare. CT of the chest defines the radiologic features precisely. Small nodular opacities are seen in the regions of maximal disease and also in areas away from the predominant site of the disease. Bronchietatic changes are present adjacent to apical cavities in *classical* form. In nonclassical form of disease bronchiectasis is bilateral and widespread. Disseminated form of disease may not show any radiologic abnormality or exhibit bilateral infiltrates. It may be associated with hilar or mediastinal adenopathy and/or pleural effusion. The radiologic abnormalities are more likely produced by coexistent conditions in AIDS patients.

Since NTM may colonize the respiratory tract of patients with preexisting lung disease, their isolation from sputum, bronchial washings or lung biopsy may not establish the infection. The appearance of NTM at microscopy is generally indistinguishable from that of *M. tuberculosis*. NTM are identified by their pattern of pigmentation, microscopic appearance, biochemical reactions and growth characteristics. The NTM are traditionally classified as rapid and slow growers on the basis of growth.

Other bacteriological investigations which are employed for identification include the biochemical tests and serotyping protein electrophoresis. The newer molecular methods, such as the gene probes and gene amplification (polymerase chain reaction) are now available for the detection of NTM, such as *M. avium, M. intracellulare* and some rapid growers. More advanced techniques, such as DNA fingerprinting are sometimes used for characterization of NTM. DNA sequencing of variable genomic regions provides a rapid and accurate method to identify NTM.

Nontuberculous mycobacterium (NTM) infections cannot be differentiated histopathologically from tuberculosis. Immunodiagnostic techniques, such as the regions of difference (RD) antigens, encoded proteins have been used for the diagnosis of both latent and active tuberculosis.

Treatment

The disease produced by NTM makes a slow progress, though it may remain stable for long periods. The disseminated form of disease has a rapid fatal course. NTM except *M. kansasii* exhibit a high degree of *in vitro* resistance to many of the standard antituberculosis drugs.

Treatment of NTM infection is indicated only if the organism is responsible for the disease and is not simply a colonizer. Multiple antimicrobials are required for prolonged periods. The infection from *M. kansasii* is treated with a combination of isoniazid, rifampicin and ethambutol (15 mg/kg) for 18 months. Pyrazinamide is ineffective.

The treatment of infection due to *M. avium* complex is difficult. Multidrug therapy is indicated in those exhibiting a progressive course or is severely ill. Treatment consists of a macrolide, rifampicin and ethambutol given three times weekly for noncavitary disease and daily with or without an aminoglycoside for cavitary disease. Disseminated lesions due to *M. avium* complex in AIDS patients may be treated with rifampicin, ethambutol, clofazamine and ciprofloxacin. Those exhibiting stable disease are observed and the underlying pulmonary disease is treated with bronchodilators, antibiotics if sputum is purulent and smoking cession. Mycobacterial disease may get eradicated without specific therapy.

When specific treatment is initiated it consists of isoniazid, rifampicin and ethambutol (25 mg/kg for the first 2 months followed by 15 mg/kg) with an initial supplementation of streptomycin for 3–6 months. Treatment has to be given for 18–24 months. Those exhibiting an extensive disease and those who fail to show sputum conversion on the four-drug regimen, cycloserine and ethionamide are to be added to the therapeutic regimen. Drug-drug interaction is an important treatment consideration especially in the elderly age group. Inhaled amikacin has been used in some patients with treatment-refractory NTM disease.

Surgical resection of the lesion may be undertaken in those having a localized disease. Some newer agents that may be active against NTM are rifabutin, clarithromycin, azithromycin and ofloxacin. *M. chelonae* is generally resistant to the antituberculosis drugs and other conventional antibiotics. It shows susceptibility only to amikacin, cefexitin and imipenem.

SUMMARY

In summary, an increased trend of NTM infections is recognized, especially in patients with HIV infection or with other causes of immunosuppression. Pulmonary manifestations and lymphadenitis are most common, while disseminated forms, skin and soft tissue involvement may also occur. Diagnosis is established on the basis of clinical features, radiological and microbiological investigations. Treatment is somewhat difficult requiring multiple drugs for prolonged periods.

CHAPTER 17

Community-acquired Pneumonia

Charles Feldman, Ronald Anderson

INTRODUCTION

Community-acquired pneumonia (CAP) is described as a lung infection, acquired in the community, most commonly bacterial in nature, associated with the inflammation of the lung parenchyma, distal to the terminal bronchiole, with clinical and radiological evidence of consolidation of part or parts of one or both lungs. The overall mortality of CAP varies from less than 1% in outpatients to approximately 14% in cases admitted to hospital and to 50% or more in patients requiring intensive care unit admission.

MICROBIAL ETIOLOGY

A wide variety of pathogens can cause CAP but by far, the most common pathogen is *Streptococcus pneumoniae*, which accounts for some 20–80% of cases and remains the most common pathogen even among cases requiring intensive care unit admission. In HIV-infected patients, as in nonimmunocompromised cases, *S. pneumoniae* remains the most common pathogen in CAP.

It is also becoming increasingly recognized that cases of CAP due to both seasonal and pandemic influenza may be complicated by secondary bacterial infections, most commonly due to the *Pneumococcus*. In this regard, it is interesting to note that during the occurrence of the recent H1N1 pandemic influenza infections, a substantial number of patients with CAP, particularly those requiring hospitalization or developing critically illness, were documented to have secondary bacterial infections.

RISK FACTORS

There are a number of risk-factors responsible for CAP. These include extremes of age, comorbid diseases, such as diabetes, chronic obstructive pulmonary disease (COPD), cardiovascular disease and HIV infection. Excessive alcohol consumption, tobacco smoking, malnutrition, obesity and immunosuppressive treatments are also important risk factors. The exact mechanisms by which these conditions actually predispose to pneumonia is unclear, but in general terms, they may predispose to an increase in bacterial colonization of the airway, and/or allow direct access of the bacteria to the lower respiratory tract, and/or be associated with impairment of normal host defenses and/or clearing mechanisms.

Cigarette smoking plays as a major risk factor for CAP, in both HIV-infected and uninfected individuals. The exact mechanisms by which cigarette smoking predisposes to pneumonia are uncertain, but are almost certainly multifactorial and cigarette smoking has multiple effects on host defenses. Nasopharyngeal colonization by microorganisms, such as the *Pneumococcus* is an essential first step in the pathogenesis of pneumococcal infections. Cigarette smoking may also enhance the risk of CAP because of its association with COPD. Passive smoking in the home is also a risk factor for CAP in the elderly. Most importantly in current smokers who have pneumococcal CAP, there is a greater risk of development of severe sepsis, the patients require hospitalization at a younger age with fewer underlying comorbid conditions, there is an increased 30-day mortality independent of smoking-related or other comorbidity and age.

PATHOGENESIS WITH PARTICULAR REFERENCE TO THE *PNEUMOCOCCUS*

Pneumococcus has a polysaccharide capsule which is responsible for the virulence of the organism. It promotes resistance by opsonophagocytosis as well as entrapment of mucopolysaccharides present in the mucus. The presence of protein virulence factors in the *Pneumococcus* further contributes to suppression of host defenses. The virulence factors neutralize both innate and adaptive immune responses. All these mechanisms promote pneumococcal attachment to the airway epithelium through enablement of bacterial adhesions.

The first step in the causation of invasive pneumococcal disease is nasopharyngeal colonization. Colonization also activates host defense, therefore protecting against severe infection. Innate and adaptive immune responses triggered by the aforementioned virulence factors, as well as cell wall components, such as lipoteichoic acid (LTA) and proteoglycans, if efficiently mobilized, can control and eradicate pneumococcal colonization. The immune-mediated specific protection is attributed to the IgG and secretory IgA antibodies against the polysaccharide capsule of the *Pneumococcus*.

In summary, the inhalation of *Pneumococcus* into the nasopharynx may result in several possible outcomes:
- Eradication by the host defenses
- Carrier state
- State of persistence
- Acute infection.

During persistence state, the bacteria encased in biofilm, lie dormant. Both carrier and persistence states may get activated during immunosuppression or a concurrent viral infection.

DIAGNOSTIC TESTING

A vast number of studies have been undertaken over many years to assess the value of the various microbiological techniques that are available for the diagnosis of likely microbial etiology in patients with CAP. The commonly employed tests include sputum smear examination with Gram's stain, culture and pneumococcal antigen detection. Blood culture, serological investigations and urinary examination for *Legionella* and pneumococcal antigens may also be done. Fiberoptic bronchoscopy is sometimes required to obtain bronchial secretions or lavage fluid for investigations. One technique that has significantly improved the rapid sputum diagnosis of pneumococcal pneumonia is the real-time quantitative polymerase chain reaction (qPCR), with detection of the *pneumolysin (ply)* gene appearing to be useful in patients who have already received antibiotics.

Other recent innovations in CAP-related molecular diagnostics include multiplex PCR procedures which enable the simultaneous detection of a range of bacterial and viral pathogens in bronchoalveolar lavage, sputum, saliva and nasopharyngeal swab specimens. While isolation of microorganisms from blood culture is considered a *gold standard* for the diagnosis of likely etiology of CAP, a number of studies have indicated that there is a low yield from blood cultures and that even a positive result does not frequently result in a change in antibiotic management, or subsequent cost saving, particularly in non-severely ill cases.

There is considerable debate about the routine need for a chest radiograph in all patients with CAP, particularly in cases not apparently severe enough to require hospital admission. Some have suggested that it remains an *essential initial test* in the diagnosis of CAP that is recommended in most guidelines, certainly for hospitalized cases. The chest radiograph is unhelpful in suggesting likely microbial etiology and is performed in order to confirm the presence of pneumonia, to delineate the extent of the pulmonary involvement, as an indicator of the severity of infection, to delineate the presence of underlying disorders and to determine the presence of any complications.

The assessment of oxygenation is recommended in both outpatients and inpatients and can be undertaken by pulse oximetry, particularly in outpatients or by arterial blood gas analysis. Routine hematological and biochemical testing do not help determine likely etiology, but will assist in the assessment of comorbid illness, and influence decisions regarding need for hospitalization, severity of infections and choice and dosage of initial, empiric antimicrobial therapy.

PROGNOSIS

The outcome of CAP is influenced by a number of factors, including host factors, bacterial factors and antibiotic factors. Among the host factors, older age, the presence of underlying comorbid illness and various genetic characteristics of the host, all are potentially associated with the increased risk of pneumonia, as well as a worse outcome. Severity of illness on its own may impact negatively on pneumonia outcome, even in the absence of any of these other risk factors. A number of severity of illness indices and various scoring systems have been developed to assist in severity assessment, among which the PSI and the CURB-65 score (derived from the British Thoracic Society rules) are the most commonly used.

The subject of severity of illness assessment and the various tools that are available, including the various scoring systems and the various biomarkers, are reviewed extensively elsewhere. The PSI score comprises of 20 variables that include details of demographic characteristics, comorbidity, clinical features and results of laboratory and radiographic investigations.

The CURB-65 score stands for confusion (mental), blood urea (>7 mmol/L), respiratory rate (>30 breaths/min), blood pressure (systolic <90 mm Hg, diastolic $\leq$60 mm Hg), age $\geq$65 years). CURB-65 is used to diagnose patients with severe CAP at high risk or mortality while PSI identifies low-risk patients who can be managed at home. CRB-65 (without the need for blood urea) is the modified version of CURB-65 with equal results.

There are also a myriad of biomarkers that have been studied with regard to their utility in the assessment of severity of CAP. These have been extensively reviewed elsewhere. These biomarkers are probably more appropriate for use in the more severely ill, hospitalized patient with CAP and appear to be a promising area for future research. However, it is important to remember that neither severity of illness scoring systems, nor biomarkers can replace sound clinical judgment and should be seen as adjuncts to decision making.

Among the bacterial factors that may impact on the outcome of pneumonia, are the nature of the infecting microorganism, its associated virulence factors and its susceptibility to commonly prescribed antibiotics. Significant consideration also needs to be given to the potential impact of antibiotic resistance, particularly pneumococcal resistance to beta-lactam agents on the outcome of pneumonia.

Among the antibiotic factors, choice of agent, dosage and duration of therapy and time to the initiation of antibiotics from the time of presentation of patients to hospital, all potentially play a role in the outcome of pneumonia. Importantly, new strategies recommended for antibiotic management, for example, the use of combination antibiotic therapy in more severely ill hospitalized cases with pneumonia, including the subset of patients with bacteremic pneumococcal infections, have been said to have a positive impact on pneumonia outcomes. The most commonly used combination therapy, which has been shown to be beneficial, is the addition of a macrolide to standard beta-lactam therapy, although benefit has also been shown with other combinations.

One aspect of patient prognosis that requires special consideration is the presence of cardiac changes/complications, such as cardiac failure, cardiac arrhythmias, and even myocardial infarction, as a complication of the pneumonia, even in patients with no previous underlying cardiac condition. These events tend to occur quite early in the course of the infection and are associated with an increased short-term mortality. Their occurrence in patients with CAP also highlights the potential benefit of CAP prevention using pneumococcal and influenza vaccination.

TREATMENT

The mainstay of therapy for CAP is the use of antibiotics. Empirical antibiotic therapy should particularly take into consideration severity of illness, likely etiological agent, resistance patterns among commonly identified pathogens, especially *S. pneumoniae* and underlying comorbidities. An additional consideration in the developing world is the cost of the individual drugs. Antibiotic therapy should be commenced as soon as possible after diagnosis.

A number of guidelines, both in developed and developing worlds, recommend the use of oral therapy with amoxicillin for outpatients. Macrolide monotherapy has been suggested as an alternative, particularly for patients allergic to penicillin. Other oral agents, such as amoxicillin/clavulanate, second-generation cephalosporins and fluoroquinolones can be used.

For more severely ill, hospitalized cases, most guidelines recommend the use of a beta-lactam/macrolide combination or monotherapy with a respiratory fluoroquinolone. For cases requiring ICU admission, additional agents are recommended; for example, the addition of an aminoglycoside to a beta-lactam/macrolide combination to provide additional cover for suspected gram-negative infection. If a fluoroquinolone is used for an ICU patient, it is commonly recommended that it should be combined with another agent, such as beta-lactam. The CAP guideline from India recommends, in this setting, the use of a beta-lactam/macrolide combination in patients not at risk of *Pseudomonas aeruginosa* with various recommendations for those with suspected *P. aeruginosa* infection.

Caution must be exercised with the routine use of fluoroquinolone monotherapy for patients presenting with CAP in regions where tuberculosis is endemic, since such cases may actually be infected with *M. tuberculosis* for which fluoroquinolones have excellent in vitro activity. In this situation, fluoroquinolone use may be associated with delays in the diagnosis of tuberculosis with the masking of this infection. Consequent to this is the potential for patient morbidity and even mortality, as well as ongoing secondary transmission. Furthermore, there are additional concerns that fluoroquinolone monotherapy used in this situation may result in fluoroquinolone-resistant tuberculosis.

Adjunctive Therapy

General support for patients with CAP includes attention to nutrition and hydration, analgesia and supplemental oxygen. Macrolide antibiotics and corticosteroids are important adjunctive therapies which have been frequently used. Addition of a macrolide to the antibiotic therapy adds to the antiinflammatory and immunomodulatory actions. These actions help augment host responses as well as attenuate the virulence of bacteria. Corticosteroid use is most commonly recommended in patients with severe CAP in association with septic shock.

Prevention of Infection—Vaccination

An important aspect to consider in the overall control of CAP, and in particular pneumococcal pneumonia, is the prevention of infection using vaccination. Currently two pneumococcal vaccines are commercially available, namely the polyvalent polysaccharide vaccine (PPV), used predominantly in adults and the pneumococcal conjugate vaccine (PCV), used predominantly in children. Evidence points to a lower, but not insignificant protective effect, even in nonbacteremic pneumonia, such that this should not preclude the more widespread use of the vaccine. Furthermore, recent studies also point to a significant beneficial effect in preventing pneumococcal pneumonia and decreasing disease severity, even in the vaccinated elderly. Lower rate of pneumonia and improved outcome have also been seen in HIV-infected adults who have received PPV previously.

Even more compelling is the evidence for the use of the PCV in the safe prevention of pneumococcal infection in children in both low income and industrialized countries, including HIV-infected individuals, meeting international criteria of cost-effectiveness even for lower income countries. PCV has been effective in lowering the rate of invasive pneumococcal disease not only in vaccinated children, particularly those below the age of 2 years, but also in nonvaccinated children and even in adults and the elderly in the community. As such the vaccine appears to have both direct immune benefits in those vaccinated, as well as indirect *herd immunity* effects.

In the case of infants and very young children, PCV13 has now been included in the national immunization programs of many developed and developing countries. With respect to adults, PCV13 vaccination as a single dose is recommended by the Food and Drug Administration of the USA for adults aged ≥50 years, while in the case of those aged >19 years who have immunocompromising conditions, including HIV infection, a *prime-boost* strategy is recommended for vaccine-naïve recipients.

Influenza vaccination is also recommended in many CAP guidelines. Annual vaccination is recommended especially for individuals with comorbidities and other risk factors prone to develop influenza and other complications such as pneumonia. It is also recommended that individuals that can transmit influenza to high-risk cases, such as healthcare workers, should be immunized yearly.

CHAPTER 18

Pulmonary Fungal Infections

Arunaloke Chakrabarti

INTRODUCTION

Pulmonary mycoses can either be the primary lung involvement or be a manifestation of disseminated fungal infections. The susceptible population for pulmonary fungal infections can be divided in two groups: classical and newly recognized risk groups (Box 18.1). The growing incidences of pulmonary mycoses, which are linked to classical risk factors in the range of 3–56%. The patients usually have significant neutropenia (<500 neutrophil/µg for >10 days) as risk factor.

TYPES OF INFECTIONS

Of all pulmonary fungal infections, aspergillosis is the most important challenge. Commonly, it occurs in patients with prolonged neutropenia and recipients of organ transplants. It is also seen amongst patients with advanced stage of acquired immunodeficiency syndrome (AIDS) or chronic granulomatous disease.

Pulmonary mucormycosis is also reported in patients with uncontrolled diabetes. *Pneumocystis jiroveci* infection had frequently been reported in patients with AIDS, but recent data showed a sharp decline in incidence after chemoprophylaxis and tri-drug regimen in those patients. Yeasts are rarely reported in respiratory tract infections. Among yeasts, cryptococcal respiratory tract infections are seen more consistently. Though deep-seated infections due to black mycelial fungi are increasingly reported in recent years, they rarely cause pulmonary infections.

> **BOX 18.1:** Susceptible population for fungal respiratory tract infection.
>
> *Classical risk groups:*
> - Patients on cytotoxic chemotherapy for malignant diseases
> - Patients with hematopoietic stem cell transplantation
> - Severe AIDS (CD4 cell count <100)
> - Immunosuppressive therapy in autoimmune diseases
> - Other transplantations
> - Aging population
>
> *Newly recognized risk groups:*
> - Stay in intensive care units
> - Chronic obstructive lung disease
> - Administration of prolonged low dose of steroids
> - Cirrhosis of liver
> - Iron overload
> - Diabetes especially when poorly controlled
> - Sepsis with immunoprophylaxis
> - Malnutrition
> - Moderate-to-severe liver or kidney failure

Aspergillosis

Pulmonary aspergillosis may manifest with saprophytic, allergic or invasive presentations.

Allergic Alveolitis

Repeated exposure to *Aspergillus* antigens may lead to sensitization of exposed individuals. This hypersensitization known as *farmer's lung* or *malt worker's lung* is commonly seen amongst farmers and other farm workers working with moldy hay or stored gains. Typically, the patient will complain of cough, fever, breathlessness and other general symptoms usually about 6–8 hours of exposure.

Allergic Bronchopulmonary Aspergillosis

Allergic bronchopulmonary aspergillosis (ABPA) is an allergic pulmonary disorder caused by allergic response to *Aspergillus* hyphae without direct tissue invasion by the organism. It manifests as chronic asthma, recurrent pulmonary infiltrates, and bronchiectasis (see Chapter on ABPA).

Eosinophil-related Fungal Rhinosinusitis

Fungal involvement of nose and sinuses (fungal rhinosinusitis, FRS) is a common manifestation especially of aspergillosis. It can be either invasive or noninvasive in nature. Invasive FRS in particular erodes the surrounding structures. Noninvasive FRS may present as local fungal colonization, mycetoma (fungal ball) formation or allergic fungal rhinosinusitis (AFRS).

Saprophytic Aspergillosis

Saprophytic fungal growth usually occurs within a preexisting cavity due to old tuberculosis, bronchiectasis or cystic fibrosis. It can also develop in an emphysematous bulla or a malignant cavity. The fungal mass consists of the entangled hyphae in proteinaceous matrix. Aspergilloma may be either asymptomatic or become a cause of recurrent hemoptysis. Radiologically, it is diagnosed by Monod's sign, i.e. presence of an opacity surrounded by an air-crescent within a cavity. Filamentous fungi, such as *Pseudallescheria boydii* and *Zygomycetes* may also fungal balls in lung cavities. Such fungal balls can also develop in sinuses.

Invasive Aspergillosis

Invasive disease occurs in immunosuppressed patients and those with severe neutropenia or neutrophil dysfunction. It may however also occur in non-neutropenic patients with chronic liver disease, chronic obstructive pulmonary disease (COPD), rheumatoid arthritis and diabetes. Invasive aspergillosis may manifest with pneumonia, invasion into local structures or dissemination.

Tracheobronchial Aspergillosis

Aspergillus may colonize the tracheobronchial tree and occasionally cause tracheobronchitis. Invasive tracheobronchitis may result in severely immunocompromised patients.

Chronic Necrotizing Pulmonary Aspergillosis

Indolent infection with *Aspergillus* occurs in patients with COPD, pneumoconiosis or inactive tuberculosis. Patients may present with features of chronic bronchopneumonia refractory to standard antibiotic treatment. Evidence of fungal disease is found on biopsy. Aspergilloma formation may occur in patients with cavitating pneumonia.

Invasive Fungal Rhinosinusitis

As mentioned earlier, invasive FRS include acute invasive, granulomatous and chronic invasive. FRS depending on host immune status and geographical region. Acute invasive FRS is described by a disease course of less than 4 weeks with predominant vascular invasion occurring in an immunocompromised patient.

Mucormycosis

It is an increasingly reported polymorphic disease caused by *Zygomycetes*. The common sites of mucormycosis are the rhinocerebral area (39%), lungs (24%), and skin (19%). Pulmonary mucormycosis most commonly occurs in patients with granulocytopenia. It may variously manifest as solitary lesions, lobar consolidation or cavity formation. Disseminated disease may occasionally occur.

Fusarium and *Scedosporium* Infections

Over the past two decades, *Fusarium* spp. and *Scedosporium apiospermum* or *Pseudoallescheria boydii* (sexual stage) are emerging pathogens especially in patients with hematological malignancies undergoing chemotherapy and bone marrow transplants. The pulmonary infections caused by both agents are indistinguishable many times from that caused by *Aspergillus* spp. The organisms in tissue also resemble *Aspergillus* spp. having angular, septate dichotomously branching hyphae.

Respiratory Infections Due to Dimorphic Fungi

Dimorphic fungi such as histoplasma are often reported to cause respiratory tract infection in the Western countries. Histoplasmosis, though considered uncommon three decades back, is now increasingly reported in Asia-pacific region in many countries, especially in patients with impaired immunity. This can be partly attributed to acquired immunodeficiency syndrome. Autochthonous cases of blastomycosis are occasionally reported from this region, coccidioidomycois and paracoccidioidomycosis are rarely reported as imported disease.

Histoplasmosis usually presents as mild insignificant self-limiting respiratory disease in majority of patients from endemic areas. Both pulmonary and extrapulmonary histoplasmosis may occur especially in patients with immunosuppression. Rarely, in the presence of heavy infection, acute primary pulmonary histoplasmosis may occur even in a patient with normal immune status. In COPD, histoplasmosis may present as an indolent cavitary disease.

Pulmonary Cryptococcosis

Pulmonary cryptococcosis is generally seen in the presence of disseminated infection, more so in immunocompromised patients. Clinical features are common with any other pulmonary infection. Typical radiological findings include the presence of interstitial infiltrates, military mottling, hilar lymphadenopathy and pleural effusion. Fluffy opacities may present with a picture of acute respiratory distress syndrome.

Pulmonary Candidiasis

Primary candidal bronchopneumonia is seen in severely debilitated, neutropenic patients. Commonly, pulmonary candidiasis occurs in the presence of disseminated disease. Very low birth-weight infants are also at high risk of *Candida* infection. The presence of *Candida* in the sputum, tracheal aspiration or bronchoalveolar lavage mostly represents contamination from upper respiratory tract colonization. A definite diagnosis of *Candida* pneumonia requires histopathological proof of lung invasion. Children can also be affected by pulmonary allergic reaction due to *Candida* species.

Pneumocystis Respiratory Tract Infection

Opportunistic infection with *Pneumocystis jiroveci*, formerly known as *Pneumocystis carinii* is particularly seen in patients with AIDS. It may also occur in other immunosuppressed conditions. Common clinical features include dry cough, breathlessness, fever, tachypnea, tachycardia and hypoxemia. Chest radiology is often characteristic with bilateral diffuse infiltrates and ground glass haze.

Diagnosis of Pulmonary Mycoses

Imaging helps increase the suspicion of fungal disease. In an immunosuppressed patient, presence of a nodule, halo sign, air crescent sign, or reverse halo sign help in suspecting fungal infections. In immunocompetent patients, such signs are not available. If the patient is in ICU, think of fungal infections even when infiltrative lesion is suspected. Mycological tests should always be done to corroborate the findings of imaging investigations.

Chest radiography is not a sensitive procedure for diagnosing pulmonary mold infections at an early stage. Chest CT scan helps pick up the lesions. Fungal lesions on chest radiographs are seen as either interstitial infiltrates or macronodules. Nodular lesions may be characteristically surrounded by low attenuation, *halo* sign due to the presence of hemorrhagic inflammation especially in neutropenic patients. Air crescent may form once the nodule cavitates during the course of therapy.

Among mycological techniques, conventional procedures (direct microscopy, histopathology, and culture) are not sensitive and do not help in early diagnosis. Maximum attention has been drawn to find suitable serological or molecular diagnostic technique. Polymerase chain reaction (PCR) for detection of fungal nucleic acid in specimens, though holds promise, is awaiting further standardization and validation.

The diagnosis of pulmonary infections due to dimorphic fungi largely depends on clinical suspicion, direct examination of respiratory specimens, histopathological examination of paraffin-embedded tissue, and culture of appropriate samples. Careful examination of fungal structure on direct microscopy helps in identification of fungus as each dimorphic fungus has distinctive morphology in tissue. In an immunocompetent host, serology for antibody detection helps in diagnosis of considerable number of cases. Conversely, in immunocompromised hosts, antigen detection would be a preferable alternative. The presence of a carbohydrate antigen is useful for diagnosis of histoplasmosis and its therapeutic monitoring.

Therapy of Pulmonary Mycoses

There are a number of antifungal drugs which have now become available. Lipid formulations of amphotericin B (amphotericin B colloidal dispersion, amphotericin B lipid complex, and liposomal amphotericin B are safer than amphotericin B. Broad-spectrum antifungal triazoles (posaconazole, voriconazole), and the echinocandins (caspofungin, anidulafungin, micafungin) are newer drugs with potent antifungal effect. Voriconazole and alternatively liposomal amphotericin is the drug of choice for invasive aspergillosis. Second-line management with a lipid formulation of amphotericin B, caspofungin or posaconazole is required in patients who fail first-line therapy.

High dose of lipid-based formulation of amphotericin B (up to 10 mg/kg) is used for the first-line therapy of mucormycosis. Posaconazole is used for maintenance treatment as well as a salvage therapy. Surgical treatment involving excision of infected lesions should be done to minimize the damage to the organ. Similarly, control of underlying predisposing factors is important in management of pulmonary mucormycosis.

Fusarium and *Scedosporium* infections are also treated with voriconazole and amphotericin B (lipid based formulation) as first-line drugs with posaconazole as a salvage therapy.

Treatment of pulmonary mycoses due to dimorphic fungi depends on competency of the hosts and disease pattern. Self-limiting disease among immunocompetent hosts is managed with supportive care. Itraconazole is often used for acute pulmonary histoplasmosis or blastomycosis. Profoundly immune-compromised hosts or those with severe disease are treated with lipid formulations of amphotericin B. Pulmonary cryptococcosis in a patient with HIV infection is treated with an initial course of amphotericin B with or without flucytosine. Fluconazole is used for maintenance therapy after the initial treatment is completed. Alternatively, itraconazole may be used in patients with mild disease.

CHAPTER 19

Nosocomial Pneumonia

Vishwanath Gella, SK Jindal

INTRODUCTION

Nosocomial pneumonia is a significant problem worldwide. It is responsible for an increased mortality, morbidity, hospital stay and healthcare costs. Hospital-acquired pneumonia (HAP) is the second most common form of nosocomial infection. There is 6–20-fold increased risk of acquiring hospital-acquired pneumonia (HAP)/ventilator-associated pneumonia (VAP) in the mechanically ventilated patients.

DEFINITIONS

Hospital-acquired pneumonia (HAP) is defined as pneumonia occurring 48 hours after admission which is neither present nor incubating at the time of admission.

Ventilator-associated pneumonia (VAP) is defined as pneumonia occurring 48–72 hours after endotracheal intubation or tracheostomy.

Healthcare-associated pneumonia (HCAP): It is defined as pneumonia occurring in patients in the nonhospital settings but who have got extensive healthcare contact; it excludes HAP, VAP and CAP. HCAP is associated with the following risk factors:
- Hospitalization for more than two days in preceding 90 days.
- Residence in a nursing home or extended care facility
- Home infusion therapy
- Patients receiving chronic dialysis or home wound care

There is a lot of controversy surrounding the definition of HCAP. It is not as well standardized as HAP or VAP.

PATHOGENESIS

Nosocomial pneumonia develops when microorganisms reach the lung and overcome the lung host defenses. The main mechanism involved in the pathogenesis of nosocomial pneumonia is the colonization of oropharynx with pathogenic microorganisms and subsequent microaspiration of these contents. Predominant exogenous sources include breach of normal mucosal integrity (with numerous devices—nasogastric tube, endotracheal tube), contact through healthcare personnel, colonization of endotracheal tube biofilm. Endogenous factors that lead to increase in the gastric pH like acute illness; drugs (like proton pump inhibitors) can disrupt the sterility of the stomach and upper gastrointestinal tract, and lead to gastrointestinal colonization.

PREVENTION OF HOSPITAL-ACQUIRED PNEUMONIA AND VENTILATOR-ASSOCIATED PNEUMONIA

There are multiple risk factors for VAP which are amenable to intervention by nonpharmacological measures. All the methods that aim at preventing HAP decrease the colonization of the upper respiratory tract, oral cavity and digestive tract, thereby preventing infection.

Decontamination with Antimicrobials

- *Chlorhexidine:* Oral decontamination with chlorhexidine (2%) solution (15 mL four times daily) till after extubation has been shown to be effective in preventing VAP.
- *Selective decontamination of the digestive tract (SDD)* with topical and systemic antibiotics has been shown to be of modest benefit in preventing VAP, but not favored by all in view of the emergence of the resistant organisms.

Hand Hygiene

Healthcare personnel should do handwashing before and after contact with patients with alcohol-based solutions to prevent cross-infection between patients. Pronovost has introduced a simple checklist which has significantly reduced the incidence of central line associated infections and deaths. This checklist includes the five things to be adhered to before each central line insertion:

- Wash your hands;
- Clean the patient's skin;
- Put on a cap,
- Gown and mask;
- Avoid placing the catheter on groin; and

Airway

The care of the airway is important in preventing VAP, silver-coated endotracheal tubes have been shown to be effective in preventing VAP. Other measures which have shown to be effective are continuous aspiration of subglottic secretions (CASS); the most commonly used CASS device is Hi-Lo Evac. This device is costlier than routine endotracheal tubes.

Cuff Pressure

Endotracheal tube cuff pressure should be maintained between 20 cm and 30 cm H_2O to prevent aspiration of gastric and oropharyngeal contents directly into the trachea.

Ventilatory Circuit

Regular change of ventilator circuits has not shown to decrease the incidence of VAP, and not recommended as a measure to prevent VAP. One should avoid flushing of the condensate into the lower airway and should be emptied regularly. Closed suctioning system has not been shown to be superior to open system. It seems logical to use closed systems to avoid the risk of spraying the condensate and secretions into the ICU environment.

Use of metered-dose inhaler (MDI) for delivering aerosolized medication may reduce the risk of VAP since nebulizers get contaminated rapidly. Heated circuits are not superior to unheated circuits. Heated circuits decrease the amount of condensate; at the same time, excessive heating of inspired air can lead to drying of tracheal secretions with impending risk of endotracheal tube blockade with secretions.

Positioning

Semirecumbent position at 45° is effective in preventing VAP compared with supine position. Semirecumbent position prevents aspiration and decreases the odds of developing VAP. Regular suctioning of respiratory secretions after instilling 8 mL of normal saline showed a reduction of VAP, compared to suctioning without instilling normal saline.

Role of Proton Pump Inhibitors and H_2 Receptor Blockers

Proton pump inhibitors and H_2 receptor blockers have been shown to increase the gastric colonization and odds of VAP and HAP by increasing gastric pH. They should be replaced by sucralfate and antacids which do not alter the gastric pH in noncritically ill patients but the risks of stress ulcer bleed needs to be considered when stopping these agents as the risk of gastric bleeding increases with sucralfate though not significant.

Nasogastric and nasoduodenal tubes should be removed immediately when not required in hospitalized patients. Nasoduodenal tube feeding group has been shown to have lower incidence of VAP and achieved nutritional goals earlier compared to nasogastric tube group. Preventing intubation, reintubation and decreasing the duration of mechanical ventilation and using noninvasive ventilation, wherever possible, can help prevent VAP.

Certain components of ventilator bundles like sedation, vacation and assessment of ability to wean daily have been shown to decrease incidence of VAP. However, ventilator bundle should be hospital specific, tailored according to the available facilities.

DIAGNOSIS

Diagnosis of HAP/HCAP is predominantly based on clinical, radiological and sputum evaluation. VAP should be suspected in all intubated patients who develop new onset fever, respiratory symptoms, new chest infiltrates. In patients on ventilator, VAP is suspected from increased respiratory rate, increased minute volume, decreased tidal volume and increasing oxygen requirement. There are 2 different strategies to diagnose VAP, i.e. the clinical approach and quantitative bacteriological approach.

Clinical Approach

Clinical approach combines clinical features with semiquantitative cultures of endotracheal aspirate or sputum. In this approach, diagnosis of VAP/HAP is based on presence of new radiographic infiltrate, and presence of the following clinical criteria: fever, leukocytosis or leukopenia, purulent lower respiratory secretions, abnormal respiratory system examination, worsening oxygenation.

The specificity of clinical criteria is increased by addition of tracheal aspirate, microscopic examination and semiquantitative cultures. Microscopic examination of the tracheal aspirate for Gram stain and white blood cells will guide empirical therapy and prevent inappropriate therapy. A negative tracheal aspirate for Gram stain, inflammatory cells and semiquantitative cultures in the absence of recent change in antibiotic therapy within 72 hours has a strong negative predictive value (94%) for VAP suggest the need to rule out other noninfectious causes of pulmonary infiltrates.

CPIS (clinical pulmonary infection score) increases the specificity of clinical diagnosis. It incorporates clinical, radiological, physiological (PaO_2/FiO_2 ratio) and microbiological data into a single numerical value. When CPIS score exceeded 6, a good correlation was found with pneumonia diagnosed by quantitative cultures of samples obtained by bronchoscopic and nonbronchoscopic methods. A CPIS score of ≤/=6 at 72 hours has been used to stop antibiotics without adversely affecting mortality and ICU stay, thereby preventing inappropriate use of antibiotics.

Clinical responses after 48–72 hours in combination with semiquantitative cultures are taken into consideration to decide the further course of action regarding antibiotics.

CPIS is simple and easy to perform at bedside. It is a useful tool not only in diagnosing VAP with modest sensitivity and specificity but also in evaluating the clinical response to treatment and determining the appropriate duration of treatment.

Failure to initiate treatment in cases of VAP as soon as the diagnosis is suspected will lead to increased mortality. All the patients suspected to have VAP will receive broad-spectrum antibiotics according to risk factors and local microbiological epidemiology after lower respiratory tract secretions are sent for culture. The initiation of antibiotics should not be delayed for obtaining cultures especially in hemodynamically unstable patients. Other mimics of pulmonary infection like atelectasis, pulmonary thromboembolism (PTE), hemorrhage and congestive heart failure which can present with similar clinical manifestations should be ruled out before considering a diagnosis of VAP/HAP. Clinical approach may sometimes lead to excessive antibiotic treatment if other mimics are not ruled out before labeling a patient as having VAP.

Bacteriological Approach

In this approach, patients are only treated after culture results arrive, and if cultures of the respiratory samples show growth above a threshold level. The Achilles heel of this approach lies in avoiding overtreatment and thereby preventing resistance to antibiotics. Quantitative cultures on the other hand are more specific with variable sensitivity and differentiate colonization from infection when a specific threshold is taken for diagnosis of VAP. The lower respiratory tracts secretions obtained through bronchoscopic bronchoalveolar lavage (BAL) and protected specimen brush (PSB) are highly specific. Mini-BAL and blind endotracheal aspirate (nonbronchoscopic) quantitative cultures have high sensitivity and low specificity retaining the diagnostic accuracy.

A combined approach shown in the algorithm (Flowchart 19.1) is better in view of the shortcomings of both the approaches and will address most of the issues.

Response to Therapy

Response to therapy occurs in 48–72 hours in most (75%) of the patients. Response can be assessed by the improvement in fever, oxygen requirement, tracheal secretions, leukocytosis and radiological picture. Most importantly, fever and oxygen requirements improve after 48–72 hours other things may take time to improve. Radiological resolution generally lags behind, although there may be initial deterioration in radiological picture. Resolution is slower in elderly, patients with COPD and patients with associated endobronchial obstruction. The presence of the following radiological features indicates rapid deterioration:

- Multilobar involvement
- >50% increase in infiltrates in 48 hours
- Development of cavitary or necrotizing pneumonia
- Development of large pleural effusion

Flowchart 19.1: Algorithm of a combined approach for ventilator-associated pneumonia management.

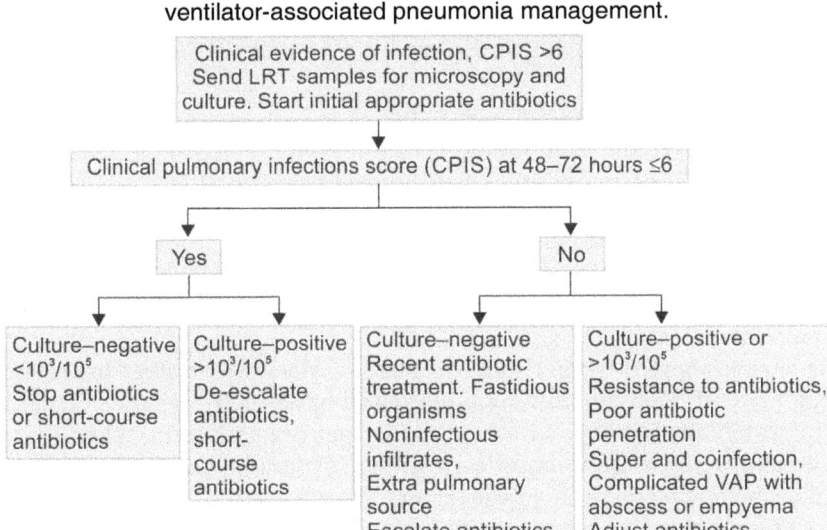

Antibiotics should not be changed in the initial 48–72 hours unless there is evidence of progressive deterioration.

Therapy needs to be escalated to cover resistant organisms in nonresponding patients. Some clinicians wait for the response after changing treatment whereas others proceed with additional investigations.

TREATMENT

Appropriate and early antibiotic therapy improves survival. Inappropriate initial therapy has been shown to increase the mortality in patients with severe sepsis and VAP. The most important factor for initial inappropriate therapy is the presence of multidrug resistant (MDR) pathogens in culture reports obtained subsequently after admission and the mortality risk does not decrease even if antibiotics are changed subsequently.

Initial, empiric antibiotic treatment should be based on the individual risk factors, comorbidities and local microbiological epidemiology and should be patient specific. Broad-spectrum empiric antimicrobial regimen should be started in patients with MDR risk factors.

Drug Regimen for Multidrug Resistant Pathogens

A combination regimen containing at least 3 drugs has to be given for patients with late onset VAP/HAP and HCAP (all cases) so as to provide a broad-spectrum antimicrobial cover which should include 2 broad-spectrum drugs with anti-*Pseudomonas* cover and 1 drug with MRSA cover.
- Anti-*Pseudomonas* agents:
  - carbapenems—meropenem, doripenem, imipenem

- 3rd generation cephalosporin—cefoperazone—sulbactam, cefepime, ceftazidime
- Beta-lactam antibiotics: Piperacillin—tazobactum, ticarcillin-clavulanic acid
- Anti-*Pseudomonas* agent: Can use either an FQ/aminoglycoside:
  - Fluoroquinolone—Levofloxacin, ciprofloxacin
  - Aminoglycoside—gentamicin, tobramycin, amikacin
- Antimethicillin-resistant *Staphylococcus aureus* agent:
  - Vancomycin/Linezolid

Newer drugs for MRSA like oritavancin, dalbavancin and telavancin need to be studied in larger cohort of patients. Colistin has been used for treating MDR pathogens.

Till date, no regimen has been shown to be superior over the other. In places with high risk of *Pseudomonas aeruginosa* and other gram-negative bacilli, local microbiological bacterial susceptibility pattern should be taken into consideration before starting empirical regimen. Institution-specific guidelines should be developed taking all these factors into account.

In a broader view, for patients with early onset VAP/HAP at places where there is no increased incidence of early onset MDR pathogens, treatmemt cover should be provided for *Streptococcus Pneumoniae, haemophilus influenzae,* MSSA and the usual community acquired pathogens with beta-lactam and beta-lactamase inhibitor combinations (piperacillin-tazobactum, ampicillin-sulbactam), ceftriaxone, fluoroquinolones (levofloxacin and moxifloxacin) and doripenem.

Treatment of Ventilator-associated Pneumonia Caused by Multidrug Resistant Gram-negative Bacilli

In the past few years, the emergence of MDR Gram-negative bacteria and lack of new antibiotics has led to increased interest in an old class of drugs, *Polymyxins*. Polymyxins are an old class of cationic, cyclic polypeptide antibiotics which consist of polymyxin B and polymyxin E (popularly known as colistin). Colistin is available as colistin sulfate (for oral use) and colistimethate sodium (CMS) for parenteral use. CMS is active against aerobic gram negative bacilli–*Acinetobacter, Pseudomonas, Klebsiella* and *Enterobacter* species, MDR gram-negative bacilli. Nephrotoxicity is the most important side effect of CMS. It is dose-dependent and reversible.

CHAPTER 20

Lung Abscess

C Ravindran, Jyothi E

INTRODUCTION

Lung abscess involves localized collection of pus in a necrotic cavity in the lung parenchyma. An abscess is usually surrounded by a wall comprising fibrous tissue. Necrotizing pneumonia or lung gangrene commonly refers to the presence of a large abscess (>2 cm) or multiple small abscesses.

EPIDEMIOLOGY

Lung abscess continues to pose a major problem in the developing countries. The mortality from lung abscesses also has decreased, but remains between 2% and 10% for community-acquired lung abscess and 60% for hospital-acquired lung abscess. Most primary lung abscesses favorably respond to antibiotics with cure rates of above 90%.

Prognosis is poor in the presence of host factors such as advanced age, debilitation and malnutrition. Similarly, immunosuppression of any cause including human immunodeficiency virus (HIV) infection, diabetes and malignancy are also associated with poor outcomes, sometimes, with mortality of up to 75%.

CLASSIFICATION

Lung abscesses of less than 6-week duration are defined as acute while those of more than 6-week duration are chronic. In a healthy host, aspiration or pneumonia is the most common cause of primary abscess. On the other hand, secondary abscess occurs in host with preexisting lung disease such as bronchial obstruction or bronchiectasis. Secondary abscess commonly occurs in an immunocompromised state and may also result from extrapulmonary sites.

ETIOLOGY

Aspiration of anaerobic bacteria from the oropharynx, commonly in the presence of orogingival disease, is the most common cause of lung abscess. Aerobic gram-positive and gram-negative organisms are other common organisms. Among the aerobic organisms, *Staphylococcus aureus, Klebsiella pneumoniae, E. coli* and type III *Streptococcus pneumoniae* are frequently associated with lung abscess formation. Complicated pneumococcal pneumonia, especially with lung abscess formation was found to be a rare but important cause of lung abscess.

In the immunocompromised hosts, lung abscess may also occur due to nonbacterial and atypical bacterial pathogens. These microorganisms include *Mycobacterium* species, parasites or fungi. Parasitic abscesses with *Paragonimus* and *Entamoeba* species and fungal abscesses with *Aspergillus, Cryptococcus, Histoplasma, Blastomyces,* or others are rarely seen, especially in patients with HIV infection, malignancy and organ transplantation. The organisms are aspirated to lower respiratory tract due to many factors, which may be local or general. Other routes of the spread of infection to lungs include infected chest wall foci, infra diaphragmatic abscesses and hematogenous spread.

PATHOGENESIS

Most commonly, aspiration of oropharyngeal and gastroesophageal contents predisposes to lung abscess formation. This may happen in the presence of poor oral hygiene and orogingival infections. Aspiration also follows episodes of vomiting due to conditions such as dysphagia of any cause. State of altered consciousness due to seizures, acute alcoholic bouts, general anesthesia, head injury, cerebrovascular accidents and poisoning may also predispose to aspiration. Aspirated content in the lung forms a nidus for infection, necrosis and abscess formation.

PATHOLOGY

Aspiration lung abscess most commonly occurs in the dependent lung regions in a bed-ridden patient, such as the apical segments of the lower lobes and posterior segments of upper lobes. Lung abscess that occurs as a part of hematogenous spread may be found in any part of the lung. Multiple areas of liquefaction necrosis (*cross-country* pattern) can occur secondary to bacterial proliferation.

Liquefaction necrosis causes rapid destruction of lung tissue. On the other hand, chronic cavities such as due to tuberculosis and other indolent infections have significant bronchopulmonary fibrosis in and around the cavity.

Contiguous involvement of pleura results in empyema formation. Extension may occasionally occur in the hilar and mediastinal lymph nodes.

Metastatic lung abscesses may occur from hematogenous spread from a distant focus such as right-sided infective endocarditis which is common in intravenous drug abusers. *Staphylococcus aureus* is the most common organism in this situation. Septic embolic abscesses in patients in intensive care units may also owe their origin to the infected intravenous cannulae. They may also arise from thrombophlebitis of the deep veins of the legs or pelvis or from superficial cutaneous cellulitis. Metastatic septic abscess can also result from gram-negative infections of the urinary tract, abdominal or pelvic cavities.

CLINICAL FEATURES

Symptoms

Symptoms are either acute as in pneumonia or insidious in a chronic abscess. Fever, rigors and chills, cough and sputum production are common symptoms. Sputum is most often purulent, foul-smelling and vicious in nature. It is frequently blood stained. Chest pain and occasionally breathlessness may also occur. Sputum may not be putrid in nature in abscesses due to nonanaerobic microorganisms.

Signs

Physical signs of an abscess are nonspecific in nature. Patients usually have signs of periodontal disease or a condition causing impaired consciousness. Patients are often febrile with tachypnea. Those with an abrupt onset lung abscess are often sick. Clubbing of fingers may be present, which may develop within a few weeks and this is reversible as the abscess resolves. If the abscess is localized, there will be crackles on auscultation.

LABORATORY DIAGNOSIS

Several different laboratory investigations are required for the diagnosis of a lung abscess.

Hematological

Presence of leukocytosis is and a leftward shift on differential cell count is seen on routine hematological investigations.

Microbiological Diagnosis

Microbiological investigations such as smear examination, culture and serology are done from respiratory secretions such as sputum, bronchoalveolar lavage (BAL) and bronchial brush samples. Expectorated sputum is mostly contaminated with bacteria colonizing the upper airways. This is, therefore, not helpful to look for anaerobic infections.

Bronchoscopy is required to obtain protected brush samples or BAL from the lower airways for culture of infecting organisms. These samples are not contaminated by colonized bacteria of the upper respiratory tract. Quantitative culture can also be done on the bronchoscopic samples.

Sputum and/or bronchoscopic samples are also examined for the presence of mycobacteria and other infecting organisms including ova, parasites and fungi as and when suspected.

Blood cultures for the infecting organisms are usually negative except in severely immunocompromised patients.

Imaging Studies

Chest Radiograph

Lung abscess is usually seen as an irregular opacity with central necrosis and fluid level. Staphylococcal abscesses are frequently multiple. Pleural effusion and empyema may also be seen. The wall of the cavity can be either smooth or ragged. A cavitating carcinoma may also give appearances of an abscess. Such abscesses have more of solid component, nodular walls and eccentric cavitation.

Anaerobic abscess is usually seen in the dependent lung zones. It presents with cavitation within a dense segmental consolidation.

Computed Tomography

CT scanning helps to visualize the morphology better than the chest radiography; for example, to detect concomitant pleural involvement and empyema or lung infarction. Infected bullae may mimic an abscess especially when there is adjacent pneumonia; however, a smooth luminal margin on plain film or CT suggests the correct diagnosis.

Ultrasound Examination

Ultrasound and ultrasound-guided transthoracic aspiration is an alternative method for CT thorax and guided aspiration.

Bronchoscopy

Flexible fiber optic bronchoscopy is done to exclude bronchial obstruction for example due to bronchogenic carcinoma. It is also required to identify and remove a foreign body causing obstruction. Bronchoscopy also helps to retrieve uncontaminated specimen for culture, as well as to remove pus.

COMPLICATIONS

Empyema with or without bronchopleural fistula is a common complication in about a third of patients. Hemoptysis is a common symptom which can be occasionally massive. An abscess can occasionally spread to other parts of the same or the opposite lung. Rarely, systemic spread to may also occur to other organs, especially in the presence of comorbidities and immunosuppression. Metastatic abscesses can occur in brain, liver, spleen and other organs through hematogenous spread. An abscess can rarely rupture into the mediastinum causing acute mediastinitis and into the pericardial cavity causing pericardial abscess.

TREATMENT

It is important to know about the microbiology of the abscess and underlying comorbidities for decision making. Patient should be initiated on broad spectrum antibiotics. Antibiotics with a spectrum covering gram-negative aerobes and anaerobes are preferred. This may be modified once drug sensitivity results are available.

Antibiotic Therapy

High-dose penicillin was the drug of choice in the past. Now-a-days treatment is preferred with parenteral amoxicillin and sulbactam combination or clindamycin. Clindamycin is initially given intravenously in a dose of 600 mg thrice daily, followed by an oral dose of 150–300 mg four times a day. The antibiotic therapy is generally administered for duration of 4–6 weeks. Duration treatment is increased in the presence of empyema.

More aggressive approach is required for diagnosis of necrotizing pneumonia and abscess that develops in the nursing home facility or in a hospitalized patient. In these patients, a broad-spectrum antibiotic coverage is required. Clindamycin with or without a cephalosporin or moxifloxacin are also used in the treatment of aspiration pneumonia and lung abscess.

Antibiotic treatment is often guided by chest radiography. It is stopped only after complete radiological resolution or when the chest radiograph has shown significant resolution to the presence of a small stable lesion. Clinical improvement is seen within 3–4 days of the antibiotic therapy. Persistent fever beyond 7–10 days indicates a therapeutic failure—the cause of which should be adequately investigated. These may include underlying structural lung diseases such as preexisting sequestration, cyst or bulla. Bronchial obstruction due to a tumor or foreign body should also be looked for. Resistant bacteria, mycobacteria or fungi as causative organisms are other important causes of treatment failure. Prolonged therapy is required for a large cavity size (> 6 cm in diameter).

Surgical Care

Surgery is indicated in patients who fail to respond to medical management. It is also required in patients with suspected neoplasm or with congenital lung malformation. Lobectomy is the most commonly done; segmental resection is usually adequate for small lesions (< 6 cm diameter cavity). Lobectomy or pneumonectomy is, sometimes, required for large or multiple abscesses or for pulmonary gangrene.

Percutaneous Drainage

Percutaneous drainage is sometimes done for a complicated abscess which does not respond to medical therapy. This is especially helpful when extensive thoracic procedures cannot be done; for example, in ventilated patients. Drainage is also helpful in the following situations:
- Ongoing sepsis despite adequate antimicrobial therapy;
- Danger of rupture in a progressively enlarging lung abscess;
- Failure to wean from mechanical ventilation;
- Contamination of the opposite lung.

Percutaneous drainage compared with surgery is safe and effective. Rarely, bronchopleural fistula may develop following percutaneous drainage. These fistulae generally close with the resolution of the abscess cavity. Percutaneous drainage is especially useful to stabilize and prepare critically ill patients for surgery.

Endoscopic drainage of lung abscess is rarely attempted. It is only an additional option than replacement of percutaneous drainage or surgical resection. In selected patients in whom the abscess is nearer the central airways, the use of endobronchial catheters with laser is a relatively safe and effective option for this purpose.

PROGNOSIS

Prognosis depends on the underlying disease and other comorbidities as well as the predisposing factors. It also depends upon how early an appropriate therapy is started. A large cavity (>6 cm), necrotizing pneumonia and multiple abscesses have poorer prognosis. Similarly, the presence of immunocompromised state, extremes of age, bronchial obstruction and aerobic bacterial pneumonia also account for poor prognosis. Prognosis of amoebic lung abscess is good when prompt appropriate treatment is instituted.

CHAPTER 21

Bronchiectasis and Cystic Fibrosis

David Honeybourne

BRONCHIECTASIS

INTRODUCTION

Bronchiectasis is a chronic condition with a variable clinical course that may include acute exacerbations. Prevalence figures have varied between 4 per 100,000 population and 272 per 100,000 populations partly dependent upon the age range studied. There are sparse data on the prevalence of bronchiectasis in the Indian subcontinent.

Bronchiectasis is not infrequently misdiagnosed as chronic bronchitis and/or chronic obstructive pulmonary disease with 15–30% of patients diagnosed with COPD.

PATHOLOGY

Morphological definition has classified bronchiectasis as cylindrical or tubular, which involves dilatation of the airways and also varicose bronchiectasis. There are, in addition, focal areas of narrowing within the dilated airways. A further type is saccular or cystic bronchiectasis, which is characterized by progressive dilatation of the bronchi with collection of large clusters of cysts.

The airways in bronchiectasis show evidence of chronic inflammatory changes with high sputum concentrations of substances, such as elastase, interleukin 8 and other proinflammatory agents. It is thought that an increase in the levels of these agents is driven by recurrent bacterial infections.

PHYSIOLOGY

Classically, patients with bronchiectasis show evidence of airflow obstruction. Around 40% of cases may show significant improvement in FEV_1 after using a beta-2 bronchodilator. Also, a significant number of patients show evidence of bronchial hyperreactivity. Patients may also have a restrictive defect due to fibrotic changes associated with bronchiectasis.

ETIOLOGY (BOX 21.1)

Childhood viral or bacterial infections particularly in malnourished children are known to predispose to lung damage within the growing lung and lead to the emergence of bronchiectasis. The increasing use of immunization against whooping cough (*Bordetella pertussis*) and measles has led to a reduction in such cases. In countries where there is a high incidence of pulmonary tuberculosis, there are also likely to be many cases of patients with subsequent bronchiectasis secondary to fibrotic damage caused by tuberculosis. Other bacterial infections are known to be involved in both the early and later stages e.g. *Pseudomonas aeruginosa* and *Haemophilus influenzae*.

Atypical mycobacteria are recognized in patients with bronchiectasis and infection with these atypical organisms may initiate bronchiectasis or colonization may occur and further tissue damage is a consequence in patients with preexisting bronchiectasis.

There is some emerging evidence that there may be an association between asthma and bronchiectasis. A history of asthma usually occurs first and then evidence of bronchiectasis occasionally emerges many years later. Some of these cases may be related to ABPA.

SYMPTOMS AND SIGNS

Recurrent cough with sputum production may be an indication of underlying bronchiectasis. There should also be a high index of suspicion for underlying bronchiectasis in children with chronic respiratory symptoms. Furthermore,

---

BOX 21.1: Etiology of bronchiectasis.

Postinfectious, e.g. tuberculosis, whooping cough, pneumonia
Cystic fibrosis
Connective tissue diseases, e.g. SLE, rheumatoid arthritis,
SLE, Sjögren's syndrome, relapsing polychondritis
Allergic bronchopulmonary aspergillosis
Ciliary defects, e.g. primary ciliary dyskinesia, Young's syndrome, Kartagener's syndrome
Immune deficiency, e.g. IgA deficiency, X-linked agammaglobulinemia, common variable immunodeficiency,
Secondary to chronic lymphatic leukemia
Congenital defects, e.g. tracheobronchomegaly (Mounier–Kuhn syndrome), pulmonary sequestration
Secondary to inhalation or aspiration, e.g. due to a foreign body
Inflammatory bowel disease, e.g. ulcerative colitis

the finding of persisting inspiratory crackles over the lungs should raise the possibility of bronchiectasis.

The patient may have recurrent hemoptysis and fever at times of acute infective exacerbations. Pleuritic chest pain may also occur occasionally. Frequent respiratory infections may be associated with weight loss. Based on appearance, sputum can be classified into mucoid, mucopurulent or purulent types. A higher proportion of patients with varicose or cystic bronchiectasis have purulent sputum compared to those with tubular bronchiectasis.

Dyspnea correlates with the degree of impairment of FEV_1, sputum volume and extent of changes seen on high-resolution computed tomography (HRCT) scans. Dyspnea occurs in around 72% of cases. The absence of purulent sputum production does not exclude the possibility of underlying bronchiectasis.

A full assessment of symptoms should include the followings: An estimated or measured 24-hours sputum volume when clinically stable, a record of the number of infective exacerbations that the patient has per year, the extent of the use of antibiotics and also assessment of the effects of the symptoms on activities of daily living. The St. George's respiratory questionnaire has been used to assess the quality of life in the adult patients with bronchiectasis.

A classical sign on examination is the presence of coarse inspiratory crackles over the affected lungs especially in the lower zones, which may be present in about 70% of patients. Crackles may often extend into expiration. Coughing may temporarily lessen the crackles. Wheezing may be heard in around 45% of cases. Finger clubbing has been reported to occur in around 40% cases, although this has been less frequent in some reports.

DIAGNOSIS

Prior to CT lung scanning, bronchograms were the definitive way of diagnosing and delineating the extent of bronchiectasis. CT scanning has been shown to be the most sensitive and specific way of diagnosing the condition. In particular, the HRCT appearances may include ring-like shadows where airways are seen in cross section or a tramline appearance where airways are seen in longitudinal section. Modern high resolution CT scanners can produce 3D reconstruction of affected areas.

Nonspecific findings include focal pneumonitis, varicose constrictions or areas of atelectasis. The distribution of abnormalities seen on the CT scan may occasionally give some clue as to the underlying etiology.

Other investigations include assessment of sputum samples for bacterial, mycobacterial and fungal infections. The possibility of ABPA should be investigated by measuring the total serum IgE and looking for specific IgE and IgG to *Aspergillus fumigatus*. Immune deficiency may be detected by looking at serum IgG, IgA and IgM levels, IgG subclasses and also an assessment of functional antibody levels, particularly against *Haemophilus influenzae* and *Streptococcus pneumoniae*. In some cases, investigations for possible underlying cystic fibrosis may be appropriate. In selected patients, studies of cilial function will be appropriate particularly for primary ciliary dyskinesia. They will usually require referral to a specialist center where mucosal biopsies are examined by ultramicroscopy. Also, investigations should look for the possibility of an associated underlying connective tissue disease.

MICROBIOLOGY

Patients with established bronchiectasis may have a wide range of respiratory pathogens in the sputum. Common causes of bacterial exacerbation in bronchiectasis include *Haemophilus influenzae, Staphylococcus aureus,* Methicillin resistant *Staphylococcus aureus* (MRSA), *Streptococcus pneumoniae,* coliforms (e.g. *Klebsiella, Enterobacter*) or *Pseudomonas aeruginosa.* Assessment of sputum samples, over the course of weeks or months often provides invaluable information. Patients' airways may eventually become colonized by one or more organisms and occasionally the numbers of those organisms increase and initiate an acute exacerbation requiring antibiotics. In particular, *Pseudomonas aeruginosa* is likely to cause chronic colonization in more severe cases and may lead to progressive lung damage as part of a *vicious circle* of recurrent infection, tissue damage, predilection to further infection and then, further tissue damage.

Specific sputum testing for mycobacteria should be carried out, firstly to exclude the possibility of tuberculosis, and secondly to look for colonization and possible infection with atypical mycobacteria, such as *Mycobacterium avium-intracellulare, Mycobacterium kansasii* or *Mycobacterium abscessus.* The finding of atypical mycobacteria on two samples of sputum will then indicate the need for prolonged multiple antibiotic therapy.

TREATMENT

Treatment comprises two broad components: firstly for an exacerbation of bronchiectasis and secondly, for long-term maintenance treatment.

An exacerbation, initially the treatment depends partly on the previous microbiology results. If the patient is colonized with *Pseudomonas aeruginosa,* the treatment can be done with an oral agent, such as ciprofloxacin 500 mg twice a day; for more severe exacerbations, intravenous antibiotics may be more effective. The use of two different types of intravenous antibiotics at the same time will help in reducing the risk for emergence of antibiotic resistance. Intravenous therapy is indicated if there is a failure of improvement on oral treatment. There are currently very few oral agents available, which are effective against *Pseudomonas aeruginosa.* Ciprofloxacin is often the first choice of oral agent. Infection due to other bacterial agents, such as *Streptococccus pneumoniae, Haemophilus influenzae, Moraxella catarrhalis* or *Staphylococcus aureus,* may be treated with an oral agent, or alternatively, a single intravenous agent may be used. If the exacerbation is caused by MRSA, then two antibiotics are often recommended, either orally or intravenously.

Due to difficulties with antibiotic penetration into the damaged lung and airways, a prolonged course of antibiotics is often required. The optimum duration of such a course is unclear, however if there is a clinical improvement with a fall of serum inflammatory markers, such as C-reactive protein, this would indicate improvement and often such a course of antibiotics would last for 10–14 days.

There has been some recent evidence which suggests that physiotherapy is effective in acute exacerbations. Patients may also benefit from nebulized bronchodilators during an exacerbation. It is unclear whether a course of steroids given at the same time as the course of antibiotics has any beneficial effect. Theoretically, it may reduce the inflammatory response in the lung, but the possibility of side effects also needs to be considered.

The choice of intravenous agents for an exacerbation due to *Pseudomonas aeruginosa* includes ceftazidime, aztreonam, tazobactam, meropenem, colistin, and aminoglycosides, such as tobramycin or gentamicin. If intravenous aminoglycosides are used, then monitoring of blood levels is essential to reduce the risk of renal or auditory side effects. If tobramycin is given two or three times per day, predose and postdose levels should be measured.

It is of utmost importance to address general issues, such as maintaining adequate hydration and oxygen saturation. Noninvasive ventilation may be useful for those patients who slip into type 2 respiratory failure.

Long-term Management of Stable Disease

The general advice about stopping smoking and improving nutrition is important. Annual vaccination against seasonal influenza is advised as is pneumococcal vaccination. Patients with significant bronchiectasis should receive instructions from a respiratory physiotherapist about the choice of different airway clearance techniques and should be strongly advised to carry out home physiotherapy regularly. There is currently no good evidence to use nebulized recombinant human DNAase as a mucolytic agent, although larger studies are required. Lung function tests should be carried out before and after bronchodilators use to look for evidence of reversibility of airflow obstruction with both inhaled β-agonists and anticholinergic agents. Sometimes, exercise tolerance and symptoms may improve with these agents despite there being no significant improvement in lung function measurements.

The evidence base for using inhaled corticosteroids is limited. There have been some studies that have shown a reduction in sputum volume and an improvement in quality of life measurements without any obvious effects on lung function or exacerbation rates. Some patients may benefit from a trial of inhaled steroids for several months. Adrenal insufficiency is common in patients of bronchiectasis, but this was not associated with use of inhaled steroids.

In patients who are colonized with *Pseudomonas aeruginosa*, the use of long-term nebulized antibiotics may be helpful in reducing the bacterial load in the airways. This, in turn, may reduce chronic inflammation and hence reduce lung damage. Inhaled antibiotics, however, have the drawback of being expensive; sometimes may cause wheezing even after predosing with inhaled β-2 agonists. There is some limited evidence in the literature of benefit from long-term nebulized antibiotics in patients with more severe bronchiectasis colonized with *Pseudomonas*. On first isolation of *Pseudomonas aeruginosa* in the sputum, attempts should be made to eradicate the infection to try and stop chronic colonization.

In a small number of patients with much localized bronchiectasis, the possibility of surgery should be considered. Surgery with localized lung resection may also benefit selected patients with hemoptysis, chronic debilitating cough or a lung abscess unresponsive to antibiotic treatment. Lung transplantation may also be considered for advanced disease.

The role of long-term oral antibiotics in bronchiectasis, perhaps given as a rotation of different antibiotics, is uncertain. Recently, there has been some evidence of the potential benefit of reducing exacerbation frequency by using long-term oral azithromycin as an anti-inflammatory agent in bronchiectasis. Noninvasive ventilation can improve quality of life in some patients with chronic type 2 respiratory failure due to bronchiectasis.

COMPLICATIONS

Acute respiratory exacerbations are common and important cause of morbidity and decline in lung function. Maintenance therapy with macrolide antibiotics has been shown to be safe and effective to reduce exacerbations. Hemoptysis is a rare, but potentially a life-threatening complication of bronchiectasis. Severe hemoptysis (defined as more than 300 mL) of blood coughed up per 24-hours may occur. Whenever possible, the bleeding site should be identified by a combination of tests, such as bronchoscopy, CT lung scanning and angiography. Often, bleeding occurs from a bronchial artery and an interventional radiologist may be able to embolize the vessel. Occasionally, surgery may be necessary in a patient with severe hemoptysis. The risk of hemoptysis is shown to increase with the use of inhalers especially of beta-2 agonist agents.

Amyloidosis is an occasional complication of chronic, advanced bronchiectasis. A lung abscess may develop due to bronchiectasis, and this may be refractory to prolonged antibiotic therapy.

PROGNOSIS

The prognosis of bronchiectasis is very variable, depending upon any underlying cause, particularly immunodeficiency, the extent of the bronchiectasis and also the type of bacterial colonization. Generally, colonization with *Pseudomonas aeruginosa* is linked to a worse prognosis.

CYSTIC FIBROSIS

INTRODUCTION

Cystic Fibrosis (CF) is a disease caused by an autosomal recessive mutation on chromosome 7. In European populations, CF affects approximately 1 in

2,500 live births. There is some speculation in the literature that heterozygotes may possibly have a survival advantage when faced with other gastrointestinal infections such as cholera or typhoid. This may explain why the disease has not become gradually rarer over the centuries. However, in the Indian subcontinent, CF is less common. The exact incidence and prevalence figures are unknown.

Patients who are homozygous for delta F508 tend to have severe respiratory and pancreatic involvement although occasionally exceptions may occur. Indeed there is sometimes a discrepancy between the known genotype and the phenotype. There is increasing evidence of influence of other genes on different chromosomes, so called *modifying genes* and extensive research work is currently being carried out to identify such genes with potential implications for treatment.

The cystic fibrosis transmembrane conductance regulator (CFTR) is a 1,480 amino acid product coded for the long arm on chromosome 7. It is a glycoprotein and its function is to mediate ATP related chloride conductance. Deficiency of the CFTR causes reduced chloride conductance and consequent changes in sodium absorption by the cells. In the airways, excess sodium and water is absorbed across the cell membrane into the cell and this leads to a concentration of macromolecules and mucus in the airways. This, in turn, acts as a magnet for pathogens, such as *Pseudomonas aeruginosa*. There is also some evidence that the defective CFTR may also be proinflammatory leading to airway damage in early childhood.

Generally, groups 4 and 5 are associated with a mild phenotype. Some of these mild phenotypes may present only in adult life; in males, they may be first diagnosed in the infertility clinics.

DIAGNOSIS

Diagnosis is usually made in early childhood either by neonatal screening or by the development of symptoms, such as failure to thrive or intestinal obstruction in neonates. The diagnosis of cystic fibrosis depends upon a positive sweat test, gene analysis and also the clinical picture. Sweat testing classically involves pilocarpine iontophoresis, which is applied to the skin to stimulate sweat production, usually on the forearm. A 5 millivolt electric charge is then applied to the skin for 10 minutes and sweat is collected on a tiny piece of gauze. The chloride content of the gauze is then analyzed together with the difference in weights before and after sweat simulation.

Normally, sweat chloride levels are less than 30 millimoles/liters. The diagnostic level for classical cystic fibrosis is a chloride level of 60 or more millimoles/liter. The sodium content will also increase, although usually not to quite such a high level as the sweat chloride level. If an abnormal sweat test is recorded, it is usual to repeat the test to ensure accuracy. A small number of individuals will have a borderline sweat test between 30 and 59 millimoles/liter and this may be associated with the condition called *atypical cystic fibrosis*. These tend to be patients, who have mild symptoms and who are often diagnosed in late childhood, or as adults. Patients with atypical cystic fibrosis are less likely than classical CF patients to have pancreatic insufficiency.

CLINICAL FEATURES

Cystic fibrosis is a multiorgan disease. The lungs bear the brunt of the disorder with eventual recurrent severe respiratory infections leading to bronchiectasis. However, 85% of CF patients have pancreatic insufficiency and around 5-10% have significant cystic fibrosis related liver disease. Deficiency of micronutrients, such as vitamin A, D and E, iron, copper and zinc has been demonstrated in Indian CF children. The liver disease occurs due to chronic inflammation of the bile ducts which may eventually lead to biliary cirrhosis. Many patients with CF have a low bone mass, partly due to the effects of chronic infection, but partly due to the presence of the CFTR mutation itself. The sweat glands function abnormally and paradoxically produce a rise in sweat chloride and sodium levels, which is used (as detailed above) to diagnose the condition. Male patients are usually infertile due to inability of sperm to pass through the blocked vas deferens. With modern fertility treatments, sperm may be aspirated from the testes of such patients and *in vitro* fertilization may be possible. Generally, females with CF are fertile. Patients with CF are at increased risk of pneumothoraces.

The cystic fibrosis transmembrane conductance regulator (CFTR) abnormality leads to the development of thick and highly viscous sputum in the airways, which is very difficult for the patient to expectorate and also is an ideal area for bacterial colonization. The bacteria involved in respiratory infections in CF patients vary according to age. *Haemophilus influenzae* and *Staphylococcus aureus* are typical bacterial infections in earlier childhood. As the patient grows older, it is more likely that *Pseudomonas aeruginosa* will become the predominant pathogen and by late teens, over 50% of patients will be colonized with this organism. Chronic colonization may then lead to intermittent acute exacerbations leading to increasing shortness of breath and increased purulent sputum volume.

INFECTIONS AND TREATMENT

The cornerstone of treatment is to reduce the viscosity of sputum, improve airway clearance, treat lung infections vigorously and use anti-inflammatory agents. There is a considerable amount of research currently underway looking at the possibility of gene therapy and also drugs to influence ion transport.

An essential part of treatment is to modify and improve the nutrition of CF patients. Pancreatic insufficiency leads to poor fat absorption, which in turn, leads to abdominal symptoms of distension, diarrhea and malabsorption. Consequently, malnutrition leads to a stunting of growth and increased risk of severe lung infections.

Other pathogens in cystic fibrosis, which are less common than *Pseudomonas aeruginosa,* include the *Burkholderia cepacia* complex. The

Burkholderia complex is highly infectious and damaging to lung tissues and patients may deteriorate rapidly once they acquire this infection. Other gram-negative organisms, which may be isolated from the sputum, include *Stenotrophomonas maltophilia*, *Acinetobacter* and *Pandorea* species. Some of these relatively rare gram-negative organisms may emerge due to the long-term effects of antibiotic pressure caused by the need for recurrent courses of intravenous antibiotics in CF patients. *Aspergillus fumigatus* may cause a direct necrotizing infection in the lungs, but more commonly some patients with CF may develop allergic bronchopulmonary aspergillosis.

An increasing problem in CF patients is the appearance of atypical nontuberculous mycobacteria especially *Mycobacterium abscessus*, but also occasionally *Mycobacterium avium-intracellulare* and *Mycobacterium kansasii*. These nontuberculous mycobacteria are usually difficult to eradicate.

Specific treatments of known bacterial infections in CF are as follows: *Staphylococcus aureus* is usually treated with drugs, such as flucloxacillin or fusidic acid. Some patients acquire MRSA and may require intravenous vancomycin, teicoplanin or oral/IV linezolid. *Haemophilus influenzae* is often treated with coamoxiclav. *Pseudomonas aeruginosa* may be sensitive to oral ciprofloxacin and in some countries oral chloramphenicol is used (although there are concerns about its side effect of aplastic anemia). Often, *Pseudomonas aeruginosa* treatment requires intravenous antibiotics. The usual practice is to give at least two intravenous antibiotics together to reduce the risk of emergence of bacterial resistance.

Increasingly, long-term nebulized antibiotics are used in CF patients who are colonized with *Pseudomonas aeruginosa*. The aim is to reduce the bacterial load in the lungs and delay tissue damage. Typical examples of nebulized antibiotics that are currently in use include tobramycin and colistin.

Some older children and adults may develop abdominal distension and blockage due to distal intestinal obstruction syndrome (DIOS), previously called meconium ileus equivalent. Clinically, the patient complains of abdominal pain, bloating, vomiting or constipation. CF related liver disease can lead in severe cases to biliary cirrhosis, which may then lead to portal hypertension. There are lung complications associated with severe liver diseases, including intrapulmonary shunting, pulmonary hypertension and respiratory muscle weakness due to poor nutrition. Treatment includes the daily use of oral ursodeoxycholic acid. In severe cases, liver transplantation may be indicated.

The management of CF is based around a multidisciplinary team approach. This patient-centered approach promotes optimal treatment and improved life-outcomes. The CF team consists of doctors, nurses, physiotherapists, dieticians and clinical psychologists with additional input from specialists in diabetes, liver disease, infertility, etc.

Chest physiotherapy is essential to help the patient clear the airways and there are a variety of physical maneuvers and mechanical devices, which aid sputum production. Nebulized bronchodilators are often used to help as well.

Other Treatments

Cross infection between CF patients is a serious problem. Therefore, in outpatient clinics, both spacial and temporal separation of patients is required. Gene therapy is being investigated. The main problem has been finding a suitable vector, which enables sufficient epithelial cells to become transfected with subsequent incorporation of the normal gene into the host's genome. Initial results appear very promising.

Lung transplantation should be considered when the patient's lung function has declined with an FEV_1% predicted of 30% or less. When patients reach that level of lung function, the two year survival is around 50% and the potential advantages of lung transplantation should then be discussed with the patient.

CHAPTER
22

Anaerobic Bacterial Infections of the Lungs and the Pleura

Ashok Shah, Chandramani Panjabi

INTRODUCTION

Anaerobes as the cause of respiratory infection are infrequently recognized and rarely established. More often than not, these infections are caused by endogenous organisms that predominantly are commensals of the upper respiratory tract. Disruption of the harmonious relationship between the host and the bacteria leads to various clinic-pathologic processes that occur with anaerobic pleuropulmonary infections.

PATHOPHYSIOLOGY

Anaerobic infections of the lungs and their suppurative complications are mainly caused by aspiration of bacteria that constitute the normal flora of the oral cavity. Any breach in protective mechanisms facilitates an inflammatory process, thereby leading to disease. Aspiration is likely to occur in patients undergoing general anesthesia or having altered consciousness. The presence of artificial airways impairs glottic closure and makes the patient more vulnerable to aspiration. When aspiration is due to esophageal dysfunction or intestinal obstruction, the gastrointestinal tract is the likely source of the causative bacteria.

OTHER PREDISPOSING FACTORS

Anaerobic lung infections can also occur following dissemination from preexisting extrapulmonary infections. The classical example of this is Lemierre's syndrome which is almost always accompanied by secondary seeding, most commonly in the lungs. Necrosis of the lung tissue due to stasis is also associated with anaerobic infections. This commonly occurs in bronchiectasis, pulmonary infarction and postobstructive pneumonitis secondary to bronchogenic carcinoma or a foreign body. The other mechanisms that can cause anaerobic infections in the lungs and the pleural spaces include hematogenous and lymphatic spread, and diaphragmatic translocation from subphrenic collections. Infection via the blood stream is noted in patients with septic thrombophlebitis of the jugular or pelvic veins.

NATURAL HISTORY AND CLINICAL CLASSIFICATION

The distinct clinical categories of anaerobic respiratory infections include pneumonitis, lung abscess, necrotizing pneumonia and pleural empyema. These different pathologic entities are believed to be manifestations of different stages in the natural history of infection. By and large, the predisposing event in most anaerobic lung infections is aspiration of normal upper respiratory tract flora, seen in up to 90% of patients. The dependent portions of the lungs are most commonly involved. In the supine position, either the posterior segments of the upper lobes or the superior (apical) segments of the lower lobes are involved. When aspiration occurs in the semirecumbent posture, the basal segments of the lower lobes are chiefly affected. The right lung is twice as commonly affected as the left since the right main bronchus is more aligned with the trachea.

Acute Anaerobic Pneumonia

The earliest manifestation of anaerobic lung disease is pneumonia. The anaerobic etiology may not always be established due to similarities with acute bacterial pneumonias. Involvement of dependent segments could provide the initial hint. With appropriate therapy, the pathogenesis is arrested at this stage and the disease does not progress further towards suppuration.

Lung Abscess

Approximately 10–14 days later, necrosis and liquefaction in an area of anaerobic pneumonitis leads to the formation of a lung abscess. A thick-walled cavity greater than 1 cm in diameter, often with an air-fluid level, develops within the pneumonic infiltrate.

Necrotizing Pneumonia

Necrotizing pneumonia is characterized by suppurative lung infiltrates with necrotic areas leading to multiple small cavities (<1 cm in diameter). In comparison to a lung abscess, a greater number of pulmonary segments are involved.

Empyema

Empyemas are defined as collection of pus in the pleural cavity. They result after either an ensuing bronchopulmonary fistula or as a direct extension from subpleural segmental pneumonitis. All the three clinical entities described above can be complicated by empyema. Spread from infradiaphragmatic and subphrenic collections can also lead to the formation of empyema.

Chronic Anaerobic Pneumonitis

The term chronic anaerobic pneumonitis is used when there is no evidence of either parenchymal necrosis or pleural involvement. Histopathologic examination of such lesions reveals an intra-alveolar or an interstitial infiltrate. Inability to procure an appropriate sample for identifying the causative bacteria renders this entity to be relatively uncommon.

Septic Emboli

Another rarely encountered disease process is the occurrence of septic emboli. Like necrotizing pneumonias, diffuse and discrete infiltrates that appeared due to embolization from anaerobic thrombophlebitis were documented mainly in the first half of the previous century.

ANAEROBES AND UPPER RESPIRATORY SYNDROMES

Lemierre's Syndrome

This disease, also known as postanginal sepsis and human necrobacillosis, is a form of thrombophlebitis of the internal jugular vein predominantly caused by *Fusobacterium necrophorum*. An acute oropharyngeal infection leading to a putrid peritonsillar abscess is most often the trigger factor for this potentially destructive disease. Septicemic spread occurs primarily to the lungs and also to bones and joints. A triad of pharyngitis, neck swelling/tenderness and noncavitating lung infiltrates is described.

Ludwig's Angina

This is a periodontal infection arising from the tissues surrounding the lower third molar teeth. Although Ludwig's angina is most commonly caused by *Streptococcus*, polymicrobial infections with anaerobes have been noted in up to 40% of cases. The key features include marked local swelling over the floor of the mouth which is usually associated with pain and trismus. Submandibular cellulitis ensues leading to impairment in swallowing. In cases of glottis obstruction leading to respiratory distress, tracheotomy may be life-saving.

Vincent's Angina

This is also termed *trench mouth*, and it is heralded by an acute and sudden gingivitis. This progresses to ulceration of the interdental papillae and necrosis of the gingivae. The most common pathogen is *Prevotella intermedia*. The acute necrotizing ulcerative gingivitis may spread occasionally to cause destruction of buccal mucosa, teeth and jaw bones.

Lung Infections

Lung abscess and empyema are the two most frequently encountered forms of anaerobic pleuropulmonary infections. With the advent of antibiotics, there was a significant alteration in the microbiological profile. During the decades of 1960s and 1970s, anaerobic microorganisms accounted for up to 40% of all patients with empyema.

Community-acquired Pneumonia

The incidence of anaerobic infections in community-acquired pneumonia (CAP) has not been studied in detail. In nosocomial pneumonia, it is not easy to establish anaerobes as the chief cause since patients are already receiving broad-spectrum antibiotics before sample collection. The role of anaerobes as a cause of nosocomial pneumonia, particularly ventilator-associated pneumonia (VAP), is now well documented. Appropriate measures to minimize the chances of VAP should be advocated.

Colonization in Artificial Airways

Anaerobic bacteria, which are present in abundance in the oral flora, frequently colonize the lower respiratory tract in hospitalized patients, particularly those on mechanical ventilation. This poses a significant risk for the development of life-threatening nosocomial pneumonias.

CLINICAL FEATURES

In patients with acute anaerobic pneumonitis without any associated suppuration, the clinical findings and radiologic picture mimic acute pneumococcal pneumonia. The common features include a febrile respiratory illness, peripheral leukocytosis and absence of bacteremia. Since the natural history of cavity formation and subsequent tissue necrosis take about 7–14 days, the presentation of lung abscess and empyema is subacute and the median duration of symptoms is around two weeks.

Foul smell is considered to be pathognomonic of anaerobic infections. The putridity is believed to be due to volatile short chain fatty acids which are the end products of anaerobic metabolism. Some anaerobic cocci do not produce the volatile fatty acids. While this characteristic feature is noted in approximately 50–60% of patients with lung abscess, necrotizing pneumonia and empyema, the incidence of putrid sputum is only 5–18% in patients with acute anaerobic pneumonitis. The absence of putridness does not exclude the possibility of anaerobic lung infections.

Chronic Anaerobic Pneumonitis

Chronic anaerobic pneumonitis is an uncommon clinical entity. Patients with chronic anaerobic pneumonitis usually present as an indolent disease with a protracted course. The mean duration of illness is usually weeks to months rather than a few days. Chronic anaerobic pneumonitis can easily be mistaken for pulmonary tuberculosis in high tuberculous prevalent areas. Chronicity is attributed to the selective but paucibacillary presence of anaerobes. This is unlike other forms of anaerobic pleuropulmonary infections where there is associated polymicrobial aerobic growth.

LABORATORY DIAGNOSIS

Since the anaerobes have an inherent property of inability to survive in the atmosphere, it is not easy to obtain specimens for microbiologic examination. Appropriate specimens that have been collected stringently in order to avoid contamination should be expeditiously sent in an appropriate transport medium to the anaerobic laboratory for specific anaerobic cultures.

Cultures performed on invariably *contaminated* samples containing dense anaerobic flora of upper respiratory tract are usually futile. Growth of normal oral commensals may be an indication of anaerobic lung infection. The specimens should be inoculated on at least three different culture media to get a definitive growth of anaerobic bacteria. Quantitative cultures are applied to achieve an etiologic diagnosis in as many of the specimens thus obtained. Newer techniques like gas-liquid chromatography have helped in detecting the metabolic end products of anaerobic bacteria.

TREATMENT

Subsequent to the advent of antibiotics, the prognosis improved significantly. During the initial few decades, penicillin G was the treatment of choice for more than half of the cases. Metronidazole too showed good bactericidal activity *in vitro* against anaerobes and initial results were encouraging. Other advantages of this drug included 100% oral bioavailability and a substantially lower cost of therapy. After initial promising results, studies with metronidazole were discouraging. During the same period, better clinical efficacy of clindamycin in comparison to lincomycin was demonstrated. Clindamycin should be the initial choice for empiric treatment.

In recent times, although efficacy of several new antibiotics has been demonstrated in community-acquired pneumonia, the role of these drugs in bacteriologically confirmed lung abscess and empyema has not been systematically studied. Most of these agents show excellent activity against common aerobic respiratory pathogens including the trio of *atypical* organisms.

Amongst the fluoroquinolones, moxifloxacin and gemifloxacin have good *in vitro* activity against anaerobic organisms. Although ticarcillin and piperacillin, the semisynthetic penicillins, possess substantial anti-anaerobic properties, up to 30% of β-lactamase producing anaerobic gram-negative bacilli, especially *B. fragilis*, are resistant to this group of drugs. Imipenem, which belongs to the carbapenem group, is highly effective against β-lactamase producing *B. fragilis*.

Antibiotics should be continued until symptoms have subsided, any fluid collection has resolved or stabilized and there is appreciable radiological clearing. A minimum duration of 2–3 weeks is recommended.

Surgery

Surgical drainage is the cornerstone for management of patients with empyema. The frequency of surgery for lung abscess reduced drastically once effective antibiotics became available. In patients with lung abscess and necrotizing pneumonia without pleural involvement, the indications for surgery include failure of antibiotics and life-threatening hemoptysis. Lobectomy may also be indicated if an underlying malignancy is suspected. When surgery is contraindicated due to comorbid conditions, percutaneous catheter drainage is helpful in alleviating the symptoms.

CHAPTER 23

Bronchial Asthma Epidemiology

SK Jindal

INTRODUCTION

Asthma, although known since antiquity, remains a disease of unclear etiology, wide heterogeneity, and marked variability. There is no uniform agreement on its definition in spite of the fact that the problem is recognized and appreciated by even the layman, all over the world. For a clinician, it is characterized by episodic wheezing, breathlessness and/or cough. Functionally, there is widespread narrowing of the intrapulmonary airways and demonstrable and reversible obstruction. Pathologically, it is a chronic inflammatory disorder of the airways.

The Global Initiative for Asthma (GINA) Update (2014) describes asthma as a heterogeneous disease, usually characterized by chronic inflammation. It is defined by the history of respiratory symptoms such as wheeze, shortness of breath, chest tightness, and cough that vary over time and in intensity, together with variable airflow limitation.

The operational definition as above is fairly broad and comprehensive, but lacks precision. This is particularly difficult from an epidemiological point of view for the assessment of burden and comparative analysis. More recently, asthma is described as a syndrome consisting of many disease entities because of the presence of a wide clinical heterogeneity and overlap syndromes (Box 23.1). Further, asthma is recognized to present with a large number of systemic manifestations and other associations. Factually, asthma is now considered as a syndrome of a number of different diseases. These features make it even more difficult to define the disease and its epidemiology.

BOX 23.1: Overlap syndromes and disease entities of asthma.

- *Overlap syndromes and associations:*
  - Asthma—COPD overlap
  - Remodeled asthma
  - Asthma—obstructive sleep apnea overlap
  - Metabolic syndrome and asthma
- *Specific asthma entities:*
  - Allergic bronchopulmonary aspergillosis
  - Aspirin exacerbated asthma (Samter's triad)
  - Exercise-induced asthma
  - Churg–Strauss syndrome
  - Good's syndrome
  - Irritant-induced workplace asthma
  - Schnitzler syndrome

EPIDEMIOLOGY

The global prevalence of asthma is highly variable. In several countries, the disease prevalence is reported in about 1% to over 20% in different populations. Based on the prevalence figures, the overall global asthma burden was estimated at about 300 million patients in an earlier report.

These variations can be attributed to the differences in the environmental and climatic risk factors, the genetic predisposition and the inheritance patterns. Other important reasons, which can be counted for the difference, include the differences in the definitions used for the diagnosis of asthma, the type of sample selection and the methodologies employed in different studies.

While the prevalence of "current-asthma" from some of the European countries such as Belgium was reported as 1.2 and 3.7%, it is as high as 25.5% in Australia. The prevalence figures change according to definition used for the study; they are different for the disease when one employs the terms such as "diagnosed asthma," "recent wheeze", or "airway hyperresponsiveness (AHR)".

The mean prevalence of clinical asthma was reported as 3.5% for South Asian countries (Bangladesh, Bhutan, India, Nepal, Seychelles, and Sri Lanka) for a total population of 1.21 billion. Many of these estimates were based on limited data from selected regions; and may not, therefore, represent the overall population prevalence of a region or a country.

From India, the prevalence of as high as over 10% among school children is reported in some studies. The field prevalence of diagnosed asthma was about 5% in children and about 3% in adults. The average population prevalence was 2.4% amongst 73,605 adults of over 15 years of age, studied at four different centers in Phase I of the Indian Multicentric Study on Epidemiology of Asthma, Respiratory Symptoms and Chronic Bronchitis in Adults (INSEARCH) when a validated questionnaire and a relatively stringent definition of "ever-asthma" were used.

Phase II of the INSEARCH Study conducted at 12 different centers in a population sample of 169,575 individuals has reported a mean prevalence of 2.05% of current asthma. Another cross-sectional survey around the same period reported the prevalence of self-reported asthma as 1.8% among men and 1.9% among women. These figures point to a huge overall burden of asthma in India.

If one adds the numbers seen in children, the total number of patients could actually be higher. The estimates are likely to rise, if one uses different single criterion for diagnosis such as the "wheeze alone" or bronchial hyperresponsiveness (BHR). The prevalence in India, although somewhat lower than that described from the West, is similar to prevalence in other Asian countries. Some of the possible explanations, which have been advocated for a lower prevalence of asthma, may include the presumably protective influence of a higher incidence of childhood respiratory infections and ambient atmospheric pollution, which may partially suppress the allergic immune responses. A higher likelihood of breastfeeding in the Asian children may also be partially protective. The increasing trends in asthma prevalence, also in Asian countries, may suggest a rise in asthma burden in the near future.

Allergic bronchopulmonary aspergillosis (ABPA) is frequently recognized in about 10–15% of asthmatic individuals in India. This is an important cause of difficult or poorly controlled asthma. At the primary healthcare levels, more than half of the ABPA patients are known to have received antitubercular treatment because of the similarities in the clinical and the radiological findings before the diagnosis is established.

DISEASE BURDEN

Asthma is responsible for a significant disease morbidity. In children, the frequent absenteeism from school due to illness episodes constitutes an important cause of poor scholastic performance. Poor control may also result in irreversibility of airway obstruction and impairment of lung function later in adulthood. In adults, it results in poor work efficiency and loss of days of productive work.

There is also a huge burden from economic cost of asthma. The economic burden is related to the direct and indirect costs of management. Moreover, there are fiscal losses due to work absenteeism. The costs of "not treating" or mistreating asthma are even higher.

RISK FACTORS OF ASTHMA

The prevalence of asthma is influenced by several risk factors, which can be broadly categorized into the host and the environmental factors. The development is largely determined by host factors, while the triggering is mostly caused by environmental exposures. Some of the factors from both the host and the environmental groups may also overlap in their roles and cause asthma development, as well as the triggering of symptoms.

Host Factors

Age and Sex

Asthma is more common in children in the 5–14 years age groups.

It is twice more commonly seen in boys than girls in children of up to 14 years of age. However, the sex difference is not reported as the age advances. There is a higher incidence in women in adult age group. On an average, asthma incidence is similar in both sexes.

Genetic Factors

There is a strong family history of asthma and other allergies in the first-degree relatives of asthmatics. Genetic factors are, therefore, important in the pathogenesis of asthma. No single gene defect is identifiable in asthmatic patients. However, multiple genetic polymorphisms associated with clinical asthma and/or BHR have been identified; some of which may actually affect the bronchodilator responsiveness. Genetic factors are important determinants of susceptibility to allergic diseases and asthma. Recent studies have highlighted their role in determining the in utero development and early life susceptibility to allergies.

Other Host Factors

Asthma prevalence is different in different racial and ethnic populations. Both genetic polymorphisms and environmental exposures are likely to influence the differences in the prevalence. Nasal (allergic rhinitis) and skin (atopic dermatitis) atopies, sinusitis, and nasal polyposis are some of the common host allergies, which are strongly associated with asthma. They possibly share a common genotyping and pathogenesis. Nasal allergy in particular is said to exist with asthma as an essential companion—"one airway-one disease".

Obesity is an important risk factor recognized in several reports. In obesity, nonatopic mechanisms are more relevant in causing asthma.

Environmental Factors

Several environmental exposures, such as aeroallergens, occupational agents, tobacco smoke, outdoor and indoor air pollutants, and possibly infectious agents have been implicated in the development of asthma. Some of these agents may also act as "precipitating" or "aggravating" factors (triggers) for clinical symptoms of asthma.

Residence in the urban areas and lower socioeconomic status are other important factors likely to increase the occurrence of asthma. Tobacco smoking of all types, including the cigarettes, "bidis", and "hookah," as well as the passive exposure to environmental tobacco smoke (ETS) from other smokers may provoke asthma. Both "in utero" and childhood smoking exposure may also have an important role in the causation of asthma and BHR in children, as well as in adults. Indoor exposure at home to pollutants from combustion of domestic biomass fuel may act in a similar fashion.

Allergens

The role of allergens in asthma development is not entirely clear. House dust mites, contact with domestic pets, and exposure to a number of aeroallergens can precipitate and manifest asthma. Pollens of several plants, such as *Prosopis, Ricinus, Argemone, Amaranthus, Cannabis, Parthenium,* etc. have been implicated in the causation of asthma in India. Similarly, inhalation of several other air-borne allergens such as fungal spores, insect debris, and pet animals' dander has been recognized as risk factors for asthma. Early exposure to cat and dog dander has been reported as protective against allergen sensitization in some studies, while others suggest that it increases the risk.

Infections

Infections, especially from viruses such as respiratory syncytial virus (RSV) and parainfluenza virus are the most commonly identified triggers of asthma. This is especially so in case of children. Accordingly to some reports, early childhood infections may result in early maturation of T-helper 1 (Th1) over Th2 lymphocytes, thus having a protective effect against asthma (hygiene hypothesis). This may possibly explain the lower asthma prevalence in the developing countries, including India. This hypothesis is, however, not supported by several other reports.

The common organisms, which have been cultured from bronchoalveolar lavage samples, are the viruses (adenovirus, parainfluenza, RSV, and influenza), *Mycoplasma,* and *Chlamydia*. They may have important role in asthma development, airway inflammation, and remodeling. Of various parasites, only hookworm infestations have been shown to reduce the risk.

Occupational Exposures

Airway sensitization and increased production of IgE commonly occurs in industrial and factory workers from exposure to occupational pollutants such as chemical vapors, irritant gases, metal fumes, and other exhausts. This sensitization may clinically manifest as occupational asthma.

Occupational asthma occurs mostly in adults, generally after an exposure period of month to years in sensitized individuals. Both immunoglobulin E (IgE)-mediated and cell-mediated immunological reactions are involved.

Diet

Foods are frequently blamed to aggravate asthma. There are very few types of foods, which can be definitely identified as triggers. Fish, eggs, certain types of mushrooms, bananas, and some beans have been listed as triggers in some studies. Processed foods are also listed amongst causes of asthma in some studies. Breastfeeding during infancy is shown to be protective against asthma. On the other hand, infants fed with formula milk or soy proteins have higher incidence of asthma.

The presence of gastroesophageal reflux (GER) is considered as an important trigger especially in patients with nocturnal asthma, though the relationship of GER with asthma has recently been disputed. It was shown in a large double-blind trial that silent GER was not a likely cause of poorly controlled asthma.

SUMMARY

In summary, pathogenesis of asthma involves a complex interplay of different mechanisms, which result in a common clinical presentation of widespread airway obstruction. There are large epidemiological and clinical variations in the disease spectrum. Several of these differences are perhaps based on different inflammatory phenotypes, which are now unfolding.

CHAPTER 24

Airway Inflammation and Remodeling

Ruby Pawankar, Shu Hashimoto, Miyuki Hayashi,
Shingo Yamanishi, Manabu Nonaka

INTRODUCTION

Allergic rhinitis (AR) and asthma are considered as part of a chronic respiratory allergic syndrome, based on the unifying concept of "One airway—One disease".

Allergic asthma is characterized by the presence of immunoglobulin E (IgE) antibodies to common environmental allergens. Similarly, AR is an IgE-mediated inflammatory disease modulated by T-helper 2-type (Th2) cells. Almost 80% of asthma in children and 50% in adults are of allergic asthma origin.

Airway epithelial alterations lead to airway remodeling. This happens due to various changes such as epithelial shedding and denudation, goblet cell metaplasia and enlargement of bronchial mucous glands. Morphologically, various changes that occur in the airways include: (i) increased mucous production, (ii) subepithelial fibrosis, (iii) extracellular matrix deposition, (iv) increased airway muscle mass, and (v) vascularization.

Chronic inflammation is also responsible for tissue injury. Repair process also goes on in-between the inflammatory exacerbations. Airway remodeling is associated with poorly reversible or nonreversible airway narrowing, more severe airflow limitation and airway hyperresponsiveness in all the components of adult severe asthma.

Although much more is known in terms of the inflammatory mechanisms underlying AR and asthma, there is still a gap in our understanding of the cellular and molecular pathways involved in remodeling. Persistent eosinophilic inflammation predisposes to airway remodeling. There is also vascular remodeling possibly attributable to expression of vascular endothelial growth factor (VEGF). Vascular remodeling bears an inverse relationship with bronchodilation measured with post-bronchodilator FEV_1.

It was previously believed that airway remodeling happens later in life due to disease chronicity. It is now known that remodeling may begin early in life in children synchronously with ongoing inflammation rather than as a sequelae of inflammation.

CHRONIC INFLAMMATION IN ALLERGIC RHINITIS AND ASTHMA

Inflammatory Response

The inhaled allergens enter the airway epithelium through penetration of the mucociliary lining or via direct uptake by epithelial cells. The Th2 cells get activated by the inhaled allergens producing IL-4, IL-5 and IL-13; IgE production is then stimulated through interaction with B-cells. IgE binds to the high-affinity IgE receptors on mast cells. This cross-linking results in the beginning of a cascade of events such as the release of mediators (like leukotrienes and histamine) leading to increased vascular permeability. Continued recruitment of inflammatory cells causes release of more proinflammatory mediators.

Effector Cells of Inflammation

Mast Cells and Basophils

Mast cells are critically important in the early phases of inflammatory response as effector cells for both asthma and AR. Mast cells may also have a role in antigen presentation. They interact with airway epithelial cells to increase the production of cytokines and chemokines. Mediators such as TNF-α along with IL-4 and IL-13, increase TARC, TSLP and eotaxin production from the epithelial cells.

Basophils are also increased in nasal and respiratory secretions in AR and asthma. They also cause inflammation through binding of the allergen-specific IgE antibodies to the FceR1 receptors on basophil cell surface.

Eosinophils

Eosinophils increase in both the early and late phases of AR, correlate with nasal flow, IL-4, IL-5, IL-8 and IFN-γ, spirometric values, methacholine test positivity, percentage of predicted FEV_1 and bronchial hyperreactivity (BHR). Eosinophils are increased in symptomatic ectopics and increase in nasal, as well as bronchial epithelium and lamina propria after NAC.

Interleukin-5 plays a key role to modulate eosinophil differentiation and survival. One important therapeutic strategy for allergic asthma involves targeting IL-5 with anti-IL-5 therapy. This has been shown to result in marked reduction of peripheral blood eosinophils. But there is only partial abrogation of this response with minimal impact on clinical outcomes. Treatment with anti-IL-5 monoclonal antibody (mepolizumab) causes reduction in the levels of both peripheral blood and sputum eosinophil in patients with refractory, eosinophilic asthma. It also caused reduction in asthma exacerbations and use of oral corticosteroids. These results clearly imply that eosinophils are critical effector cells in persistent asthma and severe exacerbations at least in a subset of patients with asthma.

There is release of highly toxic granules and other derivatives from activated eosinophils which are responsible for damage to the surface epithelial cells. Subsequently loosening of their attachments causes shedding of cells into the airway lumen. The shedded cells admix with other cells eosinophils, neutrophils and mucus in the airway lumen.

T Lymphocytes

Patients of perennial AR show an increase in both activated (CD3+, CD25+) and naïve (CD45RA+) T-lymphocytes in the nasal mucosa. There is a correlation of memory T-cells with perennial AR. CD8+ T-cells correlate with mucosal mast cells in idiopathic rhinitis. There is disruption of the normal Th1/Th2 balance in both AR and allergic asthma. Some subpopulations of CD4+ T-cells (i.e. Th17 cells), which produce IL-17A, IL-17F, IL-22, TNF-α, and IL-21 may also play a role in the pathogenesis.

Neutrophils

Although neutrophils are predominantly increased in nonallergic infective rhinitis and chronic rhinosinusitis, the increased expression of activation markers on neutrophils and myeloperoxidase (MPO) levels in AR and increase in neutrophils in BAL after NAC suggests roles for neutrophils in AR. There are increased airway eosinophils and neutrophils in acute and severe exacerbations of asthma with a proportionately greater increase in neutrophils. Airway eosinophils are reduced following administration of inhaled corticosteroids. But the simultaneous increase in airway neutrophils and neutrophil chemoattractant IL-8 may cause some loss of asthma control.

Epithelial Cells

Airway epithelial cells act as a barrier against inhaled environmental allergens and other pollutants. Over the past several years, the roles of epithelial cells as effector cells have become more evident, directly via the action of inflammatory mediators, as well as via cell-cell interaction with immune cells. Moreover, its pivotal position in orchestrating airway remodeling and fibroblast proliferation is also crucial.

A number of inflammatory mediators, multifunctional cytokines and chemokines are released by the airway epithelial cells. Some of the mediators, like IL-1, IL-6, IL-8, TNF-α, GM-CSF, RANTES, eotaxin and TARC are important in the pathogenesis as well as in the migration and activation of immune cells.

Innate Lymphoid cells

It has been shown in the past that there is a role for innate lymphoid cells type 2 (ILC2s) in the development of lung inflammation from *Alternaria* species. The ILC2 may also increase airway hyperreactivity caused by influenza, and allergic sensitization due to dust mite and peanut.

Minimal Persistent Inflammation

Even when symptoms are absent in chronic inflammatory diseases like AR and asthma, a minimal level of persistent inflammation may persist. To prevent unexpected exacerbations, the treatment strategy may need to include its management. Immunotherapy and antihistamines reduce persistent inflammation by decreasing ICAM-1 expression in epithelial cells and eosinophil cationic protein in patients with mite-induced AR.

REMODELING IN ASTHMA

Airway remodeling is defined as the presence of structural change in the airways such as the epithelial fragility, reticular basement membrane thickening, increase of airway smooth muscle mass and hypervascularity. As a result, there is impairment of the normal airway function. Remodeling generally occurs in chronic and poorly controlled asthmatics with increasing severity. Some features may be recognized even in newly diagnosed or mild asthmatics. In addition, there is increase in the amount of fibroblasts and interstitial collagen, as well as mucous gland hypertrophy. These changes are more significant in the larger airways. Thickness of reticular basement membrane is the hallmark of severe asthma that is not usually seen in patients with mild asthma or chronic obstructive pulmonary disease (COPD).

Airway smooth muscles in the airways are placed in two opposing helices in a geodesic pattern. In the asthmatic airway, there is an increase in airway smooth muscle mass. There is also secretion of mediators by airway smooth muscle cells. These mediators may promote mast cell chemotaxis, proliferation and survival. On the other hand, interaction between airway smooth muscle cells and mast cells enhances activated complement-induced mast cell degranulation.

Measurement of airway function such as with FEV_1 does not give direct information on early inflammatory changes though it helps to provide indirect information on airway morphology and long-term inflammatory changes. Sometimes, inflammatory changes can also be seen in patients with asthma symptoms but normal lung function.

How Early can Remodeling Start?

Changes suggestive of airway remodeling have been studied with airway biopsies in children with difficult asthma. Both airway eosinophilia and basement membrane thickening were also seen in children with mild asthma

as well as in atopic children without asthma. Following inferences can be drawn:
- Airway eosinophilia occurs in mild as well as difficult asthma
- Airway inflammation is present before development of symptom of episodic wheezing
- Both airway inflammation and remodeling occur synchronously with ongoing and recurrent airway inflammation. Airway remodeling begins early during the disease pathogenesis, not as a complication or sequelae of airway inflammation.

CONCLUSION

In summary, remodeling in asthma involves variable degrees of inflammatory and structural alterations in the airways. There are several similarities in the inflammatory process of AR and asthma but remodeling is a feature of asthma, not present in AR. Several cells and inflammatory mediators play an active role in causing airway inflammation. In view of the similarities between inflammatory mechanisms of AR and asthma, treatment should focus on both the conditions.

CHAPTER 25

Asthma Diagnosis

Liesel D'silva, Parameswaran Nair

It is important to make a correct diagnosis of asthma for an effective disease management. A good medical history, physical examination, and spirometry are usually required for this purpose. Additional pulmonary function test (PFT), bronchoprovocation tests, measures of allergic status, chest radiography, and specific blood tests are not routinely necessary but may be useful when considering alternative diagnoses. Asthma is characterized by the demonstration of variable airflow obstruction that is reflective of a smooth muscle dysfunction. Airway inflammation may contribute to this variability of airflow but is not the defining feature. In other words, improvement in flow with steroids does not necessarily confirm the diagnosis of asthma.

CLINICAL DIAGNOSIS

Asthma is heterogeneous in character and may manifest with different clinical phenotypes. The criteria for diagnosis may vary depending upon the phenotype with which a patient may present.

Episodic symptoms of airflow obstruction or airway hyperresponsiveness are important to make the diagnosis. Airflow obstruction is at least partially reversible. It is also important to exclude the alternative diagnoses.

History in all new suspected patients should address the symptoms of cough, wheezing, breathing difficulty, chest tightness, and expectoration. Physical findings may substantiate the diagnosis, but their absence does not exclude the presence of asthma.

TESTS FOR DIAGNOSIS AND MONITORING

One cannot rely only upon the symptoms for diagnosis of asthma in view of their nonspecific nature. Following investigations are useful to substantiate the diagnosis.

Measurements of Lung Function

Spirometry is helpful to confirm the diagnosis of asthma and measures the severity, reversibility, and variability of airflow limitation. The important spirometric measurements in patients over 5 years of age include the forced expiratory volume in 1 second (FEV_1), and forced vital capacity (FVC) and peak expiratory flow (PEF). Prediction equations based on age, sex, and height are used to determine the expected values for these parameters. However, PEF has a large range of variations of its predicted values.

Caucasian prediction equations are most commonly used for the interpretation of the results of routine spirometry in India. One needs to assess the most appropriate prediction equation for use in one's own clinical practice after considering ethnic differences in spirometric values.

Spirometry

Spirometry should be accurately performed on appropriate equipment by trained personnel with monitoring of quality control. Spirometry with FEV_1 and VC values is an initial requirement and is better than PEF because it is more sensitive and discriminates between obstructive and nonobstructive ventilatory defects. FEV_1/FVC ratio less than 0.75–0.80 in adults and less than 0.90 in children suggests airflow limitation.

Normal spirometry does not rule out asthma in a patient with a history of asthma-like symptoms or in a patient taking asthma controller medications. Spirometry is often useful for excluding the possibility of chronic obstructive pulmonary disease (COPD). A low FEV_1 is also a strong predictor of a subsequent asthma exacerbation particularly in children. FEV_1 can be measured accurately even during acute asthma attacks and helps determine the need for hospitalization.

Peak Expiratory Flow

Although spirometry is the preferred method of documenting airflow limitation, PEF monitoring is valuable to confirm the diagnosis of asthma and to monitor the disease particularly in patients who are poor perceivers of symptoms, and to identify occupational causes of asthma symptoms. There are different methods of calculation for within-day variability and between-day variability in PEF. The range of predicted values derived from population studies for PEF is rather large and cannot be used for assessment of airway obstruction. Moreover, PEF also depends upon patients' effort and the peak flow meter used for the measurement. It is, therefore, advisable to use patient's own previous values for comparison.

Measurements of Airway Responsiveness

Measurement of airway responsiveness with direct or indirect bronchoprovocation challenges in patients with normal lung function.

Direct Challenges

Methacholine challenge is the most commonly employed direct bronchoprovocation test. It is a highly sensitive test performed with either the tidal breathing method or the dosimeter method. Methacholine is administered by inhalation in doubling concentrations (of up to 16 mg/mL) at 5-minute intervals. Single FEV_1 measurements are made at 30 and 90 seconds. Provocation concentration causing a 20% FEV_1 decrease is expressed as PC20 for the tidal breathing method and PD20 for the dosimeter method.

A positive bronchoprovocation test favors the diagnosis of asthma even though it cannot be considered as diagnostic. When a patient has current symptoms, a negative methacholine challenge result excludes asthma with reasonable certainty.

Indirect Challenges

In contrast to the direct challenges, the indirect challenges are more specific and thus, more valuable for confirming a diagnosis of asthma. Indirect challenge tests are the challenges of choice to evaluate individuals who may have exercise-induced bronchoconstriction and as a guide to monitor asthma treatment.

Noninvasive Markers of Airway Inflammation

A number of noninvasive measures for airway inflammation (in sputum, blood, urine, and exhaled air) have been evaluated in clinical trials, of which only exhaled nitric oxide and quantitative sputum cell counts have reached clinical practice.

Quantitative Sputum Cell Counts

Spontaneous or induced quantitative sputum cell counts provide the most valid, reliable, reproducible, comprehensive, and specific measure of airway inflammation. Sputum induction is safe and has a success rate of more than 80% in adults; however, the success rate is somewhat lower in children and induced sputum may not be possible in children of less than 8 years. Low lung function (FEV_1 less than 1 L) is a relative contraindication.

Sputum cell counts should be examined at least twice a year in stable disease and during exacerbations; quantitative cell counts should be repeated after treatment of an exacerbation with additional corticosteroid and/or antibiotic treatment. Determining the inflammatory subtypes of bronchitis with quantitative sputum cell counts will avoid the inappropriate use of antibiotics (and reduce possible antibiotic resistance) or corticosteroids (and reduce their side effects, including the potentiation of infection) and eventually lead to better management of asthma, reduce the overall cost of therapy and improve the quality of life of these patients.

Exhaled Nitric Oxide

Nitric oxide (iNOS), a marker of inflammatory response, is upregulated in the airways of asthmatics. Increased exhaled nitric oxide indicates increased iNOS activity. This is best assessed by measurement of fractional concentration of exhaled nitric oxide (FeNO). This is preferably done before spirometric maneuvers at an exhaled rate of 50 mL/second, which is maintained within 10% for more than 6 seconds. To ensure velum closure, the oral pressure of 5–20 cm H_2O should be maintained. Based on the mean of two to three values within 10%, FeNO is expressed as NO concentration in ppb.

There is an increase in the use of FeNO for assessment of eosinophilic airway inflammation in asthma. But the true relationship between FeNO and the underlying pathology in asthma remains unclear. There are both false-positive and false-negative results. Moreover, noneosinophilic bronchitis, which is frequently seen in asthma, cannot be reliably identified with FeNO measurement.

The FeNO in asthma has been used for its diagnosis, prediction of exacerbations, and tailoring the treatment. But there are ambiguities, since there are variations in the levels in the populations as well the individuals. There is a need to establish specific cutoff points for its values. It is more cost-effective to use induced sputum for FeNO measurements both as a surrogate marker for eosinophilic airway inflammation and to predict response to corticosteroids. Low values may point to the absence of airway eosinophilia and the indication to reduce the dose of corticosteroid treatment.

Exhaled Breath Condensate

Exhaled breath condensate (EBC) is an important tool for measurements of markers of airway inflammation. The condensed moisture on a cold tube from warm breath of a subject is collected and analyzed for airway pH and markers of inflammation (e.g. hydrogen peroxide, isoprostanes, and cytokines). It is a noninvasive measure, which appears quite attractive. But it needs to be standardized before its clinical application.

Measures of Allergic Status

Physicians commonly encounter patients with symptoms consistent with allergy. It can be difficult to determine that which allergen is causing symptoms from the patient's history alone. There are two main tests to look for an allergy status—(i) hypersensitivity skin tests and (ii) measurement of allergen-specific serum IgE (s-IgE). Before ordering the tests, the clinician should understand that which test to order and how to interpret the results. Avoid indiscriminate use of allergy tests, as they may be commonly associated with false-positive results. Skin and s-IgE tests should never be used as a substitute for a careful clinical history.

DIAGNOSTIC CHALLENGES

Preschool Children

Diagnosis of asthma in younger children of up to 5 years is particularly difficult. Symptoms of cough, breathlessness, and wheezing in younger children may also occur due to alternate causes, such as the following:
- Recurrent respiratory infections
- Allergic rhinosinusitis
- Recurrent aspiration due to dysfunction of swallowing reflex
- Foreign body in trachea or bronchus
- Vocal cord dysfunction
- Enlarged lymph nodes or tumor that may compress the large airways
- *Congenital problems*: Tracheobronchomalacia, tracheal or bronchostenosis, cystic fibrosis, bronchopulmonary dysplasia, congenital malformation of intrathoracic airways, primary ciliary dyskinesia syndrome, immunodeficiency, and congenital heart disease.

Tests for Diagnosis and Monitoring

There is no certain test but the following may help in making a diagnosis:
- Treatment trial
- Tests for assessment of sensitization to allergens using either skin testing or s-IgE.
- *A plain chest radiograph*: Chest radiography does not diagnose asthma but helps exclude infection (e.g. tuberculosis), congenital malformations of the airway, such as congenital lobar emphysema or other conditions.

Other Tests

Lung function tests, bronchoprovocation, and other physiological tests are difficult to perform in children with reproducible results, hence not reliable for the diagnosis of asthma in children of 5 years and younger. It is not yet clear whether exhaled nitric oxide levels can be used to differentiate different wheezy phenotypes.

Older Children and Adults

Diagnosis in this group can be often made in most cases from a careful history and physical examination together with the demonstration of reversible and variable airflow limitation by spirometry. One should, however, consider other causes of airway obstruction leading to wheeze in the differential diagnosis as well as when the patient does not respond to initial therapy. These conditions called asthma mimics may either mimic coexist with or complicate the diagnosis and management of asthma. Some of the common asthma mimics include the following.

Cough-variant Asthma

It is a subset of asthma with chronic cough as the main symptom with which the patient reports.

In addition, there is bronchial hyperresponsiveness and airway eosinophilia. Many adults with cough-variant asthma (CVA) develop typical asthma after a few years, which may imply that CVA in fact is a precursor of asthma.

Vocal Cord Dysfunction

Vocal cord dysfunction (VCD) occurs due to abnormal adduction of vocal cords during inspiration therefore causing sudden extrathoracic obstruction, choking, breathlessness, and wheezing. VCD is a distinct disorder but can occur in patients with asthma of all severity. Patients with both VCD and asthma present with nonspecific symptoms, such as dyspnea, cough, and wheeze, highlighting the need for a high index of suspicion for VCD in patients with asthma. The high prevalence of gastroesophageal reflux disease (GERD) (56.8%) raises the question of the role of acid reflux in the pathogenesis of VCD in asthmatics.

There is variable flattening of the inspiratory flow loop on spirometry; however, a normal flow–volume loop should not influence the decision to perform a laryngoscopy. Videolaryngostroboscopy (VLS) testing is required to definitively document VCD. In order to be diagnosed as VCD, the patient must demonstrate abnormal constriction during the respiratory cycle and also normal complete abduction during some portion of the examination; however, false-negative tests can occur because VCD is paroxysmal.

Gastroesophageal Reflux Disease

Typical GERD symptoms are present in about 80% of asthmatic patients who have shown positive pH probes. About 40% of patients have asymptomatic or silent GERD. Possibly, GERD may trigger asthma symptoms by direct bronchospasm and increased airway hyperresponsiveness. Alternatively, it may indirectly induce airway inflammation via microaspiration. Acid reflux may also be promoted by asthma drugs, such as beta-2 agonists and methylxanthine.

Determination of gastroesophageal pH with a pH probe is a highly sensitive test for diagnosis of GERD. However, it is not possible to say that these asthmatic patients are likely to benefit from GERD treatment.

Other Differential Diagnosis

Occasionally, several other conditions are likely to pose problems in the differential diagnostic of asthma. Some of these conditions include—congestive heart failure, pulmonary embolism, mechanical airways obstruction (benign and malignant tumors), pulmonary infiltration with eosinophilia, and drug-induced cough [e.g. angiotensin-converting enzyme (ACE) inhibitors].

Elderly Patients

The diagnosis of asthma in the elderly poses several challenges especially because of the greater chances of presence of comorbidities and difficulties in performance of tests. Greater reliance is placed on the presence of the following features—shortness of breath, chest tightness, usually dry cough, recurrent wheezing, nocturnal symptoms, worsening of disease at night, and precipitation of symptoms following exposure to cold air, exercise, or allergens.

Many older patients will have difficulty in performing PFT. Performing PFT has been shown to be feasible in up to 88% of outpatients aged 65 and older.

Occupational Asthma

It is first necessary to establish a diagnosis of asthma in a patient and then identify occupational asthma (OA). A thorough medical history and objective work-related testing usually provides a reliable diagnosis of occupational asthma. A detailed history for suspected OA includes chronological work history, job duties, exposures at work, onset and timing of symptoms, use of protective devices, presence of respiratory disease in coworkers, medication use, and past lung function.

It would be very helpful to have up-to-date material safety data sheet (MSDS) in place for every chemical or material that may pose an occupational hazard for patients. MSDS contains information that will help identify the suspect agent in the workplace.

Asthma and COPD

Airway disease can manifest with four different components, which can exist in various combinations—(i) symptoms; (ii) bronchial hyperresponsiveness; (iii) variable airflow limitation; (iv) chronic airflow limitation; and (v) airway inflammation. Both asthma and COPD are physiological characteristics— while variable airflow limitation is a characteristic of asthma, chronic airflow obstruction is seen in COPD. On the other hand, airway inflammation indicates presence of bronchitis. Overlap of different components can occur in different patients and variously manifest. These combinations can be labeled as overlap syndromes.

Airway remodeling in overlap syndrome: Subjects with severe asthma and chronic persistent obstruction have increased airway smooth muscle (15.65%) versus that (8.96%) seen in patients without chronic airflow obstruction; however, airway measurements on high-resolution computed tomographic scans revealed no differences between the groups.

Asthma and COPD overlap can be explained on the basis of the Dutch hypothesis, which considers that different types of airway diseases should be viewed as one entity with different components. The presence of one or more components is influenced by different host and environmental factors including tobacco smoke and air pollutants. Treatment in different patients is optimized depending upon the presence of different disease components.

Finally, it may be added that rapid advances in the "omics" platforms such as proteomics, transcriptomics, and metabolomics (e.g. breathomics) may provide signatures, fingerprints, or perhaps handprints of asthma that may become available for clinical use as point of care tests within the next few years.

CHAPTER

26

Control and Management of Stable Asthma

Sidney S Braman, Gwen Skloot

INTRODUCTION

Treatment protocols for the management of stable asthma have undergone considerable change over the past 60 years. Asthma is no more considered a single disease, but rather an umbrella term for multiple diseases with different phenotypes (i.e. observable characteristics) and different endotypes, each with its own unique mechanism of inflammation. Due to our increased understanding of the heterogeneity of asthma, attention has been directed to targeted therapy that addresses these differences. Better understanding of the pathogenesis and availability of new and safer drugs have made asthma management more optimistic.

GOALS OF ASTHMA TREATMENT

The short-term objectives of asthma management comprise treatment of immediate symptoms and control the fall in lung function. Long-term objectives are aimed at prevention of exacerbations. Therefore, treatment is directed toward both the objectives. There are four important components of asthma management: (i) avoidance and control of asthma triggers, i.e. respiratory allergens and irritants; (ii) careful assessment of symptoms and objective measurements of asthma control (questionnaires and physiological investigations); (iii) treatment with bronchodilator and anti-inflammatory drugs tailored to the needs of the patient in a step-up and step-down manner, and (iv) patient education.

ESSENTIAL COMPONENTS OF ASTHMA CARE

Avoidance

Environmental factors such as exposure (both indoor and outdoor) to pollutants, microorganisms and allergens are important for disease development in susceptible individuals. In particular, allergens and occupational factors are very important. It is, therefore, essential to identify the triggers and adopt avoidance measures as the first step of management.

There are a number of important household allergens that are important to avoid. House dust mites, cockroach allergens, fungi and dander of pets are most commonly identified triggers of asthma. Rodents are problematic as they excrete urine, feces, saliva and dander. House dust, a mixture of excreta of insects, mites, spores, danders, pollen grains and fibers, is highly allergenic. Removal of pets and rodents from the surroundings does not provide immediate relief since the allergen level takes months to come down.

Single-intervention efforts to improve environmental allergen control in the home are not likely to improve asthma control. Single interventions are likely to be unhelpful because most patients are sensitized to more than one allergen. Multiple-intervention environmental control studies have been conducted in high-risk urban asthmatic children with comprehensive allergen reduction methods. Interventions are required to control the moisture sources in the household to prevent the growth of molds. Control of house dust mite and insects is also important. Home visits have stressed behavioral changes such as smoking cessation, and offer an individualized approach to address pressing concerns, including asthma-related questions and social issues (e.g. poor housing, inadequate income).

Pollens of trees, grasses and weeds are important aeroallergens present in ambient air and frequently responsible for seasonal asthma. Food allergens, though frequently blamed, are not commonly involved in asthma attacks.

Asthma symptoms may also be worsened by air pollutants—both outdoor pollutants such as industrial and photochemical smog and indoor pollutants such as cooking and heating fuel exhausts, sprays and strong odors, particularly perfumes, insulating products, paints, and varnishes.

Both active and passive smoking are also blamed for worsening symptoms and deterioration of lung function. They are also reported to reduce the efficacy of inhaled and systemic corticosteroids. In children, long-term exposure to passive smoke from parents is shown to be associated with new-onset asthma.

While there is no compelling evidence that shows that emotional stress is a cause of asthma onset, there is some evidence in children and adolescents that psychological problems of the child and the caregivers can contribute to a worsening course of asthma. Interventions to reduce psychological burdens should be considered as they may improve the quality of life of patients with asthma.

Monitoring Asthma: Use Objective Measures of Asthma

Objective measurement of pulmonary function is helpful to confirm the diagnosis of asthma and to assess the disease control at various time intervals. While there is a poor correlation between the airway inflammation and lung function, physiologic measurements are extremely important in the management of asthma.

Treatment of Stable Asthma

Asthma Pharmacotherapy

β_2-adrenoceptor agonists: Selective inhaled β_2-adrenoceptor agonists are the main bronchodilator agents for the treatment of asthma, through their rapid and potent effects in relaxing airway smooth muscle. They are classified based on the duration of action into short and long acting. They produce bronchodilation by direct stimulation of the airway smooth muscle leading to relaxation via the activation of the adenylate cyclase pathway. Inhaled agents are preferred and they can be delivered by several different types of devices such as the metered-dose or dry-powder inhalers, as well as compressor-driven nebulizers.

Short-acting beta agonists (SABAs) such as salbutamol are widely used due to their acute (4-6 hours) bronchodilator effects and for the ability to protect against various triggers such as cold air, exercise and allergen. They are generally well tolerated, even with frequent use. Frequency of use is a measure of the level of symptom control. Anti-inflammatory treatment should be given when use of SABAs exceeds two times a week.

Long-acting beta agonists (LABAs), such as salmeterol and formoterol provide bronchodilation and improve bronchial responsiveness for up to 12 hours and indacaterol up to 24 hours. Like SABAs, they also inhibit the acute early allergic response, but in addition, they inhibit the late-phase response and airway hyperresponsiveness lasting up to 24 hours after allergen challenge. The use of LABAs as monotherapy should be avoided in the stable asthmatic.

Anticholinergic agents traditionally have not been part of asthma treatment plans since the short-acting agent, ipratropium, did not have the rapid onset as a reliever and was not as effective as a short-acting beta agonist. In poorly controlled asthmatics, adding tiotropium, a long-acting once a day anticholinergic, to a low-to-medium dose of inhaled corticosteroids (ICS) is as effective as adding salmeterol or doubling the dose of the ICS in an ICS/LABA combination in moderate—severe asthmatic patients. Also, long-term studies of severe asthmatics uncontrolled with an ICS/LABA combination have shown that tiotropium can improve lung function and increase the time to the first severe asthma exacerbation. Anticholinergic agents such as tiotropium, aclidinium and umeclidinium are now considered a valid therapeutic option for asthma as well as traditionally being used for COPD.

Inhaled corticosteroids: Since their introduction in the early 1970s, ICS have become the mainstay of treatment in persistent asthma. This is because of its proven efficacy, superior to other class of asthma therapy and also its lower potential for systemic side effects compared to oral glucocorticosteroids. They exert their anti-inflammatory activity via the glucocorticoid receptor complex that regulates gene transcription of proteins that inhibit proinflammatory cytokines. ICS have highly lipophilic compounds that have much higher binding affinity compared to hydrocortisone and also a highly efficient first-pass hepatic metabolism, resulting in lower systemic absorption. Clinically, they improve airway inflammation, hyperresponsiveness, airflow obstruction and symptoms in asthmatics. In the stable asthmatic with persistent symptoms, adherence to ICS treatment is of paramount importance as it has been associated with decreased risk of near-fatal and fatal asthma.

There is some evidence to suggest that higher doses of inhaled glucocorticosteroid may help to prevent progression to severe exacerbation as well as avoid the need for oral glucocorticosteroids. Use of "single-inhaler therapy" with budesonide/formoterol combination for both maintenance and relief is shown to be effective to prevent exacerbations. Side effects of ICS are both local and systemic. They are generally well tolerated especially at lower doses. One should be careful with the use of higher doses of ICS for self-management of asthma exacerbations for their potential side-effects.

Theophylline: Theophylline is usually recommended as an add-on therapy in patients who are not well controlled with ICS and LABA combination. For the patient with uncontrolled asthma, low-dose inhaled budesonide with theophylline compared to high-dose inhaled budesonide produced similar benefits and this may be achieved at theophylline concentrations below the recommended therapeutic range of 5–15 mg/dL.

Despite its attractiveness, side effects are the main limitation to its use. This is especially pronounced in the elderly where polypharmacy and potential drug-to-drug interaction are becoming more frequent. Theophylline has a rather narrow therapeutic window and unwanted effects are usually seen at plasma levels above 20 mg/dL. To avoid untoward effects, it is advisable to monitor blood theophylline levels.

Leukotriene pathway modifiers: The anti-leukotrienes may be used as first-line therapy when anti-inflammatory therapy is needed but they are generally less effective than ICS. They also have less effect compared with LABA as add-on therapy to ICS. They may, however, have special role in the aspirin sensitive asthmatic. If one is chosen, a therapeutic trial of 4–6 weeks should be allowed to determine its effectiveness. There is currently no evidence that supports its use beyond this time if there is no symptomatic improvement. The leukotriene modifiers may have an additive effect to ICS and inhaled β_2 agonist in the severe asthmatic when step-up care is needed. There is little data to suggest a role for the leukotriene modifiers for acute asthma.

Antileukotrienes are generally well tolerated. In a safety study over 3,000 patients, 4.5% developed reversible elevations of transaminases with zileuton after a few months of therapy. Reports of Churg–Strauss syndrome after initiation of zafirlukast and montelukast have also emerged, but it is likely that this has occurred as a result of systemic steroid withdrawal.

Oral corticosteroids: Systemic use of corticosteroids is reserved for patients with severe asthma, or, sometimes, as a trial of therapy to optimize lung function in patients with presence of fixed airflow obstruction despite conventional therapies. Both prednisolone and methylprednisolone are rapidly absorbed in the gastrointestinal tract. Because of the side effects of systemic corticosteroids, they should be avoided if possible in the routine treatment of chronic stable asthma even at lower doses.

Other Approaches to Asthma Treatment

Antibiotics: The role of *Chlamydia pneumoniae* and *Mycoplasma pneumoniae* in the pathogenesis of asthma symptoms and exacerbations has been suggested. As macrolides have both anti-inflammatory and antimicrobial effects that could target these organisms. The long-term safety and efficacy of macrolides for asthma care needs further study.

Biologic therapies: Biologic therapies are the newest treatments available for asthma and offer a personalized approach that can optimize outcomes and minimize adverse effects. IgE is recognized as a key component of atopic asthma pathophysiology. Omalizumab is an IgE monoclonal antibody that binds free IgE and decreases circulating IgE. It, therefore, decreases allergen-driven cell degranulation and reduces the release of preformed proinflammatory mediators and newly synthesized cytokines. This agent is used in difficulty to control asthmatics who are not responding to conventional therapy. This is also true of new anti-IL-5 agents such as mepolizumab and reslizumab that have shown benefit in patients with an eosinophilic phenotype of asthma that is identified by high levels of blood eosinophils. Multiple other biologic agents that target Th2 cytokines will likely become available to treat targeted asthmatics.

Allergen immunotherapy: Allergen-specific immunotherapy is the practice of administering gradual quantities of an allergen extract to a patient to ameliorate symptoms from subsequent exposures. Clinical evidence suggests that immunotherapy is effective to treat seasonal or perennial allergic rhinitis and asthma. It should be considered when conventional pharmacotherapy is not able to control asthma symptoms in an allergic individual. It has been shown to reduce symptoms and medication use and to improve overall asthma control, often without concomitant changes in lung function. It has also been shown to reduce the development of asthma in children with seasonal rhinoconjunctivitis.

Diet and Asthma

The relationship between dietary nutrients and asthma has been suspected but evidence from prospective and randomized trials is lacking. For example, although there is an epidemiological association between low serum levels of vitamin D and the development of asthma, asthma severity and recurrent exacerbations, recommendations cannot be made for vitamin D supplementation based on the evidence available to date. General advice for patients with stable asthma is intuitive: eat a balanced diet comprised of natural, non-processed foods with ample fruits and vegetables.

There is an association between obesity and risk for the development of asthma and, in addition, asthmatic patients with obesity generally have more severe disease with poorer control and decreased response to conventional treatment such as inhaled corticosteroid therapy.

Patient Education

Asthma management plans are designed to give the patients the skills for routine management of their disease and the ability to recognize and control exacerbations of symptoms. They are especially helpful in high-risk patients. They are usually offered by physicians and nurses but also can be taught by lay educators who have been shown to provide comparable outcomes when compared to nurse educators.

Self-management and education cause significant reduction of symptoms and improvement of quality of life. There is improvement of perceived asthma control and medication adherence. Use of glucocorticoids during the window period prior to a severe attack following a written action plan is also shown to reduce asthma mortality.

CONCLUSION

In conclusion, asthma management consists of a multi-modality approach with pharmacotherapy as the cornerstone therapy. It is important to maintain control of asthma with continued use of controller-drugs and other non-pharmacological approaches. Patient education is one of the other key component which significantly adds to the disease-control.

CHAPTER
27

Acute Asthma Exacerbations

Aditya Jindal

INTRODUCTION

An asthma exacerbation is defined as an acute or subacute worsening of symptoms and signs of disease in a patient with preexisting asthma necessitating a change in treatment. Sometimes, a patient may present simply with an acute episode for the first time or after a long period of months or years. Such an attack does not generally qualify as an exacerbated attack. An exacerbation is sometimes labeled as an "attack" or an "episode" of asthma. It also incorporates the other commonly employed terms, such as "acute severe asthma or status asthmaticus" to distinguish patients who require more intensive therapy, sometimes in a critical care unit.

TRIGGERS CAUSING EXACERBATIONS

There are a large number of environmental exposures and/or other factors, which are known to trigger acute exacerbations (Box 27.1). Not infrequently, the actual precipitating factor may remain unidentified. In some situations, more than one trigger may be responsible for an acute attack. It has been also reported that patients with more severe asthma attacks had higher trigger burden.

An exacerbation is more likely to occur in a patient with history of similar episodes in the recent past. It has been suggested that "frequent exacerbators" may constitute a distinct subphenotype of asthma with specific characteristics. Besides the asthma triggers, a number of risk factors are also identified in patients with asthma exacerbations (Box 27.2); these include—uncontrolled symptoms, poor adherence to treatment with inhalational corticosteroids

> **BOX 27.1:** Common types of triggers, which precipitate an acute asthma exacerbation.
>
> - *Respiratory tract infections:*
>   - Viral infections (respiratory syncytial virus, influenza, and rhinovirus)
>   - Mycoplasma pneumonia
> - *Environmental allergens:*
>   - Pollen
>   - Molds
>   - House dust mites
> - *Pet dander:*
> - *Tobacco smoke*
> - *Air pollutants and particulates*
> - *Exercise*
> - *Foods and drinks*

> **BOX 27.2:** Risk factors associated with acute severe exacerbations.
>
> - Uncontrolled symptoms
> - Poor adherence to inhalational corticosteroids
> - Over use of short-acting beta-agonists
> - History of recent exacerbations, hospitalization, emergency room visits, intubation, and mechanical ventilation
> - Pregnancy
> - *Comorbidities:* Obesity, major psychiatric disorder, food allergy, and rhinosinusitis
> - Poor lung function
> - Environmental exposures—smoking and allergens
> - Sputum or blood eosinophilia
> - Socioeconomic problems

(ICS), comorbidities, such as obesity, rhinosinusitis or food allergy, pregnancy, low Forced Expiratory Volume in Ist second (FEV_1), and presence of major psychiatric disorders. Some of these factors are also recognized to be associated with increased risk of asthma-related deaths; for example, the nonuse or stopping of Inhaled Corticosteroid (ICS), overuse of short-acting beta-agonists (SABA), history of near fatal asthma, previous hospitalization, emergency care visits, intubation and mechanical ventilation, and presence of comorbidities.

DIAGNOSIS AND EVALUATION OF SEVERITY

An attack may sometimes happen suddenly though more frequently it progressively develops over a few hours or days. Diagnosis is primarily made from the history of uncontrolled symptoms in spite of an increase in therapy. Characteristically, the patient complains of increasing breathlessness, cough, chest tightness, wheezing, and limitation in exercise capacity. There may be symptoms of respiratory tract infection, such as fever, sore throat, increased cough and sputum production. Nasal symptoms of excessive sneezing, rhinorrhea, and nasal blockade may also be present. Nocturnal symptoms may cause disturbance in sleep.

Physical signs may demonstrate tachypnea, tachycardia, presence of prolonged expiration, and wheezing sounds on auscultation. A severe case may present with the picture of life-threatening respiratory failure—cyanosis, headache, increased sweating, and confusion. Examination in such a case shows paradoxical pulse, low-blood pressure, hyperinflated thorax, and diminished breath sounds; wheezing sounds may not be audible in such a case.

Only urgent and essential investigations are required during an attack. Acute management should not be kept pending while waiting for the tests. Chest roentgenography is done to look for a lung infection and/or complications, such as pneumothorax and pneumomediastinum. Electrocardiogram is important to diagnose cardiac arrhythmias. Blood–gas and acid–base assessment is essential, especially for severer exacerbations. It generally shows hypoxemia, hypocapnia, and respiratory alkalosis. Normocapnia in the presence of tachypnea during an exacerbation points to a state of carbon dioxide retention, while hypercapnia and respiratory acidosis occur late in the course of severe exacerbations. Lactic acidosis is also described due to combined effects of both acute severe asthma and treatment-related effects.

MANAGEMENT

Management of Exacerbation

Management of an exacerbation depends upon the severity of an attack, the status of the preexisting functional status and the level of asthma control. The goals of management should be stratified as immediate, early, and long-term and action initiated, accordingly.

Guided Self-management

A mild exacerbation or early worsening of asthma can be recognized at home with help of guided self-management education. A written asthma-plan includes specific instructions about changes and addition of asthma drugs under appropriate medical guidance. The plan is generally helpful to abort a severe exacerbation.

Management in Primary Care

An acute exacerbation in a primary care set-up should be immediately managed. A severe exacerbation requires repetitive administration of SABAs, systemic corticosteroids, and controlled flow oxygen supplementation. While a mild exacerbation can usually be treated appropriately, a severe case requires transfer to a specialty/acute care setting.

Management in the Emergency Room/Hospital Ward

There is a serious threat of such patients worsening and entering into a life-threatening situation. Management is done according to the following principles:

- *Clinical assessment*: Besides the history of aggravating factors and essential vital signs, the objective parameters. However, management should not be delayed for any of the investigation.
- *Oxygen administration*: It is important to achieve and maintain normal arterial saturation (SaO_2 between 93% and 95%). Higher oxygen concentration of 100% may prove to be harmful and cause significant CO_2 retention. Oxygen is generally provided with the help of nasal cannulae or masks. Oxygen administration should be provided even if the facilities for arterial blood gas analysis/oximetry are not available. The treatment should be weaned off once the attack subsides and guided with the help of pulse oximetry.
- *Short-acting bronchodilators*: Bronchodilator administration is important to relieve airway obstruction and improve lung mechanics. SABAs are the first-line drugs due to the rapidity of their action. SABAs are administered either with the help of a polymeric Metered Dose Inhaler (pMDI) with spacer or through nebulization. It is generally recommended that continuous therapy with nebulization should be given for the initial period followed by intermittent on-demand administration. Salbutamol, levosalbutamol (racemic salbutamol), or formoterol is commonly employed. There is no significant difference in the outcomes seen with the use of any of the SABAs.
    - *Corticosteroids*: Systemic corticosteroids should be administered at the earliest within the 1st hour in all except mild exacerbations. Oral administration is preferred over the intravenous route. Administration of oral steroids for about a week is fairly adequate to terminate the acute attack; different dosage schedules recommended in different reports have been found to be equally effective. Patients on ICS prior to the exacerbation should not stop taking inhalational treatment. A recent study reports the additional benefit with use of nebulized high-dose budesonide in children with moderate-to-severe acute exacerbation on nebulized SABAs.
- *Other bronchodilators*:
    - *Anticholinergic agents*: Use of a short-acting anticholinergic (ipratropium) along with a SABA (salbutamol) causes greater improvement in Peak Expiratory Flow (PEF) and FEV_1. It is shown to be useful in causing a significant reduction in the number of hospitalization. However, other studies have shown no additional benefit over SABAs and systemic corticosteroids.
    - *Aminophylline and theophylline*: Intravenous aminophylline continues to be widely used in several developing countries. A meta-analysis of several studies has shown an increase in arrhythmias and vomiting with its use without any demonstrable benefit. As per the Indian Guidelines, aminophylline infusion can be used in patients with brittle asthma or when the delivery of nebulized drugs is not effective, such as in patients on mechanical ventilation with intense bronchospasm.
    - *Combined use of ICS and long-acting beta-agonists (LABAs)*: There is no clear indication to use an ICS plus LABA combination for an acute

attack. In one report, the use of high-dose inhaled budesonide and formoterol in patients who had received prednisolone showed similar efficacy as with SABA.

- *Magnesium sulfate*: There is some evidence to support the use of nebulized or intravenous magnesium sulfate ($MgSO_4$) in acute severe asthma. Intravenous infusion of 1.2 or 2 g over 15–20 minutes has been shown to reduce hospital admission in adults who fail to respond to initial treatment and persist with hypoxemia.
- *Antibiotics*: Antibiotics for acute asthma are used only in the presence of evidence of lung infection.
- *Leukotriene antagonists*: There is no significant clinical benefit with the use of either oral or intravenous leukotriene antagonists.
- *Heliox therapy*: Heliox is a mixture of helium and oxygen, which because of its lower density and higher viscosity is found to be more effective than air–oxygen mixture to administer oxygen. Heliox inhalation thereby reduces the work of breathing. As per recent review, there is a mild benefit with its use in both children and adults.
- *Noninvasive ventilation*: Noninvasive ventilation has no significant benefit except to reduce the dose of inhaled bronchodilators. Noninvasive

BOX 27.3: Indications for mechanical ventilation in acute severe asthma.

- Cardiorespiratory arrest
- Coma
- Refractory hypoxemia
- Refractory to initial management
- Drowsy, somnolent patient
- Cardiovascular compromise
- Failure of noninvasive ventilation

TABLE 27.1: Ventilator settings for acute asthma attack.

Setting	Recommendation
Mode	Volume assist-control mode ventilation
Rate	8–12/min
Tidal volume	4–6 mL/kg predicted body weight
I:E ratio	1 : 4 and higher, avoid inspiratory plateau except to measure plateau pressure
Waveform	Square waveform
Inspiratory flow	100–120 L/min
FiO_2	Titrate to maintain PaO_2 > 60 mm Hg or SpO_2 > 89%. Avoid hyperoxia
PEEP	Up to 5 cm H_2O
Plateau pressure	<30 cm H_2O
pH	>7.1 in young adults; >7.2 in elderly

(FiO_2, fraction of inspired oxygen; PaO_2, partial pressure arterial oxygen; SpO_2, peripheral capillary oxygen saturation; PEEP, positive end-expiratory pressure)

ventilation should always be administered under close supervision and continuous monitoring and should not be tried in agitated patients.
- *Sedatives*: Use of sedation should be strictly avoided because of the fear of respiratory depression, which can occasionally prove to be fatal.
- *Hospital discharge*: The patient can be discharged once he is back to his previous state of health and clinical stability is there for at least 24 hours. He should be able to eat and lie flat. He should go back to the previous inhalers and other medication.

Management in the Intensive Care Unit

A patient who deteriorates in spite of the intensive therapy in the ward should be shifted to the ICU or to a place where facilities are available for intubation and ventilation. Patient may require mechanical ventilation in the presence of refractoriness to initial treatment and other signs of persistent hypoxemia (Box 27.3).

Timely intervention helps in early recovery from the life-threatening episode. The principles of ventilatory support remain similar to ventilation in other conditions. Use of higher flow rates and prolonged expiratory time may be needed (Table 27.1).

CHAPTER 28

Allergen Desensitization

Vikram Jaggi

INTRODUCTION

The three main modalities of treatment of allergic diseases are avoidance, pharmacotherapy, and immunotherapy. Avoidance of common allergens is at best difficult and at worst impossible. Immunotherapy fills the gaps left by avoidance and pharmacotherapy. It is often effective for years after stopping the treatment. However, it is neither highly effective nor predictably effective in all patients.

DEFINITION

Allergen immunotherapy involves the repeated administration of specific allergens in low dosages to patients with immunoglobulin E (IgE)-mediated conditions. It prevents the occurrence of allergic symptoms and inflammatory reactions, which happen after natural exposure to those allergens. Presently, the preferred term is allergen immunotherapy, but it has also been referred to as desensitization (which is almost never achieved) or hyposensitization (which lacks specificity). Amongst the laymen, it has been frequently called as "allergy shots" or "allergy injections".

MECHANISMS OF ALLERGEN IMMUNOTHERAPY

Asthma is a complex disease in which many cells and cellular elements play a role. Allergen-specific immunotherapy, for the present, is the only etiology-based, disease-modifying treatment that induces rapid desensitization and long-term allergic-specific immune tolerance. The immune responses in asthma are skewed towards the abnormal T helper 2 (Th2) type responses and away from the normal Th1 type of response. Immunotherapy is shown to lead to the complex series of changes in the cellular, cytokine, and chemokine profile to steer the immune system away from the Th2 response toward a Th1 type of response. The following changes in cells and mediators have been noted with successful immunotherapy:

- *Allergen-specific IgE*: Specific IgE antibody levels may initially rise after immunotherapy followed by gradual and sustained reduction. Immunotherapy also decreases the seasonal increases in specific IgE levels that normally occur on exposure to aeroallergens.
- *Acute- and late-phase reactants*: Allergen immunotherapy blocks both immediate- and late-phase allergic response. It inhibits the recruitment of mast cells, basophils, and eosinophils that normally occur after natural exposure to allergens.
- *Blocking antibodies*: Successful immunotherapy increases the levels of allergen-specific IgA and IgG (particularly the IgG4 isotype). Allergen-specific IgG blocks IgE-dependent histamine release and antigen presentation to T cells.
- *Interleukins (ILs)*: There is an increased production of IL-12, a strong inducer of Th1 response. Increase in IL-10 levels causes reduction of beta cell antigen-specific IgE, and increase of the IgG4 levels. The proinflammatory cytokine release from mast cells, eosinophils, and T-cells is also decreased.

Although the changes mentioned above are clinically measurable, the correlation between these changes and clinical response is not consistent or strong. At present, these changes cannot be used to clinically monitor immunotherapy or its efficacy.

Indications

There are three main indications for allergen immunotherapy (Box 28.1): (1) allergic rhinitis (both seasonal and perennial), (2) allergic asthma, and (3) hymenoptera allergy.

BOX 28.1: Indications and contraindications of immunotherapy.

A. *Usual indications*:
   - Allergic rhinitis
   - Allergic asthma
   - Sting allergy

B. *Usually not indicated*:
   - Food allergy
   - Chronic idiopathic urticaria
   - Angioedema atopic dermatitis

C. *Caution required*:
   - Severe coronary artery disease
   - Unstable angina
   - Cancer
   - Unstable asthma
   - Uncooperative patients
   - Use of beta blockers

A potential candidate for allergen immunotherapy is a patient who has natural aeroallergen exposure, symptoms of upper and/or lower respiratory allergy, and demonstrable increase of specific IgE antibodies (to the clinically relevant allergens). Clinically, the ideal candidate is the patient with moderate-to-severe rhinitis and mild-to-moderate asthma induced by a few selected seasonal or perennial allergens. Allergen immunotherapy for asthma should be started only in patients with stable disease.

Selection of Allergens for Immunotherapy

A carefully taken history, knowledge of local and regional aerobiology, and corroboration with a properly performed skin prick test (SPT) will guide the physician to select the relevant allergens to be included in the immunotherapy vaccine for a given patient. SPT information is to be interpreted judiciously with caution. The results are not to be taken at their face value. For most patients, it is possible to find out less than four or five important relevant allergens. If more than one pollen from the same family has tested positive, inclusion of only the representative, one of them would suffice. Cockroach and fungal antigens have the ability to cause proteolytic degradation of other allergens, particularly the pollens. House dust mite antigen does not seem to have a similar deleterious effect on pollens, hence, can be mixed with pollens. A good allergy vaccine prescription should include comprehensive information (Box 28.2).

Schedule

The general principle is to start a dilute dose, which is gradually built up in concentration to the dose that is maximally tolerated or which gives adequate clinical response (build-up phase). This dose is then continued initially weekly, then fortnightly, and finally on a monthly basis for the maintenance phase. Certain patients would require a departure from this usual dosing schedule in that a more dilute dose is used initially and the increase in dose is more gradual.

Technique of Injections

The injections are given subcutaneously in the posterior portion of the upper part of the arm where there is maximum subcutaneous tissue. The injections can be alternated between the two arms. After the injection, heavy exercise is to be avoided for 1 hour for this can lead to rapid absorption, which may precipitate a systemic allergic reaction.

BOX 28.2: Prescription requirements of a good allergy vaccine.

- The relevant and confirmed allergens (not more than five usually; the lesser, the better)
- The starting dose (which is usually 0.1 mL of 1:5,000 dilution w/v)
- The projected therapeutic dose
- The frequency of injections (usually once or twice in a week initially in the build-up phase, then fortnightly, or monthly in the maintenance phase)

Duration of Allergen Immunotherapy

Most patients who show response to aeroallergen immunotherapy and demonstrate clinical improvement, once the maintenance dose is reached in 6–9 months time. The response is maintained during the immunotherapy. To prevent the relapse of symptoms on stopping allergen immunotherapy, it should be continued for 3 years in most patients.

Sustained clinical remission is achieved in most patients after discontinuation, while relapses may be seen in some. It is not possible to predict as to which patient is likely to relapse or maintain remission for long with the help of any test. At the end of 3 years of effective immunotherapy, a decision has to be made whether allergen immunotherapy should be continued or stopped. The decision to continue immunotherapy should be jointly made by the doctor and the patient. Immunotherapy should be continued in the presence of a good response of asthma maintained with monthly injections when there is no major inconvenience to the patient from a monthly injection. Most patients who have benefited prefer to continue monthly immunotherapy. Reasons favoring a trial to stop allergen immunotherapy to see if remission is maintained are allergic rhinitis rather than asthma; less than optimum response to immunotherapy; and a major inconvenience from the injections.

Allergic Rhinitis

A number of studies have shown a clear benefit of allergen immunotherapy in allergic rhinitis. There is significant improvement in symptoms, quality of life, medication use, and in immunological parameters.

It is also shown to prevent the development of asthma in these patients. The benefit may last for up to 3–6 years after completion of immunotherapy.

Asthma

Allergen immunotherapy is shown to be beneficial in asthma, which is stable with pharmacotherapy and is associated with rhinitis. In patients with single-allergen sensitization, allergen immunotherapy is also shown to prevent the development of new sensitization. It may also be effective in allergic rhinitis and asthma induced with house dust mite.

Bee Sting Allergy

Bee sting allergy is a "pure" reflection of a type I hypersensitivity reaction where allergy is demonstrated unequivocally to a single unambiguous allergen. Almost 80–98% of individuals will be protected from a systemic reaction upon sting challenge after achievement of the maintenance dose with venom immunotherapy. For bee sting allergy indication, immunotherapy is generally recommended for 5 years. The risk of a systemic reaction to sting is very low after discontinuation of allergen immunotherapy. The very high efficacy of allergen immunotherapy in bee sting allergy and its continued benefits even after stopping the immunotherapy is a good proof of the benefits of the therapy per se, provided allergy is clearly demonstrated, a single allergen is incriminated, and the vaccine is made using that single relevant allergen. This enhances confidence on the innate ability of allergen immunotherapy to be effective.

Side Effects and Risks

There can be local and systemic side effects. Local reactions at the injection site such as itching, redness, and swelling are quite common. The patients, in fact, welcome such reactions as an additional proof of allergy to that substance. They are generally less than 2-3 cm in diameter and subside on their own in one day. If troublesome, these can be managed by the local application of ice or with an oral antihistaminic. Such reactions generally do not require any reduction in the dose. Large reactions (greater than 2.5 cm) that occur repeatedly or after a day may predict a more serious systemic reaction; a dose reduction to the previously tolerated dose may be required.

Systemic reactions in the form of increased upper or lower respiratory allergy symptoms, urticaria/angioedema or hypotension can also occur rarely. A majority of such reactions occur within 30 minutes of the injection; hence, the mandatory 30 minute waiting period in the clinic. Most of the reasons responsible for systemic reactions are predictable and avoidable.

Very rarely, a severe reaction may occur in spite of all due diligence due to the inherent high degree of allergic sensitivity. The physician must be prepared and equipped to handle these reactions. Systemic reactions are managed in the usual way with adrenaline, injectable antihistamine, and steroid administration. Volume replacement is also required. Fatalities during allergen immunotherapy, although extremely rare, are reported.

Special Considerations in Various Patient Groups

Children Under 5 Years of Age

Immunotherapy is generally not prescribed for children of less than 5 years of age even though there are a few reports on its efficacy. It is aimed at preventing the development of asthma in these children with allergic rhinitis.

Older Children

In older children, allergen immunotherapy is effective and well tolerated. The clinical indications are similar as in adults. Response to allergen immunotherapy is generally better in children and young adults than in older adults.

Elderly Patients

Elderly patients generally respond less favorably to allergen immunotherapy. Further, presence of certain comorbid conditions like hypertension, coronary artery disease, or cerebrovascular disease makes them more prone to the risks of allergen immunotherapy. The fact that they may be taking beta blockers may make resuscitation difficult, if an allergic or anaphylactic reaction was to occur. But allergen immunotherapy can also be used in the elderly, if there is strong indication for its use.

Pregnancy

Allergen immunotherapy is effective in pregnancy. However, if an allergic or anaphylactic reaction occur in pregnancy due to allergen immunotherapy, it could have serious consequences on the continuation of pregnancy. For these reasons, the general policy is:
- Allergen immunotherapy is not initiated in pregnancy.
- If allergen immunotherapy is being given and is well tolerated, it is not discontinued in pregnancy.
- If maintenance dose has already been reached, it is continued at the same dose.
- If maintenance dose has not been reached, dose escalation is generally not done during pregnancy.

Autoimmune Disorders

There are concerns regarding allergen immunotherapy aggravating autoimmune disorders by their uncertain effects on various parameters of immune modulation. Most allergists hesitate to prescribe allergen immunotherapy to patients with autoimmune diseases.

Sublingual Immunotherapy

The conventional route of immunotherapy has been through subcutaneous administration. Sublingual immunotherapy (SLIT) is now being approved in the US after satisfactory results of trials with single-allergen immunotherapy.

Effectiveness of SLIT has been shown in both children and adults for both allergic rhinitis and asthma. It is effective against pollens (particularly grass pollen), house dust mites, and cat antigens. It generally takes longer (1-2 years) before there is improvement in symptoms. There is good theoretical support for the sublingual route for immunotherapy. The dendritic cells in the oral mucosa are different from the dendritic cells of the skin in that the oral dendritic cells have an increased expression of certain major histocompatibility complexes and costimulatory molecules, which make these cells particularly adept at antigen presentation. This may play an important role in directing subsequent immune effects.

Both subcutaneous immunotherapy (SCIT) and SLIT are effective though the SCIT has more often provided better clinical and immunological results. SLIT appears to a have a favorable safety profile as compared to SCIT. Local symptoms like itching and burning in the lips, tongue, and mouth are common. Mild gastrointestinal symptoms are also commonly seen. Rarely, aggravation of rhinitis, or even more rarely of asthma symptoms may occur. Anaphylaxis is reported, but is extremely rare. No deaths have been reported so far.

The SLIT is being widely used in Europe. There are a few questions, which remain to be answered before it is widely used—the optimum dose and dosage schedules for each allergen need to be clearly defined. Moreover, trials with mixtures of antigens are required and long-term efficacy compared to SCIT remains to be seen. With growing experience, this has the potential for greater use in allergic rhinitis and asthma.

Several modified approaches to immunotherapy have been tested to increase its benefits. These include the use of allergoids, alum precipitates, and most recently the peptides. Recombinant technology has been used to sequence proteins and produce allergens in large quantities for commercial use. Recombinant protein can also be modified to maintain its reactivity with T cells and hence preserve the efficacy, but decrease its reactivity with IgE antibodies to reduce the risk of allergic reactions.

CHAPTER 29

Patient Education in Asthma

Bharat Bhushan Sharma, Virendra Singh

INTRODUCTION

Patient education is an integral part of the treatment in almost all respiratory diseases, but its efficacy in evidence-based medicine is proved mainly in asthma. Asthma is one disease which starts in childhood and continues throughout life with marked fluctuations in severity. When a patient is sick, even to take a breath becomes a mounting task. In contrast, during symptom-free period, a patient considers himself as fit as a normal person. Patients must make day-to-day or even moment-to-moment decisions, in response to such fluctuations, mainly regarding self-medication or to ask for medical help. Factors like patient motivation, literacy and socioeconomic setup markedly influence such decisions.

GOALS OF ASTHMA EDUCATION PROGRAMS

The primary aim of asthma education is to keep the patient well and to impart ability to adjust the doses of the medicines according to an action plan. Reducing the costs is the primary aim for the healthcare services. The Global Initiative for Asthma (GINA) treatment has recommended the following issues for discussion with a patient:
- Asthma is a continuous disease
- Patient's expectation from treatment
- Patient's fears and apprehensions about asthma.

It is important to provide specific information to achieve a practical goal of a behavioral change. Review of basic principles is more useful than giving information on multiple general topics. It is also important to frequently evaluate the understanding and application of the learned behavior.

BENEFITS OF ASTHMA EDUCATION PROGRAMS

It is important to consider the following factors to decide the type of educational intervention:
- *Predisposing factors:* Patient's knowledge, attitudes, beliefs, and perceptions about the disease
- *Enabling factors:* Requirement of skills and resources
- *Reinforcing factors:* Required to make the behavior likely to be repeated or sustained over time.

METHODS AND SETTINGS

Methods

There are various methods employed in asthma education programs (Table 29.1). Written material should be provided for patient's future reference. Interactive computer programs on the internet can be individualized and used by the patients. Videotapes and other educational material may also help in individualized treatment.

As per the NAEPP guidelines, asthma education is recommended at all points of care to provide multiple chances to the patient to learn about asthma and build up self-management skills. Asthma education should be provided in the school as it helps a large number of children. Comprehensive asthma education programs in schools help improve symptom control and reduce acute-care utilization. Home-based asthma education programs significantly impact allergen control. Education on steps to decrease allergen exposure is important to reduce exacerbations, whenever allergens are considered as an important trigger.

ASTHMA EDUCATION PROGRAM COMPONENTS

It is important to use a written action plan as the most important strategy of asthma education. Patients should be taught to recognize asthma symptoms,

TABLE 29.1: Tabin Asthma education programs: Methods and benefits of asthma education

Methods	Improvements
Small group sessions	Knowledge of asthma
Individual teaching	Feelings of control
Large group lectures	Positive attitudes
Problem-solving sessions	Physical activity
Booklets	Inhaler technique
Diaries	Use of peak flow meters
Computer games	Peak flow rates
Promotion of peak flow	Asthma severity
Monitoring use	Reduction of school absenteeism
Repeated audits	Healthcare costs
Checklists	Emergency room visits/hospitalizations

understand peak flow measurements and appropriately respond to maintain asthma control.

What should be the contents of asthma education?
Patient is educated to impart skills in following aspects of asthma:
- Information on the two main components of asthma, i.e. inflammation and bronchoconstriction

Diagnosis
- Inhaler medicines and their benefits
- Difference between reliever (bronchodilators) and controller drugs (anti-inflammatory)
- Information on controller drugs which allow asthma control to be achieved and must be taken regularly instead of "on demand" basis.

Potential side effects of medicines
- Control of symptoms
- Early detection of exacerbation
- Monitoring control of asthma
- How and when to take medical assistance?

Different action plans have been shown to significantly reduce the morbidity. General counseling on nutrition, sleep, exercise and relaxation should also be given.

How to assess adequacy of teaching and understanding?
Immediate evaluation of the teaching session is done with the help of a questionnaire. Other indices of asthma control which can be used to assess the impact of education include the measurement of level of asthma control and use of healthcare services from the number of hospitalization, emergency room visits and days of absence from school or work. Assessment of quality of life and level of airflow obstruction are the other important parameters for determination of asthma education. It is important to repeat the assessment after an interval of a few weeks and every 3–6 months for long-term benefits.

PROBLEMS IN PATIENT EDUCATION

Exercise schedules and patient education are essential components of an effective respiratory rehabilitation. But there are many barriers to an effective patient education. Most importantly, these include the limited time available in the physician's office and the use of difficult medical terms which the patient does not understand. There is also a tendency to focus attention on management of the acute condition than the long-term control.

There are patient-related barriers, such as the denial of the diagnosis, stigma associated with the diagnosis of asthma and false expectations of complete cure. There are deeply ingrained beliefs about miraculous cures in some patients. Patient rarely appreciates the need of regular maintenance treatment. The fears and concerns about treatments including the inhalers especially the steroids pose special problems of counseling.

CHAPTER 30

Pharmacotherapy of Bronchial Asthma

Nusrat Shafiq, Samir Malhotra

INTRODUCTION

Two groups of drugs, controllers and relievers are used to manage asthma. In general, the controller drugs, primarily the anti-inflammatory agents are used for maintenance therapy. Reliever drugs, i.e. bronchodilators are used for symptomatic relief from acute episodes. Most of the antiasthma drugs are preferred through inhalational route.

CONTROLLERS: ANTI-INFLAMMATORY AGENTS

The major role of this class of drugs is for long-term control of asthma. These agents are not indicated when rapid bronchodilation is needed. Short-acting beta agonists (SABAs) are used for quick relief.

CORTICOSTEROIDS

Corticosteroids are amongst the most universal anti-inflammatory agents thereby reducing airway inflammation and hyperresponsiveness. Therefore, they form the cornerstone of asthma management. Both inhalational and systemic routes of administration are used in the management of asthma. Inhalational therapy is highly suitable for maintenance therapy, it needs lower doses and delivers the drug directly to the site of action minimizing the systemic adverse effects associated with corticosteroids. A large number of steroids are available for inhalational therapy. Their main differences are in pharmacokinetics, potency (budesonide > beclomethasone > flunisolide), dosing frequency and adverse effects, although most evidence suggests that they do not differ in the terms of efficacy. Systemic steroids are indicated when inhaled therapy does not work due to severe spasm during acute exacerbations, and also in chronic severe asthma. Dose should not be a deterrent, high dose must be used, usually needed only for 5–7 days. Prolonged use of systemic steroids requires to be tapered.

Pharmacokinetics

Corticosteroids are lipid soluble drugs, therefore, rapidly absorbed from the gastrointestinal tract (GIT), as well through inhalation and get widely distributed across the body tissues. They, especially the natural steroids, are the highly protein (globulin, albumin and transcortin) bound drugs. Their metabolism occurs mainly in the liver and they are excreted by the kidneys. Natural steroids are metabolized faster than the synthetic steroids, thus, have shorter half-lives, which coupled with their higher affinity for plasma proteins makes them less potent than the synthetic preparations. Many steroids have high first-pass metabolism leading to very low systemic bioavailability, for instance 10% for budesonide, 20% for fluticasone and just 1% for flunisolide.

Systemic steroids are needed for emergency management of asthma, but frequently misused for maintenance therapy. Prednisone is commonly used in asthma (30–60 mg/day) orally in the morning or methylprednisolone 4 mg/kg/day intravenously in four divided doses for severe cases. Hydrocortisone is cheaper than methylprednisolone but also has mineralocorticoid activity. Once symptoms improve, the doses can be reduced.

Adverse Effects

Corticosteroids are lifesaving drugs with an excellent risk–benefit ratio in asthma. However, they have potential to cause a large number of adverse effects, some of which can be severe, and others are serious. The adverse effect potential of inhaled steroids is lesser but may be significant. It is important to appreciate that while the dose-response curve of inhaled steroids plateaus at higher doses, the dose-systemic absorption curve is linear and continues to rise even at the high doses of inhaled steroids, with the result that even as the therapeutic effects plateau at a dose equivalent to 1,600 µg/day of beclomethasone, the probability of systemic adverse effects continues to rise with rising doses.

Systemic corticosteroid therapy is known to cause a vast number of adverse effects, their incidence and severity are directly proportional to dose (<7.5 mg/day of prednisolone is usually considered physiological) and duration of treatment, but are not dependent on the type of steroid used. The long history of their use has shown that short-course treatment (<5–10 days) even at high doses does not cause much toxicity. On the other hand, long duration of treatment even at relatively low doses is likely to cause adverse effects. The most common adverse effects during a brief course as is used during asthma exacerbations are mood disturbances, increased appetite, impaired glucose control in diabetics and candidiasis.

Steroid Withdrawal

There are two main risks of abrupt steroid withdrawal—(i) adrenocortical insufficiency and (ii) relapse of disease for which a steroid was being given. It is generally recommended to gradually taper the dose. The UK Committee on Safety of Medicines (CSMs) recommends that moderate dosage with corticosteroids (up to 40 mg daily of prednisolone or equivalent), for up to 3 weeks, may be stopped without tapering.

Drug Interactions

Enzyme inducers like barbiturates, carbamazepine, phenytoin, primidone, or rifampicin increase their metabolism, leading to decrease in their effects. An increased risk of hypokalemia occurs with concomitant use of potassium-depleting diuretics, amphotericin B, xanthenes and β-2 agonists. Concurrent administration with nonsteroidal anti-inflammatory drugs (NSAIDs) leads to increased incidence of GI bleed and peptic ulcers. Reduced efficacy of antidiabetics and antihypertensives may need dose adjustment.

In asthma, inhaled steroids are the drugs of first choice for prophylaxis and maintenance treatment in patients whose symptoms need regular use of beta-2 agonists. Their regular use decreases bronchial reactivity, provides symptomatic relief, reduces the requirement for inhaled beta-2 agonist "rescue" and also has "systemic steroid sparing effect". Their effects are apparent within a few days to a week, but maximum effects need months of use. Despite these advantages, they cannot be considered as curative drugs; however, there is clinical trial evidence to show that discontinuation of steroids leads to disease exacerbation.

Fixed-dose combinations of steroids with long-acting beta-2 adrenergic agonists are also available, for instance budesonide plus formoterol and fluticasone plus salmeterol. The combination has been shown to be synergistic and provides several advantages; the molecular mechanisms for the same have now been elucidated. It has been shown inhaled beta-2 agonists lead to the increased localization of steroid receptors in the nucleus and provide the additive suppression of release of inflammatory mediators.

LEUKOTRIENE RECEPTOR ANTAGONISTS

Leukotrienes, the products of arachidonic acid metabolism are highly potent bronchoconstrictors, the action is primarily mediated via LT1 receptors. While montelukast, zafirlukast and pranlukast are cysLT1 receptor antagonists, zileuton is lipoxygenase inhibitor; both the approaches are effective in asthma with decreased frequency of exacerbations (as effective as steroids) and improved asthma control seen in randomized trials. They have been shown to reduce symptoms, increase airway caliber, improve bronchial reactivity and decrease airway inflammation, but to a lesser degree than steroids. The response to therapy is less homogeneous as compared with other antiasthma drugs and patients can be classified into responders and nonresponders; only in responders can these drugs be considered as alternatives to steroids.

There are case reports of Churg-Strauss syndrome (systemic eosinophilia) with its use. It is recommended to discontinue treatment, although the causality has remained questionable. In some patients it had occurred after steroid withdrawal, which had led to speculation that asthma might have been a part of some undiagnosed vasculitis, which got unmasked by steroid withdrawal. Others have contended that Churg-Strauss syndrome may have been a precursor of severe asthma. Lastly, similar systemic eosinophilias have been observed in patients taking fluticasone and cromoglycate, a finding that points toward a nondrug cause. On the contrary, Churg-Strauss syndrome has been seen with other leukotriene antagonists, montelukast and pranlukast as well, which points toward a class effect.

Montelukast

Montelukast is probably the most commonly used compound of this class. It reaches peak plasma concentration in 3–4 hours after oral dose. It is similar to zafirlukast in most aspects, but has a longer duration of action. It is also licensed for use in children in reduced doses.

These drugs have been tried with varied success in several other indications, such as in rhinitis, bronchiolitis, cystic fibrosis, eczema, eosinophilic esophagitis, graft-versus-host disease, mastocytosis, sleep-disordered breathing and urticaria. The adverse effect profile is similar to that of zafirlukast. Suspected postmarketing adverse effects reported to the regulatory agencies include edema, agitation and restlessness, allergy (anaphylaxis, angioedema, urticaria), chest pain, tremor, dry mouth, vertigo, arthralgia, depression, suicidality and anxiousness.

Zileuton is an orally active 5-lipoxygenase inhibitor for use as an alternative adjuvant to long-acting beta agonist and corticosteroids in chronic management of asthma. The most common adverse effects are headache, pharyngolaryngeal pain, gastrointestinal disturbances, myalgia and sinusitis. Rarely, hypersensitivity, urticaria, rash, and leukopenia have occurred. Elevated liver enzymes and severe hepatic injury may rarely occur. It is, therefore, advisable to monitor liver function once monthly particularly in the first 3 months of therapy. It may increase the plasma levels (leading to toxicity) of warfarin, propranolol and theophylline.

Leukotriene inhibitors inhibit early and late bronchoconstrictor responses to antigens, not suitable for the acute attacks of asthma. Recently, it has been shown in a randomized trial in adults with acute asthma that intravenous montelukast plus standard treatment produced significant relief of airway obstruction (FEV_1) with an early (10 min) onset of action. These drugs are particularly useful for asthma induced by NSAIDs, cold air and exercise. They can be used along with inhaled steroids in patients with moderate persistent asthma and may have a steroid-sparing. Montelukast has been shown to improve both asthma control and asthma-related quality of life in patients insufficiently controlled with inhaled steroids or inhaled steroids plus LABAs.

MAST CELL STABILIZERS

Two drugs in this category, cromolyn and nedocromil probably act by several mechanisms: Inhibition of the release of mediators from mast cells, inhibition of white blood cell trafficking in airways, reversal of increased leukocyte activation, antagonism of substance P, inhibition of the effects of platelet-activating factor (PAF) and suppression of the effects of chemotactic peptides on blood cells. There is enough clinical evidence to show that pretreatment with these agents blocks allergen-induced bronchoconstriction making them suitable for use before exercise or allergen exposure. Moreover, their long-term use reduces the severity of symptoms and the need for bronchodilators. They are not as effective as inhaled steroids, but combination with steroids improves asthma control. Like anticholinergics, an N-of-1 trial for 4 weeks can help identify individual patients that respond best (or do not respond) to this class of drugs.

The first agent in this class, cromolyn is available in inhalational forms, administered in a dose of 2 mg four times daily. The dose may be increased to six or eight times daily, if poor control is a problem. Cromolyn is not indicated for the treatment of acute asthmatic attacks. Its withdrawal may lead to recurrence, should therefore be attempted under steroid cover if steroid doses were reduced because of its use. Also, the dose should be gradually tapered over a period of 1 week.

Nedocromil sodium is similar to cromolyn in most aspects, generally considered to be its alternative except that its duration of action is somewhat longer. It is usually started in dose of 4 mg (inhaled) four times a day. The other uses are similar to cromolyn. It has poor systemic bioavailability from the GIT. The adverse effects are mild, infrequent, mostly transient and do not require the discontinuation of therapy. Paradoxical bronchospasm is rare.

The major indication for the use of mast cell stabilizers is to prevent asthmatic attacks in patients with mild-to-moderate asthma. Nedocromil is not approved for use in patients less than 12 years of age while cromolyn is approved for use in adults, as well as children.

Anti-immunoglobulin E Monoclonal Antibodies

Monoclonal antibodies, which bind to the site on immunoglobulin (Ig)E antibody to prevent its binding to receptors (FCεR1 and FCεR2) present on mast cells and other inflammatory cells, are a new class of drugs approved for use in certain cases of asthma. Omalizumab is the prototype of this class of "biological drugs".

Omalizumab

It is a recombinant humanized monoclonal antibody targeted against IgE. Once it binds to IgE receptors on inflammatory cells, it prevents interaction of IgE with these inflammatory cells and prevents their release. It is produced in Chinese hamster ovary (CHO) cells in cell culture. It is approved for prophylactic use as add-on therapy to standard treatment in adult patients with moderate to severe, persistent, allergic, IgE-induced asthma. It decreases exacerbations, improves quality of life and reduces steroid requirements. It does not have a bronchodilator effect, has no role during acute exacerbations.

The dose is variable, ranging from 75–300 mg every 4 weeks to 225–375 mg every 2 weeks. The dose depends on the patient's body weight and pretreatment serum IgE concentrations. It is administered subcutaneously, it is not recommended to give more than 150 mg at one site. Injection site reactions, including erythema, stinging, bruising and induration are the most common adverse effects. Generalized pain, fatigue, arthralgia, dizziness, earache, GI disturbances, headache and alopecia are some other adverse effects. Flu-like syndrome and an increased incidence of infections (parasitic, viral) have been seen. Rarely, Churg–Strauss syndrome, hypersensitivity reactions, including urticaria, dermatitis, pruritus and anaphylaxis are reported. The temporal relation of anaphylactic reactions to omalizumab is unpredictable. The side effects may occur after the first dose or within a few days after a dose, or even more than 1 year after a patient is on regular therapy. Severe thrombocytopenia and an increased incidence of cancer are two other potentially serious adverse effects with its use.

Mepolizumab

Mepolizumab, a monoclonal antibody against IL-5, has received an orphan drug status for the management of hypereosinophilic syndrome. When given as an infusion to patients with refractory eosinophilic asthma with a history of recurrent exacerbations, mepolizumab reduced the number of blood and sputum eosinophils, had steroid-sparing effect in patients who had asthma with sputum eosinophilia despite prednisone treatment.

RELIEVERS—BRONCHODILATORS

The treatment of asthma achieved a landmark in 1897 when John Abel was able to prepare crude adrenal extract (*epinephrine*). Subsequently, in 1920s and 30s, many epinephrine analogs were synthesized, including isoproterenol. However, its beta selectivity was not known. Its use became widespread only in the middle part of the 20th century. Development of isoprenaline in inhalational form was a big step, but tragically caused thousands of deaths during the 1960s.

Bronchodilators are broadly classified as below:
- *Beta-2 adrenergic agonists*: Short-acting, long-acting and ultra-long-acting
- Methylxanthines
- Anticholinergic agents.

BETA-2 ADRENERGIC AGONISTS

Beta-2 adrenergic agonists are the most efficacious and widely used bronchodilators. They can be used by inhalation, or systemically provide excellent smooth muscle relaxation and rapid bronchodilation with relatively few side effects, thus providing excellent risk–benefit ratio. The most preferred route when using these drugs is inhalational because the mast cells are located close to the airway lumen and more easily accessible to this route. However, less than 10% of the inhaled drug reaches the site of action, the remainder is swallowed. In order to reduce systemic adverse effects, the stress is on developing drugs that have low systemic bioavailability [poor absorption from the gastrointestinal tract (GIT) or high first-pass hepatic metabolism]. Another strategy is to increase the drug delivery to lungs and simultaneously decrease the amount of drug reaching the GIT; for example, by attaching a spacer to the metered-dose inhaler (MDI).

Mechanism of action: Human lungs contain both alpha and beta adrenergic receptors; alpha receptors are not known to play any significant role in the regulation of the airway smooth muscle (ASM) tone. On the other hand, beta adrenergic receptors, subtype-2, are the most important regulators of airway smooth muscle tone. Traditionally, the mechanism of action of beta-2 adrenergic agonists has concentrated on airway smooth muscle relaxation mediated through elevated cAMP levels. Additionally, beta-2 adrenoceptors are expressed in inflammatory cells like mast cells, macrophages, neutrophils, eosinophils, as well as in type I and II alveolar cells. Activation of beta-2 adrenoceptors leads to the inhibition of these cells. This may additionally contribute to the benefits obtained with beta-2 adrenergic agonists.

Short-acting Beta-2 Agonists

The agents of this group are used by inhalational route mainly. They are considered the most effective agents for relieving acute bronchospasm. They are also indicated for preventing exercise-induced bronchospasm. If SABAs are needed more than twice per week, it is considered to indicate the inadequate control of bronchial asthma. Use of more than one SABA canister for quick relief of bronchospasm in a period of 1 month indicates an increased possibility of emergency department visit.

Salbutamol: Salbutamol (albuterol) is the prototype SABA. It is given by inhalation, orally and parenterally (but not in all countries). The preferred route of administration is inhalation, even though only 10–20% of the administered dose reaches the site of action while the rest is swallowed or left behind in the device. Salbutamol, unintentionally, but invariably swallowed from the inhaler device or taken orally as tablet, is readily absorbed from the GIT. Tremors and nervousness are the most common adverse effects, they are dose-dependent and seen in up to 20% of patients. Headache (7%), palpitations, tachycardia (5%), muscle cramps (3%), elevated blood pressure, insomnia, restlessness, weakness, nausea, dizziness, and chest discomfort/heartburn are also observed. Throat irritation or sore throat and nosebleeds can also occur. Other rare adverse effects, which are occasionally seen are: allergic reactions, rash, hives, throat irritation itching; difficulty in breathing; tightness in the chest; swelling of the mouth, face, lips or tongue; chest pain; ear pain; fast or irregular heartbeat; new or worsened troubled breathing; pounding in the chest; red, swollen, blistered or peeling skin; severe headache or dizziness; unusual hoarseness; and wheezing, swelling, bronchospasm or anaphylaxis (shock). Worsening of diabetes and lowering of potassium have been also reported. In a rare patient, inhaled salbutamol can paradoxically precipitate life-threatening bronchospasm.

Salbutamol should be given with caution in hyperthyroidism, myocardial insufficiency, arrhythmias, susceptibility to QT-interval prolongation, hypertension and diabetes mellitus. Hypokalemia should be kept in mind in severe asthma as the hypoxia associated with the condition and the concomitant drugs used in the situation may exacerbate hypokalemia. There are reports of abuse of salbutamol among both asthmatic and nonasthmatic (especially) young persons.

Drug interactions: Though pharmacokinetic interactions are not remarkable, pharmacodynamic interactions may be of concern. Concomitant use with other beta-2 agonists, corticosteroids, diuretics and xanthines may cause increased risk of hypokalemia. A propensity to cause hypokalemia increases the predisposition to digitalis induced arrhythmias. There may be adverse cardiovascular additive effects such as hypertension and tachycardia (if combined with tricyclic antidepressants or monoamine oxidase inhibitors). Similar interaction can occur with other stimulant sympathomimetic drugs, especially in patients with underlying coronary heart disease. Beta-blockers (especially nonselective) block salbutamol effects and bronchospasm may occur.

Use in asthma: For the relief of acute bronchospasm, 1 or 2 inhalations of salbutamol 100 µg may be given from a conventional metered-dose aerosol as required, up to four times daily. Two inhalations may also be given just before the exertion for the prophylaxis of exercise-induced bronchospasm. A dose, double to that of conventional aerosol is often required when the drug is administered in the powder forms. Long-term use of beta adrenergic agonists is known to reduce the efficacy of the agents. This has been attributed mainly to the process of receptor desensitization.

- *Bitolterol:* A long-acting beta-adrenergic agonist, it is the prodrug of colterol—a long-acting beta-adrenergic agonist synthesized mainly in the lungs. Although it has a long duration of action (>5 hours), unlike other long-acting beta-adrenergic agonists, it can be given for acute exacerbations of bronchospasm because of its rapid onset of action (about 2 minutes).
- *Orciprenaline:* Also known as metaproterenol, it is less selective for beta-2 receptors than salbutamol, therefore causes more adverse effects. When given by inhalation, its onset of action is 30 minutes and duration 1–5 hours. Because of its nonselective action, it has been used orally or by slow intravenous (IV) infusion in the treatment of bradycardia (like isoprenaline).
- *Pirbuterol:* It is a selective beta-adrenergic agonist with properties similar to that of salbutamol. The onset occurs in 10 minutes and the action lasts for 5 hours.

- *Terbutaline*: It is similar to salbutamol in most aspects except that its half-life is longer (16–20 hours). It is given mainly for the relief of acute exacerbations. It is available for inhalational, parenteral and oral administration.
- *Fenoterol*: It has a rapid onset (5 minutes) after inhalation. It was implicated in the asthma-related epidemic (increased morbidity and mortality) in New Zealand in 1970s and 1980s.
- *Oral beta agonists*: Oral preparations of beta-2 agonists have the disadvantage of a worse side-effect profile compared to inhaled preparations. A brief course of albuterol or metaproterenol syrup may be considered in the children of less than 5 years of age who cannot manipulate MDIs and yet have occasional wheezing. In occasional patients with severe asthma exacerbations, in whom the aerosol delivery causes worsening of cough and bronchospasm; oral forms of albuterol, metaproterenol or terbutaline may still be effective.

Long-acting Beta-2 Adrenergic Agonists (LABAs)

Long-acting beta-2 adrenergic agonists as well as ultra-long-acting agents are used for the maintenance therapy of asthma. The mechanism of action is similar to that of SABAs.

- *Salmeterol:* This LABA (duration of action 12 hours) is used for maintenance therapy in conjunction with corticosteroids. The onset occurs at 10–20 minutes, but the peak effect is delayed making it unsuitable for the treatment of acute spasm. The current practice in chronic asthma is not to use salmeterol as a substitute to inhaled steroids, but to add it to inhaled corticosteroid rather than increasing the dose of inhaled corticosteroid.
- *Formoterol:* Formoterol is a partial agonist, touted for lesser propensity to desensitization of the beta-agonist activity. Experimental studies, however, have demonstrated that at equally effective doses, all beta-2 agonists may be equally susceptible to desensitization. Like salmeterol, it has to be used in conjunction with corticosteroids. Addition of long-acting beta-adrenergic agonist to low or high dose of inhaled corticosteroids reduces the risk of asthma exacerbation compared to inhaled corticosteroid given alone. Inhaled formoterol is rapidly absorbed after inhalation. The plasma half life of the drug after administration is around 10 hours. Due to its rapid onset and long duration of action it is used both as a reliever and as a controller (in combination with corticosteroids).
- *Bambuterol:* Bambuterol metabolizes to terbutaline, the active metabolite. As result of slow metabolism, its approximate duration of action is around 24 hours. It may cause an increase in nonfatal heart failure in elderly patients.
- *Clenbuterol:* It is used in the dose of 20 μg twice daily, by inhalation. It is being widely abused by sportsperson for improving performance and also by farmers for improving the muscle mass of livestock. These effects remain unproven.

Ultra (Very) Long-acting Beta-2 Adrenergic Agonists

Attempts to further increase the duration of action of beta-2 agonists have been made so as to get compounds suitable for once daily administration, which by improving compliance, may also improve the outcomes. Most of these compounds are R,R-enantiomers of existing drugs since it is likely that these isomers will have less desensitization. Arformoterol, the R,R-isomer of formoterol has been shown to have duration of action of 24 hours. However, studies have also indicated that clinically important difference may not exist between the duration of action of formoterol and arformoterol. Carmoterol is another ultra long-acting beta-agonist with the structural elements of both formoterol and procaterol. In clinical trials, it has been shown to be as effective as formoterol, but is not yet approved. Clinical trials have also demonstrated safety and efficacy of another ULABA, indacaterol. It has, in addition to prolonged duration of action, a quick onset of action. Some of these agents are likely to be marketed soon. Many of the beta-2 adrenergic agonists are available as fixed dose combinations with inhaled corticosteroids while some are available as fixed-dose combinations with once-daily long-acting muscarinic antagonists (LAMAs).

METHYLXANTHINES (XANTHINES)

Theophylline, theobromine and caffeine are three important methylxanthines (some nonmethylated xanthines are under development). Aminophylline (theophylline-diamine) is a commonly used derivative of theophylline. The exact mode of action of xanthines is not known. The primary action (although at high concentrations, in vitro) is through inhibition of phosphodiesterases group of enzymes (PDEs), which in turn prevent breakdown of cAMP and cGMP, leading to their accumulation and effects such as relaxation of smooth muscle, stimulation of cardiac function, and inhibition of release of cytokines and chemokines (TNF-alpha, leukotrienes).

Although xanthines are nonselective inhibitors of PDEs (of which at least five types are known), the enzyme most likely responsible for their action is PDE4 (to a lesser extent, PDE5), located on bronchial smooth muscle and inflammatory cells. Attempts to make selective PDE4 inhibitors (designer xanthines) have not been successful, the development of at least three selective PDE4 inhibitors (roflumilast, cilomilast and tofimilast) has been stopped due to various toxicities seen at low doses.

The second important mechanism of action of xanthines is through competitive inhibition of adenosine receptors. Adenosine can modulate adenyl cyclase activity, cause bronchial smooth muscle contraction and histamine release leading to bronchoconstriction. In conclusion, xanthines have both bronchodilatory and anti-inflammatory effects, but which one is more important remains unclear. The other effects of xanthines include central nervous system (CNS) stimulation (especially with caffeine), positive chronotropic and inotropic effects on heart, stimulation of gastric acid and intestinal enzyme secretion, mild diuretic effect (especially with theophylline), and stimulation of skeletal muscle (including the diaphragm) contraction.

Theophylline

It is the prototype drug of the class available for oral and parenteral administration. Dosage of modified release formulations should be titrated for an individual patient. Parenteral preparations are seldom used. Elimination is primarily hepatic, the metabolites as well as the unchanged drug (10%) are excreted in urine except in neonates (50% excreted unchanged). Therapeutic drug monitoring (TDM) may be needed with its use, it being a narrow therapeutic index drug and having multiple interactions. An optimum therapeutic concentration is generally considered to be between 10 µg/mL and 30 µg/mL. Toxicity has been seen with the rapid intravenous administration of therapeutic doses of aminophylline resulting in cardiac arrhythmias.

The adverse effects commonly encountered with theophylline and xanthine derivatives irrespective of the route are gastrointestinal irritation and stimulation of the CNS. Serum concentrations of greater than 20 µg/mL are associated with an increased risk of adverse effects. Overdosage may also cause agitation, diuresis, repeated vomiting, cardiac arrhythmias, hypotension, electrolyte disturbances (such as hypokalemia, hyperglycemia, hypomagnesemia), metabolic acidosis, rhabdomyolysis, convulsions and death.

Aminophylline

It is a prodrug of theophylline (joined with ethylenediamine), releases theophylline in vivo. It is given slowly intravenously by slow injection (or infusion) in acute severe bronchospasm, at a rate greater than 25 mg/min. It is important to elicit drug history of the patients before the administration of intravenous aminophylline. In patients already on xanthine medication, it is safe to omit the loading dose or if possible, serum concentration estimated and the required dose calculated. It is also administered orally and rarely, rectally absorption from the latter route is erratic. Besides asthma, it is also used in the management of COPD, neonatal apnea and erectile dysfunction (local application). It has been also tried in motor neuron disease, methotrexate-induced neurotoxicity, and for removal of fat (locally).

Diprophylline

Unlike theophylline, diprophylline is largely cleared unchanged renally (half-life 2 hours) and does not need dose modification in patients with hepatic dysfunction. Unlike theophylline, drug interactions are uncommon. It is used in doses of 15 mg/kg, three to four times a day.

Caffeine

Caffeine is a xanthine that is more widely acknowledged as a CNS stimulant. It increases alertness and reduces sleep. In doses of 5–10 mg/kg, it has a bronchodilator action that is weaker (40%) compared to theophylline, which is why it is hardly used in asthma.

Xanthines (particularly theophylline and aminophylline) were used as first-line bronchodilators in the past, but their position was taken by steroids and beta-2 agonists. Xanthines are less efficacious and have greater potential for adverse effects. There has been a resurgence of their use for their anti-inflammatory properties and because of the availability of slow-release preparations for nocturnal control.

ANTICHOLINERGIC AGENTS

Airway smooth muscles express both M2 and M3 muscarinic receptors. Besides in airway smooth muscles, muscarinic receptors are also present in glandular and surface epithelial cells, endothelial cells and various inflammatory cells in the airway. Acetylcholine produces bronchoconstriction predominantly by acting through M3 muscarinic receptors. While the agents are useful in acute asthma, there is insufficient evidence for their role in chronic asthma. Specifically, they were shown to cause significant reductions in hospital admissions with favorable symptom scores, particularly in the respect of daytime dyspnea and daily peak flow measurements. These drugs may be used to provide additive benefit to SABA in moderate-to-severe asthma exacerbations or may be used as alternative bronchodilators for patients who do not tolerate SABA.

Ipratropium Bromide

It is a quaternary ammonium antimuscarinic agent. When given by inhalation, it causes direct bronchodilatation. Ipratropium bromide provides additive benefit to SABAs in moderate-to-severe asthma exacerbations, leads to somewhat higher and prolonged effect compared to either agent used alone. It may also be used as an alternative bronchodilator for patients who do not tolerate SABAs. When ipratropium is used alone, the bronchodilation by onset is slower, the magnitude is lesser and more variable as compared to SABAs. The exact cause of variability in response to ipratropium is not known, may be related to the intrinsic parasympathetic tone in a particular patient as well as the contribution of parasympathetic system in causing bronchoconstriction.

Being an anticholinergic, it is associated with the dryness of mouth, constipation (rarely paralytic ileus), tachycardia, palpitations and arrhythmias. Rarely, it can cause urinary retention (especially in the presence of prostatic hyperplasia) and precipitation of angle closure glaucoma. Patients with glaucoma should be advised to be careful while using these agents to avoid the mist entering the eyes. Antimuscarinics cause impaired drainage of aqueous humor while beta-2 agonists increase the production of aqueous humor; their concomitant use (which is routinely done) may be potentially harmful in susceptible patients. Rarely, paradoxical bronchospasm (seen also with other bronchodilators, may be attributable to some preservative) and hypersensitivity reactions (urticaria, angioedema, rash and anaphylaxis) have been reported.

Tiotropium Bromide

It is a long-acting quaternary ammonium anticholinergic agent (duration of action 24 hours) available for aerosol administration. About one-fifth reaches systemic circulation after dry powder inhalation and about one-third after inhalation of the solution. It should not be used for the initial treatment of acute bronchospasm, primarily used in the maintenance treatment of COPD, as well as of asthma. It is used once daily as two inhalations of 2.5 µg from the MDI. Besides the adverse effects seen with other antimuscarinics, pharyngitis, sinusitis, rhinitis and epistaxis have been reported.

Recent advances in anticholinergics have focused on the development of agents with lower systemic absorption and thereby having lesser adverse drug reactions, as well as on oral formulations. Aclidinium bromide is a long-acting anticholinergic agent selective for M3 receptors. The drug is being evaluated mainly for COPD and was shown to have bronchodilator effect lasting for 24 hours in healthy volunteers challenged with methacholine. With better efficacy observed when anticholinergics are used in conjunction with beta-adrenergic agonists, certain fixed-dose combinations have been recently approved, several others, particularly with tiotropium, are under development.

CHAPTER 31

Allergic Bronchopulmonary Aspergillosis

Ritesh Agarwal

INTRODUCTION

Aspergillus and other fungi frequently colonize the respiratory tract of healthy individuals. In hypersensitive individuals, it can be responsible for a number of respiratory conditions such as hypersensitivity pneumonitis, *Aspergillus*-sensitized asthma, severe asthma with fungal sensitization, and allergic bronchopulmonary aspergillosis (ABPA). Formation of fungal balls (Aspergilloma) generally occurs in preexisting chronic cavities. In a few patients, usually with immunosuppression and comorbidities, aspergillus colonization may progress to chronic pulmonary aspergillosis, invasive airway aspergillosis and invasive pulmonary aspergillosis.

Allergic bronchopulmonary aspergillosis (ABPA) is the most important clinical manifestation of pulmonary aspergillosis. It is attributed to the hypersensitivity to different antigens released by *Aspergillus fumigatus* usually in patients with bronchial asthma and cystic fibrosis (CF). Many fungi other than *A. fumigatus*, can also cause a picture similar to that of ABPA, known as allergic bronchopulmonary mycosis (ABPM). In countries with high prevalence of tuberculosis, almost a third of ABPA patients are initially misdiagnosed.

EPIDEMIOLOGY

An increase in *Aspergillus*-specific IgE levels (or an immediate-type cutaneous hypersensitivity to commercial or an indigenously prepared extract of *Aspergillus*) may occur in the absence of asthma which is defined as *Aspergillus* sensitization (AS), or *Aspergillus* hypersensitivity. ABPA, on the other hand, is defined by the presence of asthma along with features of AS. ABPA may develop in a small proportion of patients with AS in due course of time. ABPA is present in 1–2% of patients with bronchial asthma and in 2–15% of patients with CF in the population. Various studies from India generally report a higher prevalence of ABPA in asthma. In India, the total burden of ABPA has been estimated at about 1.38 million in adult asthmatic population of about 27.7 million at an assumption of 5% population prevalence of ABPA complicating asthma.

PATHOGENESIS

Exposure to high concentrations of *A. fumigatus* spores from garbage dump sites, agricultural conditions, bird droppings, and smoking moldy marijuana have been reported to cause ABPA. Not all asthmatics exposed to the same environment develop ABPA. Due to defective clearance in patients with asthma and CF, inhaled conidia of *A. fumigatus* and occasionally other fungi, are able to germinate. Consequently, there is growth of hyphae in mucus plugs. The immune response in AS/ABPA is a Th2 CD4+ T-cell response which is quantitatively increased in ABPA than AS. This aberrant response is currently believed due to the genetically susceptibility to the disorder, and several defects have been described in innate and adaptive immunity. Familial occurrence of about 5% has been documented in ABPA.

The fungi release antigens and exoproteases that compromise mucociliary clearance, stimulate and breach the airway epithelial barrier, and activate the innate immune system of the lung, including the epithelial and the alveolar production of several inflammatory cytokines. This leads to influx of inflammatory cells including the neutrophils and the eosinophils with resultant early- and late-phase inflammatory reactions. The inflammatory cells (partly contributed by fungal proteases) lead to tissue injury and the characteristic pathology of ABPA.

PATHOLOGY

The finding of proximal bronchiectasis i.e. involvement of segmental and subsegmental bronchi with sparing of the distal branches is typical of ABPA. The bronchi are filled with thick tenacious mucus plugs of dense eosinophilic material with many cells and granular debris. Histopathological examination shows the presence of mucus, fibrin, Curschmann's spirals, Charcot-Leyden crystals and inflammatory cells. Scanty hyphae are also demonstrable in the bronchiectatic cavities. The bronchial wall is usually infiltrated by inflammatory cells, mostly the eosinophils. The peribronchial parenchyma contains a mixed chronic inflammatory response, with conspicuous eosinophilia.

Recurrent or transient parenchymal opacities are generally the result of eosinophilic pneumonia. Occasionally, fungal growth in the lung parenchyma can occur in some patients with ABPA. Patients can also demonstrate a pattern similar to that of bronchiolitis obliterans with organizing pneumonia. Noncaseating granulomatous inflammation containing eosinophils and multinucleated giant cells, i.e. bronchocentric granulomatosis is present in the airways. Fungal hyphae may be identified in the centers of some granulomas in the peribronchial tissue. The pathologic appearance is quite distinct from that of necrotizing pneumonia with vascular invasion described in patients with invasive aspergillosis. In patients with ABPA and localized tissue invasion, the host response seems to be able to limit the growth of the fungus and severe tissue destruction does not occur. Rarely, cases of invasive aspergillosis complicating the course of ABPA have been described in the literature.

CLINICAL FEATURES

The most common clinical presentation is that of poorly controlled asthma. Patient may have symptoms of low-grade fever, wheezing, hemoptysis or productive cough. Bronchial hyperreactivity is frequently present. Expectoration of solid, brownish-black mucus plugs is a characteristic symptom seen in 31–69% of patients. Presence of hemoptysis, expectoration of brownish-black mucus plug, and history of pulmonary opacities all point towards the diagnosis of ABPA. However, patients with ABPA can be surprisingly asymptomatic.

Physical examination often reveals the findings of polyphonic wheeze but can be normal in some cases. Clubbing is seen in about 16% of patients, usually in patients with long-standing bronchiectasis. Coarse crackles can be heard in about 15% of patients. Physical examination is also important to detect complications of pulmonary hypertension and/or respiratory failure. During exacerbations of ABPA, localized findings of consolidation and atelectasis can occur. Clinical assessment alone may not be enough. Immunological investigations are generally required for the differential diagnosis.

LABORATORY FINDINGS

Aspergillus Skin Test

An immediate cutaneous hypersensitivity to *A. fumigatus* antigens using either a skin prick test or by intradermal injection of the antigen is a characteristic finding of ABPA. A positive reaction is characterized by development of a wheal and erythema within one minute which reaches a maximum after 10–20 minutes, and resolves within 1–2 hours. Intradermal tests are generally more sensitive than skin prick tests (SPTs).

Serum IgE Levels

A normal total serum IgE level excludes ABPA as the cause of patient's current symptoms, if the patient is not taking glucocorticoids. After treatment with glucocorticoids, the serum IgE level starts declining. In most patients, however, the levels do not reach normal values.

Serum IgE Antibodies Specific to *A. fumigatus*

A. fumigatus-specific IgE >0.35 kUA/L is the most sensitive investigation in the diagnosis of ABPA, and is currently the preferred test for ABPA screening.

Radiological Investigations

There is a wide spectrum of radiographic abnormalities seen in ABPA: transient or fixed pulmonary opacities often described as consolidation; mucoid impaction presenting as *finger-in-glove* opacities or presence of tramline shadows. Some patients may show characteristic finger-in-glove opacities and toothpaste shadows on their X-rays. In later stages, there may be fibrosis and collapse mainly affecting the upper lobes. This stage is frequently suggestive of the development of chronic pulmonary aspergillosis (CPA).

High-resolution computed tomography (HRCT) of the chest (1–1.5 x 5–15 mm) has high sensitivity and specificity to detect abnormalities that are not visualized on chest radiograph and allows better delineation of the extent and type (cylindrical, varicose, cystic) of bronchiectasis. Bronchiectasis, mucoid impaction, mosaic attenuation, presence of centrilobular nodules and tree-in-bud opacities are some of the important findings seen on HRCT scans. Bronchiectasis in ABPA extends to the periphery in up to 40% of the lobes involved by bronchiectasis. The ABPA working group has thus removed central from the bronchiectasis in ABPA. Further, bronchiectasis has been considered a complication and not a diagnostic criterion of ABPA.

Mucus plugs in ABPA can be normo-, hypo- or hyper-dense; hyperdense mucus is seen in up to 20% of patients. High-attenuation mucus (HAM) is a pathognomonic finding in patients with ABPA. It is radiologically diagnosed when the mucus is visually denser than the paraspinal skeletal muscle (Fig. 31.1). The presence of HAM was shown to have 100% specificity for diagnosis of ABPA. Thus, the presence of HAM confirms ABPA as the cause of underlying bronchiectasis. HAM is not only associated with an immunologically severe disorder but is also a marker of recurrent relapses. Some of the ABPA patients show uncommon findings such as miliary nodular opacities, perihilar opacities, pleural effusions, pulmonary masses and whole lung collapse.

Serum Precipitins (or IgG Antibodies) Against *A. fumigatus*

Present in almost 69–90% of patients with ABPA, they probably indicate the continued growth of fungus in bronchi or body tissues. These precipitins are however, not specific as they are also present in 1–10% of normal subjects, hospitalized patients, and other pulmonary disorders including asthma, SAFS and CPA. *A. fumigatus* specific IgG with titers >27 mgA/L is highly specific in the diagnosis of ABPA. The detection of IgG against *A. fumigatus* by enzyme immunoassay is preferred to precipitin detection by the traditional double-diffusion method.

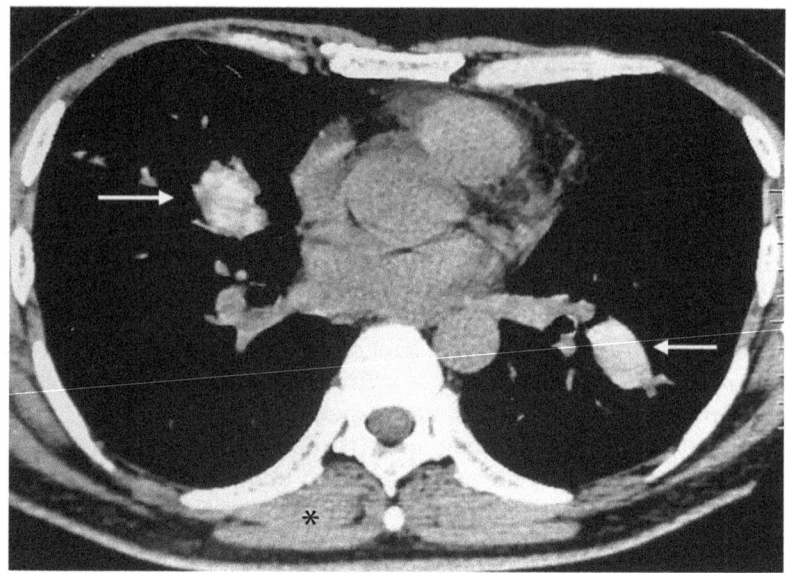

Fig. 31.1: Computed tomographic image of high-attenuation mucoid impaction (arrows).

Peripheral Eosinophilia

The total peripheral blood eosinophil count more than 500 cells/μL is commonly seen in patients with ABPA. However, a low eosinophil count does not exclude ABPA.

Sputum Cultures for *A. fumigatus*

Growth of *A. fumigatus* in the sputum supports the diagnosis of ABPA. But it is valuable only if cultures are obtained before starting antifungal therapy, and when susceptibility testing and/or real-time molecular testing for resistance of any isolates are performed. Sputum cultures are not required in routine care, if they are solely being employed for the diagnosis of ABPA.

Pulmonary Function Tests

These tests have no diagnostic value in ABPA. They are, however, extremely beneficial in monitoring. Spirometry can be used to assess and categorize the severity of asthma and/or the underlying lung disease. The pulmonary function tests generally show obstructive physiology with varying severities and reductions in diffusion capacity.

Role of Specific *Aspergillus* Antigens

Crude extracts from *Aspergillus* often used for testing of ABPA lack reproducibility and consistency. Moreover, there is cross-reactivity with other antigens. Recombinant antigens may find a more valuable role for diagnosis of ABPA.

DIAGNOSIS AND DIAGNOSTIC CRITERIA

The Rosenberg–Patterson criteria, that are a constellation of clinical, radiological and immunological features, are most often used for diagnosis of ABPA; the International Society for Human and Animal Mycology (ISHAM) ABPA working group, has recently proposed new criteria so as to simplify the diagnosis of ABPA (Box 31.1). The new criteria are simpler, more objective and thus beneficial in clinical research studies as they will facilitate a uniform diagnosis across the centers.

MANAGEMENT

There are two important aspects of management of ABPA:
- Initiation of immunosuppressive therapy (primarily glucocorticoids) to control the immunologic activity, and

---

BOX 31.1: Criteria used for the diagnosis of allergic bronchopulmonary aspergillosis.

Rosenberg–Patterson criteria (1977)

Major criteria
Bronchial asthma
Immediate cutaneous hyperreactivity to *Aspergillus* antigen
Elevated serum IgE levels
Elevated levels of *A. fumigatus*-specific IgG and/or IgE in serum
Central bronchiectasis
Fleeting pulmonary opacities on chest radiograph
Peripheral blood eosinophilia
Elevated serum precipitins against *Aspergillus*

Minor criteria
Expectoration of brownish-black mucus plugs
Delayed cutaneous hypersensitivity to *Aspergillus* antigen
Presence of *Aspergillus* in sputum

ISHAM (International Society of Human and Animal Mycology) ABPA (Allergic bronchopulmonary aspergillosis) Working Group Criteria (2013)

Predisposing conditions
Bronchial asthma
Cystic fibrosis
Obligatory criteria
Elevated total IgE levels (more than 1000 IU per milliliter)
Elevated IgE and/or IgG levels against *A. fumigatus* (>0.35 kUA/L)
Other criteria (at least three of five)
Immediate cutaneous hypersensitivity to *Aspergillus* antigen
Presence of serum precipitating antibodies against *A. fumigatus*
Radiographic pulmonary opacities (fixed/transient)
Absolute eosinophil count more than 1000 cells per microliter
Central bronchiectasis on HRCT

- The use of antifungal agents to reduce the fungal burden due to fungal growth in the airways. The goals of therapy include asthma control, prevention and treatment of ABPA exacerbations and prevention of the onset/progression of bronchiectasis and thus CPA.

Systemic Glucocorticoid Therapy

Oral corticosteroids are currently considered the treatment of choice for ABPA. They are used to suppress the immune hyperfunction as well as to control the activity of both asthma and ABPA because of their anti-inflammatory effect. The clinical effectiveness of steroid therapy is reflected by clinicoradiological improvement and decrease in patient's total serum IgE levels. There does not seem to be any correlation between serum levels of *A. fumigatus*-specific IgE levels and disease activity. The goal of therapy is not to attempt normalization of IgE levels but to decrease by 25%, which in most cases, is associated with complete clinical and radiographic improvement.

Inhaled Corticosteroids

Inhaled steroids achieve high concentrations in the tracheobronchial tree in these patients. They are also associated with minimal systemic side effects, and thus have been evaluated in ABPA as a systemic steroid-sparing therapy.

Oral Azoles

Almost 50% of patients experience exacerbations when steroids are tapered and around 20–45% become glucocorticoid-dependent. Adverse effects related to chronic steroid therapy are also common. The use of specific antifungal agents in ABPA is based on the principle that removal or reduction of fungal burden and thus the antigenic stimulus would mitigate the immune response. Pooled analysis has shown that itraconazole can significantly decrease the IgE levels by 25% or more when compared to placebo but did not cause significant improvement in lung function. Itraconazole may have interaction with several other drugs as well as erratic gastrointestinal absorption, The therapy should ideally be monitored by drug levels to ensure adequate bioavailability. Suboptimal blood levels of the drug have been correlated with clinical failure and possible development of azole resistance. Newer antifungal agents including voriconazole, and posaconazole have also been shown to be efficacious. These drugs are usually used in patients who are intolerant to itraconazole or fail to respond to itraconazole. Long-term voriconazole and other azoles therapy have several adverse effects including skin cancer.

Other Therapies

Numerous other therapies have been tried in ABPA. They can be tried in individual patients such as those with treatment-dependent ABPA who develop drug-related adverse reactions, but should not be used as a routine measure. Nebulized amphotericin and inhaled steroids have also been used for treatment of ABPA. There are a few reports on use of omalizumab, a humanized monoclonal antibody against IgE, as a potential therapeutic approach. Severe exacerbations of ABPA are sometimes treated with pulse doses of intravenous methyl prednisolone and methotrexate. They have also been used for treatment as a steroid-sparing strategy.

ALLERGIC BRONCHOPULMONARY MYCOSIS

Allergic bronchopulmonary mycosis is defined as an ABPA-like syndrome due to non-*Aspergillus fumigatus* fungi. Several other fungi are reported to cause this syndrome although the incidence is far less than that of ABPA. The diagnosis is made on demonstration of sensitization to the specific fungi in addition to the other criteria similar to that for ABPA.

CHAPTER
32

Burden of Chronic Obstructive Pulmonary Disease

Monica Barne, Sundeep Salvi

INTRODUCTION

Chronic obstructive pulmonary disease (COPD) is a leading global cause of morbidity and mortality. COPD prevalence, morbidity and mortality varies across countries and regions of the world and largely depends upon the exposure to various risk factors, mainly smoking, exposure to indoor air pollution, occupational exposure to particulate matter and other noxious agents and poor socioeconomic status. The world needs to take cognizance of the impending epidemic of this and take appropriate measures to curb this increasing burden.

MORTALITY DUE TO CHRONIC OBSTRUCTIVE PULMONARY DISEASE

Global Mortality

World Health Organization (WHO) estimates about 3 million deaths due to COPD worldwide, which corresponds to almost 5% of all deaths globally. The Global Burden of Disease Study 2010 (GBDS) report states that although the number of deaths dues to COPD has declined over the past two decades from 3.1 million to 2.9 million, COPD is still the 3rd largest cause of mortality. COPD is now the 3rd leading cause of deaths worldwide; almost 90% of deaths from chronic obstructive pulmonary disease occur in low- and middle-income countries. India and China alone are responsible for 63% of deaths due to COPD. The estimated deaths due to COPD in India in 2002, were over half a million, second only to China which was responsible for an estimated 1.3

million deaths. The mortality rates were then projected to increase by over 30% every decade. But whereas the number of deaths in China has declined from 1.3 million to 0.93 million in 2010, India has overshot this 30% prediction and mortality due to COPD in India has increased from 0.59 million in 2002 to 0.91 million in 2010 making it the biggest contributor to the up-scaled ranking of COPD.

Mortality in India

Chronic respiratory diseases (namely chronic obstructive pulmonary disease or COPD, asthma and other respiratory diseases) are the second leading cause of deaths among Indian adults between 25 years and 69 years of age and are responsible for about 10.2% of deaths in this age group. According to the Government of India-Medical Certification of cause of Death report for the year 2010, chronic respiratory diseases were the third largest cause of deaths and have shown a steadily increasing pattern over the past few decades whereas infectious diseases which were the second largest cause of certified deaths, had shown a steady decline. The death rate due to COPD in India has doubled in the past decade.

PREVALENCE OF CHRONIC OBSTRUCTIVE PULMONARY DISEASE

Global Prevalence

Two hundred ten million people across the world are believed to suffer with COPD. Prevalence of COPD varies from country to country and within the country from region to region not only due to the different levels of exposure to risk factors but also due to the remarkable variation in the survey methods, diagnostic criteria and analytical approaches. Several studies have estimated the prevalence of COPD in the past, but the tools for diagnosis of COPD have been largely ill-defined. On one hand, prevalence based on self-reported symptoms (chronic cough, sputum, etc.) most likely overestimated the true burden of COPD while physician's diagnosis in absence of spirometry usually underestimates true COPD.

The variations in prevalence rates may not necessarily be only due to the actual difference in prevalence in various countries but also likely depends upon the fact that the diagnostic and research tools vary from study to study. The tools used to define COPD have included respiratory symptoms, doctor diagnosed self reported COPD and spirometry defined COPD (ratio between FEV_1 and FVC measured either before bronchodilator or after bronchodilator). Moreover, the cut off value for the forced expiratory volume/forced vital capacity (FEV_1/FVC) ratio has also varied from study to study. There is considerable within study variation in the prevalence of COPD depending upon the criteria for defining COPD. For example, using the European Respiratory Society (ERS) definition of COPD gives a prevalence of 11.0% which increases to 40% if the American Thoracic Society (ATS) criteria is used to define COPD.

Considering this wide variation in the study methodology, and definitions of COPD, a worldwide study called Burden of Obstructive Lung Diseases (BOLD) was initiated in 2002 which had attempted to determine the prevalence of COPD using a standardized validated respiratory questionnaire and spirometry. For diagnosis of COPD, the investigators used the Global initiative for Obstructive Lung Disease (GOLD) criteria i.e. post bronchodilator FEV1/FVC <70% on spirometry. The prevalence of stage II or higher COPD was reported in 10.1% of population (11.8% for men, and 8.5% for women). There was an increase in prevalence with age and smoking. BOLD investigators used lower limit of normal (LLN) as the cut off to define COPD i.e. $FEV_1/FVC<LLN$ instead of the FEV_1/FVC <0.7. This was done to minimize known age biases.

A systematic review of articles published between 1990 and 2012 estimates the number of COPD cases to about 26.3 million (18.5-43.4 million) cases of COPD which is an estimated 31.5% increase as compared to the prevalence rates in 2,000. The only BOLD study conducted in South Africa which defined COPD by airflow obstruction on post bronchodilator FEV_1/FVC reported a prevalence of 22.2% in men and 16.7% in women aged ≥40 years. This was by far the highest country rates reported within the global BOLD study till 2011.

Prevalence in India

An extensive review of all data published on COPD prevalence in India from 1964 to 1995 has provided the backbone for the estimation of morbidity and mortality and projected economic burden of COPD. This review showed that there is a wide variation in the prevalence of COPD in different parts of India, the highest being reported from North Indian rural population (9.4%). This wide variation was explained by the wide variety in the exposure to risk factors like smoking, environmental tobacco smoke, biomass fuel, occupation and socioeconomic status.

Another review assimilated data from 16 studies on chronic bronchitis and COPD conducted after 1980 and presented the prevalence of COPD in different geographical, socioeconomic conditions in racially and culturally different populations in India, which are exposed to different risk factors like tobacco smoke, indoor air pollution due to use of biomass fuel and outdoor air pollution. Despite the heterogeneity of these studies in their study population, methodology, study tools used, risk factors assessed and outcomes, the study concludes that the existing estimates of general prevalence of chronic bronchitis in rural areas was between 6.5% to 7.7%.

Indian Study on Epidemiology of Asthma, Respiratory symptoms and chronic bronchitis (INSEARCH), the large multicentric field survey that was conducted with the help of a structured and validated questionnaire in both the urban as well as rural populations at 16 different centers across India revealed overall prevalence of about 4%. Prevalence of COPD in smokers was 2.65 times higher than in nonsmokers, and amongst the smokers, the prevalence was higher amongst bidi smokers as compared to cigarette smokers. Exposure to Environmental Tobacco Smoke (ETS) was associated with a 40% increased odds of COPD which increased to 57% amongst those concomitantly exposed to biomass fuel. A questionnaire-based study amongst 12,000 slum dwellers from Pune city in Maharashtra is also notable for the fact that probably for the first time, this study showed that amongst those diagnosed with COPD, 69% were never smokers. The overall prevalence of questionnaire-diagnosed COPD amongst the never smoker males was 6.8% and females was 4.4%.

The National Commission on Macroeconomics and Health in its Background Papers on the Burden of Diseases estimated that out of the 65 million cases of chronic respiratory diseases in India in 2005, about 17 million were due to COPD. The morbidity due to COPD was projected to increase to 22.2 million by the year 2016. But if we apply the current prevalence rate of about 7% to the population in India which is above 45-years, the estimated number of COPD patients in India would be about 25 million already.

DISABILITY ADJUSTED LIFE YEARS (DALYS) DUE TO CHRONIC OBSTRUCTIVE PULMONARY DISEASE

Disability adjusted life years (DALYs) represent the morbidity that is caused by the illness taking into account the years lived with disability (YLD) and the years of life lost (YLL) due to premature mortality. According to the Global Burden of Disease study (2010), COPD is responsible for 76.8 million DALYs, 33% of these DALYs are contributed by India alone. COPD ranks 3rd in DALYs globally due to the huge numbers contributed by China and India but though China leads in the number of deaths, the DALYs due to COPD are 16.7 million, much lesser than the 25.8 million DALYs from COPD in India.

Economic Burden of Chronic Obstructive Pulmonary Disease

Global Economic Burden

There are high costs involved in the management of COPD. Besides the very high direct costs, i.e. personal and family expenditures spent for the diagnosis and treatment of the disease, there are huge indirect costs or economic losses attributable to the loss of work, premature morbidity and mortality. Moreover, there are added cost of attendants and caregivers as well as the family costs resulting from the illness. The healthcare costs for patients with COPD also increased with time due to market trends and newer forms of treatment which become available. For example, the direct costs had increased by 38% between 1987 and 2007. There is a continued increase of about 5% every year between 2006 and 2009. The costs of hospital admissions remain the largest contributor to this increased expenditure.

Different studies have shown a trend of direct cost growth in the elderly population, which is stated to be mainly due to more frequent use of acute healthcare services, especially for managing COPD exacerbations. A large amount of this expenditure can be curbed by early diagnosis, effective management of the stable condition and prevention of exacerbations of COPD. The appropriate use of maintenance therapy has been shown to reduce the incidence of exacerbations and has the potential to reduce overall costs associated with the management of patients with COPD.

The Global initiative for Obstructive Lung Diseases also states that in developing countries, direct medical costs may be less important than the impact of COPD on the workplace and home productivity. Because the healthcare sector may not provide long-term supportive care services for severely disabled individuals, COPD may force two individuals to leave the workplace—the affected individual and a family member who must now stay home to care for the disabled relative. Since human capital is often the most important national asset for developing countries, the indirect costs of COPD may represent a serious threat to their economies.

Economic Burden in India

There is no recent data on the economic burden from expenditures on management of COPD. The direct cost estimates were earlier assessed in an ICMR sponsored project in 1998. It only involved expenditures on daily treatment and exacerbations (indoor/outdoor treatment). The assessment was an underestimation considering the facts that the State's expenditures on treatments and healthcare infrastructure were not accounted for. Importantly however, the costs reflected an important financial burden of about 30% of the patient's income. There has been no assessment of the losses attributed to premature morbidity and mortality. COPD being a chronic, progressive disease poses a huge economic burden on the patient as well as the healthcare systems. At individual level, it frequently proves to be financially ruining some for families with average income. A large part of this expenditure is because of delayed diagnosis and improper management and is preventable if we follow proper guidelines for diagnosis and management.

CONCLUSION

In conclusion, the incidence and prevalence of COPD are fast increasing due to the ever increasing smoking epidemic compounded by poor socioeconomic status. It has been estimated that almost 50% of smokers may develop COPD. In addition; nonsmoking COPD caused mainly due to exposure to smoke from biomass fuel, occupational exposure to dust and gases, poor socioeconomic status, etc. is fast emerging as an entity that is causing considerable morbidity and mortality amongst nonsmokers too.

CHAPTER 33

Risk Factors for Chronic Obstructive Pulmonary Disease

Sneha Limaye, Sundeep Salvi

INTRODUCTION

Chronic obstructive pulmonary disease (COPD) is the result of an interaction between genetic and environmental factors. This is also influenced by the presence of comorbid diseases. Tobacco smoking is the most established risk factor. There is enough evidence to suggest the role of risk factors other than smoking. It is important to identify the risk factors as an important step to develop strategies for prevention and treatment. The presence of various risk factors also helps in making the diagnosis of COPD.

TOBACCO SMOKING

Tobacco smoking was first associated with the risk of developing COPD in the 1950s. Since thereafter; several prevalence as well as intervention studies have focused on COPD mostly amongst smokers.

Tobacco smoking is more prevalent in the developed countries, although the number of smokers is now declining slowly. The prevalence is particularly high in Russia, China, Eastern Europe, Southeast Asia and South America. On the other hand, the number of smokers in the developing countries is increasing rapidly. There are an estimated 1.1 billion smokers worldwide and India's contribution is 110 million. Interestingly India has the second largest number of female smokers in the world (12.1 million) after USA, although the prevalence is low, but rising in the cities.

The prevalence of smoking in the Indian population is 28.5% in men and 2.1% in women. It is estimated that by 2030, tobacco consumption in any form will account for 10 million deaths per year, half of them aged 35–69 years.

Almost 82% of world's smokers reside in the developing countries, and nearly 17% of world's smoking population resides in India. There is a wide range of the prevalence rate of smoking from the lowest of 13.9% in Punjab to the highest of 49.4% in Mizoram. *Bidi* is the most common form of smoking, more so in the rural areas. Different forms of tobacco smoking prevalent in India are cigarette, *bidi*, hookah and chillum smoking. In India and other Southeast Asian countries, *bidi* smoking is more common than cigarette smoking.

Tobacco smoking increases the risk of COPD by 2–3 folds, although not all smokers develop COPD. Some of the earlier reports estimated that only 15% of smokers develop COPD. New evidence suggests that up to 50% of smokers developed COPD. Growing amount of evidences has associated hookah smoking as a risk factor for various diseases including COPD. The hookah smoke consists of 0.15–1 per puff, an average hookah session lasts 20–80 min which is equivalent of smoking 100 cigarettes or more. The Indian study on Epidemiology of Asthma, Respiratory symptoms and chronic bronchitis (INSEARCH) study reported hookah smoking was associated with higher odds of having chronic bronchitis in comparison to cigarette smoking. These findings are consistent with studies from other parts of world.

ENVIRONMENTAL TOBACCO SMOKE

Environmental tobacco smoke (ETS) exposure (passive smoking) is also shown to cause COPD both in smokers and nonsmokers. There is an increasing body of evidence to show this association of ETS exposure with COPD in nonsmoking wives and colleagues of smokers. The association between ETS and COPD has been shown to be consistent across various cross-sectional and longitudinal cohort studies. Both temporal and dose–response relationship have been established in studies that evaluated cumulative lifetime exposure. ETS has also acute negative effects on pulmonary function. For example, restaurant workers experience a substantive fall in spirometry after a single work shift in a smoky environment.

HOUSEHOLD AIR POLLUTION

About half the global population (3 billion people) use biomass fuels for cooking and heating purposes. Burning of biomass solid fuel (includes wood, twigs, crop residues and animal dung) emits very high levels of indoor air pollutants, both particulate matter and the gaseous pollutants. Many of these homes are poorly ventilated, exposing these individuals to very high levels of indoor air pollutants.

Women, young girls and small children are exposed for the longest duration because they spend more time in close vicinity to the biomass smoke. During their lifetime, women are exposed for around 30–40 years, equivalent to 60,000 hours of exposure to biomass smoke or inhaling a total volume of 25 million liters of highly polluted indoor air. Exposure to biomass smoke induces the same amount of risk of COPD as tobacco smoke.

MOSQUITO COIL SMOKE

Of the available forms of mosquito repellents, mosquito coils are the most widely used repellents in Asia, Africa and South America as they are cheap, easy to use and readily available. An estimated 29 billion mosquito coils are sold every year and are used by 2 billion people across the globe; in South India, about 73% of people living in rural areas and 42% of people living in urban areas are reported to burn mosquito coils at home.

The bulk of the coil is made up of wood powder, coconut shell powder or joss powder, along with binders, dyes, oxidants and other additives which allow the coil to smoulder for around 6-8 hours during the night. Both short-term and long-term animal exposure studies with mosquito coil smoke have shown significant adverse impacts on lung histology, including epithelial cell damage, interstitial cellular accumulation, pulmonary edema and emphysema.

OUTDOOR AIR POLLUTION

Ambient urban air pollutants (both gaseous and particulate matter) are associated with an increased risk of respiratory symptoms, asthma, COPD, allergic rhinitis, lower respiratory tract infections and lung cancers. Respiratory morbidity and cardiovascular mortality are significantly more in adults exposed to high levels of ambient air pollutants. Residents of areas along the highways with heavy motor vehicular traffic have significant impairment of lung function and increased prevalence of COPD. High levels of respirable ambient air pollutants may also cause worsening of and exacerbation of preexisting COPD.

CHRONIC OBSTRUCTIVE PULMONARY DISEASE ASSOCIATED WITH OCCUPATIONAL EXPOSURES

Occupational exposures are known to cause COPD for over four decades. Exposures to toxic gases at workplace, grain dust in farms, and to dust and fumes in factories were reported to be strongly associated with COPD in several earlier studies. Longitudinal studies have also documented the association of COPD with other occupational exposures amongst miners working in coal and hard rock miners as well as workers engaged in tunnel construction and concrete manufacturing. The effect of heavy exposure to dusts is detrimental even more than cigarette smoking. Risk of death due to COPD is significantly higher among construction workers and those engaged in brick manufacturing, gold mining as well as iron and steel foundries. There is prolonged exposure to silica dust in these occupations where average respirable dust levels reach up to 10,000 µg/m^3.

CHRONIC OBSTRUCTIVE PULMONARY DISEASE ASSOCIATED WITH PULMONARY TUBERCULOSIS

Pulmonary tuberculosis has been shown to be associated with chronic airflow obstruction. The amount of airflow obstruction is related to the extent of the disease, the amount of sputum produced and the duration after the diagnosis or completion of treatment. Air flow obstruction results from fibrosis as well as enhanced airway inflammation following tubercular infections.

CHRONIC ASTHMA

Chronic persistent and severe asthma especially when poorly treated can cause irreversible airway obstruction similar to that seen in COPD. There are marked similarities in the airway inflammation seen in severe asthma and COPD. Both these conditions have increase in the number of neutrophils and IL-8, increased proteases and oxidative stress. Moreover, there is reduced responsiveness to corticosteroids. Poorly treated chronic persistent severe asthma may present with features of COPD in the subsequent years.

GENETIC FACTORS

Recent studies have indicated that COPD can run in families, and several potential genes have been identified. Several gene polymorphisms have been implicated in COPD, but the functional genetic variants known to influence the development of COPD are not known.

Deficiency of α_1 antitrypsin is the best known genetic factor linked to COPD. This recessive trait is most commonly seen in individuals of Northern European origin in about 1–3% of patients. Tobacco smoking and exposure to other pollutants, further add to the risk of developing panlobular emphysema in patients with low concentrations of this enzyme.

Various other genetic syndromes have been suggested to have some role in development of COPD in nonsmokers. There is a clear association of cutis laxa, a rare inherited connective tissue disorder with emphysema in adolescents and childhood even in some nonsmoker patients. This is mostly caused by mutations in elastin genes.

Facial Wrinkling

Facial wrinkling is known to be associated with cigarette smoking and increases with the number of pack years smoked. The exaggerated skin wrinkling seen in smokers with COPD than in normal smokers has been associated with increased MMP-9 expression by keratinocytes. It has been suggested that there may be a common mechanism and a common genetic susceptibility. Cigarette smoking (that is a proven risk factor for COPD) also results in cellular senescence.

SOCIOECONOMIC STATUS

Several of risk factors of COPD are more commonly present in people with poor socioeconomic status. These include poor nutrition, crowded housing conditions, and childhood respiratory tract infections. There is increased prevalence of exposures to tobacco smoke, biomass smoke, other air pollutants, and occupational exposures. However, poor socioeconomic status is also shown to be independently associated with COPD.

In summary, there exist a host of risk factors important in the development of COPD. The environmental exposures such as the tobacco smoking and air pollution are most commonly identifiable. The genetic predisposition may play an equally important role, but remains an investigational issue at present.

CHAPTER
34

Pathophysiology of Chronic Obstructive Pulmonary Disease

Bill Brashier, Sundeep Salvi, Baishakhi Ghosh

INTRODUCTION

The pathology of chronic obstructive pulmonary disease (COPD) is characterized by certain morphological and cellular changes occurring in the airways and lung parenchyma due to ongoing chronic inflammatory processes. Further, the inflammation of COPD also causes lung parenchymal changes, such as destruction and enlargement restricted to the respiratory bronchiole and the central portion of the acinus (centriacinar emphysema), destruction and enlargement uniformly involving the whole acinus (panacinar emphysema) and infiltration of CD8+ T lymphocytes.

INFLAMMATORY CHANGES

The basic pathophysiologic consequences of COPD inflammation consist of increased resistance to airflow and loss of elastic recoil. These changes are responsible for a decrease in expiratory flow rates. There is also disruption of alveolar walls and increased apoptosis of alveolar epithelial cells. Consequently, more effort is required for the air to be exhaled, which happens mostly due to narrowed airway and pressure changes in the thorax. These physiological changes cause earlier closure of small airways resulting in more air trapped in the lungs. Further, there is flattening of the diaphragm and expansion of the rib cage due to hyperinflated lungs. These anatomical alterations place the respiratory chest wall muscles and the diaphragm at a mechanical disadvantage causing impairment of their force-generating capacity. Thus there is an increase in the metabolic work of breathing causing heightened sensation of dyspnea. All these changes occur due to inflammatory cells and mediators which are increased in COPD.

Role of Neutrophils

The neutrophil has been highly acclaimed as a key effector cell in the pathogenesis of COPD, to a degree that COPD has been characterized as neutrophil-mediated disease. Moreover, neutrophilic inflammation has been primarily implicated in steroid nonresponsiveness in COPD. In COPD, there is a quantitative increase in lung neutrophils the reason for which is still elusive. There is also increased expression of adhesion molecules such as intercellular-cellular adhesion molecule-1 (ICAM-1) and endothelial adhesion molecules (E-selectin) in both the endothelium as well as neutrophil cell surface which can enhance neutrophil stickiness to the capillary endothelium and assist their migration into the lungs.

An imbalance between neutrophilic proteases and local antiproteases has been highly implicated in the COPD pathogenesis. There is also evidence to suggest that the neutrophils from the COPD subjects have greater chemotactic responses and greater ability to digest the surrounding tissue than the neutrophils of normal subjects. The primary role of these proteolytic enzymes is to generate a pathway for the movement of leukocytes into the tissue and in this process they unsparingly degenerate the elastic connective tissue of the lung parenchyma leading to emphysema. Restoring balance between proteases and antiproteases in the lungs of COPD seems to have promising prospects for future therapy in COPD management.

Role of T Lymphocytes

Inflammation of COPD involves both innate and adaptive immune mechanisms. Infiltration of CD8+ and CD4+ cells occurs not only in the alveolar wall and small airways but also in the adventitia of pulmonary vasculature. The pulmonary vascular infiltration, in addition to the other alterations may lead to the development of pulmonary hypertension. It is the CD8+ cells which are more predominant and more likely involved in pathophysiology of COPD.

Intriguingly, an antigenic mechanism is required to stimulate the T-cell inflammatory response. These inflammatory changes appear in mild COPD and increase markedly with increasing disease severity. They persist even after the triggers such as air pollution or tobacco smoke are removed. This self-perpetuation of the adaptive immune system confers further understanding as it may explain the persistence of inflammation in the lungs of COPD patient. It is possible that the inflammatory and oxidative stress injury can create endogenous autoantigens in the lungs augmenting continued CD4/CD8 response in the lungs. There are also antigens in the tobacco smoke which may also induce the response.

Another possibility is that increased colonization of the lower airways and airway infections could either costimulate or mimic as antigens and provide a persisting antigenic stimulus that maintains the inflammatory processes. The association between recurrent childhood viral infections and the development of COPD in adult life indicate that viruses and bacteria recruit lymphocytes into the lungs as a part of the adaptive immunity.

T Helper 17 Cells

Th17 and related cytokines such as IL-17A, IL-17F and IL-22 and IL-23 has been linked to various autoimmune diseases such as rheumatoid arthritis and psoriasis. The presence of Th17 cells in the inflammatory pool of COPD has also been implicated in association with autoimmune anti-elastin immunological response.

Macrophages

In chronic obstructive pulmonary disease (COPD), macrophages may increase by almost 20 times. Lung macrophages have potential to produce higher levels of antiapoptotic proteins that not only prolong the life of macrophages, but also cause accumulation of macrophages in COPD lung. The cell wall of macrophages is provided with wide array of CD receptors which when triggered can induce production of various cytokines and chemokines, oxidation products, hormones such as leptin and enzymes such as MMPs, serine proteinases, and neutrophil elastases and many more, which then trigger the inflammatory cascade of COPD.

Second and one of the prime functions of COPD is phagocytosis which is a process of recognition and removal of foreign particles or microbes from the host and efferocytosis which is a process of engulfment of cellular debris of the local apoptotic bodies. Counteracting oxidative stress with N-acetyl cysteine has shown to improve phagocytosis in COPD macrophages *in vitro* models. Procysteine improves efferocytosis in COPD macrophages. Clinical trial with azithromycin has also shown to improve efferocytosis in the COPD macrophages.

Role of Oxidative Stress

Oxidative stress has a very significant role in every stage of the pathogenesis in COPD. Increased oxidative stress in the airspaces can initiate a number of early inflammatory events in the lungs. The free oxidant radicals in the lungs and systemic circulation arise from the sources of air pollutants such as cigarette smoke and biomass fuel, and also inflammatory cells such as neutrophils and macrophages.

Reactive oxygen species are also released from activated inflammatory leukocytes such as neutrophils and macrophages, which are known to present in increased numbers in the lungs of cigarette smokers. The inflammatory mediators released by these cells permanently switch on the oxidative stress mechanisms, providing a continuous source of free oxidant radicals which not only confine to the lungs but also spill into the systemic circulation and affect other body organs with particular predilection to the heart and skeletal muscles.

Nuclear Factor Erythroid 2-related Factor 2

There is burgeoning evidence to indicate that there is a depletion of nuclear factor erythroid 2-related factor 2 (NRF2) in the COPD lungs. NRF2 is a key transcription factor that regulates the expression of antioxidant response element (ARE)-regulated antioxidant and cytoprotective genes. Experimental studies have shown that cigarette smoke can enhance expression and production of NRF-2. On the other hand, depletion of NRF-2 can enhance susceptibility to develop emphysema, propagate inflammation, enhance neutrophil elastase activity, enhance oxidative stress and also increase the sensitivity to oxidative stress-related injuries.

Apoptosis

Enhanced programmed cell death (Apoptosis) of structural tissues is cardinal to various chronic inflammatory diseases. In COPD, apoptosis is independent of inflammation and has implicated the pathogenesis of emphysema. Endothelial cells, epithelial cells, interstitial tissue and inflammatory cells such as neutrophils and lymphocytes, have shown to demonstrate enhanced apoptosis. Usually, apoptosis is compensated with cellular proliferation to replace the dying cells. However, the evidence indicates that there is a presence of pertinent imbalance between cell death and cell proliferation as hallmark in COPD development.

Apoptotic byproduct which is normally phagocytosized by macrophages fails to effectively clear the apoptotic material (efferocytosis) from the lungs. The perpetual presence of apoptotic debris could be the trigger for an ongoing inflammation cascade. Currently, the pharmacological interventions that have the potential to reduce apoptosis and enhance apoptotic clearing mechanisms in the macrophage are being explored in new advancement of COPD treatments.

NEW INSIGHTS INTO SMALL AIRWAY OBSTRUCTION

Until now, it has been largely believed that small airway obstruction in COPD is secondary consequence to destruction of alveoli and adjoining elastic tissue leading to kinking of small airways, in conjunction with small airway structural changes. However, microimaging computed tomography (CT) studies indicate that terminal bronchioles undergo obliteration or apoptosis much before emphysema develops. This has generated a possible hypothesis that loss of terminal bronchiole could precede emphysema in development stages of COPD pathologies.

CHRONIC OBSTRUCTIVE PULMONARY DISEASE AS A DISEASE OF SYSTEMIC INFLAMMATION

Chronic obstructive pulmonary disease has been now recognized as a multicomponent disorder, associated with systemic inflammation and extrapulmonary manifestations. It has now been well documented that the inflammation that develops in the patient does not confine to the lungs but spills into the systemic circulation through the pulmonary vessels and predisposes almost every organ system in the body with particular predilection to the heart, as the heart is the first organ that receives all the blood from the pulmonary vasculature. More than 20% of cases of COPD suffer with chronic heart failure, while up to 70% of patients have osteoporosis independent of steroid treatment or decreased physic activity. Also, almost 50% of COPD patients have one or more component of metabolic syndrome.

These inflammatory makers along with persistent hypoxia increase the basal metabolism in the body leading to catabolic changes such as reduced muscle mass, wasting of skeletal muscles and diaphragmatic weakness. Notably, interventions such as regular exercise and physiotherapy have been shown to reduce systemic inflammation. There has also been a strong association between depression and COPD. There is emerging evidence indicating insulin resistance in some COPD patients due to systemic inflammation and recently an association with diabetes and COPD has been demonstrated.

Systemic Manifestations and Comorbidities of Chronic Obstructive Pulmonary Disease

SK Jindal, PS Shankar

INTRODUCTION

Chronic obstructive pulmonary disease (COPD), characterized by progressive airflow limitation, is now considered a systemic disease with widespread extrapulmonary manifestations. While some comorbidities are caused by COPD itself, the others result because of the common risk factors such as tobacco smoking or due to chronic systemic inflammation possibly as a spillover of the inflammation in the airways and lung parenchyma.

PATHOGENESIS

The pathological changes in the lungs include peribronchial fibrosis, airway narrowing, alveolar walls destruction, and loss of elastic recoil. All these changes cause airway narrowing and airflow limitation. Besides inflammation, there is an imbalance between oxidants and antioxidants, which plays an important role in the pathogenesis of COPD. There is a marked oxidant-antioxidant imbalance in smokers and during acute exacerbations of COPD. The reactive oxygen species generated by the neutrophils are responsible for damage to different organs. An increased oxidative stress is also likely to cause changes in fibrinolysis contributing to atherosclerosis, in the coronary and cerebral arteries.

The mechanisms of systemic manifestations are not completely understood. The various pathogenic mechanisms, which initiate in the lungs, also affect the other target tissues. The following mechanisms have been postulated to explain the pathogenesis of systemic manifestations of COPD.

Mediators and Cytokine Spillover from Lungs

The circulating levels of a number of cytokine mediators are increased in patients with COPD. These include interleukin (IL)-1-beta, IL-6 and tumor necrosis factor (TNF)-alpha, and interferon (IF)-gamma and leptin. These cytokines and chemokines are responsible for migration and activation of inflammatory cells. These mechanisms are regulated by epithelial cells, endothelial cells, smooth muscle cells, fibroblasts, and different inflammatory cells. The systemic effects are possibly caused by low-grade systemic inflammation due to the presence of numerous inflammatory mediators and cytokines released from the lungs into the systemic circulation, i.e. lung to plasma spillover.

Attempts have been made to study their role through analyses of exhaled air condensates. Inflammatory cytokines have been isolated from sputum, exhaled breath condensate and bronchoalveolar lavage (BAL) fluid from COPD patients. Unlike in asthma, the findings in COPD have not been very helpful. Inflammatory markers in the blood [e.g. IL-6, C-reactive proteins (CRPs), and fibrinogen] have also been studied.

Peripheral Blood Inflammatory and Other Cells

The evidence from other cross-sectional studies shows no clear association between lung and systemic inflammation, which suggest that the systemic inflammatory response is not caused by the "spillover" or overflow of inflammatory mediators from the pulmonary circulation, but by the systemic peripheral, inflammatory cells such as the neutrophils and lymphocytes. There are several other cells including the macrophages and the mononuclear cells, which are attracted by mediators such as CCL2 and CCL3. Involvement of T-lymphocytes, especially the cytotoxic CD8+ cells has also been postulated.

The presence of hypoxia in severe COPD may also be responsible for an increased production of cytokines, which activate TNF-alpha and soluble TNF-R. It is also possible that the inflammatory mediators are produced by the muscle cells or other extrapulmonary cells located in the endothelium and fatty tissue.

While it is likely that different systemic manifestations are explained by different mechanisms, the concept of inflammation as responsible for multisystem involvement has been established. The understanding of these pathogenic mechanisms is expected to change the clinical practice and pharmacotherapy of COPD.

SYSTEMIC MANIFESTATIONS

There are a large number of systemic features and comorbidities seen in COPD (Box 35.1). Interestingly, some of the general clinical features, such as weakness, weight loss, anxiety, depression, and others earlier considered as "vague" or nonspecific in nature, are now identified as more definitive and significant manifestations of nonpulmonary systemic involvement.

> **BOX 35.1:** Important systemic manifestations of chronic obstructive pulmonary disease (COPD).
>
> - *General:* Wasting and weight loss, nutritional anomalies, anemia
> - *Musculoskeletal:* Skeletal muscle dysfunction, osteoporosis, reduction in exercise tolerance and performance
> - *Cardiovascular:* Pulmonary vascular disease/chronic cor pulmonale, ischemic heart disease—acute cardiac events, cardiac failure, stroke
> - *Endocrine:* Diabetes, metabolic syndrome, dysfunction of pituitary, thyroid, gonads and adrenals
> - *Neuropsychiatric:* Depression, disordered sleep, anxiety, cognitive function decline

Wasting and Weight Loss

Muscle wasting and weight loss are common manifestations of COPD. Weight loss is attributable to increased basal metabolic rate and an increased work of breathing. Increased metabolic rate is also due to inhaled beta-2 agonists, altered amino acid composition, and tissue hypoxia. The increased breakdown of cell proteins, especially in muscles, occurs due to several different factors such as the presence of acidosis, infection, changes in intermediate metabolism or inadequate caloric intake. Most of these changes are especially marked during acute exacerbations of COPD. There is also significant loss of skeletal muscle mass, especially so in the lower limbs. Quadriceps muscle weakness in patients with advanced disease is also attributed to physical inactivity.

Weight loss and muscle wasting are likely to involve an imbalance in an ongoing protein degradation and replacement. Alterations in the relative levels or activities of endocrine hormones such as insulin, growth hormone, testosterone, and glucocorticosteroids are also responsible for those complications.

Skeletal Muscle Dysfunction

Skeletal muscle dysfunction in COPD occurs from sedentary lifestyle, tissue hypoxia, and systemic inflammation. It is characterized by muscle atrophy, loss of strength, and reduction in exercise capacity. This is particularly so in case of diaphragm, which has to constantly work against an increased load. Other skeletal muscles suffer dystrophy due to patient inactivity.

The activities and the exercise capacity of patients with COPD get limited due to weight loss and skeletal muscle dysfunction. Therefore, the quality of life (QOL) is significantly impaired. There is worsening of exercise tolerance and performance, increased healthcare utilization, and increased mortality. Muscle weakness is recognized to contribute independently to poor health status. Some of these manifestations, i.e. body mass index, degree of air flow obstruction, dyspnea, and exercise capacity (the BODE index), have been used as measures of disease severity and mortality risk in COPD.

Cardiovascular Problems

The link between COPD and cardiovascular disease (CVD) has been shown in a large number of epidemiological, clinical, and pathogenetic studies. Cardiovascular system has a complex interaction with the respiratory system. Pulmonary vascular abnormalities are common in the presence of a chronic lung disease such as COPD. Pulmonary hypertension, right ventricular dysfunction, and chronic cor pulmonale have been recognized since long. It is now known that structural changes in pulmonary arteries can occur early in COPD before the onset of hypoxemia. Systemic inflammation, atherosclerotic coronary heart disease, and cardiovascular deaths are known as important complications of COPD.

The burden of cardiovascular as well as the cerebrovascular disease is high in COPD patients. There is significant evidence to support the COPD–CVD association. There was a significant relationship of CVD with COPD associated with a marked impairment of functional capacity and QOL indices. Presence of other comorbidities, such as psychiatric problems, alcohol abuse, and diabetes along with CVD, is important determinant for QOL impairment. The CVD in COPD was significantly more common in the presence of diabetes mellitus.

Cardiac failure was seen in 10–46% of patients of COPD, while 40% of patients with cardiac failure showed some evidence of COPD, about half of whom were not earlier recognized. A large population of patients who present with acute heart failure and concomitant COPD had different clinical characteristics than those without the presence of COPD. There is enough data from epidemiological and other studies to show that atherosclerosis and coronary artery disease are associated with decline in forced expiratory volume in 1 second (FEV_1). The risk for cardiovascular death was 75% greater for patients who had a lower FEV_1.

Arrhythmias in COPD are common, but rarely fatal. The right ventricular arrhythmias are more often seen in the presence of chronic cor pulmonale. There is increased occurrence of arterial fibrillation, atrial flutter, and nonsustained ventricular tachycardias. The occurrence of both COPD and coronary artery disease is possibly due to the shared risk factors, such as tobacco smoking, as well as to the similar pathogenic mechanisms, i.e. systemic inflammation.

Inhaled long-acting beta-agonist (LABA) and inhaled corticosteroids (ICS) reduce arterial stiffness measured with aortic pulse wave velocity (aPWV). This is an important determinant of cardiovascular events and mortality in COPD. It is also possible that the lower levels of vitamin D are associated with increased total and CVD mortality.

Endocrinal Disorders

A number of endocrine functional disorders have been described in COPD. Derangements of pituitary and thyroid function, gonads and adrenals have been seen in some studies. Hypogonadism in men has been reported in

22–69% of patients; testosterone replacement is associated with modest improvement in fat-free mass and limb muscle strength. Diabetes along with other manifestations of metabolic syndrome has been described, especially in the presence of CVD. The presence of CVD disease in COPD is higher in the presence of type II diabetes mellitus.

Several mechanisms have been proposed to cause endocrine dysfunction—hypoxemia, hypercapnia, systemic inflammation, and glucocorticoid administration for airway obstruction. The presence of endocrine imbalance increases the overall morbidity and cardiovascular risks. The decreased protein anabolism and increased catabolism affect the body mass and also account for muscle dysfunction. Altered renin-angiotensin-aldosterone function affects the blood flow, fluid balance, and the renal function. Other systemic effects of endocrinal disorders include the disturbances of control in breathing, worsening of respiratory mechanics, and impairment of cardiac function.

Neuropsychiatric Derangements

Depression and anxiety are more common in COPD than in healthy age-matched controls. Psychiatric comorbidities and alcohol abuse were strong determinants of health-related QOL in COPD patients. Disordered sleep is commonly ascribed to hypoxemia, hypercapnia, and diminished ventilatory responses. It is further aggravated by the concomitant presence of nocturnal respiratory symptoms, anxiety, and depression. Obstructive sleep apnea is present in about 10–15% patients of COPD ("overlap syndrome"). Other sleep disturbances seen in more than half of the COPD patients include the diminished arousal responses, longer latency in falling asleep, more frequent awakenings, or generalized insomnia. The sleep disturbance increases with the disease severity.

Impairment of intellectual function is also common. The cognitive decline, along with other neuropsychiatric problems, is attributed to the presence of hypoxemia and has shown to improve with long-term oxygen therapy in some small studies.

Osteoporosis

Osteopenia and osteoporosis were reported in 68% of patients with COPD. It is characterized by low bone mass and microarchitectural destruction of bones. Osteoporosis may lead to generalized bony pains, compression fracture of the spine, and compromised lung function due to kyphosis and thoracic vertebral compression. Corticosteroid therapy, including inhaled steroids, is generally considered responsible for osteoporosis; although in one study, compression fractures were reported in 49% of the patients who had COPD and had never received steroids. Other common risk factors for COPD and osteoporosis include the older age, tobacco smoking, vitamin D deficiency, and systemic inflammation.

THERAPEUTIC CONSIDERATIONS

The recognition of systemic features has made the greatest impact on clinical course, complications, and therapy of COPD. The variable host response and subsequent clinical phenotyping have made it possible to develop a targeted treatment with the help of a multisystem approach. COPD treatment is no longer limited to inhalational and oral bronchodilators and ICS alone, but a multimodality treatment for multiple comorbidities. Some of the treatment failures are possibly due to the phenotype heterogeneity of COPD and its different systemic manifestations. The future treatments with statins, angiotensin-converting enzyme inhibitors, and anti-inflammatory drugs, and targeting the comorbid conditions may help to change the natural history of COPD and improve the mortality.

Lastly, it is shown that the elderly patients who are at an increased risk of almost all the comorbidities of COPD discussed earlier, may benefit from the treatment of concomitant comorbidities. Further, development of anti-aging molecules, such as sirtuin agonists, can be helpful and may also reduce the risk of lung cancer. It should, however, not be overlooked that aging alone is not an exclusion criterion for pulmonary rehabilitation and other treatment of COPD. Assessment and appropriate treatments of COPD and the comorbid conditions has been shown to provide similar benefits of management.

CHAPTER 36

Treatment of Chronic Obstructive Pulmonary Disease

Peter J Barnes

INTRODUCTION

Though the asthma management has significantly advanced in the last 10 years or so, developments in the management of chronic obstructive pulmonary disease (COPD) have been rather few. Most of the current treatments do not significantly slow the progression of airway obstruction. Treatment is largely based on changes in lifestyle and use of bronchodilators to improve the lung function. The current pharmacological management provides only limited benefit.

RISK FACTORS AND THEIR PREVENTION

Environmental Risk Factors

The most important treatment strategy is avoidance of environmental risk factors, wherever possible, to prevent disease progression. Smoking cessation strategies constitute the primary focus of attention.

Stopping Smoking

Smoking cessation is the only intervention that reduces the accelerated rate of decline in lung function and the number of exacerbations. The strategy is important even in the elderly patients (Fig. 36.1). It also reduces the mucous hypersecretion as well as the risks of associated atherosclerosis and cardiovascular disease. Smoking cessation is more effective early in the course of disease becomes less effective as the disease progresses to severe and very severe disease.

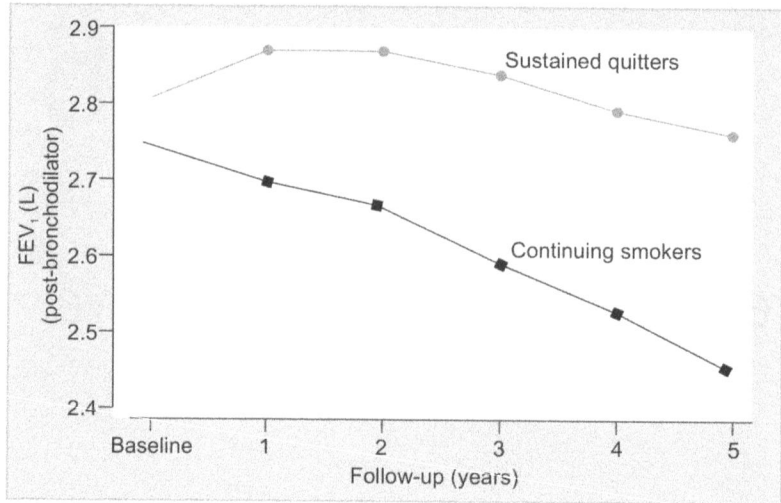

Fig. 36.1: Smoking cessation reduces the rate of decline of lung function in patients with chronic obstructive pulmonary disease (COPD), if instituted early in the course of the disease. (FEV_1, forced expiratory volume in 1 second)

Gradual reduction is usually not successful. There are several methods of smoking cessation. Psychological counseling, group therapy, behavioral therapy, and several other measures are reported to be useful. Nicotine used as chewing gum, skin patches, nasal spray, or an inhaler may double the long-term (6–12 months) abstinence rates. Bupropion is reported to double the quit rate of nicotine replacement therapies. More recently, varenicline, which is a partial nicotinic agonist, has been introduced and shown to be the most effective way of quitting smoking. Varenicline is usually given for 12 weeks and is well tolerated but some patients develop nausea, insomnia, and depression.

Avoiding Biomass Fuel Exposure

This may be addressed by using alternative fuels, such as liquefied petroleum gas (LPG) or natural gas, ethanol or biogas, although this may not be available or affordable in poor rural communities. Improving ventilation of the cooking area, reducing cooking time, or cooking outdoors may also help. Substitution of traditional open fires with locally produced improved stoves has been shown to improve respiratory health in women and to improve lung function and disease progression.

PHARMACOTHERAPY

Bronchodilators

Bronchodilators remain the mainstay of drug therapy for the present. The degree of bronchodilatation is typically about 5% improvement in forced expiratory volume in 1 second (FEV_1). Bronchodilators cause improvement in dyspnea and exercise tolerance without any significant effect on spirometry or lung hyperinflation (air trapping). Bronchodilators may also help reduce respiratory muscle fatigue (controversial) and improve mucociliary clearance. The choice of bronchodilator will partly be determined by patient preference and cost. The preferred bronchodilators include the long-acting beta-2-agonists (LABA—formoterol, salmeterol, indacaterol) and/or long-acting muscarinic antagonist (LAMA—tiotropium bromide, glycopyrronium, aclidinium). Several bronchodilators are available for COPD (Table 36.1).

Anticholinergics

Airflow obstruction of COPD is predominantly attributed to increased vagal cholinergic tone, which appears to be the only reversible element in management. Anticholinergics are probably the most effective bronchodilators in its treatment.

Clinical use: Short-acting anticholinergics, such as ipratropium bromide and oxitropium bromide are administered three or four times daily, whereas the long-acting tiotropium bromide is given once daily. All of them are used through inhalational route. Tiotropium even when added to other therapies is effective in improving lung function and quality of life at all stages of COPD. Tiotropium also reduces severe exacerbations and hospital admissions, as well as mortality from COPD and cardiovascular disease. In addition to tiotropium,

TABLE 36.1: Bronchodilators for chronic obstructive pulmonary disease (COPD).

Drug	MDI (µg)	Nebulizer (mg)	Oral (mg)	Duration (h)
Beta-2-agonists:				
Salbutamol	100–200	2.5–5.0	4	4–6
Terbutaline	250–500	5–10	–	4–6
Indacaterol	150–300	–	–	24
Formoterol	12–24	–	–	12
Salmeterol	50–100	–	–	12
Bambuterol	–	–	10–20	12
Anticholinergics:				
Ipratropium	40–80	0.25–0.5	–	6–8
Oxitropium	200	–	–	7–8
Tiotropium	18	–	–	>24
Glycopyrronium	50	–	–	24
Aclidinium	400	–	–	12
Theophyllines:				
Theophylline SR	–	–	200–400	12–24
Aminophylline SR	–	–	200–400	12–24

(MDI, metered dose inhaler)

there are other LAMAs now available or in late clinical development including glycopyrronium and umeclidinium, which are once daily and aclidinium, which is twice daily.

Anticholinergic drugs may have additive bronchodilator effects with beta-2-agonists so may be given together. For short-acting drugs, ipratropium-salbutamol inhalers are popular, whereas once daily combination inhalers containing tiotropium with formoterol are also available.

Side effects: Inhaled anticholinergic drugs are usually well tolerated. There are very few systemic side effects since systemic absorption is insignificant. There is no detectable reduction of airway secretions with inhaled ipratropium bromide, even in high doses, may precipitate glaucoma is reported in some elderly patients due to nebulized ipratropium bromide. This is, however, attributed to the direct effect of the nebulized drug on the eye and can, therefore, be avoided by use of a mouthpiece rather than a face mask. About 5–10% of patients on LAMA complain of dryness of mouth. Mostly, it does not require discontinuation of treatment.

Beta-2-Agonists

Short-acting beta-2-agonists are used mainly for symptom relief. They can be sometimes used on a regular basis. LABAs are preferred therapy for COPD as they give better control of symptoms and are used as a maintenance therapy. These drugs act on airway smooth muscle causing a relaxation in large and small airways. They act as functional antagonists and reverse bronchoconstriction irrespective of the cause. There is some evidence that beta-2-agonists may increase the ventilatory drive to hypercapnia (but not to hypoxia).

Side effects: Side effects are not usually a problem; excessive use does not appear to be dangerous, even in patients with hypoxia and with cardiovascular disease.
- Muscle tremor more commonly seen in the elderly patients is attributable to direct effect on skeletal muscle beta-2-receptors.
- Tachycardia occurs due to direct effect on atrial beta-2-receptors as well as due to the reflex effect from increased peripheral vasodilatation via beta-2-receptors.
- Hypokalemia, usually mild, is the direct effect on skeletal muscle uptake of potassium ions via beta-2-receptors.
- Restlessness
- Hypoxemia may result due to increased V/Q mismatch due to pulmonary vasodilatation.

Short-acting beta-2-agonists: Short-acting inhaled beta-2-agonists, such as salbutamol and terbutaline, are recommended for the immediate relief of symptoms. Ideally, they should not be used regularly (as tolerance to their protective effects occurs), although in patients with severe COPD, regular nebulized beta-2-agonists may be indicated.

Long-acting inhaled beta-2-agonists: Salmeterol and formoterol give bronchodilatation and protection against bronchoconstriction for over 12 hours. Indacaterol is a once daily LABA that is approved for use in COPD. Other once daily LABAs, including vilanterol and olodaterol, are also becoming available. There is compelling evidence that these LABAs are useful as bronchodilators in patients with COPD and that once daily drugs are more effective than twice daily drugs. These drugs may improve symptoms, quality of life, and exercise performance and reduce air trapping through relaxant effects on small airways. They have a similar efficacy to anticholinergics, but together there have additive effects.

Oral beta-2-agonists: Although inhaled beta-2-agonists are preferred, some elderly patients have problems with using inhalers. Slow release oral beta-2-agonist preparations, such as bambuterol and slow release salbutamol, are available. Side effects are more frequent than with inhaled preparations. Bambuterol is a prodrug, which is slowly metabolized to terbutaline and is effective as a once daily preparation.

Theophylline

Theophylline is a useful additional bronchodilator in patients with severe COPD. This effect is seen with plasma concentration of 10–20 mg/L. Moreover, the oral administration has the advantage of treating small airways. It may have additional benefits due to its effects on mucociliary clearance and respiratory muscles. Anti-inflammatory effect, specifically to reduce neutrophilic inflammation, is seen with lower doses of theophylline (plasma concentration 5–10 mg/L). Low-dose theophylline is also shown to reduce exacerbations of COPD.

Side effects: Side effects are mainly due to phosphodiesterase (PDE) inhibition and include:
- Nausea and vomiting
- Headache
- Restlessness
- Gastroesophageal reflux
- Diuresis
- Cardiac arrhythmias (usually plasma concentration >20 mg/L and due to adenosine receptor antagonism)
- Epileptic seizures (usually plasma concentration >30 mg/L and due to adenosine receptor antagonism).

Doxofylline: It is a methylxanthine with similar bronchodilator properties to theophylline. It is not an adenosine receptor antagonist, so there is reduced risk of cardiac arrhythmias or seizures. It does not significantly inhibit PDE isoenzymes, which may also contribute to its better safety profile. In addition, there are fewer drug interactions.

Corticosteroids

Maintenance treatment with oral corticosteroids should be avoided as there is no evidence of benefit and a high risk of side effects in COPD populations. There is not much evidence to suggest the beneficial role of inhaled corticosteroids (ICS) in patients with pure COPD. Oral corticosteroids are found to useful in about 10% of patients who are likely to suffer from coexisting asthma (asthma-COPD overlap—ACO). This group of patients should, therefore, receive regular ICS.

There is reduction (20–25%) in rate of exacerbations in patients with severe disease on high doses of ICS. But ICS do not reduce the progression of COPD (measured by annual fall in FEV_1). Similarly, there is no reduction in mortality with corticosteroid use.

Side Effects

High-dose ICS may be responsible for systemic side effects, such as osteoporosis more commonly seen in the nonambulatory and poorly nourished elderly population. High-dose ICS are also associated with cataracts and an increased risk of diabetes. There is also an increased risk of pneumonia in these patients. Lower doses of ICS will have less risk of side effects and budesonide may be less likely to have adverse effects than fluticasone propionate. Slow withdrawal of inhaled steroids in patients, even with severe disease and a history of exacerbations, is not associated with increased exacerbations and a small fall in FEV_1.

Phosphodiesterase Inhibitors

Several selective PDE4 inhibitors have been tested in COPD and most failed because of insufficient clinical efficacy or unacceptable side effects (most commonly nausea, vomiting, diarrhea, and headaches). Roflumilast is the only PDE4 inhibitor approved for COPD, which provides modest clinical benefit in COPD patients with severe disease, and frequent exacerbations. Some improvements in lung function and a small (~20%) reduction in exacerbation frequency are reported. But there are no improvements in clinical symptoms and quality of life. However, many patients develop side effects and discontinue therapy. It may be indicated for patients with frequent exacerbations instead of high dose ICS.

Combination Inhalers

Several fixed combination inhalers are now available and several more in development for COPD patients. These combinations are more convenient and may improve adherence. Several studies have demonstrated a benefit of combination inhalers containing a corticosteroids and a LABA. Most of the benefit is provided by the LABA component. Any superiority of combination inhalers over LABA alone in reducing exacerbations may be counteracted by the higher risk of side effects due to the corticosteroids component. ICS-LABA combination inhalers improve symptoms and reduce exacerbations with a reduction in all cause mortality, although this does not quite reach statistical significance.

Several LABA–LAMA combination inhalers have been developed. These are based on the additive bronchodilator effects of LABA and LAMA that have been demonstrated in several studies. In one study, a maximally effective dose of indacaterol was given and since LABA inhibit all bronchoconstrict or mechanisms, including cholinergic tone, no further bronchodilatation should be possible. Addition of glycopyrronium in combination with indacaterol doubles the bronchodilator response. Other LABA–LAMA combination inhalers include vilanterol/umeclidinium (Anoro) and olodaterol/tiotropium (once daily), formoterol/glycopyrronium and formoterol/aclidinium (twice daily).

SUPPLEMENTARY OXYGEN

Supplementary oxygen to correct hypoxemia is an important component of therapy. This is required for all acute exacerbations in all hospitalized patients. Controlled oxygen (24%) is preferred for the treatment to avoid the excessive CO_2 retention. On the other hand, long-term oxygen therapy (LTOT) is also referred to as domiciliary oxygen is indicated in selected patients. Careful assessment should be done before prescribing LTOT because of the risk of precipitation of respiratory failure due to CO_2 narcosis, if supplementary oxygen is used in patients with CO_2 retention.

The LTOT has been shown to provide several beneficial effects:
- Improvement in exercise capacity (increased endurance)
- Reduction in dyspnea
- Reduction in pulmonary hypertension, by reducing hypoxic pulmonary vasoconstriction
- Reduction in hematocrit by reducing erythropoietin levels
- Improved quality of life and neuropsychiatric function
- Reduction in severe desaturation episodes during sleep.

Domiciliary oxygen therapy can be provided in three different ways:
1. Long-term and low-dose oxygen for patients with chronic respiratory failure
2. Portable oxygen therapy for exercise-related hypoxia and dyspnea
3. Short-burst oxygen therapy for temporary relief of symptoms.

Selection of Patients for LTOT

All patients should be assessed by a pulmonary specialist.

Absolute indications are:
- Stable COPD with hypoxemia and edema
- FEV_1 less than 1.5 L, forced vital capacity (FVC) <2.0 L
- Arterial partial pressure of oxygen (PaO_2) less than 55 mm Hg (<7.3 kPa), arterial partial pressure of carbon dioxide ($PaCO_2$) more than 45 mm Hg (>6 kPa)
- Stability demonstrated over 3 weeks on optimal therapy.

Relative indications are:
- As above but without edema or $PaCO_2$ more than 45 mm Hg
- Palliative (symptom relief).

Portable oxygen is indicated in patients who desaturate during exercise and its efficacy needs to be assessed during a treadmill or 6-minute walk test with patients wearing the portable oxygen cylinder. Portable oxygen may also be indicated in patients with severe exercise limitation irrespective of oxygen desaturation. Portable oxygen may also be needed in such patients during commercial airline flights (provided by airline).

ANTIBIOTICS

Infection is often the cause of progression or acute deterioration in patients with COPD, the combating of infection by the appropriate use of antibiotics is an important part of therapy. In fact, the organisms causing pulmonary infections are often the same as those found normally in the upper respiratory tract. It may be difficult to know, if a pathogen isolated from the sputum is responsible for the exacerbation. The common bacterial organisms responsible for exacerbations of COPD include *Streptococcus pneumoniae, Haemophilus influenzae, Moraxella catarrhalis,* and *Mycoplasma pneumoniae* (less common). The choice of antibiotic depends upon the likely organisms, the likely sensitivity of the organisms in the community, the tolerance of the patient for the drug, and the response to treatment. Since many strains of *H. influenzae* are now beta-lactamase producers and hence resistant to ampicillin/amoxicillin, the choice for initial therapy commonly lies between:
- Amoxicillin/clavulanic acid (Augmentin)
- Erythromycin or other macrolides (clarithromycin and azithromycin)
- A cephalosporin, e.g. cefaclor
- A tetracycline, e.g. doxycycline.

Macrolide antibiotics (erythromycin and azithromycin) reduce exacerbations of COPD, but it is not certain whether this is an antibiotic or an anti-inflammatory effect of the macrolide. Since long-term antibiotic treatment may have adverse effects (cardiovascular risk and deafness) and increase bacterial resistance, they may be only indicated in selected patients, such as those with coexistent bronchiectasis who have persistently purulent sputum.

OTHER DRUG THERAPIES

Mucolytics

Different mucolytic therapies have been used to increase the ease of mucous expectoration and reduce mucous hypersecretion in an effort to improve lung function:
- *Stopping smoking,* the most effective way
- *Anticholinergics*
- *Beta-2-agonists* and *theophylline*

- *Steam inhalation* (with or without aromatics). This may provide symptomatic relief, but there is no evidence to suggest that it improves lung function or long-term symptom control.
- Several drugs, such as *bromhexine* and *ambroxol*, reduce mucous viscosity in vitro. But, there is little evidence to recommend these drugs as well as the expectorants, such as *guaifenesin* and *potassium iodide* as a routine therapy.
- *Recombinant human DNase* (alpha dornase, Pulmozyme) has beneficial effects in some patients with cystic fibrosis, but its role in COPD is not yet clear.

Antioxidants

Oxidant damage plays an important in the pathophysiology of COPD. Therefore, antioxidant therapy seems quite logical. N-acetyl-cysteine (NAC) and carbocisteine, originally developed as mucolytics, have well-documented antioxidant effects. But their role in the management of COPD is not established.

Vaccines

- Influenza vaccine is recommended as patients with COPD are subject to severe exacerbations with infection and there is evidence for a reduction in acute exacerbations and hospital admissions. Influenza vaccination reduces all-cause mortality. It should be given prior to the winter season.
- Polyvalent pneumococcal vaccine is used in many countries to protect against the development of pneumococcal lung infections. Pneumococcal vaccination does not reduce mortality and there are no convincing large trials to show a reduction in exacerbations.

Neuraminidase Inhibitors

Inhibitors of neuraminidase, such as zanamivir (inhaled) and oseltamivir (oral), speed the recovery from influenza. However, there are no specific trials in patients with COPD and it is not yet certain whether this treatment is cost-effective.

Treatment of Dyspnea

Breathlessness is the most distressing symptom in many patients, particularly in those with severe emphysema. Drugs, which may reduce the sensation of dyspnea, include nebulized opiates, slow-release morphine, dihydrocodeine, and benzodiazepines. But their effect of depressing the ventilatory drive is potentially dangerous. They are better avoided, particularly during exacerbations.

Antitussives

Cough is another troublesome symptom of COPD, which is frequently refractory to most treatments. Cough, however, may also have a protective effect in clearing secretions. The regular use of antitussives is therefore not recommended in COPD.

NONPHARMACOLOGICAL TREATMENTS

Several nonpharmacological approaches are useful as an important component of a comprehensive rehabilitation program. This is particularly useful in the elderly patients.

Surgery

Surgical techniques are useful for more severe emphysema. These include heart–lung transplantation or single lung transplantation for disabling emphysema. Lung volume reduction surgery has been used with variable success rates. This procedure involves excision of severely affected emphysematous lung and found to be effective in highly selected patients. This is generally done in patients with bilateral, predominantly upper lobe emphysema and evidence of air trapping. It has shown to result in sustained improvement in lung function, reduction in symptoms and exacerbations. Bronchoscopic lung volume reduction can be also employed to avoid the surgical morbidity and mortality of lung volume reduction surgery (LVRS). Several devices, including one-way valves, coils, sealants, airway bypass stents, and bronchoscopic thermal vapor ablation, designed to collapse and remodel hyperinflated lung are currently being tried in clinical trials.

CHAPTER
37

Acute Exacerbations of Chronic Obstructive Pulmonary Disease

Raja Dhar, AG Ghoshal

INTRODUCTION

Exacerbations of chronic obstructive pulmonary disease (COPD) may occur despite adequate disease control. Most patients experience episodes of exacerbations at least one or more times during their lifetime and many suffer with these episodes at least one to three times a year. These episodes may vary immensely in terms of frequency and severity. COPD exacerbations have a major impact on the physical, emotional, and economic condition of the patient.

COPD EXACERBATION

An acute exacerbation of COPD (AECOPD) occurs in the natural course of COPD. It is characterized by an acute change in the patient's clinical condition. There is increase in breathing difficulty, cough, and/or sputum production, which is more than the routine day-to-day variability requiring a change in management. There are no universally agreed criteria to categorize acute exacerbations. The following operational classification can help to classify the clinical severity of the event and its outcome.

- *Level I*: Treated at home
- *Level II*: Requiring hospitalization
- *Level III*: Leading to respiratory failure and intensive care unit (ICU) admission.

Causes of COPD Exacerbations

Lower respiratory tract infections are responsible for about 50% of COPD exacerbations. Other causes may include the exposure to indoor or outdoor air pollutants, changes in weather conditions, and several other host factors such as poor compliance to therapy. The established etiologies of AECOPD have been precised in the acronym—ABCDEFGX:
- *A*irway viral infection
- *B*acterial infection
- *C*oinfection
- *D*epression/anxiety
- *E*mbolism (pulmonary)
- *F*ailure (cardiac, or failure of lung integrity—pneumothorax)
- *G*eneral environment
- *X* (unknown).

Symptoms of COPD Exacerbation

Usually, patients present with one or more symptoms of acute exacerbation. During clinical assessment, several clinical elements should be considered such as the severity of the underlying COPD, the presence of comorbidities, and the history of previous exacerbations. The physical examination should include evaluation for the effects on cardiac hemodynamic and respiratory systems. The diagnostic investigations include the chest radiography, sputum and blood examination, spirometry, and other relevant tests.

Management of COPD Exacerbation

Both the subjective evaluation and the objective criteria (Table 37.1) should be considered to decide whether a patient should be treated at home or in the hospital. However, the decision to treat at home or at hospital can changed rapidly in the presence of a sudden deterioration of condition.

Primary Care

In patients with an exacerbation managed in primary care, it is not generally recommended to send sputum samples for culture; it is not in routine practice. On the other hand, pulse oximetry may be especially in the presence of clinical features of a severe exacerbation.

Prognostication: The CRB65 score, a risk stratification method validated for use in community-acquired pneumonia, has recently been shown to have utility in AECOPD. Serum procalcitonin has recently been advocated for use in deciding regarding antibiotic treatment in patients with AECOPD. However, recent studies show that procalcitonin is useful in COPD patients for alerting clinicians to invasive bacterial infections such as pneumonia, but it does not distinguish bacterial from viral and noninfectious causes of AECOPD. Serum uric acid is increased in respiratory disease, especially in the presence of

TABLE 37.1: Clinical factors that determine whether the patient should be treated at home or hospital.

Factor	Indication to treat at home	Indication to treat at a hospital
Able to cope at home	Yes	No
Severity of breathlessness	Mild	Severe
General health condition	Good/satisfactory	Poor/deteriorating
Level of activity	Good	Poor/confined to bed
Cyanosis	No	Yes
Worsening peripheral edema	No	Yes
Level of consciousness	Normal	Impaired
Already receiving LTOT	No	Yes
Social circumstances	Good/adequate support	Living alone/not coping
Acute confusion/altered mental status	No	Yes
Rapid rate of onset	No	Yes
Significant comorbidity (particularly heart disease and insulin-dependent diabetes)	No	Yes
$SaO_2 < 90\%$	No	Yes
Changes on the chest radiograph	No	Present
Arterial pH level	>7.35	<7.35
Arterial PaO_2	>7 kPa	<7 kPa

(LTOT, long-term oxygen therapy; SaO_2, arterial oxygen saturation; PaO_2, arterial partial pressure of oxygen; pH, potential of hydrogen)

hypoxia and systemic inflammation. High-uric acid levels (>6.9 mg/dL) in AECOPD were an independent predictor of 30-day mortality, but not of 1-year mortality. Poor outcome is predicted from elevated cardiac biomarkers such as B-type natriuretic peptide (BNP) or troponin.

Patients Referred to Hospital

In all patients with an exacerbation referred to hospital:
- A chest radiograph should be obtained.
- Arterial blood gas tensions should be measured and the inspired oxygen concentration should be recorded.
- An electrocardiogram (ECG) should be recorded to exclude cardiac comorbidities.
- A full blood count should be performed; urea and electrolyte concentrations should be measured.

- A theophylline level should be measured in patients who are on theophylline therapy at admission.
- If sputum is purulent, a sample should be sent for microscopy and culture.
- Blood cultures should be taken, if the patient has fever.

Outpatient Management for COPD Exacerbation (Level I)

The treatment of exacerbation has to be based on the clinical presentation of the patient.

The essential components of treatment include the following:
- *Bronchodilators*: Short-acting beta-2-agonist and/or ipratropium by metered dose inhaler (MDI) with spacer or hand-held nebulizer as needed. Consider adding long-acting bronchodilator, e.g. formoterol (by metered dose inhaler plus spacer or nebulized route).
- *Corticosteroids (the actual dose may vary)*: Oral prednisone 30–40 mg per OS QD for 10 days; consider using an inhaled corticosteroid.
- *Antibiotics*: May be initiated in patients with altered sputum characteristics; choice should be based on local bacteria resistance patterns (amoxicillin/ampicillin, cephalosporins, doxycycline, macrolides).
  If the patient has failed prior antibiotic therapy, consider—amoxicillin/clavulanate or respiratory fluoroquinolones.
- *Patient education*: Check inhalation technique, consider use of spacer devices.

Inpatient Management of COPD Exacerbation (Levels II and III)

The decision to admit a patient is decided on the basis of clinical features, the severity of dyspnea, presence of respiratory failure, and emergency room therapy. The presence and severity of cor pulmonale, complicating severe bronchitis, pneumonia, and other comorbid conditions are also considered while making the decision for admission.

General consensus supports the need for hospitalization in patients with severe acute hypoxemia or acute hypercarbia. Less extreme arterial blood gas abnormalities, however, do not assist decision analysis. Other factors that identify "high-risk" patients include a previous emergency room visit within 7 days, the number of doses of nebulized bronchodilators, use of home oxygen, previous relapse rate, administration of aminophylline, and the use of corticosteroids and antibiotics at the time of previous emergency room discharge.

Pharmacological Management

It constitutes the mainstay of treatment of COPD exacerbation. Following drugs are most commonly employed:
- *Inhaled bronchodilators*—preferably nebulized.
- *Systemic corticosteroids*: Inhaled or oral corticosteroids:
  - Prednisolone (30–40 mg per day) should be prescribed for 10 days. If the patient cannot tolerate oral intake, consider equivalent dose by intravenous (IV) route.

- Prolonged therapy with corticosteroids has no advantage. It is, therefore, recommended that the course of corticosteroid treatment need not be longer than 14 days.
- Patients, particularly those discharged from hospital, should be given clear instructions about why, when, and how to stop their corticosteroid treatment.

- *Antibiotics*: Antibiotics are required, if there is any history of purulent sputum production, change in sputum color, consistency and volume, presence of clinical symptoms of pneumonia and/or consolidation on chest radiograph. Choice of antibiotics is made on the basis of local bacteria resistance patterns. However, when this information is not available, macrolides or second-generation cephalosporins can be used.
- *Theophylline and other methylxanthines*: Intravenous theophylline should only be used as an adjunct to the management of exacerbations of COPD, if there is an inadequate response to nebulized bronchodilators. Care should be taken when using intravenous theophylline because of its interactions with other drugs (e.g. ciprofloxacin, clarithromycin, allopurinol, phenytoin, etc.) and potential toxicity, if the patient has been on oral theophylline. Within 24 hours of starting the treatment, the theophylline levels should be monitored to maintain within therapeutic range (10-20 μg/mL). Thereafter, monitoring should be done as frequently as indicated by clinical circumstances.
- *Respiratory stimulants*: It is recommended that doxapram is used only when noninvasive ventilation is either unavailable or considered inappropriate (e.g. hypersensitivity, pulmonary embolism, severe hypertension, cerebral edema, epilepsy, hyperthyroidism, etc.).
- *Oxygen therapy*: Oxygen therapy is always required for the relief of severe respiratory distress in patients with exacerbations. It is also needed for prevention of tissue hypoxia by maintaining arterial oxygen saturation (SaO_2) at more than 90%. Oxygen therapy should be controlled at low flows without causing worsening or precipitating hypercapnia and respiratory acidosis. Mechanical ventilation may be necessary, if pH falls below 7.35 (acidemia).

Noninvasive positive pressure ventilation (NIPPV) should be offered to patients with exacerbations when, after optimal medical therapy and oxygenation, respiratory acidosis (pH < 7.36) and/or excessive breathlessness persist. All patients considered for mechanical ventilation should have arterial blood gases measured. Mechanical ventilation is a mode of assisted or controlled ventilation using mechanical devices that cycle automatically to generate airway pressure. Intubation should be considered in patients with NIPPV failure, presence of severe acidosis (pH < 7.25), hypercapnia [$PaCO_2$ > 8 kPa (60 mm Hg)], tachypnea > 35 breaths/min, and/or presence of complications such as metabolic abnormalities, sepsis, pneumonia, pulmonary embolism, barotrauma or massive pleural effusion].

De-escalation of Therapy

Patient's recovery should be monitored by regular clinical assessment of their symptoms and observation of their functional capacity. During recovery from an exacerbation from COPD, daily performance of forced expiratory volume in 1 second (FEV_1) or peak expiratory flow is not advised, since the magnitude of change is small as compared to the variability of measurement. Discharge should be planned once there is significant improvement and clinical stability of the patient.

CHAPTER 38

Pulmonary Rehabilitation

Rachael A Evans, Roger S Goldstein

INTRODUCTION

Patients with chronic obstructive pulmonary disease (COPD) commonly present with exertional breathlessness and fatigue and typically they become less active to avoid these symptoms. This reduction in activity can lead to loss of confidence, depression, loss of work, or inability to perform hobbies and social isolation, resulting in substantial disability. Abnormalities in gas exchange as well as the restrictive ventilatory limitation associated with hyperinflation contribute to the symptoms of exertional breathlessness and diminished exercise capacity.

In addition to the primary pulmonary pathology, there are secondary alterations in skeletal muscle function, nutrition, bone density, gonadal hormones, hemoglobin, and mood, many of which influence exercise tolerance and health-related quality of life.

The spiral of inactivity is also affected by symptoms of anxiety and depression experienced by many patients with COPD. The sensation of dyspnea generates feelings of anxiety, but anxiety itself can manifest as dyspnea. Low mood is frequently reported by patients with COPD related to their disability and loss of function, but may also be a preexisting phenomenon predisposing to smoking. Unfortunately, the effect of low mood on motivation and self-esteem further impact on inactivity.

ROLE AND DEFINITION OF PULMONARY REHABILITATION

The term "rehabilitation" refers to the process of restoration of function despite physical or psychological disability. Pulmonary rehabilitation (PR) programs have developed over the last few decades as a therapy targeted at the secondary alterations of COPD, aiming at improving both the functional and psychosocial aspects of an individual. It is now recommended as an integral part of the clinical management of patients with COPD and has a strong, supportive evidence base demonstrating a reduction in dyspnea, and improvements in both exercise tolerance and health-related quality of life.

According to the American Thoracic Society (ATS) and the European Respiratory Society (ERS), PR is defined as—"a comprehensive intervention based on a thorough patient assessment followed by patient-tailored therapies that include, but are not limited to, exercise training, education, and behavior change, and designed to improve the physical and psychological condition of people with chronic respiratory disease and to promote the long-term adherence to health-enhancing behaviors".

Pulmonary rehabilitation programs include several evidence-based components and should not be mistaken for more general programs of activity promotion, convalescence, or pure self-management programs.

CHANGING PULMONARY REHABILITATION POPULATION— WHOM TO REFER?

Patients with COPD are the traditional target population for PR. However, the spiral of inactivity also applies to other chronic respiratory diseases, providing a rationale for rehabilitation, which has been reported to be beneficial in other conditions including pulmonary fibrosis, post-tuberculosis lung disease, thoracic restriction, bronchiectasis, cystic fibrosis, asthma, pulmonary hypertension, pre- and postoperatively for lung resection, volume reduction, or transplantation.

The predominant clinical inclusion criterion, for referral for PR, is exertional dyspnea that interferes with function as assessed by the Medical Research Council (MRC) Dyspnea Scale. This is a simple, self-assessed scale, which can easily be used to screen those who may benefit from rehabilitation. International guidelines suggest referral for PR for patients with Grades III-V scale. There is evidence to suggest that patients with milder levels of breathlessness may also benefit. The Global initiative for Obstructive Lung Disease recommends rehabilitation for any symptomatic patient with GOLD stage II and above [forced expiratory volume in 1 second (FEV_1) < 80% predicted].

Both the primary respiratory disease and existing comorbid conditions should be optimally managed prior to enrolment. Patients with obstructive disease should receive optimal airway care. Any preexisting depression should be addressed as it is known to be associated with poor compliance and response to rehabilitation. Diagnostic assessment and optimizing management should occur prior to commencing PR.

Patients need to be able to participate in endurance exercises and those with a predominantly orthopedic, neurological, or peripheral vascular limitation to exercise, are commonly excluded. Safety criteria should be adhered to, for example, a myocardial infarction sustained within 3 months, unstable angina, moderate-to-severe aortic stenosis, or uncontrolled blood pressure will all exclude patients from being enrolled. Patients with unstable cardiovascular disease must be assessed and treated appropriately prior to inclusion to a program. Nonclinical factors may be pivotal. These include a reasonable level of comprehension, realistic expectations of the program, motivation to improve, an ability to follow instructions, acceptable health literacy, and a supportive home and family.

The assessment should systematically address the inclusion and exclusion criteria and further inform the patients about the process of PR. An assessment of dyspnea, exercise performance, and health status is standard and can inform both individual progress and program quality.

OUTCOME MEASURES

Full Cardiopulmonary Exercise Tests

The gold standard measurement of exercise capacity is peak oxygen consumption. Typically, tests are performed on a cycle ergometer providing a stable platform, but a treadmill can also be used particularly, if cycling is not familiar. Endurance tests can be performed using the same equipment set at an intensity relative to the peak performance.

Six-minute Walk Test

The most commonly used field test is the 6-minute walk test (6MWT). The test is completed over a 30-meter flat course. It is self-paced and standardized instructions are given. The 6MWT can be influenced by encouragement— which is, therefore, standardized. It is likely closer to peak exercise capacity although the distance walked is referred to as a measure of functional capacity. The 6MWT distance is highly correlated with other outcomes of COPD such as mortality and is featured in the multidimensional severity index; the BODE index. It is reliable, valid, and interpretable, all important qualities for its use in clinical research.

Incremental Shuttle Walk Test

The incremental shuttle walk test (ISWT) is a symptom-limited, externally paced test, conducted along a 10-meter course, and reflects maximal exercise capacity. The walking speed increases every minute until the patient is too breathless or fatigued to continue or can no longer maintain the required speed. The result is presented as the total distance achieved. It is reproducible after a single practice test.

Endurance Shuttle Walk Test

The endurance shuttle walk test (ESWT) was developed as a test of submaximal exercise capacity. It is similarly symptom-limited, externally paced and uses the same 10-meter course as the ISWT.

Health Status

Health-related quality of life (HRQL) has become an important outcome for assessing chronic disease interventions. Most disease-specific questionnaires have components that assess dyspnea and activity limitation. The two most commonly used and therefore the best understood are the Chronic Respiratory Questionnaire (CRQ) and St George's Respiratory Questionnaire (SGRQ). They are both reproducible and evaluative, but the SGRQ has the advantage of also being discriminative. Generic questionnaires such as the Medical Outcomes Short Form-36 Questionnaire (SF-36) can also be used.

Dyspnea

The MRC scale is often used as an outcome measure for dyspnea. It is a valid and reproducible instrument, but not designed to be an evaluative tool. It is, however, a valuable guide to staging the severity of COPD. The Baseline Dyspnea Index and the Transition Dyspnea Index (BDI–TDI) are disease-specific, valid, reproducible, and interpretable. Together with the SGRQ and the CRQ, the BDI–TDI is among the most frequently employed measures of outcome in PR.

Clinical Important Difference

For many of the outcome measures described a "clinically meaningful" change has been evaluated. This adds to clinical interpretation of results from an intervention. If achieved, it provides a rationale for introducing or withdrawing a management intervention.

CORE COMPONENTS OF A PULMONARY REHABILITATION PROGRAM

The core components of a program include the following:
- *Exercise training*: Exercise training is an essential component to PR and has the largest supporting evidence base of all the other components.
  - *Lower-limb endurance training*: Lower-limb endurance training is mandatory for individuals who wish to improve exercise tolerance and reduce dyspnea on exertion. It is individually prescribed, based on an assessment exercise test and progressed throughout the program. High-intensity training is recommended in the healthy population for achieving cardiorespiratory fitness. Walking and cycling are both effective training modalities. Although interval training has a good rationale for allowing the muscles to recover during the lower intensity periods, studies have not identified interval training as being more effective than constant load training for those with COPD.
  - *Resistance training*: Resistance (strength) training has received much attention over the last two decades and is recommended by international guidelines. Although muscle strength is improved compared to endurance training alone, this has not translated to additional improvements in

exercise tolerance or health status. Upper limb resistance training is commonly performed using free weights and currently unsupported endurance exercises are recommended in the guidelines.
- *Multidisciplinary education*: Examples of typical education topics are shown in Box 38.1. Education is commonly delivered in a group setting, but should be supplemented with individual support and other ongoing educational materials such as computer-based and online learning modules. Psychological support is a core component of PR, as many patients experience symptoms of anxiety or depression.

Self-management can be taught within or outside of PR. It increases patients' involvement and control of their disease and improves their sense of wellbeing. It has been shown to reduce resource utilization—especially that attributable to unscheduled visits to the hospital. Patients learn to cope and react to their disease.

A minimum of three supervised sessions per week for 6 weeks is recommended, but due to recognized financial and time constraints, two supervised sessions with at least one other home session is acceptable. Additional home training alongside the supervised sessions should be commenced from the outset.

MAINTENANCE

Follow-up and maintenance are required to sustain the benefits of PR in keeping with the principles of long-term chronic disease management. A close relationship between primary and specialist care is also important as the majority of patients with COPD will be managed by their primary care physician or nurse practitioner.

As adherence to the exercise protocol decreases, the level of exercise achieved is often reduced. This is especially the case following a respiratory exacerbation. There are many approaches to the frequency and location of the maintenance process including whether it is necessary for this to be institutionally based or whether effective programs can be accessed through community centers. Repeat modified (short-term) programs result in similar short-term gains in exercise tolerance, but without an overall long-term benefit.

BOX 38.1: Example of topics for the education component.

Multidisciplinary education:
- Exercise
- Nutritional advice
- Relaxation
- Devices and oxygen therapy
- Benefits advice
- Energy conservation
- Travel
- Sexual intercourse advice
- Disease education
- Pharmacology

Oxygen

Supplemental oxygen during exercise may be required for safety reasons in those who exhibit profound desaturation. Under laboratory and field exercise conditions, oxygen can improve exercise performance by reducing the ventilatory requirements.

MOBILITY AIDS

Although walking sticks can improve balance and posture, rollators provide more stable support, improve balance, and enable the user to sit comfortably on the seat provided. These benefits are sustained, if the patients continue to use the rollator at home. Rollators also have the advantage of being able to carry oxygen or other small items such as groceries.

REHABILITATION TEAM

The multidisciplinary team should encompass the skills of respiratory physiotherapists, occupational therapists, nurses, assistants, and physicians. It is often not possible to have the complete range of disciplines in person, but the skill set should be available. Team members should all have basic and intermediate life-support skills and at least one member in the exercise sessions should have advanced life support.

SETTING

Pulmonary rehabilitation programs have been hospital based for stable disease both as inpatient and outpatient settings. There are limitations with this approach namely transport and accessibility. As in most countries, the provision of PR does not reach the demand, and community and home-based programs are sometimes available.

EXACERBATIONS

Exacerbations are the real enemy of PR, as all the components that improve with PR—dyspnea, exercise tolerance, muscle strength, and health-related quality of life are all reduced following an acute exacerbation. Many patients do not reach their pre-exacerbation level of functioning and clinical practice is of repeat referral for a shorter (booster) program. There is the evidence that undergoing PR immediately postexacerbation is beneficial and not associated with adverse effects.

PERFORMANCE ENHANCEMENT

Several approaches to enhancement have been evaluated. Calorie supplementation appears to help normal weight patients, but not those with cachexia. Creatine supplementation has not been demonstrated to impact on exercise performance. Anabolic agents are not currently recommended. Patients should be optimally managed pharmacologically prior to entry into PR and the addition of a long-acting anticholinergic has been shown to improve PR compared to placebo.

CONCLUSION

In summary, a clearer understanding of adherence to rehabilitation requires an understanding of self-efficacy, behavioral adaptations, and other determinant factors. Maintenance programs are necessary for comprehensive long-term management of chronic respiratory diseases, just as they are for nonrespiratory conditions. The frequency, content, and duration of maintenance programs need to be better defined. Frequent exacerbations are likely to remain a large healthcare burden for patients with COPD and particular attention should be given to integrating exercise therapy early in the recovery period.

CHAPTER
39

Bullous Lung Diseases

Aditya Jindal, Gyanendra Agrawal

INTRODUCTION

A bulla is an air-containing space of more than 1 cm diameter in the distended state within the lung parenchyma. In surgical lung specimen, a bulla causes a local protrusion from the surface of the removed lung. Of various bullous lung conditions, bullous lung disease is characterized by the presence of bullae in one or both the lung fields, with normal intervening lung while bullous emphysema is a condition in which bullae occur in conjunction with the emphysematous changes in the non-bullous lung. Sometimes, the bullae are big to occupy more than one-third of the hemithorax, a condition called giant bullous lung disease. In such cases, there is compression of the surrounding lung parenchyma. It is a rare form of bullous lung disease which may frequently need differential diagnosis from pneumothorax.

There are subtle differences between the terms bulla, bleb and cyst. A bleb is a small space containing air which is lined by the elastic lamina and lies between the two layers of visceral pleura. A bulla lies within the connective tissue septa of the lung present deep to the internal elastic layer of the visceral pleura. It has no formal wall of its own. On the other hand, a cyst is a separate structure lined by epithelium which is present within the lung parenchyma or the mediastinum.

PATHOGENESIS

Bulla arises from destruction of alveolar walls resulting in dilatation and confluence of airspaces distal to terminal bronchioles. A bulla is surrounded by attenuated and compressed lung parenchyma. There are many hypotheses to explain the development of bullae. Most likely, the bulla arises due to the underlying paraseptal emphysema. The structural weakness of the interalveolar septa caused by elastolysis, which itself may be secondary either to a constitutional disorder or to enhanced proteolysis is the predominant mechanism for the development of paraseptal emphysema. Airspaces in paraseptal emphysema may become confluent and develop into bullae, which may be large. Airway obstruction caused either by loss of airway support or by inflammatory changes in the walls of small airways, also, contribute to progressive enlargement of these airspaces; ultimately resulting in the formation of bullous emphysema.

The pressure in bullae is normally negative and same as that of pleural pressure. The bulla is more compliant than the surrounding lung. Therefore, the bulla gets easily inflated with lesser pressure than that required for the surrounding lung. During inspiration, when bullae and the adjacent lung parenchyma are subjected to same negative pleural pressure, bulla fills preferentially than the surrounding lung like a *paper bag*. This *paper bag compliance* is seen up to a critical lung volume, after which they become stiff and much less compliant than lung.

Chronic marijuana smoking is also believed to cause bullae formation through microscopic injury to the airways or other unknown mechanisms.

ETIOLOGY

Bullae may form in a number of diseases and other settings (Box 39.1). Tobacco smoking is the most important risk factors for bullous emphysema. Alpha 1-antitrypsin deficiency and other hereditary conditions of rare familial disorders can also cause lung bullae and emphysema. The cause cannot be

BOX 39.1: Causes of bullae in the lungs.

- Extraneous/environmental
  - Tobacco smoking
  - Marijuana smoking
  - HIV infection
  - Post-tubercular fibrosis
- Rare familial disorders
  - Alpha-1 antitrypsin deficiency
  - Fabry's disease
  - Cutis laca
  - Ehlers–Danlos syndrome
  - Marfan's syndrome
  - Neurofibromatosis
- Miscellaneous
  - Ankylosing spondylitis
  - Sarcoidosis
  - Langerhans' cell histiocytosis
  - Idiopathic pulmonary fibrosis
- Idiopathic bullous disease

ascertained in a subset of patients with bullous disease, they are labeled as idiopathic bullous disease.

CLINICAL PRESENTATION

Small bullae usually produce no symptoms, signs or significant alterations in pulmonary function; they are detected during routine chest radiography. Spontaneous pneumothorax can occur due to rupture of one or more bullae. Most of the causes of bullae formation are therefore responsible for recurrent pneumothoraces.

The most common presenting symptom in bullous lung disease is of gradually progressive exertional dyspnea. Occasionally, they may develop sudden severe increase in breathlessness either due to pneumothorax or over distension due to air-trapping. Chest pain may occur in a patient with bullous lung disease. This is also due to overdistension of the large bullae or development of pneumothorax. Overdistension causes a diffuse dull aching type of chest pain, usually located retrosternally. Hemoptysis is an uncommon presentation, and usually indicates hemorrhage inside the bullae. Increase in cough and sputum production, in patients with known bullous disease, usually point to the presence of infection in a bulla. Occasionally, giant bullae may cause localized hyperresonant note and decreased breath sounds. Giant bullae may commonly present with vanishing lung syndrome.

RADIOLOGIC FEATURES

Small bullae are not usually seen on the plain chest radiographs but are easily visible on computed tomography. Apical bullae may sometimes be misinterpreted as cavitation on plain radiographs. They can be differentiated if it is remembered that cavities are centered within areas of consolidation and they do not merely overlap them.

High resolution computed tomography (HRCT) is almost diagnostic as it can locate the bullae with considerable accuracy even when not suspected on clinical findings and plain radiography. HRCT is also helpful to define the extent and sites of bullae as well as the presence of other lung parenchymal abnormalities, such as diffuse nonbullous emphysema, bronchiectasis, infected cysts, pleural disease and pulmonary hypertension. Computed tomography scans can help in differentiating bullous lung disease from bullous emphysema. The intervening lung parenchyma is normal in bullous lung disease as opposed to changes of emphysema seem in emphysematous bullae.

PULMONARY FUNCTION TESTS

Spirometry in patients with bullous lung disease usually shows restrictive defect. This is presumably due to loss of lung tissue and compression of the intervening normal lung by the bulla. On the other hand, a predominant obstructive defect is seen in patients having bullous emphysema. The diffusing capacity is reduced to a greater extent in bullous emphysema as compared to bullous lung disease. Unlike most other tests, diffusion capacity correlates better with morphologic estimates of emphysema. The diffusing capacity fails to increase normally during exercise.

In patients with bullous lung disease, the lung volumes should be assessed by both the helium dilution technique and body plethysmography. The volume of the bullae is determined by the difference in total lung capacity (TLC) measured by body plethysmography and that by the helium dilution technique.

Respiratory muscle strength assessed by the measurements of maximal inspiratory and transdiaphragmatic pressures improves after bullectomy in patients with bullous emphysema. But in some patients, the resting pulmonary artery pressures are increased and get further exaggerated during exercise due to reduction in the pulmonary vascular bed.

NATURAL HISTORY

Systematic long-term studies on the natural history of bullous lung disease are lacking. Patients should be monitored at regular intervals by chest radiography. Bullae may enlarge at a variable rate over several months and years. Sometimes, sudden expansion may follow a period of relative stability. In some patients, often young men, there may be the inexorable progression of idiopathic giant bullous disease. The alternative name given for the devastating nature of this condition is *vanishing lung syndrome*. In some patients, bulla may disappear either spontaneously or following infection and hemorrhage, or with medical therapy alone.

COMPLICATIONS

The main complications of bullae are pneumothorax, infection or hemorrhage. When infected, bullae usually contain fluid and develop an air–fluid level. Air fluid levels within the bullae are relatively uncommon. Fluid may be frequently resorbed, and cause complete resolution of the bulla. An infected bulla differs from an abscess in that the patient is less ill, the wall of the ring shadow is thinner and has a sharp margin, and there is less adjacent pneumonitis. Sometimes, there is colonization of a fungus within the bulla, i.e. mycetoma or fungal ball, most commonly with *Aspergillus*. Hemorrhage inside the bulla is a less common complication and it manifests as hemoptysis or decrease in hemoglobin level. Pneumothorax may occur due to the rupture of the bulla in pleural cavity or as a complication of paraseptal emphysema.

TREATMENT

An asymptomatic patient diagnosed to have bullous lung disease should be reassured and educated about the disease. All attempts should be made to quit smoking. The patients should be asked to avoid activities that promote rupture of bulla like *scuba-diving*. Appropriate treatment for the associated disease like asthma or chronic obstructive pulmonary disease (COPD) should be given. There are case reports of spontaneous resolution of progressively enlarging giant bullous emphysema after medical therapy for COPD was instituted. Appropriate antibiotics and chest physiotherapy should be started as soon as the diagnosis of infected bullae is established.

Because of the impairment of respiratory function, and the higher incidence of coexisting infection and cancer, the giant bulla should be resected in all patients, even if they are asymptomatic. Enlarging bullae causing incapacitating dyspnea or chest pain or impending respiratory insufficiency also need to be resected. Any lung mass associated with bullae should be considered as an indication for surgery. Other indications of bullectomy include infected bullae and that causing recurrent pneumothorax.

Thoracoscopic bullapasty performed in fully awake patients is reported to be well tolerated and effective. Antilogous pleural reinforcement of staple line in surgery is another safe and cost effective measure. Thoracoscopy carries a lower mortality and complication rates than the other surgical approaches.

Lung volume reduction surgery (LVRS) involves the resection of 20–30% of emphysematous lung from each side. Other treatment approaches for giant bullae include reduction pneumoplasty and Brompton's procedure (endocavitary aspiration with sclerosis and pleurodesis); the latter is preferred in patients with poor pulmonary function.

Resection of giant bullae provides significant relief even in the absence of widespread obstructive lung disease. But there is less certain therapeutic advantage of surgical lung resection in generalized emphysema. As a rule, surgical intervention is avoided in bullae associated with either obstructive or fibrotic lung disease, unless life-threatening complication arises.

CONCLUSION

In conclusion, bullae in the lungs may arise due to various conditions. It is important to distinguish between widespread obstructive airways disease with concomitant bullae and primary bullous lung disease. Clinical presentation and management approach significantly differ in different situations. Progressive bullae formation is associated with significant morbidity and mortality.

CHAPTER

40

Upper and Central Airways Obstruction

VR Pattabhi Raman

INTRODUCTION

Upper airway obstruction (UAO) can be classified as acute and chronic, and the causes for both are quite different. Chronic UAO poses a diagnostic dilemma, and is frequently misdiagnosed and managed as bronchial asthma. On the other hand, acute UAO poses a therapeutic challenge and is best managed in a well-equipped setting that has physicians trained in difficult airway management. UAO is defined as the obstruction of the airways at or proximal to carina, including the nose, mouth, pharynx, and larynx. The pressure that affects the caliber of upper airways in the extrathoracic region is atmospheric pressure while the intrathoracic pressure is the pleural pressure.

PHYSIOLOGICAL CONSIDERATIONS

The classification of UAO on the basis of the anatomical landmark, i.e. the thoracic inlet has also got physiological significance and helps in the understanding of the differences that one sees when one assesses the flow-volume loops of extrathoracic and intrathoracic obstruction. Also, the nature of obstruction, whether it is stiff or pliable, determines whether there will be changes in severity in relation to changes in the transmural pressure. A stiff lesion, as in some cases of postintubation tracheal stenosis (PITS), does not allow dynamic differences in the diameter of the stenosis and in the airflow between inspiration and expiration. This is called fixed airway obstruction.

In cases of bilateral abductor palsy of vocal cords, there are differences in the caliber and the airflow during the respiratory cycle. Because of the extrathoracic nature of the obstruction, inspiration worsens and expiration lessens the obstruction. This is an example of variable airway obstruction. Based on these parameters, UAO can be divided into fixed obstruction, variable extrathoracic obstruction and variable intrathoracic obstruction.

CLINICAL FEATURES

Acute airway obstruction usually presents as severe breathlessness and agitation. Stridor is the usual diagnostic sign. Stridor is frequently audible unaided and stethoscope is seldom required.

Chronic obstruction is frequently misdiagnosed and managed as asthma and/or chronic obstructive pulmonary disease (COPD) for a variable period of time before the recognition of upper airway problem. The patient may also present very late in the course of the disease. Tracheal lumen of less than 8 mm usually produces symptoms after exercise and of less than 5 mm produces stridor.

High index of suspicion is usually required in chronic UAO. Diligent history taking, including the history of intubation and of thyroid surgery could serve as a clue. Many cases of chronic UAO have periods of worsening, which get better with antibiotics and steroids, further delaying the diagnosis. Certain features, such as hemoptysis, and relative refractoriness to asthma treatment should alert the physicians about the possibility of UAO and the need for further investigations.

DIAGNOSIS

Radiology

Plain X-ray is seldom useful. It may show obvious mediastinal lymphadenopathy or sometimes a tracheal tumor with extramural extension. At times, the penetrated film may show the site of obstruction. Computed tomography (CT) is very valuable to diagnose airway obstruction. In particular, the reconstructed images (Fig. 40.1) provide relevant details about the site, the extent, and the nature of obstruction. Some patients with very severe stenosis may not be able to lie down flat and hold their breath for the study. Magnetic resonance imaging (MRI) is not very commonly sought. It may give valuable information by its superior contrast resolution.

Spirometry

With UAO, flow at higher lung volume may be limited by obstruction. UAO causes more pronounced decrease in peak expiratory flow (PEF) than in the forced expiratory volume in 1 second (FEV_1). An increased ratio of FEV_1 (mL) divided by PEF (L/min) should alert the clinician to the need of an inspiratory and expiratory flow–volume loop. This ratio is called as Empey's Index, the value of more than eight suggest the presence of central or UAO. Poor initial effort by the patient can also increase the index. Hence, it is very important that the patient's inspiratory and expiratory efforts are maximal and the

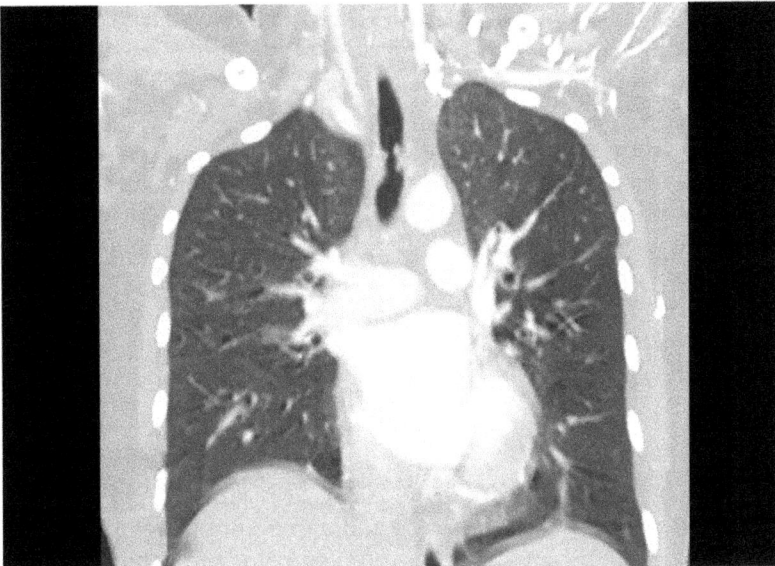

Fig. 40.1: Reconstructed computed tomography image of a patient with tracheal stenosis.

technician should confirm this in the quality pattern of repeatable plateau of forced inspiratory flow.

Bronchoscopy

Bronchoscopy, which provides the most useful information in UAO, is the procedure of choice. It is useful to have an idea about the lesion with a CT done before bronchoscopy, so that planning could be better. The cause of the anatomical obstruction can be diagnosed in the case of an intramural pathology like a tumor. Care, however, has to be taken while passing a flexible bronchoscope through a very narrow lumen; even a minor hemorrhage can become catastrophic by causing critical airway narrowing. It is wise to employ rigid bronchoscopy in such a case of severe obstruction.

In cases of extrinsic obstruction, bronchoscopy could be valuable in assessing the mucosa, if there is a transmural invasion. It also helps in assessing the extent of involvement to guide a definitive therapy. In cases of functional obstruction, such as in tracheomalacia (TM), bronchoscopy is mandatory.

ACUTE UPPER AIRWAY OBSTRUCTION

Foreign Body

Typically seen in children aged between 2 years and 4 years, aspiration of foreign bodies can be also seen in older children and the elderly individuals. In the elderly patients, it commonly occurs in the presence of comorbidities with depressed consciousness and poor swallowing reflex. In pediatric population, choking is the most common symptom followed by a protracted cough. Radiography is useful only in the case of radiopaque foreign bodies or when there is expiratory hyperinflation. Normal chest X-ray does not exclude foreign body aspiration.

Early intervention is important, especially when vegetable matter like groundnut or bean is aspirated since granulation happens rather rapidly and at times, so profusely that it may not be visible in bronchoscopy. Also, delayed removal may not result in complete healing of the granulation tissue. Groundnut is probably the most common foreign body among children in India. Though rigid bronchoscopy is considered the gold standard for the retrieval of an aspirated foreign body, there is a definite role for flexible pediatric bronchoscopes for both diagnosis and retrieval of pediatric foreign bodies.

Acute Laryngeal Edema

Acute laryngeal edema may happen in following anaphylactic reactions causing life-threatening angioedema—prototype being the penicillin allergy or nonsteroidal anti-inflammatory drugs (NSAIDs) allergy in aspirin-sensitive asthma. The deterioration is rapid and early intervention is crucial. Parenteral administration of adrenaline can be lifesaving. This has to be distinguished from a rare autosomal-dominant condition called hereditary angioedema. This condition happens secondary to deficiency of C1 inhibitor enzyme due to mutations of its gene.

Localized swelling that is self-limiting can happen at any site of the body including the skin, genitalia, and the gastrointestinal tract. The angioedema is life-threatening when it happens in the larynx, especially if untreated. The attacks are not precipitated by allergy, but by trauma and stress. The age of presentation is variable. Prophylaxis is useful, if started early (with tranexamic acid) or attenuated with androgens like danazol. In patient's refractory to prophylaxis of danazol, pasteurized plasma-derived C1 inhibitor (pC1-INH) concentrate has been found to be useful in reducing the recurrence. In acute attacks, pC1-INH concentrate (intravenous dose of 20 U/kg) and newer drugs like icatibant—bradykinin receptor-2-antagonist (30 mg subcutaneous injection) have been shown to provide rapid relief.

Infection

Infection as a cause of acute UAO typically occurs in children. This may include infections, such as acute epiglottitis caused by either *Haemophilus influenzae* or beta-hemolytic streptococci, and Ludwig's angina characterized by a rapidly progressing cellulitis involving submandibular space. The treatment involves rapid airway stabilization, antibiotics, and surgical drainage of the pus.

Viral croup often caused by parainfluenza virus is managed by nebulized adrenaline and parenteral corticosteroids. Bacterial tracheitis is usually caused by *Staphylococcus aureus* infection. Bronchoscopic appearance shows the presence of erythema, edema, thick secretions, and at times, plaques in the trachea.

CHRONIC UPPER AIRWAY OBSTRUCTION

Vocal Cord Dysfunction

This is a syndrome in which the vocal cords adduct during inspiration producing UAO-like features. Patients are usually females in the age group of 20–40 years. It masquerades the diagnosis of refractory asthma with multiple attacks is usually managed as asthma.

The "wheeze" typically appears at lower lung volumes since the obstruction happens during the inspiration and for the same reason, the chest X-ray does not show hyperinflation. Spirometry done during the episode may show the classical loop of extrathoracic UAO. Flexible laryngoscopy is considered the gold standard for diagnosis, especially when done during the episode. The classical description during the inspiration consists of adduction of the vocal cords with a small diamond-shaped chink in the posterior region of the vocal cords. Reassurance and breathing exercises may reduce the intensity during the acute episode and interestingly, rapid shallow breathing (like panting) has been found to be useful. Speech therapy, psychological counseling, and avoidance of triggers would help in long-term management.

Tracheobronchomalacia

Tracheomalacia refers to the weakness of tracheal walls, frequently due to reduction, and/or atrophy of the longitudinal elastic fibers of the pars membrane; or cartilage integrity, such that the airway is softer and more susceptible to collapse. TM may be localized or diffuse and usually affects intrathoracic portion of trachea. If main bronchi are also involved, it is called tracheobronchomalacia (TBM).

Pediatric Tracheomalacia

Tracheomalacia is the most common congenital abnormality of trachea. There is a strong association with prematurity, mucopolysaccharidosis, tracheoesophageal fistula, and some congenital heart diseases. There is a male preponderance. Acquired causes include long-standing tracheostomy and pressure from vascular slings. Congenital TM is usually self-limiting and the children outgrow the disease by the age of 2–3 years. Severe cases are managed by the use of continuous positive airway pressure (CPAP), or by surgical procedures like aortopexy.

Adult Tracheomalacia and Tracheobronchomalacia

Tracheomalacia in adults is predominantly seen in the middle-aged male individuals who are also smokers. Adult cases most commonly happen following the trauma, including after intubation, tracheostomy, external chest trauma, and after lung transplantation. Emphysema, chronic bronchitis, chronic inflammation like relapsing polychondritis (RP), and chronic extrinsic compression of the trachea are the other important reasons.

Acquired TM is commonly seen in association with long-term intubation and tracheostomy. It is usually a short-segment stenosis. A comprehensive in-depth review on TM describes that the length of malacic segment secondary to postintubation in usually less than 3 cm. More than 50% decrease in airway caliber occurring during expiration is diagnostic of TM.

Symptomatic cases need to be treated depending on the etiology. Focal TM in postintubation or post-traumatic cases should be respected, if possible. Alternatively, it can be managed with tracheostomy, if the segment can be bypassed. The advantages of tracheostomy in such a situation are that the tube acts like a stent. Long-flange tracheostomy tubes are available for the purpose. The tracheostomy can also be an interface for CPAP application. However, tracheostomy can also predispose to TM of a different segment of trachea.

Polychondritis

Relapsing polychondritis is a rare and interesting disease. It is a multisystem disorder with unknown etiology, and characterized by recurrent progressive inflammation and degeneration of the cartilage and the connective tissue. Clinical features depend on the cartilage that is involved. It is important to understand that apart from cartilaginous structure of the external ear, nose, peripheral joints, larynx, and tracheobronchial tree, other proteoglycan-rich structures can become involved including the heart, blood vessels, and inner ear. The usual symptoms include progressive dyspnea, cough, stridor, hoarseness, chest discomfort, and features of respiratory failure.

Bronchoscopic techniques, such as balloon dilatation, and tracheobronchial stenting used alone or in combination might give some respite from symptoms for patients with airway complications. Interventional procedures provide a good short-term relief. However, long-term outcome is quite variable.

Tracheopathia Osteochondroplastica

It is a rare, slowly progressive disorder of unknown etiology. Endoluminal projections of bony and cartilaginous nodules arise from the submucosa of the trachea. The nodules characteristically spare the posterior membrane but may be present in the proximal, main bronchi also. The presentation is usually with chronic cough, dyspnea in advanced cases, and minimal hemoptysis due to the ulceration of the overlying mucosa. Diagnosis is based on typical bronchoscopic appearances, and biopsy is not generally needed. There is no definitive treatment. Severe obstruction may warrant therapeutic interventions.

Tracheobronchial Amyloidosis

Tracheobronchial amyloidosis (TBA) is very rare and characterized by endoluminal accumulation of abnormal proteins in the form of fibrils, which cause obstructive symptoms. Dyspnea, cough, hemoptysis, and hoarseness are usual presenting symptoms. Diagnosis is made by bronchoscopy and biopsy with specific congo red staining. Response to medications like steroids and melphalan is suboptimal, severe obstruction warrants debulking.

Tuberculosis

Endobronchial tuberculosis (TB) is not an uncommon problem in the developing world. The true incidence in patients with sputum-positive pulmonary TB is difficult to estimate because bronchoscopy is usually avoided. Endobronchial TB is seen more commonly in females, perhaps because they tend to retain the infected secretions in the bronchial tree and avoid expectoration. It is also more common in the left than the right side bronchi probably because the left main bronchus is narrow and lengthy and hence the infected sputum may remain in contact with the bronchi for a longer time. The disease is quite refractory to chemotherapy alone. Hence, early identification by bronchoscopy is encouraged in a suspected patient. Suspicion arises, if a patient with TB develops wheeze or breathlessness. Surgery is ideal, if the involved segment is small. If the disease is extensive, balloon dilatation or thermal désobstruction followed by silicone stenting can be tried.

Sarcoidosis

As in TB, an airway abnormality in sarcoidosis is often overlooked. Endobronchial involvement is usually seen in the elderly age groups, smokers during advanced stages of parenchymal involvement, and with thickening of bronchovascular bundles on high resolution CT. It carries a relatively poorer prognosis. Obstructive sleep apnea syndrome is seen more often in patients with sarcoidosis, especially lupus pernio. Tracheal obstruction secondary to sarcoidosis is very rare.

The classic endobronchial sarcoidosis is characterized by mucosal islands of waxy yellow mucosal nodules, measuring 2-4 mm in diameter. The nodules are sparse in the trachea, but abundant in the main, lobar, and segmental bronchi. Other changes are mucosal erythema, granular mucosa, cobblestone mucosa, mucosal plaques, bronchial stenosis, airway distortion due to cicatricial changes in parenchyma, bronchiectasis, extrinsic compression due to mediastinal lymphadenopathy, or airway hyperresponsiveness.

Tracheal Stenosis

Tracheal stenosis is an important cause of UAO. It may happen secondary to trauma to trachea, following prolonged intubation, i.e. PITS and after tracheostomy, i.e. post-tracheostomy tracheal stenosis (PTTS). Idiopathic stenosis is rare.

Mechanical ventilation has made a great difference in the outcome of many sick patients with respiratory failure, but the use of endotracheal tube have resulted in a group of diseases that have become more common than before.

Despite the use of low-pressure cuffs, which have reduced the incidence of tracheal stenosis significantly, the incidence of PITS and PTTS is high, i.e. 0.6–21%. It is seen predominantly in females, presumably because of smaller tracheal lumen and hence, prone to injury.

Usage of high-cuff pressure in an intubated patient predisposes to mucosal ischemia, which also worsens in the presence of hypotension when the capillary pressure is lower. Pressure necrosis and chondritis result, which lead to either the development of cicatricial tissue and membranous type of stenosis or to the cartilage damage which results in weakening and a complex stenosis.

Bronchoscopic management is sufficient in a majority of cases of membranous stenosis and can be very useful as either a standalone therapy or as a bridge to surgery in very sick patients. Bronchoscopy is used both for achieving and maintaining an effective lumen. Some of procedures to tackle membranous stenosis can be done with a flexible bronchoscope, but it is important that the bronchoscopist is trained in rigid bronchoscopy as well.

In membranous stenosis, stent is not required after dilatation, since the cartilage is not involved and the stability of airway is not affected. In complex stenosis, however, the underlying cartilage is damaged and collapsible. Therefore, despite achieving a good lumen by bronchoscopic means, it has to be followed by leaving a stent at the end of procedure.

Tumors

Primary tracheal tumors can arise from the respiratory epithelium, salivary glands, and mesenchymal structures of the trachea. Squamous and adenoid cystic carcinoma account for about two-thirds of tumors from trachea. Benign tumors of the trachea include tumors from surface epithelium like papilloma, papillomatosis, tumors from glands, and tumors from mesenchymal structures. Endotracheal metastases are much less common than endobronchial metastasis.

Other Causes

Bilateral vocal cord palsy can happen secondary to thyroid malignancy or thyroid surgery. Others include the neurological diseases or idiopathic causes. Cases of bilateral vocal cord palsy have been reported following nasogastric tube, systemic lupus erythematosus (SLE), and esophageal surgeries.

THERAPEUTIC CONSIDERATIONS

As is true with many other conditions in medicine, treating the primary cause of the UAO is important. However, it is also important to manage the obstruction. Obstruction can occur due to intrinsic pathology as in the case of tumors or tracheal stenosis, and extrinsic compression as in compression from thyroid swelling or esophageal cancer. Functional obstruction without significant anatomic narrowing can happen secondary to TM. In cases where surgery is feasible, especially in short-segment complex stenosis or tracheal tumors, it should be offered. Several other interventional approaches provide a good quality of life in most of the conditions.

In the cases of intramural pathology, achieving a patent lumen is accomplished by techniques like rigid bronchoscopy, laser, electrocautery, and argon plasma coagulation, while airway stenting is necessary for extramural compression or TM where maintaining lumen is the key issue. Silicone stents are preferred over metallic stents because the latter are difficult to remove after deployment.

CHAPTER 41

Interstitial Lung Diseases

Nagarjuna V Maturu, Dheeraj Gupta

Diffuse interstitial lung disease (ILD) encompasses a group of disorders of diverse etiologies with common feature of generalized involvement of lung interstitium. It includes over 200 different diseases which, in spite of their heterogeneous nature, have several common clinical, radiological, and histological manifestations.

ETIOLOGY AND CLASSIFICATION

Interstitial lung disease is broadly grouped as—(1) primary, when the cause is unknown, and (2) secondary, when there is an identifiable disease responsible for the interstitial involvement (Box 41.1).

Primary Interstitial Lung Disease

Primary ILD is idiopathic in origin. No secondary cause or association is identifiable. The latest American Thoracic Society/European Respiratory Society (ATS/ERS) update (2013) classified idiopathic interstitial pneumonias (IIP) based on clinicoradiological, pathological features, the incidence, and natural course of the disease (Box 41.1). An ILD is considered to be idiopathic only after a carefully history and focused investigations have ruled out secondary causes of the same.

Secondary Interstitial Lung Diseases

Most forms of secondary ILDs have either a known etiological cause or an association with another disease of known (or unknown) etiology (Box 41.1). An ILD secondary to another illness factually represents the pulmonary involvement of the primary disease rather a separate entity.

BOX 41.1: Important causes of interstitial lung disease.

1. *Primary or idiopathic interstitial pneumonias:*
   – *Major idiopathic interstitial pneumonias:*
     - Idiopathic pulmonary fibrosis
     - Idiopathic nonspecific interstitial pneumonia
     - Respiratory bronchiolitis-associated interstitial lung disease
     - Desquamative interstitial pneumonia
     - Cryptogenic organizing pneumonia
     - Acute interstitial pneumonia
   – *Rare idiopathic interstitial pneumonias:*
     - Idiopathic lymphoid interstitial pneumonia
     - Idiopathic pleuroparenchymal fibroelastosis
   – *Unclassifiable idiopathic interstitial pneumonias*

2. *Secondary:*
   – Known causes:
     - Infections:
       - Tuberculosis (miliary)
       - Bacterial (atypical pneumonias)
       - Fungal
       - Parasitic
       - Viral
     - *Noninfectious causes:*
       - Hypersensitivity pneumonitis
       - Pneumoconioses
       - Drug induced
       - Radiation induced
       - Malignancies
       - Systemic vasculitides
   – *Association with diseases of unknown etiology:*
     - Sarcoidosis
     - Connective tissue disorders:
       - Systemic sclerosis
       - Rheumatoid arthritis
       - Polymyositis and dermatomyositis
       - Systemic lupus erythematosus
       - Sjogren syndrome
     - Chronic eosinophilic pneumonia
     - Miscellaneous:
       - Histiocytosis
       - Eosinophilic granuloma
       - Lymphangioleiomyomatosis
       - Tuberous sclerosis

It is important to understand that the clinicoradiological and pathological features of primary and secondary ILDs may be similar. It is only the identification of an antecedent cause, which shall differentiate secondary from primary ILDs. For example, nonspecific interstitial pneumonia (NSIP) pattern can occur due to drugs and several connective tissue diseases (CTDs). When no cause is identified, it is labeled as idiopathic NSIP. Similarly, the usual interstitial pneumonia (UIP) pattern can either be idiopathic or secondary to CTDs like rheumatoid arthritis (RA) or chronic hypersensitivity pneumonitis (HP). When idiopathic, it is called as idiopathic pulmonary fibrosis (IPF).

EPIDEMIOLOGY

The exact incidence and prevalence of ILD are unknown. Most reports suggest that the disease comprises about 15% of a pulmonary physician's practice. IPF is the most common ILD. The prevalence of IPF is most common (175 per 100,000) in the elderly in individuals more than 75 years of age; almost two-thirds of patients with IPF are over 60 years of age at diagnosis. Given that the population is aging globally, ILDs are likely to be encountered with increasing frequency.

PATHOLOGY

A number of diseases of diverse etiologies cause pulmonary inflammation and/or fibrosis, which serve as the final common pathways to lung damage. Characteristically, there is cellular infiltration and thickening of pulmonary interstitium and of alveolar walls, as well as the presence of mononuclear cells in the alveolar lumen. The cellular exudate comprises primarily of alveolar macrophages, but lymphocytes, neutrophils, eosinophils, and plasma cells are also present. Although the total collagen component of lungs remains normal, the ratio of type I to type III collagen is increased. The interstitial involvement progressively encroaches upon the alveolar spaces, the terminal bronchioles and also the overlying pleura. Therefore, the ILDs are better referred to as "diffuse parenchymal lung diseases" (DPLDs). In advanced-stage disease, there is presence of extensive fibrosis, obliteration of the alveolar lumen, and formation of multiple cystic spaces, which give the appearances of a honeycomb. Even though the ILDs significantly involve the airways and the vessels, they should be distinguished from airway and vascular diseases.

PATHOGENESIS

Chronic inflammation, recurrent epithelial injury, and impaired wound repair are some of the possible reasons of pulmonary fibrosis. Pulmonary fibrosis is considered to result from an aberrant defense reaction with failure of mechanisms, which are normally responsible for repair. It is now recognized that there is persistent and/or repetitive injury responsible for inflammation followed by recruitment of a host of inflammatory cells.

As per the recent concepts, ILD (IPF) should be considered as a neoproliferative disorder of the lung. Both IPF and cancer are characterized by genetic alterations and carry a poor prognosis. Like the cancers, there is a response to growth and inhibitory signals and resistance to apoptosis. Moreover, the myofibroblast origin and behavior, altered cellular communications, and intracellular signaling pathways are all fundamental pathogenic hallmarks of IPF.

DIAGNOSTIC APPROACH

The final diagnosis of ILDs essentially rests on the evaluation of clinical, radiological, and pathological features. The various steps, which are needed include—(1) a good history to include demographics, family history, occupational, and environmental exposures; (2) physical examination; (3) chest radiographs; (4) high-resolution computed tomographic scans (HRCT); (5) blood tests; (6) fiberoptic bronchoscopy with bronchoalveolar lavage (BAL) or transbronchial lung biopsies (selected patients); (7) surgical lung biopsy (selected patients).

Clinical History

The clinical signs and symptoms are generally not specific. Most commonly, the patient presents with progressive dyspnea on exertion and dry cough. The various factors in history, which need to be taken into consideration while framing a differential diagnosis, include:
- Age at diagnosis
- Progression of the disease
- Sex of the patient
- Smoking status
- Associated symptoms
- Family history
- Occupational history
- History of drug intake.

Physical Examination

The bi-basilar dry and end-inspiratory "velcro" crackles are quite characteristically heard in most patients of IPF. These crackles are attributed to the opening up of collapsed alveoli when equalization of pressure occurs between the alveolar spaces and the proximal bronchiole during inspiration. Finger-clubbing is present in about one-third of patients. Hypertrophic osteoarthropathy is rarely seen. Breath sounds are vesicular and quite distinct. Bronchovesicular or bronchial breathing is heard in the presence of a consolidation, a cavity, or an advanced disease. Cyanosis is generally absent at rest but desaturation occurs and cyanosis appears after even mild exercise. Patients with secondary ILD may also have signs of the underlying disease. Patients with CREST syndrome (calcinosis, Raynaud's phenomenon, esophageal dysfunction, sclerodactyly, and telangiectasia) or mixed connective tissue disease (MCTD) may present with pulmonary hypertension as the primary manifestation.

Chest Radiography

The interstitial infiltrates are seen as discrete linear, nodular, or reticulonodular shadows diffusely distributed in both the lungs. The individual nodular shadows are usually of less than 2 mm in diameter. Presence of diffuse mottling or ground-glass appearances may suggest an active stage of diffuse alveolitis. In advanced disease when fibrosis is extensive, the lungs get shrunken and reduced in volume. Small, uniform sized, quadrangular cystic spaces, which represent patent bronchioles give the typical appearances of a honeycomb lung.

HRCT of the Chest

Recognition of the pattern on HRCT is of utmost importance, while approaching patients with ILD. The presence of symmetrical, bibasilar (apicobasal gradient), and subpleural intralobular septal thickening with or without honeycombing is considered characteristic of UIP pattern. Diseases such as sarcoidosis, histiocytosis, and lymphangitis have more characteristic patterns. HRCT is also of some help in making a quantitative assessment of pulmonary fibrosis. Spiral CT scan gives an even better resolution, especially in a patient with tachypnea who cannot hold his breath.

Pulmonary Function Tests

Most ILDs demonstrate a restrictive defect on spirometry and pulmonary function test (PFT) cannot help in differential diagnosis. They are important, however, for functional assessment and to monitor therapy. Tidal volumes are generally small and both the vital capacity and the total lung capacity are reduced. Expiratory flows are normal or even "supranormal". Airway obstruction, characterized by reduced forced vital capacity (FVC) and forced expiratory flows, can occur in certain ILDs, which can have concomitant small airway involvement like hypersensitivity pneumonias, sarcoidosis, Pulmonary Langerhans Cell Histiocytosis (PLCH) and lymphangioleiomyomatosis (LAM). Reduced diffusing capacity (DLCO) and arterial hypoxemia (reduced PaO_2) may not be present in the early stages. Some degree of arterial hypoxemia on exercise is almost always demonstrable.

Bronchoalveolar Lavage

Bronchoalveolar lavage (BAL) is more often used to rule out the differentials to ILD like infections and malignancy. BAL is helpful to diagnose infections (e.g. tuberculosis, histoplasmosis, coccidioidomycoses, and endemic fungal infections) and some other noninfectious diseases. Increases in BAL lymphocytes may suggest the diagnosis of sarcoidosis, HP, or other granulomatous processes. Infective microorganisms such as the mycobacteria, fungi, or *Pneumocystis jiroveci* can be isolated from BAL fluid. Presence of lymphocytosis in the BAL fluid is shown to predict a better response to corticosteroid therapy.

Other Investigations

Although nonspecific, hematological investigations provide useful information. Unexplained anemia is seen in diffuse alveolar hemorrhage and CTDs. Mild-to-moderate leukocytosis is common in both primary and secondary ILDs. Eosinophilia is more characteristically seen in eosinophilic pneumonias, vasculitides, sarcoidosis, and drug-induced lung disease. Occasionally, there is leukopenia and/or thrombocytopenia.

Abnormal liver or renal function tests suggest the involvement of these organs. Elevated calcium may be seen in sarcoidosis and malignancies. Increased enzymes such as creatinine phosphokinase and aldolase are present in polymyositis and dermatomyositis. Increased serum angiotensin-converting enzyme (SACE) in sarcoidosis is quite characteristic but may be seen in silicosis, hypersensitivity pneumonias, and other diseases like tuberculosis.

A number of immunological parameters are described in connective tissue disorders and other ILDs. Hypergammaglobulinemia, positive serum autoantibodies (e.g. the antinuclear factor) and circulating immune complexes may be seen. Antibasement membrane antibodies in Goodpasture's syndrome, antineutrophil cytoplasmic antibody (C-ANCA) in Wegener's granulomatosis, Churg–Strauss syndrome and systemic necrotizing vasculitis, and anti-Jo-1 antibody in polymyositis and dermatomyositis are generally considered characteristics.

Radionuclide scanning using gallium and positron emission tomography (PET) scans with 18F-FDG glucose isotope has a place to identify disease activity and to predict response to therapy. Similarly, the clearance of aerosolized technetium-99m diethylenetriaminepentaacetic acid (DTPA) is markedly increased in patients with inflammatory lung diseases including sarcoidosis.

Lung Biopsy

Lung biopsy is required only when the clinicoradiological findings are atypical to exclude an infection, vasculitides, or malignancy. It may also help to predict the response to treatment and prognosis of a patient. For patients with IPF and other IIP, transbronchial lung biopsy (TBLB) with the help of fiberoptic bronchoscopy is less rewarding. Whenever, there are atypical features, transthoracic or open surgical approach provides a better option to obtain lung tissue. Surgical lung biopsy achieves three purposes—(1) establishes a precise diagnosis; (2) assesses the extent of inflammation and fibrosis; (3) identifies a histopathological pattern for IIPs.

TREATMENT

Treatment options for ILD are limited, especially for IIPs, particularly IPF. It is important to identify and establish a clear and potential etiology to determine appropriate therapeutic interventions. In the absence of a satisfactory and definitive treatment for IPF, most objectives are achieved with supportive and symptomatic therapy. Several different groups of drugs have been tried in its treatment. Supportive treatment is provided for respiratory failure, pulmonary hypertension, cor pulmonale, and congestive cardiac failure, wherever indicated. Long-term pulmonary vasodilators have not shown to prevent the development of pulmonary hypertension.

Anti-inflammatory Therapy

Anti-inflammatory therapy has remained the mainstay of treatment for several different groups of ILDs. The IIPs, which respond to corticosteroids/immunosuppressants, include the NSIP (the cellular variant), cryptogenic organizing pneumonia (COP), desquamative interstitial pneumonia (DIP), and lymphoid interstitial pneumonia (LIP). Acute interstitial pneumonia also responds to steroids in up to 50% of the patients. Corticosteroids also form the initial line of management for CTD-ILDs, eosinophilic pneumonias, hypersensitivity pneumonias (along with trigger avoidance), and sarcoidosis. Many times, corticosteroid-sparing agents such as azathioprine may be needed, especially when the treatment is needed for a prolonged duration. Severe forms of ILDs may need concomitant agents like cyclophosphamide.

The role of corticosteroids and other anti-inflammatory drugs in fibrotic ILDs like IPF and the fibrotic NSIP is limited. The recent guidelines on IPF recommend not using any of these drugs for managing patients with IPF. The only indication for the use of corticosteroids in patients with IPF is an acute exacerbation of the underlying disease.

Antifibrotic Agents

There is a greater trend to rely on antifibrotic drugs for the treatment of fibrosing ILDs. Of the several antifibrotic agents, which had been tried, pirfenidone, an orally administered pyridine, is the only drug, which has shown clinical promise. It has antifibrotic, antioxidant, and anti-inflammatory properties. It has been used in doses ranging from 1,200 mg/day to 2,400 mg/day. The common side effects of pirfenidone are gastrointestinal intolerance, skin rash, and hepatotoxicity. Nintedanib (BIBF 1120), a multiple tyrosine kinase inhibitor (VEGF, FGF, and PDGF), also has antifibrotic properties and is the other drug to have shown some clinical promise.

The other drugs, which have been tried, include colchicine, D-penicillamine, interferon gamma, and others. None of these agents are currently recommended for clinical use.

Other Treatments

Antioxidants, such as N-acetyl cysteine (NAC) to reduce oxidative stress, are shown to offer some clinical advantage when used along with antifibrotic agents. The role of NAC in managing patients with IPF is debatable. Drugs targeted to prevent or reduce apoptosis, angiogenesis, and coagulant activity may find some use in the future. Presently, no drug from these groups is available for clinical use. It is a better option to resort to symptomatic palliative therapy and withdraw immunosuppressive drugs in case there is no response in the initial 3–6 months of use and for end-stage disease.

Transplantation

Lung transplantation is the only hope for the advanced end-stage disease. Single lung transplantation is recommended in most patients. A 5-year survival is reported in up to 40–60% of patients. The common post-transplant complications include the risk of rejection, multiple opportunistic infections in an immunosuppressed host and organizing pneumonias. The lack of availability of organ for transplantation and very high costs involved in the procedure are the limited factors. Living donor lobar lung transplantation (LDLLT) is an evolving option for patients with end-stage lung disease.

Other Supportive Measures

The primary goal of management of a patient involves his restoration to the highest possible functional state. Pulmonary physical rehabilitation program should be, therefore, encouraged. Daily walks or use of a stationary bicycle are useful. Supplemental oxygen should be provided in patients with hypoxemia at rest or during exercise. Higher flow rates may be frequently required than those needed in chronic obstructive pulmonary disease (COPD). Dry cough is a highly distressing symptom. Antitussive agents should be used in adequate dosages. Low-dose opioids are effective and fairly safe for the palliative management of dyspnea in terminally ill IPF patients.

Pulmonary hypertension, cor pulmonale, and right heart failure should be appropriately managed as and when diagnosed. Phosphodiesterase type 5 inhibitor sildenafil causes preferential pulmonary vasodilation and may improve gas exchange in patients with severe lung fibrosis and secondary pulmonary hypertension. But no improvement is demonstrated in exercise tolerance, the primary endpoint. Other vasodilator agents, which have been tried in managing patients, include bosentan, ambrisentan, and macitentan.

ACUTE EXACERBATION OF ILD

Acute exacerbation of idiopathic pulmonary fibrosis (AE-IPF) is characterized by rapid deterioration of lung function and other clinical parameters during the course of disease that is not due to infections, pulmonary embolism, or heart failure. This condition needs to be differentiated from acute interstitial pneumonia (earlier described as Hamman–Rich syndrome), which occurs in patients with no underlying lung disease. The simplified 2007 consensus criteria for the diagnosis of AE-IPF include—(1) previous or concurrent diagnosis of IPF; (2) worsening of dyspnea over the last 30 days; (3) new onset infiltrates (ground glass opacities or consolidation) on computed tomography (CT) chest; and (4) absence of infection and other causes of deterioration including pulmonary edema and pulmonary thromboembolism.

The true etiology and pathogenesis are not known but the massive lung injury occurs due to some unknown etiologic agent. Acute exacerbation in a patient with preexisting IPF is characterized by diffuse alveolar damage. High-resolution CT is helpful in both management and prognostication. After excluding infections and other possible causes of worsening, treatment is tried with enhancement of immunosuppression giving pulse doses of methyl prednisolone and cytotoxic agents. Acute exacerbation of the underlying ILD can also occur in fibrotic NSIP and CTD-related ILDs. The approach and the management are the same as that of AE–IPF.

PROGNOSIS

Prognosis of ILDs, secondary to systemic diseases or other causes, is determined by the natural course of the underlying disease. While NSIP, COP, DIP, and Respiratory Bronchiolitis-associated Interstitial Lung Disease (RB–ILD) respond better, the IPF is progressive and fatal. The median survival of IPF is about 4 years. Both acute exacerbation of IPF and acute interstitial pneumonia are rapidly fatal. The patient may sometimes die in a course of a few weeks or months.

Given the age of many with ILD, patients are at risk for other age-related diseases and need close follow-up with their internists. There are several factors, which determine survival. Survival is worse for males with age of onset of more than 50 years at the time of diagnosis. Other factors for poor survival include—moderate/severe dyspnea on exertion, history of tobacco use, and moderate loss of lung function (TLC < 45%, DLCO < 40%). Similarly, presence of neutrophilia/eosinophilia on BAL, honeycombing on HRCT, lack of response to corticosteroids or moderate/severe fibrosis, and fibroblastic foci on histology are bad prognostic signs.

CHAPTER 42

Idiopathic Interstitial Pneumonias

H Shigemitsu, Ngozi Orjioke, Carmen Luraschi-Monjagatta

The idiopathic group of interstitial lung disease (ILD) is labeled as idiopathic interstitial pneumonias (IIPs) further classified as follows—usual interstitial pneumonia (UIP) or idiopathic pulmonary fibrosis (IPF), idiopathic nonspecific interstitial pneumonia (NSIP), respiratory bronchiolitis–interstitial lung disease (RB-ILD), desquamative interstitial pneumonia (DIP), cryptogenic organizing pneumonia (COP), and acute interstitial pneumonia (AIP); the rare idiopathic pneumonias include lymphoid interstitial pneumonia (LIP) and idiopathic pleuroparenchymal fibroelastosis (PPFE); and finally the unclassifiable IIPs. Nearly two-thirds of patients with IPF are men above 60 years of age. Reports from India suggest that age at presentation is almost a decade earlier though there is a trend toward increasing incidence of IPF with advancing age.

DIAGNOSIS (FLOWCHART 42.1)

Nonproductive cough and progressive dyspnea with exertion usually prompt the patient to seek medical attention. The onset and progression can be variable, thus a detailed history of onset and duration of symptoms and associated features must be obtained. Detailed history of tobacco use, family history of lung disease, current and prior drug use to rule out medication-induced lung fibrosis, and occupational exposure history must also be carefully elucidated. When the clinicoradiological features are atypical of IPF, lung tissue obtained by surgical biopsy or bronchoalveolar lavage (BAL) with transbronchial biopsy (TBBx), preferably transbronchial lung cryo-biopsy (TBCL) based on available modalities to evaluate the histopathology may be helpful to rule out other possible etiologies as infections or diffuse alveolar hemorrhage. Laboratory

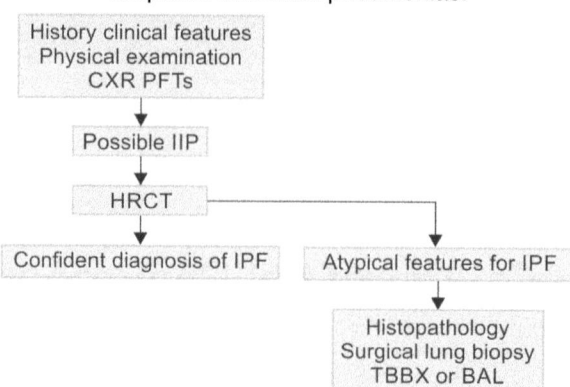

Flowchart 42.1: Simplified algorithm for diagnosis of idiopathic interstitial pneumonias.

(HRCT, high-resolution computed tomography; IIP, idiopathic interstitial pneumonia; PFT, pulmonary function test; TBBx, transbronchial biopsy; BAL, bronchoalveolar lavage; IPF, idiopathic pulmonary fibrosis; CXR, chest X-ray)

tests for autoimmune disease, vasculitides, and immunological response to organic inhalational exposure may assist in directing the clinician to various etiologies that are known to cause IIPs.

HISTOLOGICAL FEATURES

Histopathological examination of lung is helpful in the diagnosis of IIPs. The patterns have been shown to correlate with the clinical course and response to treatment. In IPF, the characteristic injury pattern is UIP. The hallmark of UIP is fibroblastic foci, which consist of dense eosinophilic fibrosis with scattered foci of young myxoid fibrosis and fibroblasts. These foci represent the advancing or progressive edge of disease and are required to be a major component of the histological pattern for a confident diagnosis. The injury is predominantly seen in the subpleural region and consists of a pattern of temporal heterogeneity; the areas of injury with fibroblastic foci and honeycombing are seen adjacent to relatively unaffected tissue.

IDIOPATHIC PULMONARY FIBROSIS

Epidemiology

Idiopathic pulmonary fibrosis alone accounts for over 50% of all IIPs. It shows UIP pattern on surgical lung biopsy. It is predominantly seen in the elderly men with a median age of 66 years at time of diagnosis.

Etiology

The cause of IPF is unclear, but it is increasingly becoming clear that it represents in part a response to injurious agent(s) in genetically predisposed individuals, followed by deregulated inflammation, repair of the interstitium and alveolar epithelium. The possible risk factors for alveolar injury include but are not limited to cigarette smoking, environmental exposures (metal and wood dust, farming, and other inorganic particles), infections (viral), and gastroesophageal reflux disease (GERD) with microaspiration. Eventually, chronic inflammation and an imbalance in the production of various cytokines, growth factors, and profibrotic agents result in inexorable fibrotic response with collagen deposition.

Signs and Symptoms

Paroxysmal nonproductive cough associated with progressively worsening of shortness of breath are the most common symptoms. These symptoms have an insidious onset and are often present for months prior to the diagnosis. End-inspiratory crackles are present on lung examination, with finger clubbing in 25–50% of patients. In late stages of disease, signs attributable to pulmonary hypertension or right heart failure may be present.

Diagnosis

The high specificity of the high-resolution computed tomography (HRCT) of chest in many instances allows a reasonably confident diagnosis without a lung biopsy. The typical findings on HRCT scan consist of predominantly peripheral, subpleural, bibasilar reticular abnormalities; traction bronchiectasis and subpleural honeycombing (Table 42.1). If ground–glass opacities appear to be the predominant radiographic finding, an alternate diagnosis other than IPF must be strongly considered.

TABLE 42.1: High-resolution computed tomography (HRCT) criteria for usual interstitial pneumonia (UIP) pattern.

UIP pattern—needs all four features	Possible UIP—needs all three features	Inconsistent with UIP, if any, of the seven features
Subpleural, basal predominance	Subpleural, basal predominance	Upper or mid-lung predominance
Reticular abnormality	Reticular abnormality	Peribronchovascular predominance
Honeycombing with or without traction bronchiectasis	Absence of features listed as inconsistent with UIP	Extensive GGO or > reticular abnormality
Absence of features listed as inconsistent with UIP		Profuse micronodules
		Discrete cysts
		Diffuse mosaic attenuation/air trapping
		Consolidations

(GGO, ground–glass opacity).
Source: Raghu G, Collard HR, Egan JJ, et al. An official ATS/ERS/JRT/ALAT Statement: idiopathic pulmonary fibrosis: evidence-based guidelines for diagnosis and management. Am J Respir Crit Care. 2011;183(6):788-24.

Treatment

Treatment is targeted at resolution and slowing down the progression of disease. There is no treatment that improves survival in IPF. The new ATS/ERS/JRS/ALAT guidelines of 2011 make emphasis against treatment with monotherapy with steroids, colchicine, cyclosporine A, interferon gamma, bosentan, and etanercept, since none those medications improve survival nor slow the progression of the disease. A phase-3 trial of pirfenidone for 52 weeks and a randomized trial of nintedanib (intracellular inhibitor of tyrosine kinase), at several centers including the United States, has showed slow decline in forced vital capacity (FVC) and progression-free survival providing hope for better treatment options.

Supportive care with supplemental oxygen, immunizations, prompt treatment of infections, and pulmonary rehabilitation help to improve the quality of life. In spite of these therapies, IPF portends a poor prognosis with a median 5-year survival of less than 50%. Lung transplantation becomes the only option for treatment for eligible patients, although this is not readily available in many developing countries.

Prognosis

The general clinical course is variable, some patients stay with stable lung function for many years, while others show slow progression of impairment and some may report even accelerated progression. Acute worsening of function due to acute IPF exacerbations, infections, or other comorbidities can be part of this disease behavior. Factors associated with increased risk of mortality include level of dyspnea, severity on baseline diffusing capacity of the lungs for carbon monoxide (DLCO) or percentage of worsening, extension of honeycombing, worsening of fibrosis on HRCT, desaturation less than 88% on 6-minute walk test (6MWT) as well pulmonary hypertension.

NONSPECIFIC INTERSTITIAL PNEUMONIA

Idiopathic nonspecific interstitial pneumonia is more commonly associated with other clinicopathological conditions, such as connective tissue disorders, drug toxicity, hypersensitivity pneumonitis, and human immunodeficiency virus (HIV) infection. It may, however, occur as a distinct clinical entity in the absence of any other systemic disease. The mean age of onset (40–50 years) is about a decade earlier than in IPF. It has been also reported in the pediatric population. It occurs equally in both men and women, and has unknown association with cigarette smoking.

Etiology

Unlike IPF, the etiology of NSIP may be more evident with autoimmune diseases, hypersensitivity pneumonitis, and certain inhalational exposure. The etiology in a significant number of patients with NSIP remains elusive and coined as idiopathic NSIP, which has unique features than other forms of NSIP.

Signs and Symptoms

Onset is gradual and some patients have associated constitutional symptoms, such as fever and weight loss in addition to respiratory symptoms, such as chronic cough and dyspnea. Finger clubbing is less common than in IPF can occur in 8% of patients. Inspiratory crackles are usually present on lung examination.

Diagnosis

Clinical features in the presence of a restrictive pattern and a reduction in DLCO suggest the diagnosis of an interstitial pulmonary disease. Histologically, NSIP consists of varying degree of inflammation and involvement; it can be further separated into cellular and fibrotic NSIP. In cellular NSIP, mild-to-moderate homogeneous interstitial chronic inflammation is the predominant feature, unlike fibrosing NSIP where uniformly dense fibrosis is the prominent feature. Temporal uniformity, the paucity of fibroblastic foci and honeycomb lesions are the features that histologically differentiate NSIP from UIP.

Radiographically, cellular NSIP, in contrary to IPF, shows diffuse symmetric interstitial infiltrates and ground-glass opacities with subpleural sparing. In fibrotic NSIP, the radiographic signs of fibrotic disease are similar to those of IPF.

Treatment/Prognosis

There are three subgroups of NSIP based on the degree of inflammation and fibrosis on histopathology—(i) group 1 primarily with interstitial fibrosis; (ii) group 2 with both inflammation and fibrosis; and (iii) group 3 primarily with fibrosis. Patients with cellular NSIP usually respond well to corticosteroids unlike fibrotic NSIP. Thus, the prognosis is good in cellular NSIP, as opposed to fibrotic NSIP, which has been shown to mirror that of IPF, given the similarities in histology and clinical features.

DESQUAMATIVE INTERSTITIAL PNEUMONIA

Etiology

Desquamative interstitial pneumonia is a rare IIP primarily seen in smokers in the 4th–5th decades of life. In at-risk patients, tobacco induces injury to the bronchiolar and alveolar epithelium. As in patients with pulmonary Langerhans cell histiocytosis, abnormal T-cell proliferation and increased secretion of peptides have been described. It is likely that this disorder like other cigarette smoking-related lung diseases, occurs in susceptible individuals following initial injury to the pulmonary epithelium.

Signs and Symptoms

Dyspnea at rest or on exertion is the most common presenting symptom. Onset is insidious with cough which cough may be dry or productive of nonpurulent sputum. Systemic symptoms are usually absent, digital clubbing is seen in some patients. Physical examination shows crackles in less than 50% of patients.

Diagnosis

Typical radiographic findings include patchy ground-glass opacification with a predilection for the lower zones; in rare cases, it can even be normal. The pulmonary function tests (PFTs) can show a combined obstructive and restrictive defect, often with a decrease in DLCO. Histologically, the pattern is characterized by chronic interstitial inflammation. There is significant presence of numerous intra-alveolar mononuclear cells or macrophages, thought to be desquamated epithelial cells. It is also common to find multinucleated giants cells.

Treatment

There is clinical response to smoking cessation alone or in combination with corticosteroid therapy, as well as some possible spontaneous resolution. In some cases, in spite of clinical stability, abnormal radiographic features may persist.

RESPIRATORY BRONCHIOLITIS-ASSOCIATED INTERSTITIAL LUNG DISEASE

Respiratory bronchiolitis-associated interstitial lung disease is a variant of DIP with a patchy distribution rather than a diffuse process. It commonly occurs in smokers in the 3rd–4th decades of life.

Signs and Symptoms

Most patients are either asymptomatic or have mild symptoms of dyspnea and cough of an insidious onset. Inspiratory crackles are present on lung examination, digital clubbing in up to 25% of patients.

Diagnosis

On spirometry, a combined defect with abnormalities of gas exchange is often seen. Ground-glass opacities and attenuation may be seen on chest imaging, and associated with thickening of walls of central and peripheral airways. These findings are ultimately associated with the pathological lesions of respiratory bronchiolitis consistent with macrophages infiltration with more peribronchiolar distribution than intra-alveolar as in DIP.

Treatment

The only proven therapy for RB-ILD is smoking cessation. Only those who continue to be symptomatic in spite of smoking cessation should be considered for corticosteroid therapy. Prognosis is good and patients usually improve with smoking cessation. To date, there are no documented cases of respiratory failure or death directly attributable to RB-ILD.

CRYPTOGENIC ORGANIZING PNEUMONIA

Cryptogenic organizing pneumonia, previously known as bronchiolitis obliterans with organizing pneumonia (BOOP), often presents with a flu-like illness of subacute onset (weeks to a few months). It is often the result of a nonspecific response to lung injury.

Etiology

Organizing pneumonia is termed cryptogenic when the triggering agent or the disease process is not identifiable. Possibly, both the lung injury and inflammation are initiated and perpetuated by inflammatory cytokines produced in situ by alveolar macrophages.

Signs and Symptoms

Cryptogenic organizing pneumonia often presents clinically as a flu-like illness of subacute onset (weeks to a few months). Fever, dry cough with malaise, anorexia, and weight loss are often present with mild dyspnea, especially on exertion. Physical findings are sparse, inspiratory crackles are present on lung examination.

Diagnosis

The diagnosis should be considered in patients with features of nonresolving pneumonia. Chest X-ray shows patchy migratory, unilateral, or bilateral airspace disease with predominantly peripheral distribution. On CT scan, the opacities range from ground glass to dense peribronchial consolidation with multifocal and subpleural involvement. These radiographic findings can also be seen in other conditions. Less commonly, radiographic features of diffuse interstitial opacities and solitary focal lesions may be seen.

Treatment/Prognosis

Most patients respond well to corticosteroids, but relapses can occur, requiring chronic steroid therapy. Cytotoxic drugs and steroid-sparing agents are used in addition to corticosteroid where there is slow response to steroids alone. A small group (10–15%) may progress to pulmonary fibrosis and one-third of patient can relapse. Factors that may predict poor outcomes include the lack of lymphocytosis on BAL, predominantly interstitial pattern on imaging and histological features of scarring and remodeling of lung parenchyma.

ACUTE INTERSTITIAL PNEUMONIA

Acute interstitial pneumonia, characterized by diffuse alveolar damage (DAD), is a rare and frequently fatal disease. It is generally encountered in previously healthy individuals following an episode of acute respiratory illness. The mechanisms responsible for AIP are not clearly understood; however, there is diffuse acute lung injury resulting in acute respiratory failure.

Signs and Symptoms

The presentation is similar to that of acute respiratory distress syndrome (ARDS). There is no predilection for age and sex, but are mostly seen in adults. The onset is acute and often preceded by symptoms suggestive of viral upper respiratory tract infection followed by widespread pneumonia. Hypoxemia develops early followed by respiratory failure requiring mechanical ventilatory support. There is no association with smoking.

Diagnosis

The criteria include rapidly progressive clinical course (>2 months) leading to respiratory failure; exclusion of infectious, toxic, autoimmune, or any other cause of ARDS; DAD with hyaline membranes in early or exudative stages, observed on biopsy specimens; radiological findings consistent with ILD as bilateral ground-glass opacities with consolidation; and absence of chronic lung disease. Bilateral airspace disease seen on radiography correlates with DAD seen on histology. BAL is not helpful in diagnosis, but it is useful to rule out other possible etiologies, such as infections, acute eosinophilic pneumonia, and diffuse alveolar hemorrhage.

Treatment

Since there is no proven treatment, supportive care with oxygen supplementation and mechanical ventilation is indicated. Early corticosteroid therapy and combination therapy with intravenous cyclophosphamide and vincristine have been reported. Newer agents, such as inhaled nitric oxide, anticytokine antibodies, and surfactant, may be useful.

Prognosis

Mortality is greater than 60%. Based on the morphology of lung parenchyma on CT, some authors report that this may help differentiate fulminant forms of AIP. Those who survive may have no residual lung damage, residual pulmonary fibrosis, or recurrent disease.

LYMPHOID INTERSTITIAL PNEUMONIA

Etiology

Lymphoid interstitial pneumonia is a rare IIP, which most commonly affects the women in the 5th decade of life. It can, however, occur at any age. LIP possibly represents a lymphoproliferative disorder confined to the lungs. LIP has also been described in association with systemic diseases, most notably HIV infection [or acquired immunodeficiency syndrome (AIDS)] although some cases remain idiopathic. It has also been described in post-bone marrow transplantation.

Signs and Symptoms

It is slow in onset with increasing cough and breathlessness. Constitutional symptoms, such as fever, weight loss, and arthralgias, may be prominent features. Chest examination often reveals bibasilar crackles with digital clubbing being rare.

Diagnosis

Chest X-ray may show an alveolar pattern predominantly at the bases or a diffuse disease with honeycombing. The predominant cell type on BAL is lymphocyte with a restrictive pattern on lung function tests. Histology reveals dense interstitial lymphoid infiltrate.

Treatment

Some patients improve spontaneously without any treatment. Clinical improvement to corticosteroid therapy has been reported. In some cases, cytotoxic agents, including cyclophosphamide, azathioprine, and cyclosporine have been used. Supplemental oxygen therapy and treatment of pulmonary infections may be necessary.

IDIOPATHIC PLEUROPARENCHYMAL FIBROELASTOSIS

Idiopathic pleuroparenchymal fibroelastosis is a new and rare IIP characterized by predominant pleural and subpleural upper lobe fibrosis.

Diagnosis and Treatment

The PPFE, a rare disease, is seen more frequently in the 4th and 5th decades of life, with a median of 57 years of age. Exertional dyspnea and nonproductive cough are the primary symptoms. Pneumothorax is frequent. It is associated with decrease anteroposterior diameter of the thoracic cage known as *"flattened thoracic cage".*

High-resolution CT chest shows pleural thickening along with nodular and reticular opacities in bilateral upper lobes. Restrictive physiology with increased Residual Volume/Total Lung Capacity (RV/TLC) can be found on PFTs. Intra-alveolar fibrosis, septal fibroelastosis of the visceral pleural with lymphoplasmacytic infiltrates and fibroblast foci can be observed in the histology.

The PPFE appears to be resistant to any kind of immunosuppressive therapy. The disease is progressive with a poor prognosis close to 50% survival at 10 years.

UNCLASSIFIABLE IDIOPATHIC INTERSTITIAL PNEUMONIA

Unclassifiable category is applied to those cases where there is discrepancy in the clinical, radiological, or histological characteristics, or where previous treatment of the patient modified the primary findings or the new histological patterns are found. Multidisciplinary discussion is essential in these cases to determine the best course of further diagnostic and treatment approaches.

CHAPTER 43

Sarcoidosis

Dheeraj Gupta, Sahajal Dhooria, Om P Sharma

Sarcoidosis is a multisystem granulomatous disorder of unknown etiology. The disease occurs worldwide and affects young- and middle-aged adults of both genders. The lungs are the most frequently involved organs, but its chameleon-like presentation can involve any organ including the eyes, skin, bones, heart, liver, and the brain.

ETIOLOGY AND RISK FACTORS

Genetic Predisposition

Clustering of sarcoidosis occurs in families. The familial clustering, more commonly seen among the white, mostly involves only parent–child pairs or sibling pairs. More complex pedigrees are rather rare. Many of class II major histocompatibility complex (MHC) alleles have been implicated for different manifestations of sarcoidosis. Also, new predisposing genes have been identified with genome-wide association studies (GWAS). Newer advances in molecular techniques like large-scale and systematic genetic sequencing will further help in discovering new risk loci.

Environmental and Occupational Risk Factors

Possibly, a number of environmental and occupational exposures to various inflammation-evoking stimuli may trigger sarcoidosis-like manifestations. There is an increased risk among workers with industrial exposure to organic powders, building materials, hardware, and gardening material. Occupational exposures (wood-burning stoves, fireplaces, and consumption of water from wells), living or working on a farm, exposure to metals at work, and working in humid places with musty smells have also been blamed amongst the risk factors. On the other hand, there is some evidence to suggest that tobacco smoking is protective for sarcoidosis.

Infectious Agents as Risk Factors

Identification of structures similar to microorganisms such as *Leptospira* species, *Mycoplasma* species, and *Propionibacterium* species on examination of the sarcoid granuloma on electron microscope and immunohistochemical techniques supports the role of infecting organisms in the etiopathogenesis. Herpes virus, retrovirus, *Chlamydia pneumoniae*, *Borrelia burgdorferi*, *Rickettsia helvetica*, and *Pneumocystis jiroveci* are other organisms, which have been reported. However, there is strongest evidence for *Propionibacterium* and the *Mycobacterium*.

There are several strong points to suggest that sarcoidosis is in some way related to tuberculosis ever since sarcoidosis was first described, for example, histopathologic appearances of granulomas, reports on mycobacterial disease before, during, or after sarcoidosis, and the finding of mycobacteria in occasional granulomas of sarcoidosis support the mycobacterial relationship. Possibly, the presence of mycobacterial infection or bacillus Calmette–Guérin (BCG) vaccination may result in the development of autoimmunity in a genetically predisposed host. It is also possible that the cell wall-deficient L-form of mycobacteria, which is difficult to isolate, is responsible for sarcoidosis.

PATHOGENESIS AND IMMUNOLOGY

Granulomatous inflammation, the central feature in the pathogenesis of sarcoidosis, is a protective response to an inciting agent. It limits inflammation and protects the tissue. Though the exact antigen inciting this response in sarcoidosis is yet unclear and it may, in fact, be different in different patients and different demographic areas. The granulomatous inflammation in sarcoidosis is characterized by an altered balance of T helper 1 (Th1)/Th2 responses. While Th1 cytokines [interferon (IFN)-γ and interleukin (IL)-2] are expressed dominantly, there is a low level of expression of Th2 cytokines (IL-4 and IL-5). Oxidative stress may also play some role in the pathogenesis of sarcoidosis.

Depression of delayed type hypersensitivity (anergy) is an important clinical phenomenon, which, in fact, is frequently used as a diagnostic test. The anergic state is possibly due to a subgroup of CD4 T cells, which abolishes IL-2 production and inhibits T-cell proliferation.

PATHOLOGY

Presence of noncaseating, compact, and "naked" granulomas is the characteristic feature of sarcoidosis on histopathology. A sarcoid granuloma typically comprises lymphocytes, macrophages, well-differentiated epithelioid cells, multinucleated giant cells, fibroblasts, and mast cells. There are CD4 T cells in the center and CD8 T cells and B lymphocytes in the periphery. Histological findings differ with the stage of the disease. Fibrinoid necrosis may sometimes be seen in nodular and necrotizing sarcoid granulomatosis. Nonspecific cytoplasmic inclusions such as asteroid bodies, Schaumann bodies, Hamazaki-Wesenberg bodies, and calcium oxalate crystals are sometimes seen. Granulomatous inflammation is known to quickly resolve with or sometimes even without therapy. But granulomas are also known to persist and show hyalinization. Fibrosis and scarring may occur in chronic sarcoidosis.

CLINICAL FEATURES

Almost, any part of the body can be affected in sarcoidosis, but the lung is the most common site of organ involvement.

Pulmonary Involvement

Almost, 20–50% of patients are asymptomatic or present with nonspecific symptoms. The most common clinical signs and symptoms include dry cough, chest pain, and dyspnea. Chest pain may sometimes point to the presence of a complication such as pleuritis or pneumothorax, or even pulmonary embolism, due to antiphospholipid antibody syndrome associated with sarcoidosis on rare occasions.

Radiographic Findings

The chest radiographic abnormalities are seen in more than 90% of patients. Frequently, the diagnosis of sarcoidosis is first suspected on routine chest roentgenography done for an incidental indication, sometimes, in an asymptomatic individual for medical examination. The presence of symmetrical bilateral hilar and mediastinal lymphadenopathy is the characteristic finding seen in about 50–85% of cases. Lymph nodes are generally bulky and sharply defined, with a clear line of translucency between the mediastinal shadow and the nodes—classically described as "potato nodes". Hilar adenopathy is occasionally seen. Around 25–60% of patients show pulmonary parenchymal infiltrates, which are typically bilateral and symmetrical, present most commonly in the upper and mid-lung fields. A chest radiographic staging system for sarcoidosis is as given in Table 43.1.

Nodules in sarcoidosis are typically present along the bronchovascular bundle and subpleural regions. Mass-like lesions may sometimes form due to the coalescence of these granulomata. Occasionally, there are small nodules surrounding the conglomerate nodules giving an appearance of "sarcoid galaxy sign". Contrast-enhanced computed tomography (CT) scan shows more extensive lymphadenopathy than the typical hilar and paratracheal nodes seen on chest radiograph. The presence of ground-glass attenuation may suggest acute alveolitis due to granulomatous inflammation. "Reverse

TABLE 43.1: Chest radiographic staging of sarcoidosis.

Stage	Features
Stage 0	No involvement
Stage 1	Bilateral hilar adenopathy, often with right paratracheal adenopathy
Stage 2	Stage 1 + pulmonary infiltrates
Stage 3	Pulmonary infiltrates without adenopathy
Stage 4	Advanced parenchymal lung disease, including fibrosis, honeycomb lung, traction bronchiectasis, cysts, bullae, and emphysema, with or without adenopathy

halo" sign typically described with invasive fungal infections has also been reported in sarcoidosis.

Functional Abnormalities

Pulmonary function abnormalities are present in 20-40% patients with a normal chest radiograph. Pulmonary function is, however, impaired in 50-70% of cases when the chest skiagram shows abnormal. Typically, the abnormalities include reductions in the vital capacity, diffusing capacity, arterial partial pressure of oxygen (PaO_2) and lung compliance. Spirometry often reveals a restrictive pattern, though an obstructive defect may also be there.

Other Intrathoracic Manifestations

Pleural involvement (including effusions and thickening) is uncommon but reported in 5-10% of patients. Pleural effusions seen in 1-3% of patients with sarcoidosis and are more commonly seen in stage 2 and 3 disease.

Extrapulmonary Involvement

Extrapulmonary organs are involved in about two-thirds of the patients. Constitutional symptoms (fever, night sweats, weight loss, fatigue, myalgia, and arthralgia) occur more frequently with extrathoracic sarcoidosis. Skin and eye are most commonly involved. Any organ can be involved in sarcoidosis, cardiac, and neurological involvement being the most serious forms.

Skin

Common skin lesions include erythema nodosum (EN), subcutaneous nodules, plaques, lupus pernio, and maculopapular eruptions. Granulomatous inflammation can be demonstrated in the specific lesions of sarcoidosis on biopsy. EN presents as tender nodules on the extremities is the most common nonspecific lesion. Löfgren's syndrome is a typical subset of sarcoidosis, which presents with EN and hilar lymphadenopathy (sometimes also with polyarthropathy and nongranulomatous uveitis). Lupus pernio is the most severe form of skin manifestation. These lesions are sometimes destructive and erode into the cartilage and bone of the face.

Eye

Uveitis, retinal perivasculitis, retinal scarring, and glaucoma can occur in sarcoidosis. Symptoms may vary depending upon the site of involvement. Commonly, a patient may have blurred vision, red eye, painful eye, or photophobia in anterior uveitis to vision loss in posterior uveitis. About one-third of patients with anterior uveitis are asymptomatic (a "quiet eye"). Dry eyes may occasionally occur due to the involvement of lacrimal glands. Rarely, optic neuropathy can result in rapid and permanent loss of vision.

Cardiac

Both cardiac and neurologic sarcoidosis, though rare, may be life-threatening in nature. Cardiac sarcoidosis can cause left ventricular dysfunction, heart block, and arrhythmias that can sometimes result in sudden death.

Neurosarcoidosis

Facial palsy due to the involvement of seventh cranial nerve is the most common manifestation of neurosarcoidosis. This may sometimes precede the diagnosis of sarcoidosis. Sarcoidosis can affect any part of the nervous system and present with clinical features as per the site of involvement. Rarely, it may behave like multiple sclerosis.

Other Extrapulmonary Organ Involvement

Sarcoidosis may affect the upper airways, and the gastrointestinal, hematological, endocrine, genitourinary, and musculoskeletal systems. Asymptomatic histological involvement of liver may be seen in 50-65% patients. Similarly, spleen may also be involved with minimal or no symptoms. Peripheral lymphadenopathy may be seen in about 10% of patients. Sarcoidosis of the upper respiratory tract with involvement of nasopharynx, hypopharynx, larynx, and sinuses is underappreciated. Rarely, vocal cord palsy may also occur.

Typical bone lesions usually consist of small cysts or cortical defects in the small bones of the hands or feet. Joints, if involved acutely, as is often seen in patients with Lofgren's syndrome, carry a good prognosis. Chronic sarcoid arthritis is rare but can progress to cause joint deformities.

Abnormalities of Calcium Metabolism

In sarcoidosis, hypercalcemia has been reported to occur in 2-63% of patients; hypercalciuria is three times more common than hypercalcemia. These abnormalities can lead to nephrolithiasis and renal failure. Rarely, hypercalcemia may cause acute pancreatitis.

DIAGNOSIS

The diagnosis of sarcoidosis rests on a triad of clinical, radiological, and histological criteria. Although the diagnosis of sarcoidosis can be reached with a high level of confidence in up to 80% of patients using clinical data and High-Resolution CT (HRCT) imaging, it is imperative that a histological diagnosis should be obtained in all patients as far as circumstances permit (except in those with the classic **Löfgren's syndrome**). This is especially so in tuberculosis-endemic areas, because the clinical and radiological picture of the two diseases may be overlapping.

Histological Diagnosis

Biopsy of the skin or peripheral lymph nodes, if enlarged, may yield the diagnosis in a few cases. However, most patients having thoracic or internal organ involvement would require a sampling of the mediastinal lymph nodes, the airway mucosa, and/or the lung parenchyma. Granulomatous inflammation may be encountered in lung biopsies even in stage I sarcoidosis.

Endobronchial ultrasound (EBUS) is a novel bronchoscopic modality, which helps to improve the yield of Transbronchial Needle Aspiration (TBNA). EBUS-guided TBNA (EBUS–TBNA) has an average yield of around 80% (range: 54–93%) in the diagnosis of sarcoidosis.

The characteristic findings on biopsy is the presence of compact noncaseating epithelioid cell granulomas, however, an alternative diagnosis has to be excluded. A general differential diagnosis of granulomatous inflammation is given here (Box 43.1).

Tuberculin Skin Test

A negative tuberculin test is heavily relied upon for diagnosis of sarcoidosis. A positive tuberculin skin test (TST) in a patient suspected to suffer from sarcoidosis should alert the treating physician for a thorough workup for tuberculosis.

Miscellaneous Investigations

Bronchoalveolar Lavage

Bronchoalveolar lavage (BAL) has a high positive predictive value but the samples require more than 15% lymphocytes on cell count to be useful for the diagnosis of sarcoidosis. Diagnosis is favored by an elevated ratio of CD4/CD8 in BAL fluid.

Serum Angiotensin-converting Enzyme

A rise in serum angiotensin-converting enzyme (SACE) activity seen in active sarcoidosis is neither sensitive nor specific as a diagnostic tool. It may be normal in sarcoidosis. On the other hand, there may be elevated SACE levels in other disorders such as diabetes mellitus, cirrhosis, acute hepatitis, chronic renal disease, silicosis, Gaucher's disease, leprosy, asbestosis, and berylliosis.

Gallium Scanning

Gallium uptake associated with specific findings in sarcoidosis indicates the presence of inflammation. While "lambda sign" indicates uptake by the hilar

> **BOX 43.1:** Common pathological differential diagnosis of sarcoidosis.
>
> *Mycobacterial*:*
> - Tuberculosis
> - Atypical mycobacteria
>
> *Fungal infections*:*
> - Cryptococcosis
> - Aspergillosis
> - Histoplasmosis
> - Coccidioidomycosis
> - Blastomycosis
> - Pneumocystis
>
> *Bacterial:*
> - Mycoplasma
> - Brucella
>
> *Hypersensitivity pneumonias*
>
> *Drug reactions**
>
> *Pneumoconiosis:*
> - Beryllium (chronic beryllium disease)*
> - Titanium
> - Aluminum
>
> *Malignancy:*
> - Lymphoma*
>
> *Others:*
> - Wegener's granulomatosis (sarcoid-type granulomas are rare)
> - Chronic interstitial pneumonia (UIP, LIP)
> - Necrotizing sarcoid granulomatosis (NSG)
> - Granulomatous lesions of unknown significance (GLUS syndrome)
>
> *Source:* Adapted from Joint ATS/ERS/WASOG statement on sarcoidosis.
> *Note:* Conditions marked with (*) can also present with hilar and mediastinal lymphadenopathy.

and right paratracheal nodes, the lacrimal and salivary gland uptake results in the "panda sign".

18-Fluorodeoxyglucose–Positron Emission Tomography (18FDG–PET) Scanning

It acts as an adjunct to the routine investigations in assessing disease activity, especially in extrapulmonary sites, and monitoring treatment response, and also helps to identify occult sites for biopsy.

TREATMENT

Patients having moderate-to-severe symptoms, a decrement in the quality of life, or significant physiological impairment, should be treated. The following may serve as guiding principles of treatment of pulmonary sarcoidosis according to the radiological stage:

- *Stage 0 or I*: Asymptomatic patients with stage 0 or stage I disease nearly always remain free of symptoms without treatment, hence do not require treatment. Nonsteroidal anti-inflammatory drugs (NSAIDs) may be used for fever and joint pains. Sometimes, a short course of prednisone 15–20 mg/day is necessary in patients who do not respond to NSAIDs.
- *Stage II*: Treatment is required for patients with symptoms (cough, dyspnea, chest pain, and effort intolerance). Treatment is also needed for patients with significant lung function impairment.
- *Stage III*: These patients mostly have symptoms along with lung function impairment. They almost always need treatment. Treatment is also needed for asymptomatic stage III patients who show progressive pulmonary function impairment.
- *Stage IV*: These patients often show extensive fibrosis and bullae formation. Their response to corticosteroids and immunosuppressive therapy is rather poor.

Patients with severe extrapulmonary manifestations (ocular, neurological, cardiac, upper airway involvement, lupus pernio, and those with hypercalcemia) should always be treated with immunosuppressive therapy. In both neurosarcoidosis and cardiac sarcoidosis, higher initial doses of steroids (1 mg/kg/day) are required. Atrioventricular conduction blocks and left ventricular function generally show recovery, while the data on ventricular tachycardia and mortality are sparse. Asymptomatic hypercalciuria and hypercalcemia can cause nephrocalcinosis and renal failure. They should always be looked for and treated with steroids (apart from hydration, diuretics, and low-calcium diet).

The options for nonsteroidal treatment (also called disease-modifying antisarcoid drugs [DMASDs]) are cytotoxic drugs, antimalarials, biologics, and other agents. Barring the anti-TNF-α drugs, most of these agents take a few weeks to months to be effective. Therefore, steroid treatment should not be tapered for at least a month after the addition of an alternative agent, unless the steroid adverse effects are major.

Cytotoxic Drugs

These include methotrexate, azathioprine, leflunomide, mycophenolate mofetil, cyclophosphamide, and chlorambucil and constitute the most promising alternative to corticosteroids. Methotrexate (MTX) is the preferred second-line drug for steroid refractory cases and can be used as a steroid-sparing drug as well. Occasionally, it may be used as a first-line agent in combination with steroids. The recommended initial dose is 10–15 mg once a week along with folic acid 5 mg weekly or 1 mg daily. Azathioprine (2 mg/kg/day) may also be used as a steroid-sparing agent. It is equally efficacious as methotrexate, but results in a higher risk of infections.

Antimalarials such as chloroquine and hydroxychloroquine act as immunomodulators and have been successfully used for cutaneous sarcoidosis involving the paranasal sinuses, sarcoid-related hypercalcemia, and neurosarcoidosis. Hydroxychloroquine in a usual dose of 200–400 mg daily is effective in treating chronic pulmonary sarcoidosis. The third-line treatment involves the use of biological agents. Infliximab is typically administered as an intravenous infusion of 3–5 mg/kg on weeks 0 and 2, with repeat dosing every 4–8 weeks thereafter. There are chances of relapse in more than half of the patients after discontinuation of treatment. Adalimumab can also be used and is administered subcutaneously. Allergic reactions are lower than with infliximab, since it is a fully humanized antibody. Use of TNF-α inhibitors may be responsible for opportunistic infections and an increased risk of reactivation of latent tuberculosis. There are concerns about a possible increase in malignancy, such as lymphoma, new onset and worsening of congestive heart failure, and demyelinating diseases.

The duration of treatment in each patient is individualized and is gauzed on the basis of symptoms, organ involvement, and response to therapy. There is frequent relapse of symptoms when the treatment is tapered off. Prolonged treatment is recommended for the continued suppression of disease activity. Management of complications of disease, adverse events due to different treatments and of comorbid conditions is also important.

PROGNOSIS AND MORTALITY

Prognosis of sarcoidosis is linked to the severity of the disease. Sarcoidosis is usually a benign disease. Many patients may remain asymptomatic as well as spontaneous remission is common. In 10–30% of cases, the disease may follow a chronic course, sometimes leading to significant deterioration in lung function. Extensive fibrosis and pulmonary hypertension may develop in some patients with progressive disease. A sharp drop in respiratory functions and other complications should alert the clinician.

CHAPTER 44

Pulmonary Eosinophilic Disorders

Subhash Varma, Aditya Jindal

INTRODUCTION

Eosinophilia and lung disease is currently recognized to be either secondary to known causes or a primary involvement. Eosinophilic lung disease, therefore, includes conditions known to involve the lung that are associated with peripheral and/or pulmonary eosinophilia.

EOSINOPHILS

The mature eosinophil varies from 12 to 17 μm in diameter and has a bilobed nucleus in an eosinophilic cytoplasm. It is characterized by the presence of primary and secondary granules in the cytoplasm, which are clearly visible on electron microscopy. Primary granules are rounded, membrane limited structures and contain Charcot Leyden crystal protein. The secondary granules are somewhat oval and consist of a dense core clearly visible in a less dense matrix. The core of these granules is formed by major basic protein (MBP) while the matrix contains various other enzymes, such as eosinophil-derived neurotoxin (EDN), eosinophil cationic protein (ECT) and eosinophil peroxidase. Additionally, dense lipid bodies that are not membrane bound and contain enzymes for metabolizing arachidonic acid, are present. These serve as sites of eicosanoid synthesis.

Eosinophils have a diurnal variation in response to the level of endogenous steroids with higher levels in the morning. Pyogenic infections lead to eosinopenia, while parasitic infestations and drugs cause eosinophilia. Eosinopenia can also occur in response to exogenous steroids, estrogens and epinephrine.

Pulmonary Eosinophilic Disorders

As a part of the human leukocyte system, eosinophils have a variety of functions to perform. They are especially important in the defense against helminthic infestations—eosinophilic products are lethal to the larval stages of these parasites. The role of eosinophils in allergic disorders, parasitic and neoplastic diseases, tissue inflammation or idiopathic eosinophilia as a result of their proinflammatory and cytotoxic effects is also now better understood. These effects are related to the release of preformed granule constituents and inducible lipid mediators, cytokines and oxidative products. The role of eosinophils in tissue injury has been elucidated by the demonstration of protein constituents of primary and secondary granules in the tissues involved in eosinophilia-related disorders.

A large number of conditions are associated with the development of eosinophilia (Box 44.1) with manifestations in different organ systems necessitating a careful search for the cause.

BOX 44.1: Pulmonary eosinophilic disorders.

Primary pulmonary eosinophilia
- Predominant involving lung
    - Acute eosinophilic pneumonia
    - Chronic eosinophilic pneumonia
- Systemic disease with lung disease
    - Churg–Strauss syndrome
    - Idiopathic hypereosinophilic syndrome

Secondary pulmonary eosinophilia
- Infections
    - Parasitic infestations
        - *Transient passage (Löffler's syndrome)*: Ancylostoma, Ascaris, Strongyloides
        - *Tissue resident*: Paragonimiasis, echinococcosis
        - Heavy hematogenous seeding
            - Trichinella
            - Visceral larva migrans
            - Disseminated strongyloidiasis
            - Schistosomiasis
    - *Fungal infections*: Coccidioidomycosis, histoplasmosis
    - *Other infections*: Tuberculosis, brucellosis
- Tropical pulmonary eosinophilia
- Allergic bronchopulmonary aspergillosis
- Hypersensitivity pneumonia
- Drugs, toxins and radiation

Lung disorders with associated eosinophilia
- *Interstitial lung disease*: Sarcoidosis, idiopathic pulmonary fibrosis, Langerhans cell histiocytosis, connective tissue disease
- Asthma
- Bronchiolitis obliterans—organizing pneumonia
- Neoplastic disorders—hematological malignancies, solid organ tumors
- Postlung transplant

PULMONARY EOSINOPHILIC DISORDERS

A holistic approach to pulmonary eosinophilic disorders involves understanding the place of lung diseases associated with eosinophilia in the overall gamut of eosinophilic disorders. In recent years, a significant evolution in classification and differentiation has taken place. Broadly, eosinophilic disorders are divided into the following categories:
- Hypereosinophilic syndromes (HES) previously considered idiopathic for which the causes are now known—these include PDGFRA-associated myeloproliferative neoplasms and lymphocytic variants of HESs.
- Organ restricted eosinophilic syndromes—pulmonary eosinophilic disorders and eosinophilic gastrointestinal disorders
- Syndromes in which eosinophilia and eosinophil-associated pathogenesis are central to the diagnosis—Churg-Strauss syndrome
- Hereditary disorders characterized by eosinophilia.

Löffler's Syndrome

The original description was of a syndrome consisting of no to minimal respiratory symptoms along with fleeting pulmonary opacities and peripheral eosinophilia. A similar syndrome may be seen secondary to drug reactions. There is no age or sex predilection and the patients typically present with an acute, self-limiting disease comprising of low-grade fever, dry cough, dyspnea and rarely, hemoptysis. Blood examination shows moderate-to-marked eosinophilia; respiratory secretions may also show eosinophilia. The chest X-ray will show transient, migratory, nonsegmental interstitial or alveolar infiltrates. The symptoms typically resolve within 1–2 weeks.

Acute Eosinophilic Pneumonia

Acute eosinophilic pneumonia is an acute onset rapidly progressive disorder that occurs in the previously normal young adult population and causes acute onset, severe respiratory failure. The median age at onset is approximately 30 years and has a slight male preponderance. The exact cause in the majority of individuals is not known though it has been associated with unusual activities, such as cave exploring and wood working. This has led to a hypothesis that AEP is due to a hypersensitivity reaction to fungal antigens; though nothing has been proven as yet. Also, cases have been reported in individuals who have recently taken up smoking; interestingly, cases have been reported recently after exposure to e-cigarettes and to secondhand smoke.

The clinical presentation is that of acute onset disease with rapid progression to acute respiratory distress syndrome (ARDS) over 2–3 days. Patients may present with fever, cough, myalgias, dyspnea, pleuritic chest pain that progresses to frank respiratory failure. A somewhat characteristic feature is the absence of any multisystem involvement despite severe respiratory failure. A possibility of acute eosinophilic pneumonia should always be kept in mind during the evaluation of any ARDS patient.

Investigations typically show leukocytosis with initial absence of peripheral blood eosinophilia, though the IgE levels may be moderately increased. The chest X-ray shows bilateral patchy reticular infiltrates that progress rapidly to an ARDS like picture with diffuse alveolar or interstitial infiltrates. The computed tomography (CT) scan shows ground glass opacities and/or consolidation which may patchy or diffuse in nature and smooth interlobular septal thickening distributed in a random manner without any zonal predominance. Bilateral pleural effusions may also be seen while pleural fluid analysis shows marked eosinophilia and high pH. Pathologically, the main finding is that of a diffuse alveolar damage syndrome, with marked eosinophilic infiltration in the interstitium and in the alveolar spaces. Fibrinous membranes are commonly seen; airway involvement with mucous plugs has also been described. AEP is not characterized by either formation of granulomas or by alveolar hemorrhage. Pleural eosinophilic infiltration has been noted in 10% of cases.

Despite its severe clinical presentation, AEP is highly responsive to corticosteroids. Mechanical ventilation may be required for severe cases, with ventilation strategies as for ARDS. The mortality rate is low with prompt treatment that results in a rapid and sustained response and infrequent relapses. The diagnosis requires a high index of suspicion and is made only after exclusion of all other causes.

Idiopathic Chronic Eosinophilic Pneumonia

The disease generally has an insidious onset and indolent course. Predominant symptoms are low-grade fever, drenching night sweats and weight loss. Associated productive or nonproductive cough, dyspnea and wheezing are the other presenting features. Dyspnea is generally mild, but at times may progress to a point that mechanical ventilation may be required. Extrapulmonary manifestations other than fever, asthenia and weight loss occur rarely; they include arthralgias, joint pains and heart failure. In fact, presence of significant extrapulmonary symptoms should necessitate a search for other systemic disorders such as vasculitis or hypereosinophilic syndrome.

There is usually a moderate leukocytosis with an elevated eosinophil count; the platelet count may also be elevated. However, the absence of peripheral eosinophilia should not preclude the diagnosis. BAL fluid also shows marked eosinophilia ranging from 12% to 95% of the total. Serum IgE levels are moderately elevated in about half of the cases.

The radiographic features of CEP are quite variable. Characteristically, infiltrates are dense, patchy, bilateral, peripheral and symmetrical, involve the upper and mid zones and are progressive in nature. They may be subpleural in location. The characteristic "photographic negative of pulmonary edema" that occurs following involvement of extensive areas or whole lung is seen in less than 25% of cases. Pleural effusions are uncommon though reported. HRCT shows bilateral involvement with areas of ill-defined consolidation and ground glass opacification, areas of patchy consolidation with atelectasis and septal thickening. There may be mediastinal lymphadenopathy and nodular infiltrates.

Histopathologic examination reveals infiltration of the interstitium and alveoli by eosinophils, lymphocytes, macrophages and plasma cells with disruption of the local architecture. Evidence of proliferative bronchiolitis obliterans, microangiitis and microabscesses may also be seen.

There is a dramatic response to corticosteroids in CEP with symptoms decreasing within 6–48 hours and radiological clearing within months. Oral steroids with dose ranging from 0.5 to 1 mg/kg/day can be used and treatment in low doses is maintained for at least 6–12 months or longer. Relapse occurs in half to two-thirds of treated patients after discontinuation of steroids. However, currently no risk factors indicative of relapse are recognized. The relapse can usually be controlled by reinstitution of steroids which may need to be given for prolonged periods of time. The dose of oral steroids can be brought down by the addition of inhaled corticosteroids. The use of omalizumab, an anti-IgE antibody, has been described recently as a steroid sparing agent in CEP with good results.

Churg–Strauss Syndrome (Eosinophilic Granulomatosis with Polyangiitis or EGPA)

It has now been defined as an eosinophil-rich and necrotizing granulomatous inflammation often involving the respiratory tract, and necrotizing vasculitis predominantly affecting small to medium vessels, and associated with asthma and eosinophilia. It can affect any age group with peak incidence between 30 years and 50 years, without any sex predilection.

The underlying pathology is believed to be an immune hypersensitivity, accounting for the presence of antinuclear cytotoxic antibodies (ANCA) and nearly universal finding of an atopic state in these individuals. The presence or absence of ANCA allows the differentiation of these patients into two subgroups. The group with ANCA positivity has more frequent mononeuritis multiplex, glomerulonephritis, purpura and alveolar hemorrhage while the ANCA negative group has more frequent cardiomyopathic features and lung infiltrates.

Eosinophilic granulomatosis with polyangiitis has been associated with the use of leukotriene inhibitors, montelukast more than zafirlukast. The onset of the disease is variable from 2 days to 12 months after the initiation of therapy and it occurs almost exclusively as corticosteroids are being tapered off. This is considered to be an unmasking of the underlying disease rather than the result of drug use. There have also been reports of EGPA occurring after the use of omalizumab.

Eosinophilic granulomatosis with polyangiitis is commonly diagnosed when a patient with long-standing asthma develops symptoms suggestive of vasculitis, i.e. mononeuritis multiplex, purpura, etc. along with peripheral eosinophilia and lung infiltrates.

The respiratory manifestations of EGPA include upper respiratory tract disease, asthma, pleural effusions and Löffler's like syndrome. The upper respiratory tract is involved in approximately 75–85% of cases and manifests as allergic rhinitis, sinusitis and nasal polyposis.

Asthma is the predominant feature of EGPA. It may be present for many years before the diagnosis of EGPA is made. It is usually predominant in the prodromal and eosinophilic stages of the disease and may subside with the onset of the vasculitic phases. A short interval between the onset of asthma and that of vasculitis is considered a sign of increased severity.

The cardiovascular system is commonly involved and is the leading cause of mortality. Patients may develop coronary vasculitis leading to myocardial infarction and ischemic cardiomyopathy or congestive cardiac failure secondary to eosinophilic myocardial infiltration. Acute and chronic constrictive pericarditis and pericardial tamponade may also occur. The development of coronary vasculitis is associated with high risk of mortality of around 60%.

Systemic manifestations may be prominent, include fever, weight loss, arthralgias and arthritis, lymphadenopathy, splenomegaly, urological and ocular disease. These generally herald the onset of extrapulmonary disease. Neurological manifestations are seen in up to two-thirds of patients include mononeuropathy and polyneuropathy, cranial neuropathy especially optic neuritis, mononeuritis multiplex, seizures, cerebrovascular accidents and subarachnoid hemorrhage.

Gastrointestinal tract manifestations generally consist of eosinophilic gastroenteritis or vasculitis causing abdominal pain, bleeding, diarrhea, intestinal obstruction, bowel perforation, gastric ulcers and liver function test abnormalities. Dermatologic manifestations like palpable purpura, nodules, ulcers, maculopapular rashes and livedo reticularis may occur. Renal involvement consists of interstitial nephritis, focal segmental glomerulosclerosis, hematuria and hypertension following renal infarction. However, chronic renal failure is unusual in EGPA as compared to other forms of vasculitis.

Overall, about 40% of patients have ANCA positivity; this is generally perinuclear (pANCA) with specificity against myeloperoxidase. However, only 25% of patients with EGPA who have no renal disease are ANCA positive, while ANCA is positive in 75% of patients with any renal disease and in 100% with documented necrotizing glomerulonephritis.

The chest X-ray may be normal or nonspecific. Löffler's syndrome like infiltrates may be present in up to 40% of individuals and pleural effusions may be seen in one-third of cases. Other findings on radiology include noncavitatory nodules, patchy areas of consolidation or ground glass opacification, septal thickening, pulmonary artery enlargement and peribronchial thickening. Pleural fluid is acidic with high eosinophil count and low glucose levels. The choice of treatment is based on the presence of systemic involvement. The five factor score (FFS) is the most commonly used guide for treatment initiation. The five factors are: (i) proteinuria > 1 g/24 h; (ii) serum creatinine level >140 mmol/L; (iii) myocardial involvement; (iv) severe gastrointestinal involvement; and (v) central nervous system involvement. Oral prednisolone may be started at a dose of 1 mg/kg/day and continued for 6–12 weeks followed by a gradual taper to a maintenance dose, which might be continued for a year or more.

Disease activity may be followed by the disappearance of constitutional symptoms, hypertension, cardiac, renal, neurological and vasculitic disease. Laboratory markers of disease activity include ESR, IgE levels and leukocyte counts; pANCA is not useful for follow-up.

Indications for the use of cytotoxic chemotherapy include nonresponsiveness to steroids and severe systemic disease including cardiac, GIT and renal disease (proteinuria >1 g/day or renal insufficiency). Pulse cyclophosphamide is probably the immunosuppressive treatment of choice in an acute phase, whereas azathioprine may be useful for maintenance. Pulse steroids may also be used in acute settings. Other immunomodulators, such as high-dose intravenous immunoglobulin and interferon-alpha in standard dose have also been used in severe disease and so has been plasma exchange.

Hypereosinophilic Syndrome

Also known as Löffler's endocarditis and eosinophilic leukemia, hypereosinophilic syndrome (HES) is a disorder characterized by multisystem involvement and a variable presentation. It predominantly affects males and is more common from ages 20 years to 50 years, though it can occur at any age.

Hypereosinophilic syndrome is a heterogeneous disease. Its clinical manifestations are highly variable in the terms of duration, severity and organ involvement. The symptoms most often are indolent; include fever, weight loss, fatigue, anorexia, night sweats, skin rash, hepatosplenomegaly, angioedema and other system involvement.

The respiratory system is involved in approximately 40% of cases, manifested predominantly by nocturnal cough, which is usually "nonproductive". Wheezing and dyspnea also occur and occasionally the disease can progress to ARDS. Pleural effusion, pulmonary hypertension and thromboembolism may develop over a period of time.

The cardiovascular system is most common involved. There is an eosinophilic infiltration of the endocardium and myocardium leading to restrictive cardiomyopathy, endocardial fibrosis and mitral regurgitation. Intracardiac thrombus formation occurs, leading to pulmonary thromboembolism. Associated peripheral arterial or venous thrombosis has also been reported.

Neurological manifestations include encephalopathy, neuropsychiatric disturbances, memory loss, visual changes and cerebrovascular accidents secondary to thromboembolism.

Diagnosis

Blood examination shows anemia and leukocytosis (10,000–50,000/mm^3) with 30–70% eosinophils. There may be associated blood and or bone marrow neutrophilia, basophilia and eosinophilic dysplasia. Bone marrow shows an increase in eosinophils and eosinophil precursors. Eosinophilic blast transformation has been noted in 28–51% of patients. Eosinophilic infiltration of other organs is also demonstrable on histopathological examination).

Chest X-ray shows focal or diffuse nonspecific infiltrates and pleural effusions. Pulmonary function tests demonstrate an obstructive physiology. Echocardiography may show evidence of intracardiac thrombi; should be done 6 monthly in follow-up as cardiovascular disease is the major cause of mortality and morbidity in this disease.

Treatment depends upon the presence of end-organ dysfunction. In clonal and idiopathic hypereosinophilia, the aim of the treatment is to limit/reverse end-organ damage and provide symptomatic improvement. In asymptomatic patients without any evidence of end-organ damage, a careful follow-up and assessment of any end-organ damage may be a prudent policy.

Asymptomatic peripheral eosinophilia can be followed up every 3-6 months without any treatment. The first line of therapy consists of steroids, which are given orally. Prednisone, in a dose of 1 mg/kg/day for 1-2 months is followed by a slow taper to a maintenance dose, which can be continued for 1 year or longer as required. In refractory cases, treatment with hydroxyurea, vincristine, chlorambucil, cyclosporine or interferon-α can be tried. The anti-IL5 antibody, mepolizumab has also been used in patients with high IL5 levels.

Other Eosinophilic Lung Diseases

Langerhans Cell Granulomatosis

Histiocytosis X consists of three closely related disorders, occurring at different ages: Langerhans cell histiocytosis, Letterer-Siwe disease and Hand-Schüller-Christian disease. Primary pulmonary histiocytosis X, earlier known as eosinophilic granuloma of the lung, is almost exclusively found in smokers. It presents with cough, dyspnea, hemoptysis, chest pain, fever, wheezing, weight loss and recurrent, often bilateral pneumothorax. Patients also develop diabetes insipidus and bony disease. Chest X-ray shows involvement of the upper and middle zones with sparing of the costophrenic angles, reticulonodular changes, cystic lesions and bullae that may rupture to cause recurrent pneumothorax. Pulmonary function tests (PFTs) may show either a restrictive or an obstructive defect.

Treatment is based on the severity of the disease. Smoking should be stopped and patient treated with corticosteroids. Vincristine, cyclophosphamide and fludarabine have also been used. The mortality rate is less than 5% in adults.

Neoplastic Disorders

Eosinophilia may occur in association with several neoplastic conditions, both with hematological malignancies and solid organ tumors. The presence of eosinophilia may or may not be an adverse prognostic sign, depending upon the underlying disorder.

Hematological disorders associated with eosinophilia include systemic mastocytosis (in approximately 20%), nodular sclerosing Hodgkin's disease (15%), B-cell non-Hodgkin's disease, T-cell leukemia and Sézary syndrome. Of course, eosinophilic leukemia is a well-known variant of acute myelomonocytic leukemia (M4).

Solid organ malignancies include large cell cancer of the lung, squamous cell carcinomas of cervix, skin, nasopharynx, bladder transitional cell carcinoma, etc.

Tropical Pulmonary Eosinophilia

It is an important cause of marked eosinophilia, hence an important differential diagnosis.

BOX 44.2: Drugs causing eosinophilic lung disease.

- Antimicrobials:
  - Para-amino salicyclic acid
  - Nitrofurantoin
  - Penicillin
  - Tetracycline
  - Streptomycin
  - Isoniazid
  - Sulfonamides
  - Tetracycline
  - Minocycline
  - Dapsone + pyrimethamine
- Antineoplastic and immunosuppressives:
  - Bleomycin
  - Methotrexate
  - Melphalan
  - Gold salts
  - Azathioprine
  - Penicillamine
  - Beclomethasone
- Nonsteroidal anti-inflammatory drugs (NSAIDs):
  - Aspirin
  - Naproxen
  - Piroxicam
  - Nimesulide
  - Phenylbutazone
- Cardiovascular and antidiabetics:
  - Amiodarone
  - Hydralazine
  - Thiazides
  - Clofibrate
  - Sulfonylureas
- Miscellaneous:
  - Carbamazepine
  - Phenytoin
  - Dantrolene
  - Methylphenidate
  - Imipramine
  - Cocaine or heroin exposure
  - Iodinated contrast media
  - L-tryptophan.

Flowchart 44.1: Proposed diagnostic algorithm for pulmonary eosinophilic disorders.

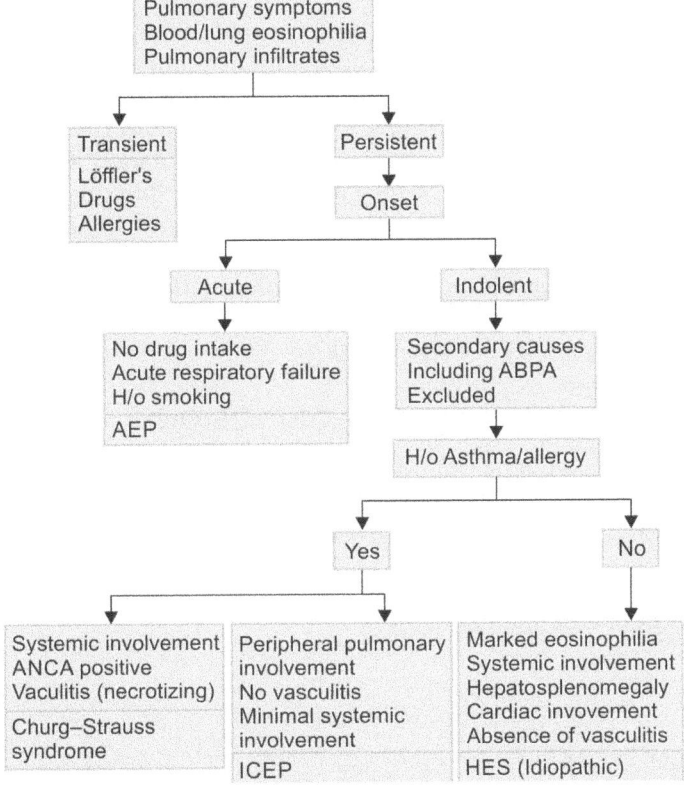

(AEP, acute eosinophilic pneumonia; HES, hypereosinophilic syndrome; ICEP, idiopathic chronic eosinophilic pneumonia; ABPA, allergic bronchopulmonary aspergillosis)

Infections

Eosinophilia occurs with a variety of infectious agents, which include bacterial, fungal and parasitic diseases. An undulating pattern of eosinophilia that corresponds to disease activity has been noted in tuberculosis. It has been shown that eosinophilia correlates with a good prognosis while eosinopenia was noted in fulminant or miliary disease.

Chronic brucellosis is also known to be associated with eosinophilia. The fungal infection most commonly associated with eosinophilia is coccidiomycosis in which it occurs as a hypersensitivity phenomenon. Other fungal infections include rare case reports of eosinophilia associated with *Histoplasma capsulatum* and cryptococcosis.

Drug- and Toxin-induced Pulmonary Eosinophilia

A variety of drugs and toxins are associated with eosinophilic lung disease (Box 44.2). The signs and symptoms of disease may manifest anywhere from a few minutes after exposure to weeks afterwards. One of the more common drugs to be implicated is nitrofurantoin, which causes acute, subacute and chronic reactions.

Symptoms, as already detailed, occur variably after exposure to the drug. These include low-grade fever, cough and dyspnea with or without wheezing. Examination might show wheezing and crackles and the peripheral blood will show eosinophilia. Chest X-ray may reveal diffuse or patchy pulmonary infiltrates; CT scans show bilateral consolidation and ground-glass opacification, both of which may be peripheral. Pulmonary function tests may either be absolutely normal, or show a reduced DLCO or a mild restrictive defect.

The syndrome usually disappears after discontinuation of the responsible drug. Corticosteroids are not universally beneficial, though their use may hasten recovery, especially in sick patients.

APPROACH TO DIAGNOSIS AND CONCLUSION

It is apparent that eosinophilic lung diseases are heterogeneous disorders that require a meticulous history taking, painstaking examination and judicious use of investigations to reach a definite diagnosis. A simplified algorithm that may be useful is given in Flowchart 44.1. It is important to reach a diagnosis because these illnesses have different course and complications and thus involve important treatment decisions.

CHAPTER
45

Infiltrative and Deposition Diseases

Pralay Sarkar, Arunabh Talwar

INTRODUCTION

There are several different diseases characterized by the deposition of abnormal materials, either endogenous or exogenous, in the pulmonary parenchyma or in other areas of the respiratory system. Although rare, they frequently pose problems in the differential diagnosis of common clinical conditions, which present with similar respiratory or other clinical manifestations.

PULMONARY AMYLOIDOSIS

Amyloidosis is a group of disorders characterized by the extracellular tissue deposition of fibrils as beta-pleated sheets, disrupting organ function. The pattern of organ involvement often depends on the nature of the precursor protein, many of which are associated with specific disease entities. Most common types of amyloidosis associated with pulmonary involvement are either AL or AA amyloidosis. Amyloidosis has association with a wide range of systemic diseases, most commonly plasma cell dyscrasias, chronic infections or inflammatory conditions.

Tracheobronchial Amyloidosis

Tracheobronchial amyloidosis is a rare disease. Here amyloid deposition typically occurs in the submucosa of trachea and main bronchi, sometimes extending to the level of segmental bronchi. Tracheobronchial amyloidosis usually occurs as an isolated airway involvement without that of lung parenchyma or other organs. Tracheobronchial amyloidosis has been associated with tracheobronchopathia osteochondroplastica though the causative relationship of these two rare conditions remains debatable.

The presentation is predictable from the site of involvement: cough, dyspnea, recurrent hemoptysis and wheezing are common symptoms. Significant narrowing of airway can happen, leading to consequences like atelectasis and recurrent pneumonia.

Nodular Pulmonary Amyloidosis

In this type of pulmonary amyloidosis, nodular deposits of amyloid occur in pulmonary parenchyma, usually bilaterally at multiple sites. Nodular pulmonary amyloidosis is usually not associated with systemic amyloidosis. Symptoms arise when a large mass produces its mechanical effects: patients present with cough and progressive dyspnea. Significant weight loss has also been reported. CXR and CT of the thorax show single or multiple pulmonary nodular opacities/masses of soft tissue density.

Diffuse Alveolar Septal Amyloidosis

In this pathological pattern of pulmonary involvement, the microscopic deposits of amyloid occur diffusely within the alveolar septae and the interstitial tissue. Interstitial/alveolar septal pulmonary amyloidosis is usually seen as a part of the systemic amyloidosis. Majority of these patients have significant cardiac involvement complicating the picture in many of these patients. Diffuse alveolar hemorrhage leading to fatality has been reported with this form of amyloidosis.

Pleural Disease

Pleural effusion is a rare manifestation of systemic amyloidosis. Cardiac involvement and congestive heart failure are common in AL amyloidosis. Pleural effusions may result from congestive heart failure; the pleural fluid in these cases is expected to be transudative in character.

Other Manifestations of Respiratory System Amyloidosis

Pulmonary hypertension has been known to develop in systemic amyloidosis with or without the presence of parenchymal lung involvement. *Diffuse pulmonary hemorrhage* has been described as a first manifestation of pulmonary amyloidosis. Amyloid angiopathy, involving small- and medium-sized pulmonary arteries, may cause *pulmonary arterial dissection*, presenting with recurrent hemoptysis.

Laryngeal amyloidosis: Laryngeal involvement causes long-standing hoarseness of voice. It may also cause airway obstruction.

Mediastinal lymphadenopathy: Mediastinal as well as unilateral or bilateral hilar lymphadenopathy can be seen in amyloidosis.

A variety of management strategies such as observation in selected cases, intermittent bronchoscopic intervention, surgical resection and external beam radiation are used in laryngotracheobronchial amyloidosis. In a given case, the choice of treatment strategy depends on the extent of involvement, the size, location and appearance of the lesions, the functional consequences of amyloid deposition and the availability of expertise in a particular institution. Bronchoscopic procedures include the mechanical debulking/resection with/without dilatation, transmucosal Nd:YAG laser treatment (for pseudotumoral mass or circumferential thickening), carbon dioxide laser ablation (for submucosal lesions) and stent placement (after establishing patency of airway lumen). Majority of the cases can be managed by bronchoscopic procedures.

LYSOSOMAL STORAGE DISORDERS

Lysosomal storage disorders (LSDs) are a diverse group of hereditary metabolic disorders caused by defects in lysosomal function. Most commonly, these disorders result from mutations in genes that encode catabolic enzymes (e.g. lysosomal hydrolases) involved in the degradation of macromolecules. Failure to degrade macromolecules causes accumulation of the same in the cells leading to cellular dysfunction and progressive clinical manifestations. More than 45 diseases have been described till date, most being inherited in an autosomal recessive manner. The clinical expression of LSDs is variable. The age of onset, the severity of symptoms and the pattern of organ involvement can vary markedly within a single disorder type or subtype. Clinical manifestations differ according to the residual enzyme function, genetic and environmental factors. Many of these disorders, e.g. Gaucher, Tay–Sachs, Pompe, metachromatic leukodystrophy, and GM1 gangliosidosis have infantile, juvenile and adult forms. Respiratory involvement can occur in various LSDs, some of whom have been also reported in adult patients.

Anderson–Fabry Disease

Anderson–Fabry disease (AFD) is an X-linked recessive disease as a result of the deficiency of the lysosomal enzyme α-galactosidase A (α-gal A). It has no ethnic predilection and occurs in about 1:117,000 live births. AFD leads to progressive accumulation of glycosphingolipids, predominantly globotriaosylceramide (GL-3), in many body tissues over a period of years or decades. Clinical manifestations include renal failure in about 30% of patients and cerebrovascular accidents in about 25% of patients.

Chest X-ray (CXR) can be normal in many patients. In keeping with the occurrence of airway disease, some of the patients have CXR changes suggestive of emphysema with or without bulla. Pneumothorax can also occur. HRCT findings of lung involvement in AFD have been infrequently reported.

Gaucher Disease

Gaucher disease is an autosomal recessive disorder as a result of the deficiency of the lysosomal enzyme glucocerebrosidase. It is the most prevalent lysosomal storage disorder. Gaucher disease leads to the accumulation of the lipid glucocerebroside within the lysosomes of the monocyte-macrophage system. Type 1 Gaucher disease patients have normal life-expectancy and may present for the first time in adult life. Type III presents in late childhood/early adolescence and has more severe and rapidly progressive visceral disease. Type II disease rarely survives beyond the age of 2 years.

Pulmonary involvement has been reported in both type I and type III Gaucher disease, is more rare in type I and more severe in type III. Clinical picture is characterized by gradual onset and progression of dyspnea that, in some cases, culminates to respiratory failure and death.

Clinical examination may show clubbing as a result of hepatopulmonary syndrome. The chest radiograph may be abnormal with or without symptoms and show bilateral diffuse reticulonodular or miliary opacities. HRCT shows bilateral irregular interlobular, as well as intralobular septal thickening.

Niemann–Pick Disease

Niemann-Pick disease (types A and B) is due to the deficiency of the enzyme acid sphingomyelinase (ASM).

Pulmonary symptoms result from alveolar lipoproteinosis. Various bleeding manifestations are common in this disease and hemoptysis and hemothorax have been reported. Cyanosis, clubbing, rales and wheezing may be present on physical examination.

No specific therapy is available for ASM deficiency. Both ERT and gene therapy have shown promising results in the mouse model. Slow and inexorable progress is the natural history of respiratory disease. Treatment with whole lung lavage has been described with clinical improvement in isolated case reports.

Hermansky–Pudlak Syndrome

Hermansky-Pudlak syndrome (HPS) is an autosomal recessive disorder characterized by the triad of oculocutaneous albinism, bleeding diathesis (secondary to defect in platelet function) and (in some cases) lysosomal accumulation of ceroid lipofuscin. HPS has been described in many different ethnic groups; HPS1 is the most frequently described subtype; it is particularly common in individuals from North West Puerto Rico and accounts for approximately 50% of non-Puerto Rican cases. Mutations in both HPS1 and HPS4 genes have been described in Indian patients.

Hermansky–Pudlak syndrome causes interstitial lung disease. Lung fibrosis typically develops in the second or third decade of life in HPS1. Clinical presentation is akin to usual interstitial pneumonia: exertional dyspnea and dry cough are the usual presenting symptoms; physical examination is conspicuous for clubbing and velcro crepitations.

The diagnosis can also be established by the genotyping of DNA samples or the demonstration of ceroid accumulation in pathological specimens. Pathological examination of the lungs shows a picture of pulmonary fibrosis, architectural distortion and diffuse lymphocytic infiltration. In addition, a distinctive feature is the presence of large vacuolated histiocytes and pneumocytes containing periodic acid–Schiff (PAS) positive fine and coarse brown pigment within areas of interstitial fibrosis.

Antifibrotic agent, pirfenidone has been tried in pulmonary fibrosis of HPS. Measures like the avoidance of smoking and environmental tobacco smoke, prompt treatment of respiratory infections, and administration of influenza and pneumococcal vaccines are recommended to preserve residual lung function. In HPS patients with end-stage lung fibrosis, lung transplantation has been used successfully. Pulmonary fibrosis in HPS is usually fatal in 4th or 5th decade and accounts for death in ~50% of HPS patients.

Lipoid Pneumonia

Lipoid pneumonia is a pattern of pathological involvement of lungs characterized by prominent deposition/filling of alveolar spaces with lipoid material. It can be called exogenous when the source of the aspirated lipoid material is from external sources and endogenous when the lipid deposition occurs without an exogenous source. Also called "cholesterol pneumonia", endogenous lipoid pneumonia typically occurs from accumulation of lipid-filled macrophages, surfactant and eosinophilic proteinaceous material derived from degenerating cells, in the alveoli distal to the bronchial obstruction. Diffuse intra-alveolar deposition of lipoprotein material, either as an idiopathic process or in the association of systemic diseases, e.g. chronic myeloid leukemia, is better termed pulmonary alveolar proteinosis (PAP).

The clinical presentation depends on the volume and acuity of the aspiration episode (s). Acute exogenous lipoid pneumonia results as a consequence of aspiration of large amount of oil/hydrocarbons, e.g. accidental poisoning in children. Here the presentation is with acute respiratory symptoms: cough, respiratory distress and low-grade fever. Repeated aspirations of small amounts of lipids result in the chronic form of exogenous lipoid pneumonia. Here the onset of symptoms is insidious with chronic cough and/or dyspnea; fever, weight loss, chest pain and hemoptysis are less common at presentation. Often the presentation is that of non-resolving pneumonia. Sometimes, the patient may be present with chronic fibrosis.

Making a diagnosis of lipoid pneumonia requires a high degree of clinical suspicion and meticulous history taking. Diagnosis is difficult as the aspiration episodes are often unrecognized and clinical and radiological features mimic many other pulmonary diseases. On CT scan, the demonstration of fat-density areas within the lesions is considered diagnostic of lipoid pneumonia. Diagnosis can be confirmed by BAL. Fat globules are found in the bronchoalveolar fluid; cytological examination of the BAL fluid shows presence of lipid-laden foamy macrophages. Lung biopsy specimens show alveoli filled with macrophages containing lipid vacuoles. Advanced lesions show larger lipid vacuoles surrounded by inflammatory infiltrates.

Prompt identification and prevention of further aspiration prevent the progression of the disease, and in some cases allow resolution. Anecdotal case reports of improvement with steroids are there; the beneficial effects in these cases may be attributed to the effect of steroids on the inflammatory process in lipoid pneumonia. Bronchoscopy with therapeutic BAL for the clearance of mineral oil from the lung parenchyma has been reported as the treatment for this condition.

Idiopathic Pulmonary Hemosiderosis

Idiopathic pulmonary hemosiderosis (IPH) is an uncommon disease of unknown etiology characterized by the repetitive episodes of diffuse alveolar hemorrhage (DAH). The causes of DAH are diverse and other causes need to be excluded before a diagnosis of IPH can be reached.

The etiology of IPH remains unknown. Familial clustering has been reported, which may suggest the inheritance of a rare genetic defect, predisposition and common exposure to environmental antigens. Suggestions of an autoimmune pathogenesis are based on indirect evidences like the presence of circulating immune complexes and the development of other autoimmune diseases in many patients of IPH who survive for more than a decade. An allergic theory has been proposed based on presence of antibodies against cow milk and coexistence with celiac disease.

The clinical presentation widely varies. Some patients have a fulminant presentation with catastrophic DAH and respiratory failure. Some patients are present with the nonspecific symptoms of chronic cough and dyspnea. Recurrent hemoptysis is yet another presentation. Patients may be present with symptomatic or asymptomatic anemia without any respiratory symptoms. All adult patients report hemoptysis at some point of time.

Investigations often reveal hypochromic microcytic anemia, a reflection of repeated DAH, binding of iron with pulmonary hemosiderin (an unusable form) and iron loss in the sputum. Plasma ferritin level does not reflect the iron-deficiency state; it is normal or elevated as a result of alveolar synthesis and subsequent release into the circulation of ferritin. During an acute phase of IPH, CXR reveals diffuse alveolar opacities and HRCT reveals bilateral ground glass opacities. After multiple episodes of bleeding, chronic changes, evident as reticulonodular interstitial shadows, are seen on HRCT. Variable amount of fibrosis eventually develops.

History of repeated episodes of cough, dyspnea and hemoptysis along with a consistent picture on CXR and HRCT, point toward the diagnosis. The demonstration of hemosiderin-laden macrophages in the sputum or in the BAL fluid confirms alveolar hemorrhage. Sometimes, the pulmonary hemorrhage is occult and the patient presents with iron-deficiency anemia only; a comprehensive investigation of the cause is required before a diagnosis of IPH is suspected and established. Serological studies for the markers of autoimmune diseases, e.g. antinuclear factor (ANF), anti-double-stranded DNA, antineutrophilic cytoplasmic antibody (ANCA, both perinuclear and cytoplasmic variants), antiglomerular basement membrane (GBM) antibody, antiphospholipid antibodies, IgG and IgE cow's milk antibodies and rheumatoid factor (RF) are negative in IPH. A lung biopsy is required to rule out other causes of DAH.

Systemic glucocorticoids remain the mainstay of the treatment. Once started during the acute phase, steroids are continued till the new pulmonary infiltrates have resolved. A slow taper-off over a few months follows, if symptoms do not recur. As maintenance therapy, various immunosuppressive agents, e.g. azathioprine, cyclophosphamide and chloroquine have been tried with or without corticosteroids, with variable success. Cyclophosphamide infusion has been tried with success as a salvage therapy in IPH exacerbation with life-threatening DAH. Gluten-free diet should be instituted in patients who have co-existent celiac disease and IPH (Lane-Hamilton syndrome). IPH patients, who had advanced chronic lung disease requiring lung transplantation, had recurrence of disease in the transplanted lung.

Intrathoracic Extramedullary Hematopoiesis

In many hematological disorders, such as thalassemia, sickle-cell anemia, hereditary spherocytosis, polycythemia vera and myelofibrosis, intense compensatory hematopoiesis leads to the formation of foci of extramedullary hematopoiesis. Extramedullary hematopoiesis can be present within the thoracic cavity, described most frequently in patients with sickle-cell anemia and thalassemia. Intrathoracic extramedullary hematopoiesis appears as paravertebral and/or paracostal masses. Formation of these masses occurs from the extrusion from the bone marrow through the cortex. The patients usually do not have any symptoms attributable to the masses. Occasional cases with symptoms due to mass effect from the large foci of extramedullary hematopoiesis and other complications, e.g. exudative pleural effusion, hemothorax have been described.

Neurofibromatosis

von Recklinghausen's disease or neurofibromatosis (NF) type 1 is an autosomal dominant disorder with characteristic neurocutaneous manifestations. Neurofibromatosis causes ILD. Most NF patients with lung involvement by ILD report dyspnea. Pulmonary function tests show an obstructive pattern with reduced DLCO. CXR and HRCT show bilateral cystic lesions with upper lobe predominance. Other radiological findings include ground-glass opacities, bibasilar subpleural reticular opacities and bullae.

CHAPTER 46

Bronchiolitis

Gyanendra Agrawal, Dheeraj Gupta

INTRODUCTION

Bronchiolitis is the nonspecific inflammation of the respiratory bronchioles and peribronchiolar alveolar sacs of variable causes, clinical manifestations and evolution. Bronchiolitis is traditionally classified as one of the interstitial lung disease (ILD).

Classification schemes have been proposed on the basis of causes and underlying diseases, radiologic features, histopathologic findings, or some combination of these parameters.

The clinical classification is primarily based on the proved or presumed etiology, related systemic diseases or other associations (Box 46.1).

GENERAL FEATURES OF BRONCHIOLAR DISORDERS

Bronchiolitis, a cellular and mesenchymal inflammatory reaction that follows damage to the bronchiolar epithelium of small conducting airways, is the most common form of disease affecting small airways. This entity is relatively uncommon in adults. Neutrophils which accumulate at the site of injury causes further damage to the airway epithelium and matrix by the release of inflammatory mediators. Depending on the disease stage, the repair process may cause narrowing and distortion of small airways (constrictive bronchiolitis) or complete obliteration (bronchiolitis obliterans).

CLINICAL PRESENTATIONS

Most commonly, the patients present with slowly progressive exertional dyspnea and dry cough. Onset of symptoms is relatively acute in bronchiolitis

> **BOX 46.1: Clinical classification of bronchiolitis.**
>
> - *Infectious bronchiolitis:* Respiratory syncytial virus, Mycoplasma pneumonia, parainfluenza, adenovirus, measles, rubella, and rubeola
> - *Drug-induced bronchiolitis:* D-penicillamine, gold, sulfasalazine, amiodarone, interferon, phenytoin, cocaine, minocycline, nitrofurantoin, carmustine, bleomycin, busulfan, Sauropus androgynus, and paraquat
> - *Inhalational injury:* Toxic fumes and gases, mineral dusts, organic dusts, volatile flavoring agents, Flock worker's lung (fine nylon fiber), grain dusts, fire smoke (World Trade Center lung)
> - *Post-transplant:* Bone marrow, heart–lung, lung
> - *Connective tissue diseases:* Rheumatoid arthritis, Sjögren's syndrome, systemic lupus erythematosus, polymyositis, and dermatomyositis
> - *Idiopathic:* Cryptogenic adult bronchiolitis, respiratory bronchiolitis, diffuse panbronchiolitis, cryptogenic organizing pneumonia, and diffuse aspiration bronchiolitis
> - *Systemic diseases:* Ulcerative colitis, chronic eosinophilic pneumonia, Wegener's granulomatosis, chronic thyroiditis, ataxia–telangiectasia, immunoglobulin A (IgA) nephropathy
> - *Other rare:* Eosinophilic bronchiolitis, lymphocytic bronchiolitis, radiation pneumonitis, primary diffuse hyperplasia of pulmonary neuroendocrine cells

from infections, inhalational injury or drugs; subacute in organizing pneumonia; and indolent and chronic in patients with post-transplant bronchiolitis. Cough with copious expectoration may be seen in infectious bronchiolitis and diffuse panbronchiolitis (DPB). Fever and constitutional symptoms are mainly seen in infectious bronchiolitis and collagen vascular diseases. Some patients may even present with pulmonary hypertension and respiratory failure in advanced stages.

Pulmonary Function Tests

Depending on the predominant physiology, pulmonary function tests (PFTs) may yield variable results. Most of the primary bronchiolar disorders and large airway diseases are associated with obstructive physiologic defects. In contrast, most of the distal acinar interstitial diseases with secondary bronchiolar involvement show restrictive or mixed pattern. Primary bronchiolar disorders show nonreversibility with inhaled bronchodilators. In addition, these patients also demonstrate reduced diffusion capacity. The obstruction of small airways results in abnormal distribution of ventilation to peripheral lung units.

Chest X-ray Findings

Chest radiography in bronchiolar disorders may be normal or demonstrate nonspecific findings like hyperinflation and peripheral attenuation of vascular markings in purely obstructive bronchiolar lesions, such as constrictive bronchiolitis. In other primary bronchiolar disorders, small nodules or reticulonodular infiltrates may be observed. Increased bronchial wall thickening may also be seen.

High-resolution Computed Tomography Findings

High-resolution computed tomography (HRCT) scan abnormalities that reflect bronchiolar diseases can be categorized into direct and indirect signs (Table 46.1). On the basis of the radiologic features, bronchiolar diseases have been classified into four dominant CT patterns: (i) centrilobular opacities with tree-in-bud pattern are seen in infectious bronchiolitis, (ii) diffuse panbronchiolitis, (iii) diffuse aspiration bronchiolitis (DAB), and (iv) immunodeficiency syndromes.

Other conditions resulting in a pattern of mosaic attenuation include connective tissue disorders, bone marrow and lung transplantation, toxic fume inhalation and drugs. Quite often many diseases will have a "mixed pattern" on HRCT. Association of tree in bud with mosaic perfusion can be seen in different entities, such as bronchiectasis and acute bronchopulmonary infections. The combination of mosaic perfusion and ground-glass opacities in the same patient, referred to as the "headcheese sign" is very suggestive of HP. HRCT findings in chemical-induced lung injuries are variable and nonspecific but may help distinguish from other forms of injuries.

Histologic Findings

Most morphological abnormalities of the bronchioles are not specific. It is difficult to recognize and classify bronchiolitis in transbronchial biopsies because of the limited sampling size, hence surgical biopsy is preferred. It is important to obtain wedge biopsies from multiple lobes because the bronchiolar pathology is often patchy.

In cellular bronchiolitis, the bronchioles' structures show an increased number of inflammatory cells. "Follicular bronchiolitis" represents hyperplasia of the mucosa-associated lymphatic tissue (MALT) and chronic peribronchiolar infiltrate along with secondary germinal centers. Respiratory bronchiolitis and RB-ILD often have accompanying emphysema.

"Diffuse panbronchiolitis" is a peculiar morphological form of cellular bronchiolitis largely restricted to the adult individuals of Japanese heritage. Its histologic hallmark is the presence of an interstitial inflammatory infiltrate containing foamy macrophages around respiratory bronchioles. Polyps of granulation tissue may partially occlude adjacent bronchiolar or alveolar lumina.

Bronchiolitis obliterans with intraluminal polyps is characterized, by intrabronchiolar polypoid protrusions of connective tissue that partially fill

TABLE 46.1: High-resolution computed tomography signs of bronchiolar disorders.

Direct signs	Indirect signs
Bronchiolar wall thickening: inflammation/fibrosis • Bronchiolectasis • Bronchiolar luminal impaction: Centrilobular nodules ± tree in bud appearance	Mosaic attenuation Subsegmental atelectasis

bronchiolar lumens. These polypoid proliferations usually extend distally in the alveolar ducts and alveoli, a pattern known as organizing pneumonia.

Constrictive bronchiolitis refers to luminal narrowing by scarring that ranges from very subtle abnormalities to complete luminal obliteration. The hallmark of this type of bronchiolitis is mural thickening by submucosal collagenous fibrosis with progressive concentric narrowing associated with luminal distortion, mucous stasis and chronic inflammation. Bronchiolar dilatation with mucous impaction and smooth muscle hypertrophy may also be seen. Peribronchiolar fibrosis and bronchiolar metaplasia are a rare condition characterized by the growth of bronchiolar epithelium into the adjacent fibrotic alveolar walls (so-called lambertosis). Inflammatory cells are scanty and usually present in the bronchiolar lumen. It represents a manifestation of previous bronchiolar injury/scarring such as viral bronchiolitis or extrinsic allergic alveolitis.

PRACTICAL APPROACH FOR DIAGNOSIS OF BRONCHIOLAR DISORDERS

The broad clinical spectrum of bronchiolar inflammatory disorders in adults can be diagnosed with the help of a practical algorithmic approach (Flowchart 46.1).

Flowchart 46.1: Algorithm for practical approach to patients with supposed bronchiolitis.

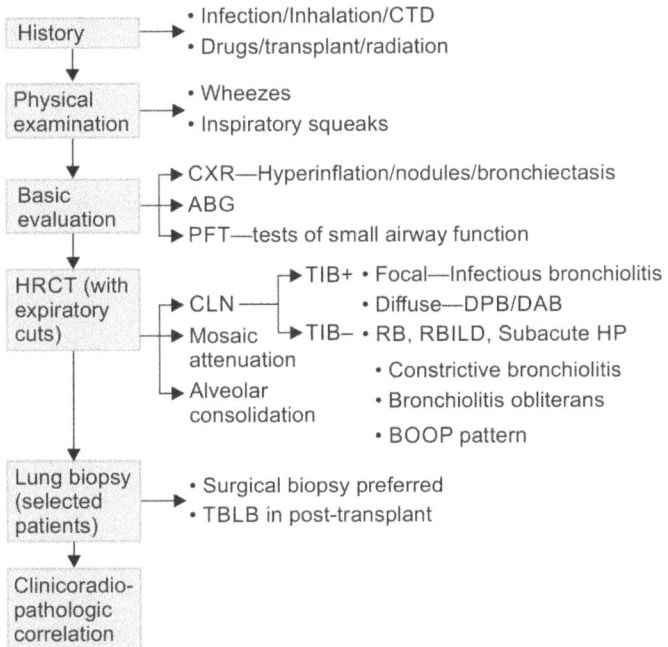

(ABG, arterial blood gases; BOOP, bronchiolitis obliterans with organizing pneumonia; CLN, centrilobular nodules; CTD, connective tissue diseases; CXR, chest X-ray; DAB, diffuse aspiration bronchiolitis; DPB, diffuse panbronchiolitis; HP, hypersensitivity pneumonitis; PFT, pulmonary function tests; RB, respiratory bronchiolitis; RB-ILD, respiratory bronchiolitis interstitial lung disease; TBLB, transbronchial lung biopsy; TIB, tree-in-bud)

A detailed history of symptoms suggestive of connective tissue disease, as well as exposure to inhalational irritants and radiation, should be elicited in order to identify a possible cause. A potential relationship with drug intake should be investigated in depth and taken into account in combination with the underlying disease. On auscultation, the presence of wheezing, inspiratory squeaks, or crackles should point to the bronchioles as the likely anatomic site involved.

After history and physical examination, posteroanterior and lateral chest radiographs (CXRs) and PFTs are typically obtained. These tests are of limited value in directing the diagnostic workup of primary bronchiolar disorders but are important to exclude large airway diseases in which secondary bronchiolar changes may be seen.

High-resolution computed tomography scanning (inspiratory and expiratory) may play a critical role in both suggesting the specific causes of bronchiolar disease and directing optimal management. In select cases, the diagnosis may be made solely using HRCT scans in combination with the history and clinical presentation, thus obviating more invasive diagnostic testing. In patients where the diagnosis of bronchiolitis and its cause is not clear, the clinical relevance of a bronchiolar lesion is best determined by identifying the underlying histopathologic pattern and assessing the correlative clinico-physiologic–radiologic context.

CHAPTER 47

High-altitude Problems

Ajay Handa

INTRODUCTION

High-altitude ascent poses multiple problems such as exposure to extreme cold temperatures, low-atmospheric pressures, and hypoxia. All of these factors lead to different altitude-related illnesses such as acute mountain sickness (AMS), high-altitude cerebral edema (HACE), and high-altitude pulmonary edema (HAPE). These illnesses compromise safety and, if unrecognized, may even be fatal. The occurrence of high altitude-related illnesses in those with pre-existing lung disease is of greater concern due to limited physiological reserve.

PHYSICAL CHANGES WITH ALTITUDE

A fall in atmospheric pressure is the most significant change with gain in altitude. Correspondingly, there is a fall in the atmospheric oxygen pressure, inspired oxygen pressure, alveolar oxygen partial pressure (P_AO_2), and arterial oxygen tension (P_aO_2). Moreover, there is a greater insensible water loss through the respiratory tract due to reduction in air density and temperature with gain in altitude. The exposure to high altitude and cold weather are also associated with cardiovascular problems such as pulmonary thromboembolism.

PHYSIOLOGICAL ADAPTATION TO HIGH ALTITUDE

The physiological changes in the respiratory, cardiovascular, and hematological systems to allow the humans to adapt and survive in high-altitude areas constitute *acclimatization*. The main changes include compensatory increase in ventilation due to the decreased P_aO_2 called hypoxic ventilatory response

(HVR). There is an increased work of breathing and respiratory muscle oxygen consumption thereby limiting exercise capacity at altitude.

Gas exchange in the alveolar capillaries is adversely affected by low P_AO_2 (reduced alveolar-capillary gradient) combined with a lower mixed venous oxygen levels, which delay alveolar-capillary equilibration. Exercise also results in an increase in cardiac output, shortening of capillary transit time, and increase in venous oxygen desaturation leading to aggravation of the physiological abnormalities and further arterial desaturation.

Despite the decrease in blood oxygen content, the delivery of oxygen to tissues is maintained by the increased cardiac output and increased red cell mass (hypoxia-induced erythropoietin secretion). The hemoglobin-oxygen dissociation curve shifts to right by production of 2,3-diphosphoglycerate (DPG) in red blood cell (RBC) and this counteracts the effects of hyperventilation respiratory alkalosis induced by high altitude.

The alveolar hypoxia triggers hypoxic pulmonary vasoconstriction (HPV) to maintain ventilation-perfusion relationship and this causes a rise in pulmonary arterial pressure. This is important in pathogenesis of HAPE and altitude-related pulmonary hypertension.

SPECIFIC ALTITUDE-RELATED ILLNESSES

Acute Mountain Sickness (AMS)

The diagnosis of AMS is essentially clinical and is based on the presence of headache plus one or more of the following symptoms—fatigue, anorexia, nausea, vomiting, giddiness, and insomnia. Occurrence of AMS increases with increase in the altitude and the rate of ascent. An initial reduction in arterial oxygen saturation (SaO_2), high body mass index (>24 kg/m^2), and cigarette smoking are other factors recognized associated with occurrence of AMS. Physical examination or laboratory studies are nonspecific for the diagnosis of AMS.

A slow ascent to high altitude is the most important step to prevent AMS. Use of prophylactic drugs such as acetazolamide and dexamethasone is also effective. Treatment requires cessation of ascent and descent to a low altitude, symptomatic treatment with non-narcotic analgesics and acetazolamide (250 mg twice daily). Both inhaled corticosteroids such as budesonide (200 µg BID) and oral dexamethasone (4 mg BID) are also shown to be effective especially for prevention of severe AMS.

High-altitude Cerebral Edema

High-altitude cerebral edema is frequently a life-threatening condition mostly seen in patients with preceding symptoms of either AMS or HAPE. It is characterized by the presence of ataxia, altered mental status (encephalopathy), or both. It is more commonly seen at altitudes above 4,000 meters. Rapid ascent to high altitudes is the most important risk factor. Same preventive measures as for AMS are helpful. Treatment requires immediate descent to lower heights. If available, recompression in a portable hyperbaric chamber along with supplemental oxygen proves beneficial. Drug treatment consists of intravenous dexamethasone (8 mg followed by 4 mg q 6 hourly). HACE can cause brain herniation and death, if the condition is not recognized in time and treated immediately.

High-altitude Pulmonary Edema

High-altitude pulmonary edema is another serious condition that affects 0.2-15% of high-altitude travelers. It is a type of noncardiogenic pulmonary edema that usually occurs at altitudes above 3,000 meters. It may develop within 2-5 days of ascent either de novo or following symptoms of AMS or HACE. It is especially common in unacclimatized lowlanders who ascend rapidly for tourism. The risk increases with the increase in altitude, the rapidity of ascent, overexertion, and exposure to cold air. Individuals susceptible to HAPE demonstrate exaggerated pulmonary vasoconstriction on exposure to hypoxia and with exercise.

Initially, the patient may complain of dry cough and decreased exercise performance. Patients with frank HAPE have dyspnea and cough on minimal activity, orthopnea, and pink frothy sputum. There may be low-grade fever, resting tachycardia, tachypnea, cyanosis, and bilateral auscultatory crackles on physical examination. It is most important to prevent the occurrence of High-Altitude Edema (HAE) through education and advice regarding importance of slow and staged ascent to encourage acclimatization and avoiding overexertion. Prophylaxis [nifedipine Sustained Release (SR) 20 mg twice daily and/or inhaled salmeterol 125 μg twice daily] should be advised for patients with a history of underlying respiratory diseases or pulmonary hypertension.

This life-threatening disorder requires immediate descent to lower altitude or recompression in a hyperbaric chamber along with supplemental oxygen along with nifedipine 10 mg stat followed by nifedipine SR 30 mg twice daily. Severe cases of HAPE can lead to severe hypoxemic respiratory failure and may require ventilatory support to correct severe hypoxemia and prevent fatal outcome. Continuous positive-pressure ventilation has been used of adjunct therapy in less severe cases.

Subacute Mountain Sickness

Sub-AMS is described in Indian soldiers posted at altitudes between 5,800 and 6,700 meters for an average of 10 weeks. Clinical manifestations consist of symptoms of dyspnea, cough, and exercise-induced angina as well as evidence of right heart failure with pedal edema, polycythemia, cardiomegaly, pericardial effusion, and ascites. Evacuation to lower altitudes usually results in rapid resolution of the illness.

Chronic Mountain Sickness

This disorder affects long-term residents with prolonged stays at high altitudes exceeding 1 year. chronic mountain sickness (CMS) is of two types—(1) Seroche-Monge's disease and (2) pulmonary hypertension without polycythemia. Monge's disease is a syndrome marked by the triad of polycythemia, hypoxemia, and impaired mental status (headache, fatigue, impaired concentration, and irritability) and clinical examination reveals clubbing and cyanosis. Vascular remodeling occurs due to prolonged hypoxic pulmonary vasoconstriction; the oxygen content of the blood is high along with increased diffusion capacity. Right ventricular failure is uncommon. Treatment includes descent and stay at lower altitudes, periodic phlebotomy, diuretics, and respiratory stimulants. The other form of CMS has pulmonary hypertension and right heart failure without polycythemia. Treatment includes descent to stay at lower altitudes as it is known to recur on altitude exposure.

EFFECTS OF HIGH ALTITUDE ON EXISTING LUNG DISEASES

Chronic Obstructive Pulmonary Disease

There are numerous physiological derangements in patients with chronic obstructive pulmonary disease (COPD), including impaired gas exchange, reduced muscle strength, and mild–moderate pulmonary hypertension. Severe COPD patients are likely to have hypoxemia and worsened pulmonary hypertension at HAA. Long-term residence at altitude has higher incidence of cor pulmonale and is associated with increased mortality.

Bronchial Asthma

The available data suggests that asthmatic subjects can travel to altitudes up to 5,000 meters without any adverse effects during short-term trips. Patients with severe asthma should be advised against travel to HAA as they are likely to deteriorate and there are lack of medical facilities at most places. Patients must continue baseline medications and carry ample supply of rescue inhalers and oral prednisolone for asthma exacerbations.

Disorders with Pulmonary Hypertension

Several reports suggest those with preexisting pulmonary hypertension (PAH) including those with altitude-related PAH are at increased risk for HAPE. The patients with PAH may develop sudden rise in pulmonary artery pressure leading to acute right heart failure or progression to sub-AMS on exposure to HAA. The advice to patients with PAH is to avoid travel to HAA. Those who cannot avoid the travel should be taught to recognize symptoms of HAPE and advised to use supplemental oxygen at high altitude. They are started on prophylaxis with nifedipine SR 20 mg BD for duration of stay. Phosphodiesterase inhibitor (sildenafil) and dexamethasone are alternatives, which can be used for prevention of HAPE.

Pulmonary Thromboembolic Disorders

There is increased risk of recurrence in patients with past history of venous thromboembolism. Majority of subjects with thromboembolic events at altitude are reported to have preexisting coagulopathy such as factor V Leiden, protein C deficiency, hyperhomocysteinemia, and use of oral contraceptive pills. Patients with preexisting thrombophilia are at an increased risk for thromboembolism at high altitude. Anticoagulation in patients with history of venous thromboembolism who travel to high altitude should continue as usual. Coagulogram should be repeated before and after return from altitude to adjust the dosages. Females on oral contraceptive use who have underlying coagulopathy should discontinue the oral contraceptives during their high-altitude exposure. An alternative strategy consists of starting low-dose aspirin during the stay at HAA.

Interstitial Lung Disease

There is little data on the effects of high altitude on patients with interstitial lung disease (ILD). Patients with ILD may report with worsening of symptoms, presence of resting hypoxemia as well as worsening of exercise-induced desaturation. Most ILD patients with some degree of pulmonary hypertension (PH) are at increased risk of HAPE. Patients with ILD need assessment for need for supplemental oxygen. The patients with P_aO_2 levels 50–55 mm Hg should receive supplemental oxygen during altitude. Patients with ILD and PH require to be started on nifedipine prophylaxis for HAPE.

Pneumothorax

Patients with pneumothorax and after thoracic surgery are advised to wait for 2 weeks before travel to HAA. Patients with persistent pneumothorax or bronchopleural fistula with chest tube or Heimlich valve can safely travel to HAA. Screening of patients with computed tomography (CT) chest in those at high risk for occult pneumothorax prior to high-altitude travel is recommended.

Ventilatory Disorders

Obese individuals are at risk of developing altitude-induced PH. Further, those with obesity hypoventilation syndrome and obstructive sleep apnea are at increased risk for developing AMS, heart failure, and HAPE. These patients should be advised to avoid travel to HAA. If the travel cannot be avoided, administer supplemental oxygen and start acetazolamide 125 mg or 250 mg BD. Patients with PH should also start nifedipine SR 20 mg BD for prophylaxis against HAPE. Patients on domiciliary continuous positive airway pressure (CPAP) therapy should continue with the CPAP devices during travel to high altitude. Necessary adjustments should be made in set pressures for machines, which lack pressure compensation.

In conclusion, the presence of lung disease does not necessarily preclude travel to high altitude. Proper evaluation should, however, be conducted before travel. Adequate prophylaxis and acclimatization should be ensured to prevent HAPE.

CHAPTER
48

Aviation and Space Travel

Ajay Handa

INTRODUCTION

Worldwide, over 1 billion passengers travel by airlines each year. The vast majority of people who travel by air are healthy individuals but approximately 5-10% of passengers have underlying diseases and respiratory ailments, including chronic obstructive pulmonary disease (COPD). The knowledge of changes in pulmonary physiology in aviation is important for pulmonary physicians to handle patients with chronic respiratory diseases.

RESPIRATORY PHYSIOLOGY WITH ALTITUDE

The fall in partial pressure of oxygen with altitude can cause hypobaric hypoxia during air travel. Commercial aircraft fly at 10,000-13,000 meter above sea level (ASL) and pressurization in the cabin is maintained to keep the level at about 2,438 meter ASL. For technical reasons, the cabin altitude cannot be maintained lower than 2,438 meter. Breathing at this altitude (15% oxygen) causes the PaO_2 to fall to 53-64 mm Hg (SpO_2 85-91%). This mild hypoxemia does not produce any symptoms and is well tolerated in healthy subjects; however, it may cause significant hypoxemia and precipitate respiratory failure in patients with chronic lung diseases. Such patients need thorough preflight evaluation and recommendation to use supplemental in-flight oxygen.

Another physical effect of ascent to altitude is the expansion of gases due to decrease in ambient pressure (Boyle's law). The expansion of gas trapped in close cavities, such as middle ear, intestine can cause discomfort. The gas within a lung bulla will expand by 30% at 2,450 m ASL and cause rupture and complications as pneumothorax, pneumomediastinum and air embolism.

Patients of COPD with emphysematous bullae are at increased risk for pneumothorax and respiratory failure during air travel and are advised to avoid air travel. Due to risk of developing respiratory distress, untreated pneumothorax is the only absolute contraindication for travel by air.

Respiratory problems account for 10% of all medical in-flight emergencies, most commonly from exacerbation of asthma and COPD.

PREFLIGHT ASSESSMENT

The aim of preflight assessment is to identify those likely to develop significant hypoxemia onboard the flight. Patients on long-term oxygen therapy (LTOT) and those with cardiorespiratory illnesses constitute important categories. Patients with severe COPD, bronchial asthma, restrictive lung diseases, past venous thromboembolism, recent pneumothorax and pulmonary tuberculosis are at high risk of deterioration during air travel and must be subjected to preflight screening. Patients with recent cerebrovascular accidents and congestive heart failure may also worsen on air travel and need to be assessed accordingly. In cardiac patients, travel on commercial airlines is fairly safe after 2 weeks of myocardial infarction without requirement of supplemental oxygen.

Preflight assessment should include detailed medical evaluation and counseling. The three methods usually adopted for preflight evaluation for oxygen supplementation include 50-meter walk test, use of prediction equations and the hypoxic challenge test. Airline medical authorities traditionally use the 50-meter-walk test for screening passengers. Those who are able to walk 50 meters are considered "fit to fly". The test is a crude assessment of cardiorespiratory status and needs to be supervised. Failure to complete the distance or developing moderate-to-severe respiratory distress should alert the physician to referral for assessment of in-flight oxygen by respiratory physician.

Nomograms and equations for predicting PaO_2 at altitude using blood gas parameters and spirometry at ground level have been developed by studies in COPD patients exposed to hypoxia (Box 48.1). In clinical practice, such equations are most frequently applied to predict fitness and requirement of on-board oxygen. Predicted PaO_2 values less than 50 mm Hg are indication of supplemental in-flight oxygen. There are no guidelines as to which of the above equation is to be used. Some authors use regression equation for calculating predicted PaO_2 at altitude. If the calculated value is 50 ± 3 mm Hg hypoxic challenge test is advised for definitive recommendations.

Considering the limited availability of facilities for hypoxic challenge tests for large numbers of patients with respiratory diseases and COPD who travel by air, the British Thoracic Society guidelines recommend that oxygen

BOX 48.1: Equations for calculating predicted PaO_2 at 2,450 m.
- PaO_2 altitude = 0.84 + 0.68 (PaO_2 ground)
- PaO_2 altitude = 0.295 (PaO_2 sea level) + 0.086 (FEV_1 % predicted) + 23.211
- PaO_2 altitude = 0.245 (PaO_2 sea level) + 0.171 (FEV_1/FVC % predicted) + 21.028

saturation measured by pulse oximetry can be used to initially screen groups of passengers. Those with SpO_2 less than 92% are advised in-flight oxygen and those with SpO_2 between 92% and 95% are prescribed hypoxic challenge test.

Those passengers who have additional risk factors, such as hypercapnia, FEV_1 <50% predicted, other diseases as lung cancer, restrictive lung diseases, comorbid cardiovascular or neurologic disease and within 6 weeks of discharge from hospital for acute exacerbation shall require hypoxic challenge testing. Those patients who are subjected to hypoxia challenge are categorized based on the measured PaO_2 after 15 minutes at FiO_2 15% and advised accordingly based on PaO_2.

PRESCRIBING IN-FLIGHT OXYGEN

Any patient with PaO_2 of less than 70 mm Hg at sea level at rest will require supplemental oxygen during air travel. Most commercial airlines will provide oxygen in-flight on advance request and physician's prescription. The expenses are required to be borne by the travelers. The oxygen supply is usually provided from cylinders so the rate of flow and duration must be specified so that adequate amount of oxygen is available during the journey. The rate of oxygen of 2 L/min is suitable for most passengers. Those on long-term oxygen therapy (LTOT) are advised to increase the flow rate 2 L/min above the usual flow rate.

Most airlines provide oxygen through simple face mask and passengers are advised to carry their nasal prongs to prevent rebreathing. The oxygen and cabin air inside the aircraft are devoid of moisture and can lead to drying of tracheobronchial mucosa and precipitation of bronchospasm. The airlines have to be informed for humidified oxygen for patients with asthma and COPD. In addition such patients must be advised to carry their medications in their hand baggage for use in emergency situations.

Airlines do not provide oxygen during waiting period and stopovers. Some airports restrict oxygen use in the airport, because of the risk of explosion. Oxygen-dependent patients must make additional arrangements for use during the waiting periods at the airports. Patients cannot use their own cylinders or concentrators, but may be able to take these items with them as baggage for use at their destination. It is also important for these patients to carry their medical documents and extradrug supplies during travel (Box 48.2).

BOX 48.2: Guidelines for oxygen-dependent patients prior to air travel

- Obtain medical certificate of fitness to fly
- Carry prescription of in-flight oxygen requirement
- Inform the airlines while booking tickets and 48–72 hours before date of journey
- Inform airlines need for oxygen before boarding and during stopovers
- Preferably take nonstop flight to destination
- Carry extratubing and personal nasal cannula
- Carry extracopies of prescriptions and medical certificate
- Carry emergency supply of medications in hand baggage

SPACE TRAVEL

The effects of gravity and its absence (in space) on respiratory physiology have intrigued scientists since time immemorial. The condition of zero gravity or weightlessness (microgravity) for assessing its effects on the human body can be achieved by two methods. These are parabolic flight in aircrafts and Space flight. The parabolic flights in commercial jet aircrafts are associated with small periods of microgravity with periods of hypergravity (increased gravitational forces) during these maneuvers. Parabolic flights are more easily available and less expensive compared to space flights. They have the disadvantage of creating motion sickness in the passengers during this "roller coaster" flight.

The flights in spacecrafts are very infrequent and extremely expensive. The advantage is that space flights have sustained periods of microgravity from 1 week to up to a year. Most research work has been done onboard Russian space station Mir and International Space Station (ISS) led by the USA. These space stations offer convenient environment for studying effects of space on human physiology. The numbers of subjects are limited to maximum of four as the crew serve as subjects and operators or both. The evaluation includes preflight and postflight testing of various parameters and comparison with data under microgravity.

MICROGRAVITY AND WEIGHTLESSNESS

There are some ground-based experiments which mimic weightlessness such as 6° head down tilt (HDT) and thermoneutral water immersion (TWI). These have been useful to study the cardiovascular and musculoskeletal responses. The significant effect of gravity on the lungs and pulmonary vasculature cannot be removed by these experiments. Further HDT and TWI caused larger reductions in resting lung volumes than microgravity, which cannot be ignored.

To understand the effect of microgravity and weightlessness in space on the respiratory system, we can take a cue from the common knowledge that even though there are no structural differences between the upper and lower parts of the human lungs, gravitational forces lead to marked functional differences between these areas. The alveoli at the top of the lung are more expanded compared with the bottom of the lung because the weight of the lungs on the lower parts. On the other hand, alveolar ventilation is higher at the bottom of the lung as compared to the apex. Gravity also influences the intrapleural pressure, parenchymal stress and pulmonary blood flow which result in regional differences in lung function. There is greater disparity in the pulmonary blood flow between the top and bottom of the lung with greater flows near the bases than the apices. This is due to the effect of hydrostatic forces on the low pressure pulmonary circulation. As a result of the profound effects of gravity on alveolar ventilation and pulmonary perfusion, ventilation perfusion ratio (V/Q) is higher at the apices than the lung bases and there are regional differences in gas exchange in the lungs.

The influence of gravity on the lung on earth and by increasing the gravitational effect has been studied. Most of the changes in lung function are attributable to gravity. The conclusions of these studies cannot be extrapolated to zero gravity conditions. A large number of studies on respiratory and cardiac functions in absence of gravity have been performed in the last decade and half.

In conclusion, the comprehensive data on changes in respiratory physiology in space have found that the effects are generally benign and unlikely to limit the activities of astronauts in space.

CHAPTER 49

Lung Disease in Coal Workers

Harakh V Dedhia, Daniel E Banks

Coal is not a pure mineral. It is formed by the accumulation of vegetable matter covered by sedimentary rock (thereby sealing it from air) and subjected to pressure and temperature over the ages. This causes the physical and chemical properties of the matter to change. The matter dries, becomes warmer and loses oxygen content, all the while increasing the relative carbon content.

CLINICAL FEATURES OF COAL DUST EXPOSURE

There is a spectrum of diseases associated with coal dust exposure. The new term to describe this is "coal mine dust lung disease" (CMDLD). Coal inhalation can result in industrial bronchitis or coal worker pneumoconiosis (CWP). CWP may present with three different clinical syndromes—(1) simple pneumoconiosis, (2) complicated CWP, or (3) progressive massive fibrosis (PMF). In addition, dust-related diffuse fibrosis and emphysema are also recognized. What determines the pulmonary presentation following exposure to coal dust is not clear.

Industrial bronchitis is a common diagnosis among workers exposed to dusts, including coal dust. It manifests as a productive cough, which persists for at least 3 months per year for at least 2 years (chronic bronchitis) associated with workplace dust exposure. In a defining autopsy study, coal dust exposure resulted in an increase in the maximal gland:wall ratio (independent of smoking), but no relationship between mucous gland size and the amount of lung dust or presence or absence of pneumoconiosis was found. These data suggest that mucous gland enlargement is related to the inhalation of larger (nonrespirable) dust particles, which present a chronic burden to the mucociliary escalator and act as irritants to the airway, whereas pneumoconiosis is related to respirable dust exposure with the internalizing of these particles into the lung interstitium.

Coal workers' pneumoconiosis results from the inhalation and deposition of coal mine dust, and the lung's reaction to its presence. Three criteria are necessary for this diagnosis. They include:
1. A chest radiograph consistent with the features of CWP
2. A work history (typically underground coal mining) sufficient in exposure and latency to result in pneumoconiosis
3. The absence of other illnesses, which may mimic CWP.

Therefore, the diagnosis of CWP can be made with confidence without histological confirmation. Clinical features, such as dyspnea, cough, and sputum production are important in addressing the degree of a miner's impairment, but are not a part of the diagnostic criteria. The radiographic appearance of CWP cannot be differentiated from silicosis, and coal miners may develop disease from exposure to both dusts.

The CMDLD is categorized as simple pneumoconiosis or PMF. The typical radiograph in simple pneumoconiosis shows small opacities, ranging in size from pinhead to 1 cm in diameter.

In addition to the typical small-rounded opacities, there is another aspect to interstitial involvement in the spectrum of coal-induced lung disease. Dust-related diffuse fibrosis, a form of interstitial disease, can be mistaken for idiopathic pulmonary fibrosis as it features irregular opacities bilaterally in the bases. Of those employed in coal mining more than 25 years with opacities, nearly 40% show irregular opacities consistent with dust-related diffuse fibrosis compared to the typical rounded nodular opacities.

Rounded nodules predominate and tend to appear first in the upper zones and then the middle and lower zones as the number of opacities increase. When the exposure is prolonged and heavy, the small opacities may coalesce and form larger nodules or masses. PMF lesions are characterized by one or more large opacities of more than 1 cm in diameter. The associated distortion of lung architecture typically includes the deviation of the trachea and major airways to the side of the most prominent area of coalescence and loss of upper zone lung volume. Other radiological abnormalities include the elevation of the hila and basilar emphysema (typically of a panacinar type). Importantly, CWP can progress after the cessation of coal mine dust exposure.

In a population comparing miners without CWP to those with CWP, respiratory symptoms and physical signs were no more prevalent in those with simple CWP. The not infrequent presence of a chronic cough and sputum production, even in the presence of CWP, is reasonably attributable to "industrial bronchitis". Alternatively, these same clinical features in a smoking miner may be partially attributable to bronchitis caused by the inflammatory stimulus of cigarette smoke. Finger clubbing is not a feature of CWP, and if noted, should prompt further investigations. Yet, when PMF is recognized on the chest radiograph, the worker frequently describes dyspnea, cough, and sputum production, although it is recognized that the degree of impairment and presence or absence of symptoms do not correlate well with the extent of chest radiographic abnormalities.

Typically, CWP is a slowly progressive illness, with radiographic features progressing over a period of many years. The appearance of a cavity in a PMF lesion or an aggressive rate of radiographic progression should prompt the examination of the sputum for mycobacterial infection. The chest radiograph in simple CWP correlates with the amount of dust in the lung at autopsy. This is not true of the complicated form of the disease, suggesting that inadequately defined host factors play a role in the development of this lesion. Hypotheses, which might explain the differences in tissue response to coal dust in those who remain with simple CWP and those who progress to PMF, include:

- Inhalation of significant amounts of silica in addition to coal in mine dust
- Infection with an atypical mycobacterial organism
- Development of specific immunologic factors, which are responsible for progression.

A special case of nodular lung reaction occurs in dust-exposed individuals who either have rheumatoid arthritis or who develop rheumatoid arthritis within the subsequent 5-10 years. This leads to discussion regarding the potential role of immunological factors in mineral dust pneumoconioses. The nodules of Caplan's syndrome vary in diameter from 0.5 cm to 5 cm and are usually multiple, bilateral, and situated peripherally. Grossly, the lesions resemble a giant silicotic nodule. Microscopically, the amount of dust in the lesion is small, there is a necrotic area in the center, and there is a surrounding cellular zone infiltrated with lymphocytes and plasma cells. In many nodules, there is a peripheral zone of active inflammation with neutrophils and a few macrophages. This observation was further enhanced when similar radiographic appearances in miners without arthritis, but in whom circulating rheumatoid factor was demonstrated.

PATHOLOGY OF COAL WORKER PNEUMOCONIOSIS

As the normal dust clearance mechanisms of the lung are overwhelmed, dust deposition increases. With the initiation and progression of fibrosis, the lung lesions increase in size and number. A focal collection of coal dust in pigment-laden macrophages around dilated respiratory bronchioles, which tapers off toward the alveolar duct, is initially apparent. This is the coal macule, the characteristic lesion of CWP. A fine network of reticulin within this collection of cells may be visible early on. Focal emphysema is a specific entity that is an integral part of the simple lesion of simple CWP. It is characterized by the enlargement of the air spaces immediately adjacent to the dust macule.

Progressive massive fibrosis is diagnosed when one or more nodules attain a size of 2 cm or greater in diameter, typically on a background of simple CWP. The 2 cm diameter is an arbitrary choice of a minimal diameter that has allowed better correlation with clinical and radiographic measurements. In other reports, nodules exceeding 1 cm are included as PMF. Gross examination of the lung in PMF reveals a solid and heavily pigmented lung, which is rubbery-to-hard in texture. These features are most common in the posterior portions of the upper lobes or the superior segments of the lower lobes. These lesions tend to occur asymmetrically, occasionally showing first in one lung and then the other, leading to a suspicion of malignancy. These lesions may also cavitate and the worker may expectorate an ink-like fluid (a clinical sign described as melanoptysis), or when these cavitary lesions are cut, they may drain ink-like fluid. Airways and vessels adjacent to the lesions are distorted and destroyed within the lesions.

Excessive silica exposures in surface coal mine drillers can also result in PMF lesions and result in "cor pulmonale" and respiratory failure.

How Coal Mine Lung Dust Disease Develops: Cellular and Immunological Factors

Coal mine lung dust disease is the result of coal dust-induced cell damage with the activation of the fibrotic process. Lapp provided a well-outlined approach to addressing how coal dust causes lung damage. The potential mechanisms include:
- Direct cytotoxicity of coal dust
- The release of oxidants, enzymes, and cell membrane constituents from alveolar macrophages (AMs) in association with cell death due to coal dust exposure
- Stimulation of cytokine release from AMs to recruit effector cells (other macrophages or neutrophils) and stimulate fibroblast proliferation and collagen synthesis in the area of coal dust deposition.

Coal dust is much less fibrogenic than silica. As an example, a mixture of 10% silica and 90% coal is far more cytotoxic to macrophages than pure coal dust. However, both dusts, when cleaved, show surface radicals by electron spin resonance spectroscopy. The free radicals generated by crushing anthracite coal are more numerous than those generated from crushing bituminous coal leading to speculation regarding free radical release from different coal ranks and the suggestion that exposure to anthracite coal increases the risk for the development and progression of disease.

Development of bronchoalveolar lavage (BAL) as a means for sampling lung cells and fluid has provided an opportunity to study the lung's response to the inhalation of various dusts. Studies of the mechanisms of inflammation and fibrosis using BAL-derived material have opened the possibility for studying at least some of the mechanisms in the pulmonary reactions in CWP. It has been suggested that constitutional differences may help to explain the variation in response to inhaled dusts, especially the attack rates and progression of CWP. One study looked at the prevalence of histocompatibility antigens in coal miners. So far, it has not been possible to confirm any definite association between these factors and CWP.

MANAGEMENT OF CMDLD

There is no proven therapy for CMDLD. The primary prevention of lung disease in miners must include continuing efforts at reducing coal mine dust exposure. Management is best directed at prevention, early recognition, and treatment of complications. The major challenges to the physician are the recognition and management of airflow obstruction, respiratory infection, hypoxemia, respiratory failure, cor pulmonale, arrhythmias, and pneumothorax.

Careful evaluation should be done for workers presenting with respiratory symptoms. The initial history and examination should be supplemented by chest radiography. Cardiopulmonary assessment as indicated should be done with spirometry, bronchodilator reversibility, diffusing capacity, electrocardiogram, echocardiogram, and resting arterial blood gas measurement. A good initial data base helps to accurately assess the worker's respiratory health and to serve as a starting point for follow-up response to therapy or disease progression.

Smoking cessation is important regardless of symptoms of respiratory disease, chest radiograph abnormalities, or pulmonary function status. Smoking cessation strategies should include physician encouragement supplemented by support from smoking cessation groups, use of pharmacological agents such as nicotine substitutes or other drugs and behavior modification techniques.

Symptomatic reversible airflow obstruction should be treated with inhaled bronchodilator therapy as indicated. Glucocorticoid therapy may be tried in patients with severe obstruction and inadequate response to the usual measures.

Hypoxemia is frequently present during exercise but can also occur at rest and during sleep. Chronic hypoxemia leads to the development of pulmonary hypertension and cor pulmonale. Other complications of chronic hypoxemia include polycythemia, and cerebral dysfunction. Therapy with low-flow oxygen is indicated when the arterial oxygen tension is less than 55 mm Hg or when clinical evidence of cor pulmonale is present.

Miners should receive appropriate immunization with influenza and pneumococcal vaccines. Bacterial and viral episodes of bronchitis or pneumonia should be promptly recognized and appropriately treated. Similarly, miners with concomitant exposure to silica dust (most often roof bolters, drillers, and motormen) deserve special attention with regard to mycobacterial infection. Symptoms of weight loss, fever, sweat, change in sputum production or malaise should be promptly investigated with a chest radiograph and examination of the sputum through stain and culture for acid-fast bacillus (AFB). Occasionally, the sputum may be negative and the infecting mycobacterial organisms can only be obtained by fiberoptic bronchoscopy with brushings and washings. Active tuberculosis in this population can be usually successfully treated with the usual drug regimens. In coal miners with a significant history of concurrent silica exposure, the treatment for tuberculosis may need to be more aggressive and long-term follow-up is indicated in view of the reports of recurrent pulmonary tuberculosis in patients with PMF after the completion of apparently adequate therapy.

Pneumothorax can be particularly troublesome in miners with pneumoconiosis. Those with bullous disease in the presence of advanced complicated pneumoconiosis are at the greatest risk. Typically, once the lung collapses, it is difficult to expand, a feature attributable to the decreased compliance associated with interstitial lung disease. Therapy with one or several chest tubes is often therapeutic; however, recurrent pneumothorax that cannot be expanded is recognized and may require an open procedure and pleurodesis.

Respiratory failure may complicate advanced PMF as it does in other chronic respiratory diseases. Ventilatory support measures are indicated when the failure is precipitated by a treatable complication. The application of ventilatory support measures should be discussed with the patient before the need arises. In general, miners with advanced pneumoconiosis are poor candidates for long-term mechanical ventilatory therapy.

Overall, improved mining methods and lower dust levels appear to be reducing exposures and the new cases of both simple and complicated pneumoconiosis. If the worker with CMDLD is unable to leave the workplace, then he/she should be encouraged to transfer from jobs with high-dust exposure to jobs with low-dust exposure. It is our opinion that any worker with simple CWP should be encouraged to leave dust exposure. Those with category 2 or great pneumoconiosis are at clear risk for progression even in the absence of additional coal dust exposure.

CHAPTER 50

Silicosis

PS Shankar, SK Jindal

INTRODUCTION

The term silicosis is applied for the lung disorders caused by inhalation of the free silica. The inhaled silicon dioxide is usually in crystalline form, most often as quartz. Since silica is colorless and nonirritant, its exposure in large amounts remains unrecognized. It does not produce any immediate effect in most instances. Chronic exposure leads to a progressive fibrosing disease. In high-pressure environment at different temperatures as found in different industrial processes, such as ceramic manufacturing and foundry process, quartz may be heated to high temperatures at high pressures.

OCCUPATIONAL EXPOSURE

Silicosis is encountered in mining and quarrying of hard rock, anthracite, coal, and metals. The sand stone industry, sand blasting, stone quarrying, and dressing, granite industry, grinding of metals, sand blasting, iron and steel foundries, brick yards, silica milling, flint crushing, glass making, ceramic manufacturing, and manufacturing abrasive soaps are some of the occupations related to silica exposure. About three million workers who are at high potential risk of silica exposure, are employed in occupations, such as mining and quarries; manufacture of nonmetallic products, such as refractory products, structural clay, and glass mica; and manufacture of basic metals and alloys, such as iron and steel, copper, ferro-alloys, aluminum, etc. The development and progression of silicosis frequently occurs after exposure to silica has stopped.

The epidemiologic studies carried out in India have shown marked variation in the prevalence of silicosis. The prevalence rate has varied from 3.5% in ordnance factories to 54.6% in the slate pencil industry. The variation is due to the fact of variability of concentration of silica in work environment of different occupations, duration of exposure and the physical properties of the silica.

Environmental Pneumoconiosis

An interesting form of nonoccupational pneumoconiosis is reported in some parts of India, mostly from the high altitude villages in Central Ladakh and Kaza in the Himalayas. Silicosis was common in the older inhabitants of villages exposed to frequent dust storms containing free silica.

PATHOGENESIS

Crystalline silica particles are inhaled while the respirable-sized particles are deposited in the distal airways and alveoli. Alveolar macrophages ingest the silica particles, migrate into the interstitium, enter the lymphatics and are transported to the regional lymph nodes.

The interaction of silica and the pulmonary alveolar macrophages is a crucial event in the development of silicosis. Macrophage injury or death will release intercellular proteolytic enzymes that are likely to take part in the lung injury. There is also the release of cytokines, which attract other inflammatory cells, such as neutrophils and T-lymphocytes. The injured macrophages and other inflammatory cells release superoxide anions and hydroxyl radicals and they cause injury to the lung tissue. Silica-activated macrophages and lymphocytes also release many inflammatory mediators, such as interleukin-1 and tumor-necrosis factor that contribute to the production of fibrosis. Silica has great fibrogenic potential and the dying macrophages liberate fibroblast stimulating factor, which causes excessive production and release of collagen by fibroblasts.

FORMS OF SILICOSIS

Silicosis has a long latency period; three different patterns of silicosis have been recognized, i.e. (i) chronic, (ii) accelerated or (iii) acute forms primarily based on the degree and duration of exposure and onset of symptoms. The clinical presentation of the disease reflects the variable intensity of exposure, rate of silica deposition in the lungs, retention of total amount of crystalline silica, latency period, and natural history.

Chronic (or Classic) Silicosis

The physiology of chronic silicosis involves chronic inflammation due to the accumulation of a variety of inflammatory mediators and fibrogenic elements. The rate of progression of the disease depends upon the rate and amount of silica deposition and retention in the lungs. The condition can be simple or complicated.

The simple chronic silicosis develops following exposure to low-to-moderate concentration of free silica over 20 years or more. Initially, there is collection of silica-laden macrophages in the loose reticulin fibers in the peribronchial, perivascular, paraseptal, and subpleural areas. Later, there is formation of silicotic nodules in which the central area gets organized with a concentric whorl-like arrangement of collagen. The lesions may have variable degrees of calcification. The nodules are seen in the pulmonary parenchyma typically in the upper lobes, and the hilar and peribronchial lymph nodes. The inflammation continues in the periphery of the nodule, which gets enlarged by including adjacent pulmonary structures. Such a stage is referred to as progressive massive fibrosis (PMF).

In complicated silicosis, the nodules coalesce to form large masses of hyalinized tissue. The masses may have a variable diameter of 2 cm or more. The blood vessels and bronchioles are obliterated. The amount of silica or inflammatory cells is negligible. They are found in the apices of the lung, and tend to be bilaterally symmetrical in distribution. There can be central necrosis and cavitation. These patients exhibit an increased susceptibility to infection with *Mycobacterium tuberculosis,* as a result of which the lesion may get cavitated.

Accelerated Silicosis

The condition is encountered in persons who are exposed to heavy amounts of silica, often over a period of 5-10 years. The rate of development and progression of accelerated silicosis is more rapid than chronic silicosis. The condition progresses even after removal of the person from the continued silica exposure. The alveolar spaces get filled with eosinophilic granular material. The collagen vascular diseases, such as systemic sclerosis, systemic lupus erythematosus (SLE), and rheumatoid arthritis (RA), are sometimes associated with this type of silicosis.

Acute Silicosis

Acute silicosis is rare, but often fatal. It is likely to occur in workers as a consequence of intense exposure to very high concentrations of silica over a period varying from several months up to about 5 years. The mechanism of injury is different from that seen in chronic silicosis. There is a stronger inflammatory response due to the presence of freshly fractured silica exhibiting abundant cleaved particle surfaces. Lungs exhibit consolidation without silicotic nodules. The lungs involved by acute silicosis show presence of hypertrophic type II pneumocytes lining the alveoli. They are responsible for the production of an excess amount of proteinaceous material and surfactant protein. The alveolar spaces are filled with eosinophilic proteinaceous material. This is referred to as silicoproteinosis. There is diffuse alveolar damage and desquamative pneumonitis.

CLINICAL FEATURES

The most common presentation of silicosis is in the form of uncomplicated chronic silicosis which develops over decades of repeated exposures to silica dust. Generally, it is asymptomatic even when the radiographic appearance suggests fairly advanced silicosis. Dyspnea on exertion is considered to be the most frequent and directly related symptom of silicosis. There can be cough and sputum production from nonspecific bronchitis or from cigarette smoking. Chest pain and hemoptysis indicate the likely complication of tuberculosis. Acute silicosis presents with dyspnea, fatigue, and cough. Other symptoms may include unexplained weight loss, fever, and pleuritic pain. Rarely, bilateral pneumothorax is also reported.

In addition to the development of pneumoconiosis in silica-exposed workers, there are several reports on increased respiratory symptoms and impaired lung function in industrial workers, miners, stone cutters, and others in the absence of a definitive radiological diagnosis of silicosis. This nonspecific symptomatology is attributed to chronic dust exposure. Stunting of lung growth is reported on long-term exposure to respirable dust in childhood and early adult life.

DIAGNOSIS

Clinical and radiological features that distinguish silicosis from other fibrotic disease include the following:
- Occupational exposure to a substantial amount of silica
- Silicotic nodule, and/or
- Involvement of hilar lymph nodes.

Radiologically, there is a close resemblance between silicosis and miliary tuberculosis. However, the size of nodules seen in tuberculosis, are less than those seen in silicosis. The radiographs of patients with silicosis usually exhibit an increased translucency as against general loss of translucency in tuberculosis.

Acute silicosis produces a homogeneous ground-glass appearance on chest radiograph. It has to be distinguished from pulmonary edema, alveolar hemorrhage, pulmonary alveolar proteinosis, pneumonia, and bronchoalveolar cell carcinoma.

The classic radiographic features of simple silicosis are rounded opacities ranging in size from 1 mm to 10 mm and occurring predominantly in the upper lung zones. They can be categorized using the International Labour Organization (ILO). International Classification of Radiographs of pneumoconiosis on the basis of size, shape, and profusion category. In addition to the size and shape of the nodules, the abundance (profusion of nodules within the parenchyma) of the lung is also important. By comparison with standard films provided by the ILO, the profusion of nodules in the patient's films can be categorized in order of increasing severity as category 1, category 2 or category 3.

Hilar lymphadenopathy is also seen sometimes in advanced nodular parenchymal shadows. There can be "egg shell" calcification of the lymph nodes, and it is strongly suggestive of silicosis. Egg-shell calcification has been also reported on X-rays of patients with sarcoidosis, scleroderma, amyloidosis, and fungal infections, such as blastomycosis and histoplasmosis. It may sometimes be seen in Hodgkin's disease especially after treatment with radiation.

With coalescence of the nodules, the upper lobes contract due to fibrosis making the conglomerate nodules to migrate toward the hilar areas. The hilar structures are pulled upward, leaving areas of compensatory emphysema at their margins and in the lung bases. With these alterations the small rounded opacities that were evident previously on the radiograph become less visible or may at times disappear. Pleural thickening and calcification are not commonly encountered, but they may be sometimes seen.

Acute silicosis may present with radiographic alveolar filling pattern leading to a ground-glass appearance, and association with conglomerate silicotic nodules is rarely seen. Pulmonary tuberculosis in the patient with silicosis may be associated with pleural effusion, localized increase in the size of opacities and cavitation.

Pulmonary Functions

Pulmonary function tests help in the evaluation of persons with suspected silicosis. There are no specific patterns of ventilatory impairment in silicosis. There can be significant airflow limitation. Both peak expiratory flow (PEF) and forced vital capacity (FVC) are reported to reduce in chronically exposed individuals. The lung function impairment is related to the degree and duration of exposure. Tobacco smoking in the presence of other dust exposure further aggravates the presence of airway obstruction. In patients with PMF, restrictive ventilatory impairment is seen in association with arterial hypoxemia.

Other Investigations

Bronchoalveolar lavage (BAL) may be undertaken when exposure history and clinical presentations are atypical. The BAL fluid of workers exposed to quartz dust will demonstrate an increased number of cells, protein and quartz in the macrophages. The amount of mineral dust in BAL fluid cells is related to the intensity of exposure and duration of employment. Lung biopsy (open or thoracoscopic) is rarely needed. It may be indicated in some clinical settings when complications are present. This is particularly important when lung malignancy is suspected as a complication.

The demonstration of tubercle bacilli in the sputum of patients suffering from silicotuberculosis is difficult in many instances. The walling in of the tubercle foci by the silicotic fibrosis prevents the elimination of tubercle bacilli in the sputum.

Complications and Comorbidities (Box 50.1)

There is an increased susceptibility to pulmonary tuberculosis and rarely to fungal infection. It is thought that macrophage dysfunction caused by the presence of silica appears to be the cause of increased susceptibility to tuberculosis and other infections. Chronic silicosis gradually leads to development of pulmonary hypertension, chronic cor pulmonale, and chronic respiratory failure. The onset of these complications is rapid in case of massive fibrosis.

Silicotuberculosis (Box 50.2)

Free silica impairs macrophage function, thereby increasing the chances of mycobacterial infection. Important predisposing factors relate to social circumstances and to living and working conditions. Tobacco smoking is an important predisposing factor. Most of these workers live in crowded and unsanitary conditions, while their jobs are in dusty environments and silica exposures are not controlled. The chances of spread of infection are higher in such surroundings. Human immunodeficiency virus (HIV) infection is reported as an important predisposition to silicotuberculosis in some of the African countries. Nontuberculous mycobacterial infections have been also seen.

Connective Tissue Diseases

There is an increased incidence of autoimmunity and diseases, such as RA and SLE in patients with silicosis. These patients exhibit positive latex fixation

---

BOX 50.1: Important complications and/or comorbidities seen in patients with silicosis.

- Pulmonary hypertension and chronic cor pulmonale
- Chronic respiratory failure
- Respiratory infections
- Silicotuberculosis
- Silicomycosis
- Autoimmune disorders
- Necrotizing nodules—Caplan Syndrome
- Scar carcinoma
- Acute/accelerated silicosis—alveolar proteinosis
- Massive pulmonary fibrosis

BOX 50.2: Characteristics of tuberculosis in silicotics.

- Frequent occurrence
- Increased risk
- Severe and persistence respiratory symptoms
- Rapid progression to fibrosis
- Poor response to antituberculosis therapy
- Necessity of longer duration of therapy

tests, antinuclear antibodies and increased levels of immunoglobulins. Necrotizing rheumatoid nodule in silicosis is a characteristic clinical picture, which is known as Caplan syndrome. Systemic vasculitis, such as microscopic polyangiitis has been occasionally reported.

PROGNOSIS

Patients with conglomerate fibrosis progress to cor pulmonale and respiratory failure. The clinical course of patients with acute silicosis is inexorably downward with the development of pulmonary fibrosis, followed by restrictive lung disease and ultimately respiratory failure resulting in death. Silicosis especially when "acute" may be complicated by secondary alveolar proteinosis with marked respiratory distress and failure.

TREATMENT

There is no specific treatment for silicosis and the therapy is directed largely at the complications of the disease. Corticosteroids, occasionally used for treatment in silicosis, have limited efficacy. Aluminum citrate has been also used with variable results. Following the diagnosis of silicosis, it is advisable to avoid further exposure to silica-containing dusts. The individual should be promptly removed from such surroundings. In advanced disease or if it has developed following a short exposure, further exposure to dust has to be avoided. The comorbid conditions, such as chronic obstructive pulmonary disease should be identified and managed. Severe airflow obstruction and cor pulmonale are treated with bronchodilators, diuretics and oxygen. Tobacco smoking, if present must be stopped.

Treatment of tuberculosis in silicosis patients poses tremendous problems. Results of standard chemotherapeutic protocols for tuberculosis in the presence of silicosis are less effective than therapy for tuberculosis alone. It is generally recommended that patients with tuberculosis should receive at least four antituberculosis drugs, such as isoniazid, rifampicin, and pyrazinamide for 2 months followed by two antituberculosis drugs (isoniazid and rifampicin) for a total of 9 months or longer. The exact duration of therapy remains debatable. Isoniazid chemoprophylaxis has been recommended for TB prevention in high risk patients. Similarly, latent TB should also be treated in such patients.

Prevention remains the main goal of silicosis. It comprises medical screening, surveillance, and dust control measures.

CHAPTER 51

Berylliosis

PS Shankar

INTRODUCTION

Beryllium (Be) is a light metal of tensile strength and is found in the Earth's crust. Beryllium-containing minerals are processed for use in aerospace manufacturing, nuclear reactors, electronics industry and manufacture of heat-resistant ceramics, fiberoptics, bicycle frames, microwave ovens, and dental alloy preparations. Mining, industrial processing, smelting and fabrication of beryllium or its alloys result in the emission of dust and fumes of beryllium to the atmosphere, surface waters, and soil. Beryllium exposure is associated with both acute and chronic manifestations. Both the acute and the chronic forms of berylliosis represent a continuum of disease involving hypersensitivity.

ACUTE BERYLLIUM DISEASE

Beryllium enters the lungs by inhalation route, and acts as a direct chemical irritant. Massive exposure induces a generalized acute inflammatory reaction in the respiratory tract and alveoli resulting in tracheobronchitis and chemical pneumonitis [acute beryllium disease (ABD), acute berylliosis]. It appears to be due to an irritative phenomenon from direct toxicity. Acute berylliosis makes people very ill. Improved industrial hygiene standards have reduced its incidence.

CHRONIC BERYLLIUM DISEASE

The chronic form of disease [chronic beryllium disease (CBD), chronic berylliosis] usually occurs after prolonged exposure of a along period to low concentrations of beryllium. The condition has a delayed onset with granulomatous response and pursues a chronic course. Long-term exposure is responsible for a mixed pattern of lung function impairment, pulmonary fibrosis, cavitary lung lesions, pneumothorax and respiratory infections.

Some beryllium may also get ingested but its absorption from the gastrointestinal tract is poor. It gets accumulated in the skeleton and gets eliminated very slowly through the kidney. Beryllium is a potent chemical sensitizer. Direct contact of soluble beryllium compounds with skin or mucosa causes allergic contact dermatitis and ulcers in susceptible persons. Chronic beryllium exposure is also reported to cause lung cancer.

PATHOGENESIS

Chronic beryllium disease is primarily an inflammatory disease due to a delayed cell-mediated immune response to inhaled beryllium particles in the lung. It is characterized by a granulomatous response with varying degrees of interstitial fibrosis. Genetic predisposition is also important in the disease pathogenesis.

Chronic beryllium disease is caused only by inhalation of beryllium in a low dose over a long period of time (10 or more years). Inhaled beryllium gets deposited in the periphery of the lung. It produces non-caseating granulomas in the pulmonary interstitium along with diffuse interstitial inflammation and fibrosis. Hilar lymphadenopathy may be present. Thus the condition will have many of the characteristics of sarcoidosis. Unlike sarcoidosis, the antigen is known in CBD.

CLINICAL AND RADIOLOGICAL FEATURES

Berylliosis can present as an allergic immune response [beryllium sensitization (BeS), acute toxic pneumonitis like reaction, or CBD] (Table 51.1). Acute berylliosis has a sudden onset and rapid development of inflammation of

TABLE 51.1: Clinical features of different types of beryllium exposure.

Type of berylliosis	Clinical features
1. Beryllium hypersensitivity	• Usually asymptomatic—sometimes skin rashes, nasal, and constitutional symptoms • Positive beryllium lymphocyte transformation test • Progresses to berylliosis
2. Acute beryllium disease	• Irritative, chemical phenomenon • Acute tracheobronchitis • Chemical pneumonitis
3. Chronic beryllium disease (berylliosis)	• Develops gradually over years • Progressively increasing dyspnea, cough, weakness, fatigue, and weight loss • Systemic manifestations • Pulmonary fibrosis, chronic cor pulmonale

the lungs causing cough and dyspnea. The more common chronic berylliosis develops very gradually with progressively increasing dyspnea, weakness, fatigue, loss of weight, arthralgia and cough with mucoid sputum. On physical examination, there may be evidence of clubbing and bibasilar crackles at lung bases. Systemic examination may show skin rashes, hepatomegaly, and lymphadenopathy.

DIAGNOSIS

Diagnosis is generally suspected on history of beryllium exposure, clinical manifestations and radiography. Radiogram of the chest shows diffuse round and reticular nodules, which later progresses to diffuse linear fibrosis throughout the lung fields or confined to the upper lobes. The hilar nodes are enlarged. It must be noted that hilar adenopathy does not occur in the absence of lung changes. High-resolution CT (HRCT) findings reveal extensive interstitial pulmonary fibrosis and pulmonary hypertension. HRCT exhibits ground glass opacification and parenchymal nodules. Pulmonary functions show a restrictive pattern and reduction in the diffusion capacity. There is hypoxemia. Occasionally, there is hyperuricemia and hypercalcemia on bronchoscopic examination.

There is an increase in number of CD4+ T cells in bronchoalveolar lavage (BAL) fluid. Presence of non-caseating granuloma on transbronchial lung biopsy specimens greatly supports the diagnosis. Blood or BAL lymphocyte transformation test is generally positive. Patients with chronic berylliosis exhibit cutaneous delayed hypersensitivity to a patch test with 1–2% beryllium nitrate or sulfate.

Beryllium lymphocyte proliferation test (BelPT) is used as a biomarker of beryllium-health effect which comprises in vitro culture of peripheral blood lymphocytes which are exposed to soluble beryllium sulfate to stimulate lymphocyte proliferation. Occurrence of beryllium-specific proliferation implies BeS which precedes the development of CBD. The course of natural history and rate of progression are not well understood. Lung biopsy reveals non-necrotizing, well-formed granulomas.

TREATMENT

The most important step in management involves the cessation of beryllium exposure. This is not only important for symptomatic treatment of beryllium hypersensitivity and acute toxicity but also for prevention of CBD. Corticosteroids constitute the mainstay of treatment for CBD. Long-term steroid therapy is helpful in suppressing granulomatous lesion and in stopping the evolution of fibrosis. Treatment is generally monitored using pulmonary function tests and HRCT of the chest. The treatment is of little help after the development of pulmonary fibrosis but for the management of cardiac and respiratory failure. Diminution in ambient levels of beryllium shows an improvement in the pulmonary status of the workers.

Most patients with acute berylliosis make full recovery in 7-10 days following initiation of therapy with steroids. Generally there are no after effects. Patients with severely damaged lungs from chronic berylliosis progress to respiratory failure, cor pulmonale, and cardiac failure.

Reduction of exposure is important in disease prevention programs. A surveillance program was found to be helpful to predict the risk of the disease employing BeLPT, among former and current construction trade workers at the governmental nuclear sites in USA.

CHAPTER 52

Metal-induced Lung Disease

Dilip V Maydeo, Nikhil C Sarangdhar

INTRODUCTION

A number of metals are associated with the development of diffuse parenchymal lung disease. Inhalation of metal dusts can cause a wide range of lung diseases, most importantly, lung fibrosis. Acute exposure to metal dusts, such as zinc oxides can cause metal-fume fever. This is an acute, but usually a short-lived response. The term hard metal lung disease (HMLD) is used to denote both the fibrotic stages like pneumoconiosis as well as nonfibrotic stages, such as asthma, bronchitis, and obliterative bronchiolitis caused by HMLD.

TYPES

- Chronic beryllium disease (CBD)
- Diffuse parenchymal lung disease due to other metals: Aluminum, cobalt, titanium, and copper.
- Hard-metal lung disease
- Metal-induced asthma and bronchitis
- Metal-fume fever: Beryllium, copper, cadmium, silver, magnesium, and zinc.
- Lung cancer: Nickel and chromium.

EPIDEMIOLOGY

Beryllium is the most extensively studied metal dust disease. There is relative paucity of information on lung disease caused by other metals, mostly confined to isolated case reports describing the disease in affected workers. It is also likely that cases are missed because the disease is not suspected and diagnosed.

Hard metal-induced asthma is an important condition described in several industries involved with metal processing and production. Cobalt asthma has been recognized in automotive manufacturing industry in recent times. Even low levels of cobalt exposure are shown to cause lung function impairment in both smoking and nonsmoking workers.

PATHOGENESIS

Metal exposure induces granulomatous reaction which predominantly comprises of clusters of lymphocytes, macrophages, epithelioid cells, multinucleated giant cells, mast cells, and fibroblasts. The chronic inflammation slowly progresses to lung fibrosis. Varying degrees of fibrosis are reported on exposure to aluminum, beryllium, cobalt, copper, and other rare metals.

Some metals are known to trigger specific immune responses. There is a delayed-type hypersensitivity response to aluminum, cobalt, gold, and zirconium in certain susceptible individuals. The skin response following an intradermal injection of the suspected agent is analogs to the reaction following purified protein derivative. Further aluminum, cobalt, gold, and titanium can also trigger in vitro lymphocyte proliferation.

The pathology of HMLD is characterized by the presence of "cannibalistic" multinucleated giant cells in the airspaces and bronchoalveolar lavage fluid. Hence, it is often referred to as giant cell interstitial pneumonia.

Metal-induced asthma and bronchitis are usually the result of allergen-induced sensitization and airway hyperreactivity, analogs to the IgE-mediated atopic reaction, though nonallergenic mechanisms may at times also be responsible.

TYPES OF IMMUNE RESPONSES IN METAL-INDUCED LUNG DISEASE

- *Antigen-specific cell-mediated immunity*: Beryllium, titanium, zirconium, aluminum, cobalt, and gold.
- *Giant-cell granuloma*: Hard metal (tungsten carbide and cobalt).
- *Foreign-body type reaction*: Copper and barium.

CLINICAL PRESENTATION AND DIAGNOSIS

High-dose exposures to metals (e.g. copper sulfate, beryllium) can cause acute pneumonitis. Symptoms typically begin with subtle onset of exertional breathlessness, nonproductive cough, fatigue and night sweats. Some patients may complain of low-grade fever, arthralgias, chest pain, and weight loss. Chest examination may reveal scattered fine crackles. Different patterns of irregular or reticulonodular infiltrates are described on chest radiography. Tuberculosis is an important differential diagnosis, especially in the developing high-burden countries.

There is presence of mediastinal and hilar lymphadenopathy in about 30% of patients with CBD. The condition is sometimes confused with sarcoidosis. On pulmonary function testing, patients with suspected CBD typically show airflow obstruction progressing to mixed patterns of obstruction and restriction. Severe restrictive pattern is seen in advanced or end-stage disease.

The clinical features of HMLD markedly resemble hypersensitivity pneumonitis. Some patients may report with episodes of work-related subacute disease and some patients may progress more or less rapidly, to lung fibrosis. Occasionally, HMLD is reported in association with other connective tissue disorders like rheumatoid arthritis or with complications like pneumothorax. The disease may sometimes occur after a short duration of exposure, thus suggesting individual susceptibility as more important factor than cumulative exposure. Thus, HMLD differs from chronic beryllium lung disease that can be diagnosed by a lymphocyte proliferation test using a beryllium salt as the antigen.

The diagnosis of metal-induced asthma and bronchitis rests on documentation of respiratory symptoms (wheeze and chest tightness) and correlation with patch tests, peak flow rates and/or bronchoprovocation tests. In patients with normal spirometry at presentation, bronchoprovocation tests, either nonspecific with either methacholine or histamine (with a PC_{20} of 8–16 mg/mL) or with specific allergen may be necessary to support diagnosis. Metal induced occupational asthma must be differentiated from bronchitis by the onset of symptoms as well as the nature of airway hyperresponsiveness.

The typical course of metal-fume fever is heralded by the development of a sweet metallic taste and dry throat along with fever, chills, myalgias and respiratory complaints like chest tightness, nonproductive, and dyspnea which occur 4–8 hours following exposure and spontaneously resolve within 48 hours. Chest radiography and pulmonary function tests are usually normal. Recurrence of symptoms on return to work after a short period of absence akin to the Monday-morning fever has also been noted. It is important to distinguish metal-fume fever from acute metal fume toxicity which develops following acute high intensity exposure to metal fumes but instead of being self-limiting progresses to fulminant respiratory distress and respiratory failure.

APPROACH

A good occupational and environmental history for exposures should be carefully obtained to identify the etiologic metal involved. Diagnosis of metal-induced lung disease can be confidently made only on clinicoradiologic-histopathologic correlation with the help of the following:
- Definitive history of exposure to metal dust
- Presence of cough and dyspnea on exertion over a long period
- Radiological findings suggestive of pneumoconiosis or interstitial lung disease
- Histopathological features of interstitial lung disease or a giant cell interstitial pneumonia pattern
- Demonstration of metallic content in lung tissue on biopsy or in bronchoalveolar lavage fluid.

It is necessary to differentiate metal-induced lung disease from other diseases with similar clinical or radiological presentation, namely tuberculosis and lung cancer, especially in the developing countries. A careful history and physical examination coupled with diagnostic efforts directed toward establishing specific diagnosis through necessary microbiological and histopathological investigations should resolve the dilemma.

TREATMENT

Treatment of metal-fume fever is mostly supportive with analgesics and antipyretics. Anti-inflammatory treatment with glucocorticosteroids may be tried for symptomatic and physiologic improvement. It is usually given for 3–6 months. Methotrexate is another anti-inflammatory drug which can be tried in patients who are either not responsive to prednisone or develop significant steroid side effects. Inhaled steroids may be used for milder disease.

Secondary consequences of hypoxemia, such as pulmonary hypertension and right-sided heart failure whenever present, should be managed with supplemental oxygen, diuretics, angiotensin-converting enzyme inhibitors and other treatments based on their clinical indication. Pulmonary rehabilitation is also helpful to improve patients' functional status and quality of life.

CHAPTER 53

Health Risks of Asbestos Fiber Inhalation

Daniel E Banks, Harakh V Dedhia

INTRODUCTION

The opinions or assertions contained herein are the personal views of the author and are not to be construed as doctrine of the US Department of the Army or the US Department of Defense.

The term "asbestos" describes six different occurring fibrous crystals (crocidolite, amosite, chrysotile, anthophyllite, tremolite, and actinolite) with a great number of industrial uses. An association between environmental or occupational exposure to asbestos and the occurrence of chest disease is well established and reported (Box 53.1). Unrecognized asbestos exposure may be indirect, occurring in the construction industry, the shipyards or when these illnesses are under consideration, a detailed occupational and family history is necessary to recognize the role of asbestos exposure in disease.

Potential work exposures occur during mining, milling, handling, manufacturing processes, and particularly, during the destruction of previously manufactured material associated with building renovation (asbestos abatement). In past decades, the major end users have been the construction, shipbuilding, and automobile and railroad equipment industry. Today, much

---

BOX 53.1: Asbestos-related pulmonary effects.

- Asbestosis (asbestos pneumoconiosis)
- Pleural plaques
- Pleural effusion (benign)
- Diffuse pleural thickening
- Pleural mesothelioma
- Lung cancer

of the insulation and friction materials are made of nonasbestos replacement fiber materials.

Asbestos is virtually indestructible and remains in the environment indefinitely. Once the fibers are incorporated into a manufactured item, there is little health risk unless the item is disrupted.

ASBESTOSIS

The term "asbestosis" refers only to parenchymal fibrosis associated with asbestos exposure. The chronic and progressive inflammation and injury produced by asbestos fibers continues from the time of exposure, through the subclinical phase, to the time when clinical disease is identifiable by the classic methods of lung function testing, chest radiography, and more sophisticated imaging such as high-resolution computed tomography (HRCT) scan.

Signs and symptoms of asbestosis are those of the other diffuse interstitial fibrotic diseases, but may not be present or only minimally noted early in the course of the illness. Dyspnea on exertion is the usual symptom of presentation, which worsens as the disease progresses and lung function declines. Nonproductive cough and chest pain are present in some cases, but occur late in the disease. When the cough is productive, it is likely attributable to bronchitis. Chest tightness and chest discomfort can be attributed to muscle pain appearing only when the cough and the dyspnea become severe. Hemoptysis is not expected and should be fully investigated as it suggests lung carcinoma. All of these symptoms may occur during the working years or even begin after exposure has ceased, becoming clinically apparent only after retirement.

The diagnosis requires a history of a sufficient exposure and latency period, chest radiographic features consistent with asbestosis, and the absence of other illnesses which might explain the radiologic features. Only in the rarest of occasions is an open lung biopsy with assessment of the mineral content of the lung necessary for the diagnosis. Disability determination is made on a clinical basis in the absence of tissue diagnosis. It is not an indication for biopsy. Although signs and symptoms of lung disease and respiratory impairment may be present, this is not a requisite for the diagnosis (Box 53.2). The chest radiograph classically shows irregular basilar opacities which, in time, may progress to honeycombing. The radiographic specificity for asbestosis, which may be identical to other diffuse fibrotic processes, is enhanced when bilateral

---

BOX 53.2: Clinical manifestations seen in some patients with asbestosis.

- Subjective respiratory complaints
- Restrictive pulmonary function tests (FVC <80% predicted)
- Finger clubbing
- Basilar crepitations
- Chest radiograph with increased basilar lung markings
- Known asbestos exposure

pleural thickening and, in particular, when pleural calcification accompanies basal parenchymal fibrosis.

High-resolution computed tomography scan has not been shown to be justified as a screening tool in the evaluation of the presence or absence of interstitial disease in asbestos-exposed workers, but it has a place in the clinical investigation of these individuals. Compared to the conventional CT scan, HRCT scan has improved our assessment of the interstitium and allows us to better appreciate interstitial and emphysematous changes.

ASBESTOS FIBERS AND THE PLEURAL SPACE

Asbestos fibers have a natural, unexplained predilection for transport to the pleura. The result is an unusual array of benign and malignant manifestations of exposure—these changes are not seen in any other disease.

Effusions attributable to asbestos exposure may be clinically manifest as being without symptoms with radiologic features of a blunted costophrenic angle as the sole manifestation of the inflammatory process to a "full-blown" bout of pleurisy with chest pain on inspiration, fever, dyspnea, and a substantial collection of hemorrhagic fluid in the affected pleural space. The effusions are exudative in nature and attribution to asbestos exposure is typically a "diagnosis of exclusion". These may be attributed to asbestos after chemical and cellular assessment of the fluid in the pleural space, as well as a sample of the pleura, provides no clear diagnosis. This may require serial chest radiographs over an observation period of 2 or 3 years as these effusions typically resolve slowly and spontaneously over a period of months. Finally, it should be noted that the "cause and effect" relationship of an exudative pleural effusion with clinical features of acute pleurisy leading to diffuse pleural thickening is often presumptive, with the effusion never recognized but thought to have occurred on a subclinical basis.

Not surprisingly, these exudative effusions leave a "scarred" pleural space as they resolve. This is manifest by the radiographic appearance of obliteration of the costophrenic angle and described as diffuse pleural thickening. Asbestos-related pleural effusions do not predict the development of lung cancer, pleural plaques or mesothelioma, although exudative effusions often accompany lung cancer as well as mesothelioma.

DIFFUSE PLEURAL THICKENING: FIBROSIS OF THE VISCERAL PLEURA

Diffuse pleural thickening is a disease of the visceral pleura. It is not specific for asbestos exposure and is often associated with fibrosis due to an inflammatory reaction caused by tuberculosis, surgery, hemorrhagic chest trauma, or drug reaction.

Diffuse pleural thickening may be responsible for dyspnea on exertion and perhaps a dry cough. Decreased respiratory excursion may be noted if the lung is "trapped" and moves little on the affected side. Diffuse pleural thickening may restrict lung function modestly if limited, but if extensive and bilateral, this may cause a significant restriction of lung function due to a "trapped lung" and result in respiratory insufficiency and failure in some instances. Although the radiographic features of diffuse pleural thickening often appear to show a more extensive pleural effect compared to the radiographic features of benign pleural plaques, data show no difference in mean exposures between workers with these two types of radiographic features. A wide distribution of exposures was recognized in both groups.

On the radiograph, diffuse pleural thickening appears as a continuous, smooth pleural opacity extending more than one-fourth of the pleural surface with blunting of the costophrenic angle. If diffuse pleural thickening is bilateral, the foremost concern is asbestos exposure. The relationship between these radiographic changes and asbestos exposure is a clinical perception and does not require histologic confirmation unless malignant pleural disease is considered. Because this primarily affects the visceral pleura in the posterior and posterolateral lower zones, the CT scan provides a better visualization than the chest radiograph. Diffuse pleural thickening can be complicated by extension of fibrosis in the interlobar and interlobular fissures to form crow's feet (a focal abnormality of the visceral pleura which appear as small, pleural, and parenchymal fibrous strands). Rounded atelectasis (the folded lung) is also known as Blesovsky's syndrome and is thought to be the result of visceral pleural fibrosis which has been "drawn back" into the lung.

PLEURAL PLAQUES: FIBROSIS OF THE PARIETAL PLEURA

One of the radiographic hallmarks of asbestos exposure is pleural plaques. These are located on the parietal pleura, are not associated with pleural adhesions, and cause no pulmonary function impairment. Workers with pleural plaques are without symptoms or signs of chest disease. How pleural plaques develop is poorly understood. First, the relationship between exposure and the development of plaques is not clear. Using chest radiographs, work from British shipyard population surveys showed that the prevalence of plaques increased with increasing doses of asbestos inhaled. In direct opposition to this conclusion, using CT scanning of the chest, there was no relationship between the plaque surface area and cumulative amount of asbestos exposure, smoking history or time since first asbestos exposure.

Grossly, plaques are firm, raised areas with a nearly white, glistening surface. Microscopically, collagen fibers are oriented in a parallel fashion in the submesothelial layers of the parietal pleura at the level of the costal margins, the diaphragms, and the paraspinal areas. Pleural calcification occurs in areas of collagen degeneration and implies that the plaque has been present for 20 or more years. Generally, neither asbestos bodies nor asbestos fibers are found in the plaques.

The earliest finding on the chest radiograph of a pleural plaque is frequently a thin line of soft-tissue density at the lateral margin of the seventh or eighth rib. This early change may be difficult to distinguish from normal "companion" shadows. The routine chest radiograph defines only 8-15% of all pleural plaques. Oblique views may assist in their recognition. The conventional CT scan recognizes plaques much earlier and at a less well-defined stage than the chest radiograph. Diaphragmatic plaques which were not always well appreciated with the conventional CT scan are better evaluated with the HRCT scan. Computed tomography scans can clearly differentiate plaques from extrapleural fat pads, a sometimes difficult distinction on the plain chest radiograph, particularly in those overweight or obese. Furthermore, in the presence of extensive and calcified pleural plaques, the CT scan permits a clearer appreciation of the lung parenchyma than the plain radiograph.

MALIGNANT MESOTHELIOMA

Although inhalation of asbestos fibers is a major risk factor for the development of mesothelioma, not all mesothelioma are associated with asbestos fiber inhalation. Exposure to amphibole fibers is much more likely to induce mesothelioma than exposure to chrysotile fibers, yet all of the commercially available fibers have been recognized to cause mesothelioma.

Clinical clues suggesting mesothelioma include symptoms which develop insidiously and include progressive dyspnea and weight loss. Most patients with mesothelioma show chest pain, often only partially relieved by analgesics, as the reason that they consult a physician. The presenting sign is usually a unilateral pleural effusion that progressively increases in size. As the disease progresses, affected supraclavicular nodes may become palpable and ribs may become tender as a result of local tumor invasion. Both superior and inferior vena caval obstruction can occur with resultant congestion, edema, and ascites. Digital clubbing may be present.

Malignant mesothelioma should be considered in differential diagnosis of all cases of unexplained exudative pleural effusion, particularly if asbestos exposure is documented. Clinical clues suggesting mesothelioma include contralateral pleural plaques and pleural calcification. In fact, among workers with asbestosis and/or asbestos-related pleural disease, there has been a significant increase in the risk for mesothelioma.

During thoracentesis, it may be difficult to enter the pleural space due to thickened pleura. The effusion is exudative, viscous and very cellular, with normal, malignant, and inflammatory cells. Cytologic examination of the fluid is often of limited diagnostic value because it is frequently difficult to differentiate benign from malignant mesothelial cells. Hyaluronic acid may be greatly elevated in effusions associated with malignant mesotheliomas. Because of rapid fluid accumulation, repeated thoracentesis, or placement of an indwelling catheter in the pleural space (depending on the clinical status of the patient), may be necessary to palliate dyspnea.

Although an open thoracotomy with pleural biopsy may well be needed to provide adequate amounts of tissue to establish a certain diagnosis, recent recommendations suggest that an earlier and equally reliable diagnosis may be gained through the use of thoracoscopy (except in cases of preoperative contraindication). Mesothelioma exhibits a high resistance to chemotherapy and only a few patients are candidates for radical surgery. To date, surgery, radiotherapy, chemotherapy, and, of late, immunotherapy or cytokine therapy, or a combination of the above, have been equally unsuccessful in curing this disease although may improve prognosis for a period of time.

LUNG CANCER

The persistence of asbestos in the lung parenchyma results in a lifelong exposure to this carcinogen. Of note, progression of asbestosis is an important risk for lung cancer. Thus, despite removal of the worker from a contaminated environment, the worker's lungs are continually exposed and the risk for cancer increased.

Our understanding of asbestos-related lung cancers in the absence of clinically recognizable asbestosis is further complicated by the multiplicative risk of smoking. In one report where asbestos exposure was high, the risk of lung cancer in cigarette smoking asbestos workers was compared to a group without asbestos exposure. Asbestos workers who smoked one pack of cigarettes per day had an 87 fold increase in the risk of developing lung cancer compared to nonsmoking, nonasbestos exposed controls. In nonsmoking asbestos workers, this risk was only fivefold. This has led to the postulate that the exposure to smoking and to asbestos causes a multiplicative risk for lung cancer.

Asbestos-related cancers are not distinct in type, nature, or their location within the lung from those solely associated with cigarette smoking.

Asbestos-related lung tumors present in the same manner as lung tumors caused by other carcinogens, except when the symptoms of asbestosis are present. In the presence of asbestosis, it is accepted that lung cancers should be compensated. In the absence of asbestosis, compensation has been debated, some refusing compensation for all cases, others favoring compensation for cases of long exposure (about in excess of 20 years).

CHAPTER 54

Occupational Asthma

PS Shankar, G Gaude

Asthma is now the most common cause of work-related respiratory disease in the industrialized countries. Occupational asthma is estimated to constitute an average of 15% of adult asthma and an even more of new-onset asthma in adults.

DEFINITION

Occupational asthma is characterized by wheezy breathlessness occurring after exposure to a sensitizer at workplace. It may also include subjects with prior asthmatic symptoms whose symptoms subsequently worsen as a consequence of sensitization. It is important to demonstrate the presence of variable airflow limitation and/or nonspecific bronchial hyperresponsiveness (NSBH) in association with exposure to a specific occupational environment. Relationship of symptomatology and airflow limitation with nonspecific stimuli outside the workplace does not qualify for the diagnosis of occupational asthma.

Workplace-related inhalation exposures can either exacerbate or induce asthma. Preexisting or concurrent asthma triggered by various work-related factors is defined as "work-exacerbated" asthma. These stimuli may include aeroallergens, irritants, or exercise at the workplace. The asthma symptoms in these patients occur at the workplace but are not caused by workplace exposures. Occupational asthma may also refer to recurrence of previously quiescent asthma (e.g. asthma in the distant past or during childhood). The current asthma in such patients may have been induced by sensitization to a specific occupational agent (sensitizer-induced occupational asthma). Similarly, exposure to an inhaled irritant at work is called as irritant-induced occupational asthma. Sensitizer-induced occupational asthma has a latency period during which the sensitization. It also includes occupational asthma usually caused by agents for which an antigen-specific immune response cannot easily be tested.

Work-exacerbated asthma and occupational asthma may coexist in the same worker. The onset of asthma at work in a person with a past history of asthma is considered more likely as the new-onset occupational asthma and not work-exacerbated asthma. It is also possible that the recent onset of asthma is unrelated to work. Reactive airways dysfunction syndrome (RADS) is a kind of irritant-induced acute onset asthma caused by a single exposure to a highly irritant material.

AGENTS CAUSING OCCUPATIONAL ASTHMA

Occupational asthma can be caused by a number of inhalational agents. Both immunological and nonimmunological mechanisms may be involved.

- *Immunological (allergic) occupational asthma:* Sensitization develops on exposure to an agent followed by a latent period of quiescence. Asthma in these sensitized subjects occurs whenever there is reexposure to even a small amount of the same agent.
- *Nonimmunological (nonallergic) occupational asthma:* It is due to an outstanding workplace irritant exposure and develops without a preceding latent period of exposure to an agent(s). This category includes irritant-induced asthma or RADS, which may occur after a single or multiple exposures to nonspecific irritants at high concentrations.

Environmental risk factors, other than the occupational exposures, are important in occupational asthma than in nonwork-related adult-onset asthma. The major risk factor for occupational asthma is the extent of exposure to the sensitizer. Atopy increases the risk of an individual becoming sensitized and contributes to an early sensitization and early occurrence of symptoms. The risk of sensitization and the development of immunoglobulin E (IgE) antibodies increase with the history of tobacco smoking.

High-molecular Weight Compounds

Exposure to high-molecular weight occupational agents (proteins, polysaccharides, and peptide compounds) is an important risk factor. There is production of specific IgE antibodies and sometimes, specific IgG antibodies. Atopic subjects are more likely affected due to IgE-dependent etiological agents.

Animal Products

Inhalation of allergens present in secreta of rodents (rats, mice, and rabbits) is a common cause of asthma in people working with these animals in the laboratories.

Plant Proteins

Exposure to various dusts of cereals amongst dock workers can cause occupational asthma. In addition, it can also cause other different syndromes, including allergen-induced airway obstruction and a febrile alveolitis-like condition.

Enzymes

Workers engaged in the manufacture of detergents and several other occupational products of plant and flower origins, beans and gums, can also cause occupational asthma.

Fish Proteins

Asthma in oyster handlers and workers engaged in processing of prawns and snow crabs occurs due to inhalation of vapors released during boiling.

Low-molecular Weight Compounds

Low-molecular weight (LMW) compounds, such as acid anhydrides, metals like platinum, some pharmaceutical products, pesticides used in agriculture, and fishing and food industry are important occupational agents causing asthma.

Wood Dusts

Western red cedar in the Pacific Northwest is the most common wood dust responsible for occupational asthma. Red cedar asthma is seen in 4–14% of the exposed population. The incidence varies with the type of industry and the level of dust exposure.

Metals

Exposure to metals is common amongst workers involved in metal mining and metallurgical industries, welding and soldering. In particular, platinum-induced asthma is a known clinical diagnosis for long. A variant of occupational asthma has been reported among potroom workers in aluminum smelters who report respiratory symptoms during a shift at work. The occurrence of nickel-induced asthma compared to contact dermatitis among exposed workers is rare. Exposure to zinc and chromium can also lead to asthma in addition to contact dermatitis.

Diisocyanates

Diisocyanates cause occupational asthma in 5–10% of exposed individuals. They are widely used in protective coatings for electric wiring, production of rigid and flexible foams, and painting of automobiles. They are commonly employed as adhesives and binders, as liners for mine and grain elevator chutes, soles of shoes, and spandex fibers. A large number of workers are therefore prone to suffer from occupational asthma.

Fluxes

Colophony obtained from pine tree is used as a flux in electronic industry. The prevalence of work-related respiratory symptoms and asthma has been reported in up to 22% of exposed electronic workers. Symptoms are related to the degree of exposure.

Anhydrides

Acid anhydrides are used in making alkyl and epoxy resins. Epoxy resins are used in adhesives and sealants for casting and coating processes. Similarly, alkyl resins constitute the base components of paints, varnishes, and plastics. Both phthalate and trimellitic anhydride exposures are known to cause occupational asthma and rhinitis. The exposure may also be associated with late respiratory systemic syndrome and pulmonary disease-anemia syndrome.

PATHOGENETIC MECHANISMS OF OCCUPATIONAL ASTHMA

Multiple genetic, environmental, and behavioral influences influence the pathogenesis of occupational asthma though the precise mechanism is not known. It is also likely that more than one mechanism, such as immunological, pharmacological, genetic, airway, and neurogenic inflammation may actually be responsible. Occupational asthma, based on its pathogenesis, is categorized as the allergic and the nonallergic variants. Allergic asthma may be either classic IgE-mediated or the polyimmunologic form. On the other hand, the nonallergic variant can be divided into RADS, pharmacologic bronchoconstriction, and reflex bronchospasm.

DIAGNOSIS

In most instances, the diagnosis of occupational asthma can be strongly suspected from the history alone, by finding a temporal relationship between symptoms and occupational exposure.

History and Physical Examination

Patients with occupational asthma may have very typical symptoms of cough, wheezing, and dyspnea and may be able to associate the onset of symptoms to a specific exposure at the workplace. As the condition progresses over several months, symptoms tend to become more severe, to start earlier and last longer, to have nocturnal symptoms, and to impinge on the weekends. Remissions initially occur on holidays, but even this feature may disappear after a sufficiently prolonged exposure.

Relationship between work and asthma symptoms should be established objectively. Specific challenge tests with the occupational agents considered to be responsible for asthma form the reference standard for the diagnosis of occupational asthma. There are no physical findings, which can be considered as specific for asthma; work-related wheezing is difficult to detect. Repeated pulmonary function testing (both during and while away from work) is usually done to make the diagnosis of occupational asthma.

Pulmonary Function Testing

Most importantly, there should be reversible airflow obstruction. Pulmonary function measured on a day away from work may be normal in up to half of those with occupational asthma. Serial measurements of spirometry when the patient has been away from work for a time and repeated when the patient returns to work, if coupled with an appropriate change in symptoms, may help confirm an association with the work environment. Preshift and postshift measures of forced expiratory volume in 1 second (FEV_1) are not generally helpful to either confirm or refute a diagnosis of occupational asthma. A serial peak flow meter recording is most frequently used and is the most easily accessible test. Changes in peak expiratory flow (PEF) from workplace exposures are best identified when the patient is as stable as possible.

Nonspecific Bronchial Inhalation Challenge

A positive challenge result supports a clinical diagnosis of asthma when baseline pulmonary function is normal. But a negative test does not rule out asthma. The test may be negative when the patient has been away from work exposure for some time. One needs to do serial measurements of airway responsiveness along with recording of PEF over a long period of time to look for the objective evidence of sensitization with the occupational agent.

Skin Test and Serology

Skin testing with common allergens, such as the house dust, danders, and grass and tree pollens may be useful in determining the atopic status of an individual. In few circumstances, especially with high-molecular compounds, appropriate extracts of potential occupational allergens are available for skin testing. The widely available nonstandardized commercial reagents can sometimes be used for skin-prick tests of food (e.g. wheat and rye extracts) and laboratory animals (e.g. mouse, rat, and guinea pig).

Total serum IgE may be useful in monitoring the patients. The use of immunologic testing in the diagnosis of allergic occupational asthma is limited. Specific antibodies, such as IgE antibodies, to various occupational allergens may be demonstrated by radioallergosorbent test and enzyme-linked immunosorbent assay. Although serologic testing is highly specific, it is often less sensitive indicator of sensitization than skin testing.

Specific Inhalation Challenge Testing

Specific inhalation challenge test is still considered the gold standard in the confirmation of the diagnosis of occupational asthma. The patient is exposed to the suspected sensitizer in a way in which he might be exposed at the workplace, although in a setting where symptoms are controlled and lung functions measured.

The most usual response to a challenge test is an immediate fall in flow rates, lasting for up to an hour. There can be immediate, delayed, or dual type of bronchial reaction. Immediate reactions show maximal response 10-30 minutes after exposure followed by complete recovery within 1-2 hours. Immediate reactions can be severe and unpredictable, hence the most dangerous. Late reactions develop slowly and progressively, either 1-2 hour (early late) or 4-8 hours (late) after exposure; they may occasionally be accompanied by fever and malaise. Late reactions mostly last for shorter duration and often respond well to an inhaled beta-2-agonist. Dual reactions contain characteristics of both early and late reactions.

MANAGEMENT

Early recognition and prompt diagnosis form the cornerstone of management. Removal of the worker from continued exposure to the inciting agent is desirable. Substitution of the agent with a less hazardous substance should be tried. Prevention and control of the exposures responsible for asthma are essential to reduce the number of incident cases. Diminution of the exposure to the inciting agent with proper engineering controls and the use of personal protective equipment may sometimes allow the continuation of work in the usual jobs in cases of workers with irritant-induced or work-aggravated asthma.

In the case of exposure to organic substances, e.g. animal antigens and wood dusts, it may be possible to combine good local exhaust ventilation, partial enclosure of processes, and respirator use to reduce exposure, sufficient enough for the person to continue to work along with the use of medication. In such situations, patients should continue anti-inflammatory agents and monitor their peak flow rates on regular basis. In cases of sensitization to LMW agents like isocyanates, acid anhydrides, and colophony, redeployment or change of job is generally required.

The management of occupational asthma does not differ significantly from the management of asthma that is not work related. Anti-inflammatory and bronchodilator therapy are required, if the patient is unwilling or unable to leave a job. The patient should be made to understand that continued exposure may lead to continued deterioration in spite of the treatment. Careful medical monitoring is important to detect persistence and/or worsening of symptoms for early interventions. Inhaled corticosteroids provide a small, but significant clinical improvement in patients with sensitizer-induced occupational asthma after withdrawal from exposure. Early administration of inhaled corticosteroids is more beneficial than later after the diagnosis is made.

Subcutaneous allergen immunotherapy is a potential option of treatment. Immunotherapy may help in occupational asthma due to one or a few specific allergens especially when avoidance of the triggering allergen is not feasible. It is, however, important that standardized allergens extracts are available for treatment. Immunotherapy helps reduce workplace symptoms, specific skin reactivity, and drug requirement; it does not improve the clinical course.

PROGNOSIS

There is significant variability in long-term sequela of occupational asthma. Symptoms may remit in case of removal of the worker from further exposure. More commonly, the occupational exposure leads to persistent symptoms and permanent bronchial hyperresponsiveness.

CHAPTER 55

Hypersensitivity Pneumonitis

PS Shankar

Hypersensitivity pneumonitis (HP) or extrinsic allergic alveolitis is a complex group of immunologically mediated alveolar and interstitial lung disorders caused by repeated inhalation of a wide variety of airborne allergens. Several different kinds of environmental, occupational, and recreational organic antigens, as well as the low-molecular weight chemical agents are responsible for hypersensitivity reactions in a significant number of affected individuals to which they have been previously sensitized. Most of these conditions exhibit similar clinical features, which develop several hours following environmental exposure.

ETIOLOGY

The inhaled antigens leading to development of HP can be classified as bacteria, fungi and their components (spores, mycelial fragments, degraded substrates, and toxins), animal proteins, and low-molecular weight chemicals. A wide variety of antigens, usually organic compounds of biological origin from bacteria, fungi, stored vegetable matters (hay, barley, and bagasse), and animal protein (avian, bovine, porcine, or insect material) and reactive low-molecular weight chemicals used in industry, such as isocyanates are responsible for initiating HP (Table 55.1).

Hypersensitivity pneumonitis induced by chemicals is relatively less common, compared to those induced by microbial and animal proteins.

TABLE 55.1: Common hypersensitivity disorders and their relationship to different exposures and antigens.

Exposure	Antigens	Diseases
Moldy hay	Thermophilic actinomycetes	Farmer's lung
Moldy bagasse	Thermophilic actinomycetes	Bagassosis
Moldy compost and mushroom	Thermophilic actinomycetes	Mushroom worker's disease
Contaminated barley	*Aspergillus clavatus*	Malt worker's lung
Compost	*Aspergillus* species	Compost lung
Esparto grass	*Aspergillus* species	Esparto dust lung
Soy sauce brewing	*Aspergillus* species	Soy sauce lung
Contaminated humidifiers, air conditioners, heating systems	Thermophilic actinomycetes	Ventilator lung
Domestic birds	Bird proteins	Bird fancier's lung
Pigeon droppings	Serum, feathers, droppings	Pigeon breeder's disease
Parakeets	Serum, feathers, droppings	Budgerigar fancier's lung
Silkworm larvae	Silkworm larvae proteins	Sericulturist's lung
Grains	Grain weevil	Grain lung
Isocyanates	Altered proteins	Hypersensitivity pneumonitis
Wood cutting	Plant protein	Woodman's disease
Contaminated metal working fluid	*Pseudomonas* species	Machine operator's lung
Detergent enzymes	*Bacillus subtilis*	Detergent worker's disease (washing powder lung)
Contaminated basement	*Cladosporium* species, *Penicillium* species	Basement lung
Contaminated hot tub water	*Mycobacterium avium* complex	Hot-tub lung
House dust	*Trichosporon asahii*	Japanese summer house hypersensitivity pneumonitis

PATHOGENESIS

Pathogenesis of HP involves a complex sequence of immunological events in a susceptible and sensitized host. It does not develop on the atopic background, the condition is neither associated with eosinophilia nor raised levels of immunoglobulin E (IgE). The sensitization results from an earlier exposure to antigen (organic dust). Following an intense re-exposure to such an antigen, there is interaction of the antigen and the "memory" system. There is formation of precipitins and complement fixing antibodies and they form immune complex aggregates of antigen–antibody to bring about systemic and pulmonary reactions.

The demonstration of precipitins against the thermophilic actinomycetes in the serum and a delay of 3–8 hours before the onset of symptoms following exposure to the antigen suggest that the pulmonary and systemic disturbances are as a result of an immune complex-mediated Arthus reaction. The immune complexes are not demonstrable in the alveolar septa or in the granuloma. A delayed type hypersensitivity reaction also to a certain extent is likely to be responsible for the development of chronic disease.

PATHOLOGY

The acute phase is mediated by neutrophils and the chronic phase by lymphocytes and macrophages in the form of a delayed-type hypersensitivity response. This is likely to lead to the formation of granuloma and progressive fibrosis. Acute HP is characterized by diffuse alveolar damage with necrosis. There is an acute inflammatory infiltrate. Pathologic abnormalities are observed in subacute and chronic forms of the disease. Subacute form is best described from a pathological viewpoint, characterized by the irregular areas of patchy consolidation with a centriacinar distribution. There are interstitial lymphocytic infiltrates, cellular bronchiolitis, and loosely formed non-necrotizing granulomas. The small and poorly circumscribed granulomas consist of the aggregates of lymphocytes, plasma cells, macrophages, and multinucleated giant cells. Presence of eosinophils and neutrophils is not characteristic. There is interstitial fibrosis with honeycomb changes in the chronic forms of the disease. These changes are similar and irrespective of the causative antigens.

CLINICAL PRESENTATION

Hypersensitivity pneumonitis presents predominantly with symptoms of dyspnea and cough. The condition may have an acute, subacute, or chronic onset. However, the manifestations frequently overlap. The manifestations are systemic and pulmonary. The systemic reactions are indistinguishable from that of infection.

Acute condition presents with fever, chills, dyspnea, myalgias, arthralgias, headache, cough, and chest tightness, 4–8 hours following a heavy exposure to the antigens. The symptoms peak in 6–24 hours following the exposure. Generally, the attack is self-limited and resolves in 1–3 days, following removal of the patient from the source of antigens. The continued exposure results in the persistence of symptoms. Physical examination usually reveals the presence of fever, tachypnea, and bibasilar crackles.

The subacute form of the disease is characterized by a slowly progressive symptomatology interspersed by discrete attacks of respiratory symptoms following heavy antigen exposure. In subacute form, the clinical features develop insidiously over a period of weeks. Cough and dyspnea are generally prominent. In some patients, the subacute form of the disease may permit the occurrence of an acute presentation especially if exposure to antigen persists.

In chronic condition, the level of antigen exposure is generally much lower and persistent. The respiratory manifestations develop slowly over months or years without any discrete attack suggesting the antigen as an offending agent. The patients suffer from increasing breathlessness, nonproductive cough, and weight loss. Fever is usually absent.

The clinical manifestations depend on the periodicity and the intensity of exposure. It may be either intermittent and heavy exposure or regular exposure in smaller dosages. The incidence of serious disability can be stopped, if the exposure is avoided or terminated. In those who expose continuously to smaller concentrations of antigen as seen in budgerigar fancier's, there is no acute history, and the features develop insidiously and progress to gross irreversible changes with fibrosis. The features of cor pulmonale and right ventricular failure ultimately supervene.

DIAGNOSIS

Diagnosis is established from history of exposure and other investigations as the following. Several criteria have been laid to make a diagnosis (Box 55.1).

Patients with acute HP exhibit polymorphonuclear leukocytosis without eosinophilia.

The chest radiograph may be normal, especially if obtained during an asymptomatic phase. In an established and symptomatic case, the radiograph shows the presence of patchy or diffuse infiltrates, fine micronodular pattern, or patchy ground-glass opacity. High-resolution computed tomography (HRCT) is highly sensitive, characteristically shows small, indistinct nodules, ground-glass infiltrates, and air trapping.

In subacute form of disease, small nodules and fine linear opacities may be seen. There is volume loss and honeycombing. These changes are predominantly noted in the upper lobes than in the lower lobes. There is evidence of pleural effusion or thickening. HRCT shows multiple, centrilobular

---

BOX 55.1: Diagnostic criteria for hypersensitivity pneumonitis.

Major criteria:
1. History of compatible symptoms that appear or worsen within hours after antigen exposure
2. Exposure confirmation based on history, environmental investigations, serum precipitin testing, and/or BAL antibody
3. Compatible abnormalities on chest radiograph or HRCT
4. BAL lymphocytosis
5. Compatible histologic changes on biopsy
6. Positive natural challenge (reproduction of symptoms and laboratory abnormalities after exposure to the suspected environment) or by controlled inhalation challenge

Minor criteria:
1. Basilar crackles on lung examination
2. Decreased diffusion capacity
3. Arterial hypoxemia at rest or with exercise

BAL, bronchoalveolar lavage; HRCT, high-resolution computed tomography

nodules throughout the lung fields. These radiological ground-glass opacities lead to volume loss and honeycombing. Emphysematous changes may be seen in the lower lung zones in nonsmokers.

Exposure to an antigen is confirmed by the presence of elevated titers of serum antibodies (IgG, IgM, and IgA). It suggests that the patient has been exposed to the suspected antigen and has mounted an immune response. The presence of antibody merely indicates the occurrence of exposure and sensitivity and not necessarily the disease.

Pulmonary function tests may be normal or show restrictive, or mixed restrictive and obstructive pattern of defects. In acute HP, there is restrictive defect with a decreased forced vital capacity, total lung capacity, and diffusion capacity. The diffusing capacity is generally decreased. Arterial hypoxemia is evident especially after exercise. Chronic HP reveals both restrictive and obstructive defects.

Skin tests demonstrate immediate or delayed type of hypersensitivity against the suspected antigens. However, it has not shown its usefulness as often there are nonspecific reactions. Inhalation challenge tests for suspected antigens may be helpful in confirming the diagnosis.

Lung biopsies from patients with chronic HP show chronic interstitial inflammation with infiltration of plasma cells, macrophages, and lymphocytes. There are poorly formed and noncaseating granulomas without any necrosis. There may be bronchiolitis, bronchiolitis obliterans, and sometimes with organizing pneumonia. In addition, there are varying degrees of interstitial fibrosis. Transbronchial lung biopsies may fail to provide sufficient material for the histopathologic study, and open lung biopsy is preferred in such a situation.

Differential diagnosis is important from few other syndromes, which may present with similar clinical manifestations. For example, inhalation of organic dusts may result in organic dust toxic syndrome (ODTS), which unlike HP, may occur in any individual without any prior sensitization. Exposure to the etiological agents of humidifier lung may also result in a non-HP syndrome, the humidifier fever. Chronic HP exhibits with features of idiopathic pulmonary fibrosis (IPF). The HP is distinguished from IPF on the basis of a detailed history of occupational and vocational history. One should make every effort to establish a link between a particular exposure either at work or at home and earlier episodes of similar manifestations.

MANAGEMENT AND PREVENTION

Hypersensitivity pneumonitis is essentially preventable by avoiding the inciting antigens. The acute episodes are self-terminating and subside, if the patient is removed from the antigen-containing environment. Avoidance of the offending antigen forms the cornerstone of the therapy. It may necessitate change in occupation and hobbies to enable complete avoidance of antigens. Efforts are made to minimize growth of an offending organism in the environment and removal of the contaminated source. The workers should wear properly fitted masks during exposure.

Persons suffering from acute manifestations respond to administration of corticosteroids. However, the utility of corticosteroids in chronic condition is not proven. A short course of corticosteroids hastens recovery and further stoppage of exposure to dust in the early stages revert the lung to the original condition. Prednisolone, 40–60 mg daily, is given to achieve an improvement. It is continued for 2 or more weeks or until there is resolution of clinical and radiological abnormalities. The dose is then gradually tapered after demonstrating objective improvement in pulmonary functions. Bedrest and supplemental oxygen inhalation are advocated. When irreversible fibrosis has developed, steroids are not helpful and the withdrawal from contact with the causative agent shows limited improvement.

PROGNOSIS

Hypersensitivity pneumonitis pursues a variable course. If the condition is recognized early, the recovery is generally expected. Generally, the manifestations of acute HP regress after a short interval following stoppage of exposure. When the acute attacks are recurrent, the symptoms may persist and lead to progressive lung impairment. The subacute or chronic HP exhibits insidious onset of symptoms. Often the conditions are recognized later in the course of illness, and it makes the prognosis unfavorable. The condition may exhibit features of emphysema in later stages. Presence of fibrosis on HRCT scan or on lung biopsy is an important predictor of higher mortality.

CHAPTER 56

Toxic Inhalations and Thermal Lung Injuries

VK Vijayan, N Goel, R Caroli

INTRODUCTION

Fires result in production of heat and smoke, both causing damage to the respiratory tract. Smoke inhalation causes a series of pathophysiological changes in the respiratory and circulatory systems. Heat exposure primarily causes damage to the upper airway passages. Inhalation of toxic gases and fumes even after a single exposure can similarly cause damage to the tracheobronchial system and lung parenchyma. Within seconds of exposure to an inhaled toxin, pathological events occur that may cause immediate distress, systemic illness lasting days, or even lead to the development of chronic lung disease. Pulmonary responses based on consequences of exposure are listed in Table 56.1.

DETERMINANTS OF INHALATIONAL LUNG INJURY

A variety of factors determine the pathological changes of a toxic inhalation, viz the size of inhaled particles, solubility of the inhaled substance in water, concentration of the inhalant in ambient air, duration of exposure, presence or absence of ventilation, and a variety of host factors (age, smoking status, comorbid diseases, use of respiratory protection, and perhaps even genetic susceptibility). In general, larger aerosolized particles are more likely to deposit in the nasopharynx via impaction and may not gain access to the lower airways, while smaller particles are able to penetrate smaller airways and effect toxicity at the level of the alveolus.

Highly soluble agents (e.g. hydrochloric acid, sulfur dioxide, ammonia, and aldehydes) have an early effect (within minutes of exposure) and cause

TABLE 56.1: Consequences of exposure.

Diseases	Common Agents
Upper respiratory tract diseases: • Rhinitis and laryngitis • Rhinorrhea • Ulceration and perforation of nasal septum	• Dust from flour, latex, pollens, SO_2, ETS, ammonia, hypochlorous acid • Cold air, carbaryl, malathion, parathion • Arsenic, copper dusts, chromic acid, and chromates
Airway diseases: • Asthma • Bronchitis • Bronchiolitis	• Acid anhydrides, aldehydes, chlorine, dust from flour, latex, pollens, isocyanates • SO_2, rock, and mineral dusts • Acetaldehyde, ammonia, chlorine
Interstitial diseases: • Pulmonary fibrosis • Alveolar proteinosis • Lipoid pneumonia • Hypersensitivity pneumonitis • Granulomatous diseases • Inhalation fever	• Asbestos, crystalline silica, talc • Fine crystalline silica dust • Oily metal working fluids • Fungi, thermophilic bacteria • Beryllium • Ameba, fungi, cotton dust, freshly generated zinc fumes
Chronic obstructive pulmonary disease: Coal dust, cotton dust, cadmium, crystalline silica, and biomass fuel exposure	
Lung cancer: Asbestos, arsenic, mustard gas, radon progeny, cadmium, and crystalline silica	

(SO_2, sulfur dioxide; ETS, environmental tobacco smoke)

acute irritant injury to the exposed mucous membranes. Those with low solubility (e.g. nitrogen dioxide, nitrous oxide, phosgene, and ozone) cause no symptoms in upper airway and predominantly penetrate into the lower airways. Hence, they cause delayed onset irritant effects in bronchi, terminal bronchioles, and alveoli.

CLINICAL PRESENTATIONS OF INHALATIONAL INJURY

Upper Airways

The initial nasal mucosal response to inhaled toxins is typically sudden and short lived. Characteristic tissue injury ranges from slight edema of the nasopharynx and larynx to epithelial ulceration and frank hemorrhage. Acute exposure to the irritant substances causes burning sensations of the nasal passages and throat, coughing, and sneezing. Sometimes, there is also copious sputum production. Burning of the eyes, profuse lacrimation, headache, and dizziness may also be present. Life-threatening airway obstruction can occur due to multiple pathophysiological effects of exposure, such as: reflex bronchoconstriction, laryngospasm/glottic closure, mucosal edema, hypersecretion, and sloughing of epithelial cells.

Epithelial injury can occur in the conducting airways by acute toxic inhalation, which exposes submucosa to dangerous effects of toxins. Mild irritant effects include tracheitis and bronchitis. Irritation and inflammation can aggravate underlying airways disease, such as chronic obstructive pulmonary disease (COPD) or bronchial asthma. The resulting edema, inflammation, and bronchoconstriction may be life threatening. The airways are also vulnerable to infections. The injury to the conducting airways may manifest as intrathoracic airflow obstruction, hours after the initial insult, and patient may present with dyspnea or chest tightness and wheezing. If individuals have a preexisting airway disease, the irritant exposure may cause more severe disease.

Reactive Airways Dysfunction Syndrome

Reactive airways dysfunction syndrome (RADS) can result following an acute, heavy exposure to a number of chemicals, regardless of the agent's potential to induce sensitization (Box 56.1). Asthma-like symptoms develop within a short period after the exposure. High-level exposure to some of the gases, such as the uranium hexafluoride gas and smokes is highly irritant. Similarly, the fumes floor sealants, spray paints, heated acids, fumigating fog, and metal coating removers may all cause the problem. There is also persistent nonspecific bronchial hyperresponsiveness following exposure. Bronchial biopsy shows inflammation and epithelial cell injury. Infiltration is present with lymphocytes and plasma cells, while eosinophils are usually absent. Chest radiographs is generally normal. Spirometry is either normal or may show mild airflow limitation. Later on, antiasthma drugs are usually required by most patients of RADS.

Irritant-induced Asthma

Patients not meeting the criteria of RADS are categorized as having irritant-induced asthma. These patients usually have history of repeated episodes of less massive exposures and develop symptoms after a lag of several days.

BOX 56.1: Diagnostic criteria for reactive airways dysfunction syndrome (RADS).
- Absence of preexisting asthma symptoms, history of asthma in remission or any respiratory disorder
- Exclusion of conditions that may mimic asthma
- History of exposure to an irritant vapor, gas, fumes, or smoke in heavy concentrations
- Onset of asthma symptoms within minutes to hours (usually <24 hours) after a single exposure or accident
- Positive methacholine challenge test
- Pulmonary function test to document airway obstruction (may or may not be present)
- Exclusion of another pulmonary disorder

Repeated exposures to irritants lasting days or weeks are required before the development of asthma.

Bronchiolitis Obliterans

Inhalational bronchiolitis obliterans develops after inhalation of an irritant gas, fume, vapor (and rarely dust), such as nitrogen dioxide, sulfur dioxide, ammonia, chlorine, phosgene, hot gases, or fly ash. Soon, this damage leads to inflammation resulting in irreversible airway obstruction. Constrictive bronchiolitis is also seen in other conditions, such as connective tissue disorders, chronic hypersensitivity pneumonitis, or following some infections, drugs and organ transplantation.

Toxic gas inhalation causes fibrous exudates and granulation tissue in the bronchi and distal bronchioles, eventually leading to obliterative bronchiolitis. There are symptoms and signs of acute chemical pneumonitis, such as chest tightness, dyspnea, and massive hemoptysis. Other fume and particulate exposures associated with obliterative bronchiolitis are sulfur mustard, nitrogen oxides, diacetyl, and alpha-diketone substitutes, multiple chemicals and incinerator fly ash released during combustion, papaverine, found in juice extracted from *Sauropus androgynus,* or katuk and fiberglass.

There are more predominant upper airway symptoms in the initial 4–6 hours of exposure to a gas, such as nitrogen dioxide, which is less water soluble. These symptoms are uncommon after exposure to a more water-soluble gas, such as sulfur dioxide. During the 2nd phase of exposure in the first 24 hours, there occurs diffuse alveolar damage, which is clinically manifest as the acute respiratory distress syndrome (ARDS). The third phase is characterized by the resolution of ARDS and presence of minimal respiratory symptoms. This may be followed by a gradual progression of shortness of breath.

Minor nonspecific abnormalities are seen on chest radiographs, which may include variable amounts of hyperinflation and peripheral attenuation of the vascular markings. Nodular or reticulonodular opacities are sometimes seen. High-resolution computed tomography (HRCT) scans show more characteristic findings, such as diffuse mosaic areas of attenuation, decreased vascularity, evidence of air trapping, and peripheral cylindrical bronchiectasis.

Acute Respiratory Distress Syndrome

Although all toxic inhalants are capable of producing distal airway disease at extreme concentration and durations, the gases most likely to do so are those with low-water solubility, such as phosgene and nitrogen dioxide, which bypass reflex bronchoconstriction and absorption by upper airway mucosa. The initial pathological events in distal airways are caused by the cellular toxicity of the inhaled agent and its derivatives, which compromise the impermeability of the alveolar–capillary interface. Profound pulmonary edema may develop that impairs gas exchange and can prove fatal. The severity of this pulmonary edema, which typically presents after a latent period of several hours following the initial insult, is likely dose related.

SYSTEMIC ILLNESSES FROM INHALED TOXINS

Systemic flu-like illness lasting for less than two days has been observed in patients exposed to organic dusts and fumes of heated metals and fluorocarbons. These are known as inhalational fevers and are of three types, viz. (i) metal fume fever (MFF), (ii) polymer fume fever, and (iii) organic dust toxic syndrome (ODTS). The course of the disease is self-limited and appears to be cytokine mediated.

Metal Fume Fever

Inhalation of a number of metal oxide fumes can cause the syndromic manifestation of MFF, which is self-limiting in nature. The history is characterized by constitutional symptoms of fever, headache, myalgia, and fatigue in association with respiratory symptoms, thirst, a metallic taste in the mouth and increased salivation. Peripheral blood examination shows neutrophilic leukocytosis. MFF is classically seen with zinc oxide fume exposure from welding galvanized steel or brass. It is also reported in association with metal pouring in brass foundries and high-temperature zinc coating processes. More rarely, magnesium and copper oxide fumes are also reported to cause MFF.

The condition is also known by a few other names—Brazier's disease, smelter shakes, brass chills, zinc chills, Welder's ague, copper fever, foundry fever, and Monday morning fever. The diagnosis is mostly based on history. Onset occurs rapidly within 3 and 10 hours after exposure. Bilateral diffuse, interstitial infiltration is seen on chest radiography. Pulmonary function tests show significant reductions in vital capacity, transfer factor, and arterial oxygen partial pressure. An increase in urine and plasma metal levels may be seen. Spontaneous recovery is usual within 24 hours. There are no known long-term complications.

Polymer Fume Fever

Polymer fume fever is a similar condition but less common than MFF. It presents with initial symptoms of dry throat, rhinitis, chest tightness, and conjunctivitis. Constitutional symptoms (fever, chills, and myalgias) may often follow exposure by about 4–8 hours, which spontaneously resolve within 1 day. Leukocytosis is often present.

Organic Dust Toxic Syndrome

Organic dust toxic syndrome is a self-limiting syndrome, which occurs due to inhalation of high concentrations of organic dust within hours of exposure. It is characterized by acute onset of fever with chills, malaise, myalgia, headache, dyspnea, chest tightness, dry cough, and nausea. ODTS typically resolves spontaneously within 48 hours following exposure.

SMOKE INHALATION LUNG INJURY

Smoke inhalation injury is responsible for severe lung-induced morbidity and mortality. Factually, respiratory failure is the most common cause of death in burn centers. The composition of smoke determines the type and severity of lung injury. Carbon monoxide inhalation is responsible for most cases of death in fires.

Inhalation of air heated to a temperature 150°C causes direct heat injury to the respiratory tract. It causes burns of the face, oropharynx, and upper airways (above the vocal cords). Heat and the chemicals in smoke produce an immediate injury to the airway mucosa causing edema, erythema, and ulceration. The gas phase of smoke also contains many long-acting oxidants, which can reach distal lung tissues. The vapors irritate the mucous membrane causing marked bronchorrhea, bronchoconstriction, and airway edema.

MANAGEMENT

The victim has to be removed immediately from the site of leakage or fire, so as to minimize the exposure and to characterize the agents involved. This is followed by thorough decontamination by removing all clothing, which has trapped chemicals. Assessment is then made for the signs of severe injury indicated by the presence of altered mental status, respiratory insufficiency, cardiovascular instability, convulsions, and unconsciousness.

Initial therapy consists of maintenance of airway patency, ventilation, and circulation. Careful examination is done for the presence of burns, trauma, and other injuries. Systemic intoxication due to certain chemicals may require treatment with specific antidotes. Diazepam, cyanide antidote kits, atropine, and pralidoxime are the most important drugs, which are helpful to manage such emergencies. Airway compromise and respiratory insufficiency may warrant high-flow oxygen, intubation, or tracheostomy. Patients going into ARDS will require mechanical ventilation as per the standard ARDS protocol. Inhaled or systemic corticosteroids and inhaled bronchodilators are useful in the management of bronchospasm.

CHAPTER 57

Drug-induced Respiratory Disease

William J Martin Jr

Drug-induced respiratory disease is sufficiently common that the clinicians need to consider in the differential diagnosis of most acute and chronic respiratory and pleural disorders.

There are more than 300 drugs associated with respiratory toxicity and the list is only going to grow as more therapeutic agents are brought to the market. Today, it is much simpler with access to the website www.pneumotox.com for an excellent and easy method to access up-to-date information on drug-induced lung reactions.

DRUGS ASSOCIATED WITH RESPIRATORY TOXICITY

Cancer Chemotherapy Agents

Cancer chemotherapeutic agents, including radiation, were among the first class of drugs or agents to be recognized as cause of respiratory toxicity (Table 57.1). Many cancer chemotherapy agents have been implicated in respiratory toxicity, not only complicating the cancer treatment regimen, but limiting additional therapeutic approaches to controlling cancer growth. Thus, the need to understand the mechanisms of chemotherapy-induced lung disease is critical to provide better strategies to maximize the antitumor effect and to minimize the pulmonary complications for the patient (Fig. 57.1).

One of the typical examples of respiratory toxicity from cancer chemotherapy occurs with bleomycin. The drug can generate oxygen radicals and damage deoxyribonucleic acid (DNA). This property makes it effective to kill cancer cells, but may also serve to injure critical alveolar lining cells and endothelial cells in the lung, which may result in acute lung injury and death.

TABLE 57.1: Cancer chemotherapy.

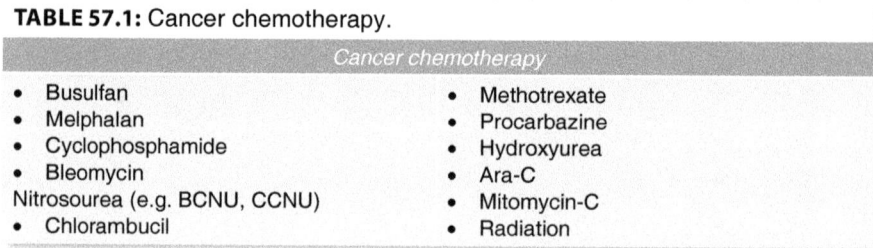

Cancer chemotherapy	
• Busulfan	• Methotrexate
• Melphalan	• Procarbazine
• Cyclophosphamide	• Hydroxyurea
• Bleomycin	• Ara-C
Nitrosourea (e.g. BCNU, CCNU)	• Mitomycin-C
• Chlorambucil	• Radiation

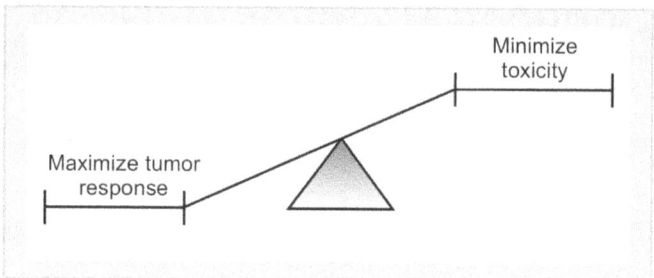

Fig. 57.1: Therapeutic strategy for cancer chemotherapy.

This process may account for the reported postoperative acute respiratory distress syndrome (ARDS) occurring in patients who have previously received bleomycin. Additionally, bleomycin pulmonary toxicity may be associated with an acute inflammatory or immune response in the lung, further comprising lung function. The ability of drugs to cause both direct toxic and indirect inflammatory-mediated lung injury is common to many drugs in the class of cancer chemotherapy agents. Each drug may be unique in how the initial injury occurs and where it occurs in the respiratory system, but the complexity of the mechanisms and the repair responses in the lung often undermine a predictable course for any given patient.

Cardiovascular Drugs

Methyldopa, commonly used to treat hypertension, was one of the first drugs associated with systemic and immunologic findings consistent with drug-induced lupus syndrome. Similarly, procainamide and hydralazine were also recognized for this side effect. Development of a positive immunologic parameter, such as the antinuclear antibody (ANA) may occur with therapy on such drugs, but this is neither necessary that a systemic drug response will occur nor does it mean that therapy should be altered. It occurs commonly with a conversion rate of 40–60% of patients on treatment. The drug-induced lupus syndrome, however, can be serious and life-threatening.

In the more recent past, the cardiovascular drug amiodarone has become an important cause of pulmonary toxicity with multiple reports and studies documenting the varied clinical presentations and findings. Amiodarone is an unusual drug as it is an iodinated benzofuran derivative and its primary metabolite is created by the liver conversion of desethylamiodarone by the removal of an ethyl group from the parent compound. The drug has a very long pharmacologic half-life of approximately 45 days and both the parent drug and its metabolite will persist long after the drug is discontinued.

For patients with a history of congestive heart failure and rhythm abnormalities, the onset of dyspnea or cough or signs of new infiltrates on a chest X-ray might easily be attributed to the underlying cardiac condition. Most typically, amiodarone pulmonary toxicity occurs insidiously with cough, dyspnea, weight loss, and evidence of progressive interstitial disease. Another form of toxicity may occur acutely with more of an alveolar pattern and can be localized or diffuse. If associated with pleuritic chest pain, the diagnosis can be confused with acute pulmonary embolism, a condition to be suspected in anyone with a diminished cardiac output. Another form of toxicity mimics bronchiolitis obliterans with organizing pneumonia (BOOP) that may present with a typical unilateral and pleural-based mass-like lesion.

Antibiotics/Antimicrobials

Pulmonary toxicity from antibiotic usage is rare, but since antibiotic or antimicrobial use is so common, it becomes one of the most important classes of drugs to consider as a cause of drug-induced lung disease (Table 57.2). Nitrofurantoin toxicity is one of the best described and oldest examples of an antibiotic that can cause severe pulmonary-pleural reactions.

Nitrofurantoin pulmonary toxicity can also occur acutely even after the first dose and this can appear with sudden onset of cough and dyspnea and a chest X-ray that has diffuse alveolar infiltrates with or without pleural effusions and may mimic the appearance of congestive heart failure. Occasionally, a patient with acute onset may have a high peripheral blood eosinophil count and this can be an important clue to the diagnosis.

In contrast, chronic nitrofurantoin toxicity may mimic the clinical and roentgenographic presentation of idiopathic pulmonary fibrosis (IPF). The concern in this case is that a missed diagnosis of chronic nitrofurantoin toxicity may result in a patient being given the diagnosis of IPF that is essentially a fatal disease over the course of a few years and for which there is no currently effective therapy outside of lung transplantation. Unlike IPF, corticosteroids hasten recovery from the fibrotic-like condition of nitrofurantoin toxicity and if instituted early in the course, the patient can expect a full recovery.

TABLE 57.2: Antibiotic agents.

- Nitrofurantoin
- Azulfidine
- Sulfonamides
- Gentamicin
- Neomycin
- Polymyxin
- Colistin
- Streptomycin
- INH, PAS
- Minocycline

Anti-inflammatory and Miscellaneous Drugs

Several anti-inflammatory agents are associated with respiratory toxicity. Classically, an overdose with aspirin can result in acute pulmonary edema and marked changes in the acid-base balance in the blood, contribute to further respiratory distress. Use of gold salts in rheumatoid arthritis remains a useful therapy for severe diseases and is well recognized as a cause of interstitial lung disease.

Penicillamine is another interesting drug that has both chelating and immunosuppressive properties. Its use, primarily as an immunosuppressive agent, in rheumatoid arthritis has been associated with different types of adverse pulmonary reactions, including: (1) Organizing pneumonia, (2) drug-induced lupus syndrome, or (3) alveolar hemorrhage.

There are excellent reviews of how illicit drugs can be a cause of adverse reactions in the respiratory system, including heroin or other narcotic drugs, cocaine and marijuana. Pulmonary toxicity includes both acute complications such as noncardiogenic pulmonary edema and long-term sequelae such as granulomatosis pneumonitis, etc. Tocolytics, such as oxytocin can induce uterine contractions and thereby prevent postpartum hemorrhage. A diverse number of drugs can cause a drug-induced lupus syndrome, which can mimic systemic lupus erythematosis, including hydralazine, penicillamine, alpha methyldopa, procainamide, various anticonvulsants and, more recently, anti-tumor necrosis factor (TNF) antibody therapy.

DIAGNOSIS AND MANAGEMENT OF DRUG-INDUCED RESPIRATORY DISEASE

There is nothing more important in the diagnosis of drug-induced respiratory disease than an accurate history and recognition that a medication or drug might be the cause of the respiratory distress. If that key-step is missed, all the subsequent testing and evaluation may not establish the link and may not make the correct diagnosis in your patient.

Obviously, chest imaging with a chest X-ray and chest computerized tomography often provide critical information regarding the pattern and extent of the disease and many provide enough information to establish a "working diagnosis" of a drug reaction. The high-resolution computed tomography (HRCT) findings of drug-induced lesions may resemble the spectrum of findings with chemical-induced lung injuries.

Pulmonary function tests (PFTs)can be helpful in confirming the typical findings of a restrictive pattern with a decrease in the diffusing capacity, although some drugs may induce obstructive changes whereas others do not affect diffusing capacity. The PFTs can also be abnormal prior to the onset of symptoms and do not necessarily indicate clinical disease or clinical progression. Many patients have more than one reasonable explanation for the diagnosis and may require a more invasive approach including a lung biopsy.

Flexible fiberoptic bronchoscopy remains a very useful tool in the assessment of patients with suspected drug-induced respiratory disease.

Bronchoalveolar lavage (BAL) can strongly suggest certain diagnoses, such as eosinophilic pneumonia or hypersensitivity pneumonitis if there is an exuberant number (>40% of total cells), representing CD8+ (suppressor/cytotoxic) lymphocytes. For example, cytological patterns of BAL fluid may help to distinguish methotrexate-induced pneumonitis in patients with cancer. In addition, bronchoscopy with transbronchoscopic lung biopsy and BAL can help in assessing the presence of other conditions, such as complicating infection, underlying respiratory disease (for which the patient might be receiving the drug) or metastatic cancer.

Even after completion of all available diagnostic tests, the clinician might remain uncertain if the patients' symptoms reflect a case of drug-induced respiratory disease. Under these circumstances, one can consider all of the information to indicate whether supportive evidence exists or whether careful assessment of the patient's status following drug withdrawal is the best approach. Many patients respond quickly to the withdrawal of a drug causing the lung reaction but if the symptoms have been present for weeks or months, the response may be slow. Under these circumstances or if the patient is severely ill, many clinicians would favor a course of corticosteroids in addition to the drug withdrawal, as it will hasten recovery and will be reassuring to both the patient and the clinician that the diagnosis was correct.

There are often no easy answers in the management of patients with suspected drug-induced respiratory disease. One must have the discipline to understand clearly the rationale for each test ordered and what you would do with the information when it is available regarding the management of the patient. Obviously, if the history, examination and chest imaging suffice to establish a "working diagnosis", then drug withdrawal with or without corticosteroids may be the best approach. In some patients, a clear definitive answer is not available even after an open lung biopsy. In such cases, clinical judgment is necessary to determine, if drug withdrawal is best to assess its impact on the patients symptoms and findings. The need for a rechallenge with a drug is rarely indicated as almost always, there are alternative therapies available for the patient and there is no justification for a rechallenge which in itself, can be life-threatening.

CHAPTER 58

Epidemiology and Etiopathogenesis of Lung Cancer

Nagarjuna V Maturu, Navneet Singh

INTRODUCTION

Lung cancer is the most common cancer which accounts for about 12.9% of all new cancers worldwide. It is also the most common cancer in men and the most common cause of cancer-related mortality in both sexes. Survival from lung cancer in India is even poorer which can be attributed to delayed diagnosis and inadequate or suboptimum treatment.

LUNG CANCER IN INDIA

The latest National Cancer Registry Programme (NCRP) 3-year report (2008–2011) of 25 population-based cancer registries has identified lung and upper aerodigestive tract malignancies as the most common cancer types in men all over the country. In women, lung malignancy is the leading cancer type only in some of the Northeastern states. A verbal autopsy analysis of 122,429 deaths from 1.1 million homes in India, lung cancer (11.4%) was the third most common cause of cancer-related mortality in men in economically productive age group (30–69 years). The age-adjusted incidence rates of lung cancer in India have shown a statistically significant increase over the last three decades (1982–2012), both in men and in women. Also, as per the NCRP estimates, the incidence of lung cancer in India is projected to increase further by 30% by the year 2020.

HISTOLOGICAL PATTERNS

The major histological types of lung cancer are: squamous cell carcinoma (SqCC), adenocarcinoma (ADC) and small cell lung cancer (SCLC). A relative increase in the incidence of ADC has been witnessed in the recent past, being the dominant histological type in most of the developed countries. Incidence rates for SqCC have declined by 30% or more among men in many countries while the decline of SCLC is less pronounced. Among females, the incidence rates for both SqCC and SCLC have shown an increase in most countries. Importantly, the incidence of ADC increased among both sexes in virtually all areas.

This histological shift in lung cancer in the developed countries is possibly linked to changes in the smoking behavior as well as to the methods of manufacturing and composition of smoking products. Use of cigarettes with low-tar and low-nicotine content as well as with filters has resulted in a tendency for deep inhalation of their smoke. As a result, the smoke carcinogens achieve a higher concentration in the peripheral areas of the lungs where ADCs tend to form. The Indian scenario is somewhat different with reference to histological patterns of lung cancer. Recent reports from some parts of the country have shown ADC as the predominant histological type of NSCLC.

An important difference in the pathogenesis of the various histological types of lung cancer occurs in relation to their site and cell of origin. The conducting bronchial airways are the sites of origin of almost all cases of SqCC and SCLC. During the process of development of SqCC, genetic, and environmental triggers lead to changes in the normal bronchial epithelium, often in a stepwise manner with formation of hyperplastic, metaplastic, and dysplastic lesions. Continuous oncogenic stimuli ultimately lead to the development of carcinoma in situ and frank SqCC. In the case of ADC, a similar mechanism is believed to be operating since atypical adenomatous hyperplasia (AAH) is a premalignant lesion and often precedes the development of overt ADC.

RISK FACTORS (BOX 58.1)

Smoking is the most important risk factor while 10–15% of lung cancers are related to factors other than active smoking.

Smoking

History of smoking is present in about 85% of non-small cell lung cancer (NSCLC) and 98% of SCLC cases. There is wide variability (1–15%) in lifetime risk of developing lung cancer amongst smokers. The risk varies with the duration of smoking (number of years smoked), age at starting smoking, intensity of smoking (number of cigarettes smoked per day), the total exposure to smoke (smoking index or pack years) and years since cessation of smoking (for reformed smokers). Smoking relationship is also modified by the presence of exposure to co-carcinogens (radon, asbestos, silica, and others) and genetic susceptibility. Several carcinogens have been identified in tobacco smoke; a few of them (including polycyclic aromatic hydrocarbons (PAH) and nicotine-derived nitrosoaminoketone), have a strong association with the development

> **BOX 58.1:** List of risk factors that have proven or possible associations with lung cancer.
>
> - Tobacco smoking (active)
> - Environmental tobacco smoke (ETS) exposure
> - Pulmonary diseases:
>   - Chronic obstructive pulmonary disease (COPD)
>   - Idiopathic pulmonary fibrosis (IPF)
>   - Systemic sclerosis-related interstitial lung disease
>   - Pneumoconiosis
> - Systemic diseases:
>   - Human immunodeficiency virus (HIV) infection
> - Air pollution (indoor and outdoor):
>   - Domestic cooking fuels
>   - Petroleum product combustion exhaust exposure
>   - Particulate matter
> - Environmental exposures:
>   - Radon
>   - Arsenic, nickel, and chromium
>   - Asbestos and silica
> - Dietary factors:
>   - Alcohol consumption
>   - Intake of vitamins, fruits, and vegetables
> - Hormone therapy
> - Genetic factors:
>   - Familial (hereditary)
>   - Specific gene abnormalities (nonhereditary)

of lung cancer. These carcinogens are responsible for the development of genetic mutations through formation of DNA adducts.

In India, the indigenous forms of tobacco are smoked more commonly than cigarette. *Bidi* smoking poses a higher risk for lung cancer than cigarette smoking. Similar to cigarette smoke, increasing intensity of exposure, increasing duration of exposure and earlier age of onset of *bidi* smoking increase the risk of lung cancer. The risk reduction following smoking cessation occurs much slower in *bidi* smokers as compared to cigarette smokers. The concentrations of several toxic and carcinogenic agents [such as hydrogen cyanide, carbon monoxide, ammonia, benz (a) anthracene, and benzopyrene] are higher in the mainstream smoke of *bidis* than in the smoke of cigarettes. Moreover, the tendu leaf used in the *bidis* is relatively non-porous with low combustibility. Therefore, the *bidi*-smoker needs to take more frequent and deeper puffs to keep it lit, making the *bidi* as more deleterious than cigarettes.

Environmental Tobacco Smoke

Environmental tobacco smoke (ETS) also known as secondhand smoke (SHS) contains all the toxic or carcinogenic agents present in mainstream smoke.

Despite ETS being established as a risk factor for lung cancer, the estimated risk has remained small (odds ratio (OR): 1.31, 95% confidence interval (CI): 1.24-1.52 in Asians) yet somehow debatable, mainly because of difficulties in exactly quantifying the exposure.

Household Air Pollution: Biomass Fuel/Coal Exposure

The International Agency for Research on Cancer (IARC) has identified coal as group 1 (known) pulmonary carcinogen and biomass fuels as group 2A (probable) pulmonary carcinogen. Duration of exposure is an important determinant with greater than 45 years exposure to indoor air pollution from use of coal or wood for cooking or heating showing an OR of 1.43 (95% CI = 0.33-6.30) for the development of lung cancer. Amongst the various biomass fuels in use, animal dung, the most common solid fuel used in India, has been shown to cause the maximum DNA damage.

Outdoor Air Pollution

Exposure to outdoor particulate matter is now identified as a group 1 lung carcinogen. Increases in both PM_{10} and $PM_{2.5}$ concentrations are associated with increasing odds of developing lung cancer even though the risk is lesser than the risk associated with active smoking. But in view of the wider population exposure to outdoor air pollution, the anticipated public health effect is likely to be huge.

Occupational Exposures

Analyses of a subsample of the European Prospective Investigation into Cancer and Nutrition (EPIC) study showed that exposure to three carcinogens [asbestos, heavy metals, and polycyclic aromatic hydrocarbons (PAH)] accounted for 14% of the socioeconomic inequalities remaining after adjustment for tobacco smoking and dietary factors. Silica and asbestos dusts, silicosis and asbestosis are associated with the development of lung cancer. Asbestos and cigarette smoke exposure act synergistically to increase the risk of lung cancer.

Arsenic has been identified as a lung carcinogen in humans. A synergistic effect of ingested arsenic and cigarette smoking on occurrence of lung cancer was also noted. Underground miners (radon exposure), textile, and wood workers are also at increased risk of developing lung cancer.

Radiation and Radon

Radon, an inert gas produced during the decay of uranium, emits alpha particles which cause DNA damage to the cells of the respiratory lining epithelium. Radon exposure in miners working underground is associated with lung cancer. Exposure to indoor radon and its decay products is also a risk factor for general population. The risk from this environmental exposure occurs in a linear dose-response relationship with no threshold. In certain areas, radon is the second important cause of lung cancer, after tobacco smoking. It is also one of the most important risk factors accounting for up to 30% of lung cancers in non-smokers.

Structural Lung Diseases

Structural lung diseases, in particular fibrosing lung diseases [idiopathic pulmonary fibrosis (IPF), scleroderma interstitial lung disease (ILD)], are considered risk factors for development of lung cancer. Patients with IPF have an increased risk of lung cancer as compared to the general population. Scleroderma-associated ILD increases the risk even in non-smokers.

Human Immunodeficiency Virus Infection

Lung cancer risk is substantially elevated in human immunodeficiency virus (HIV)-infected individuals as compared to the general population. The risk of lung cancer is unrelated to HIV-induced immunosuppression and smoking does not account for all of the increase seen in the incidence of lung cancer—the higher risk being present even after adjustment for smoking.

Genetic Factors

Familial aggregation of cases has also been documented. Several genetic polymorphisms have been shown to increase the risk of a person developing lung cancer. Some of these include polymorphisms in the genes encoding nicotinic acetylcholine receptor (NAchR), enzymes involved in xenobiotic metabolism like the glutathione S-transferase (GST), cytochrome P 450 system (CYP), and enzymes involved in DNA repair like the nucleotide excision repair gene (XPD).

Socioeconomic Status

On analysis of 64 studies, an increased risk in lung cancer incidence was observed among people with low socioeconomic profile. Lung cancer incidence was observed in three different aspects of socioeconomic profile namely (1) education, (2) occupation, and (3) income, the association being strongest for the former and weakest for the latter.

Miscellaneous Risk Factors

There is a possibility of an interaction between alcohol consumption and tobacco smoking in relation to occurrence of lung cancer. Association between hormone use and lung cancer is also likely. Divergent results were observed with a trend for higher risk among women older than or equal to 55 years and for a lower risk among women younger than this age.

MOLECULAR BIOLOGY OF LUNG CANCER

Several different molecular mechanisms may be involved in the pathogenesis of lung cancer. These mechanisms may include abnormalities in growth-stimulatory signaling pathways, tumor suppressor gene pathways, the apoptotic pathways and the epigenetic changes.

Growth Stimulatory Pathways (Tumor Oncogenes)

In some cases of NSCLC, a single specific mutated oncogene can act as the primary genetic "driver" responsible for the pathogenesis of cancer. There are three oncogenes which are of diagnostic and therapeutic interest in lung cancer (ADC); the epidermal growth factor receptor (EGFR) gene, *KRAS* gene, and the *ALK* gene.

Epidermal Growth Factor Receptor Gene Mutations

Epidermal growth factor receptor mutations are more commonly present in women, never-smokers, and East-Asians. In patients with ADC, presence of specific (sensitizing) mutations in the EGFR gene predict good response to oral EGFR tyrosine kinase inhibitors (TKIs).

KRAS Gene Mutations

KRAS mutations, known to occur in 20–30% of NSCLCs, lead to impaired GTPase activity, located downstream of EGFR. Consequently, there is constitutive activation of RAS signaling.

Anaplastic Lymphoma Kinase Translocations

ALK gene translocations are seen in up to 5% of the NSCLC, with frequency being more common (15%) in the East-Asian countries. These ALK translocations more commonly occur with 90% of the translocations seen in such patients with younger age and never or light (<10 pack years) smokers. They are seen in patients with ADC histology (solid and acinar subtypes) and in the absence of other oncogenic driver mutations such as EGFR or *KRAS*.

Tumor Angiogenesis

Angiogenesis implies the formation of new tumor-feeding blood vessels, from preexisting vasculature. It is a critical factor for the development and growth of tumors as well as for invasion and metastasis. Angiogenesis is regulated and determined by the balance between pro-angiogenic and anti-angiogenic factors released by tumor cells and adjacent host cells. With ongoing growth of tumor cells, the balance shifts in favor of the pro-angiogenic response, leading to formation of new capillaries. These new vessels are qualitatively poor (abnormal basement membranes and disorganized endothelial cells), heterogeneous and leaky.

Epigenetic Changes in Lung Cancer

Study of changes in gene expression which are caused by mechanisms other than the changes in DNA sequence is called as epigenetics. Though traditionally considered heritable, recent evidence has shown that these epigenetic changes are modifiable by environment, diet, diseases and aging. The three most common epigenetic changes are DNA methylation, modification of histone tails and the micro RNAs. These epigenetic signatures are increasingly being studied for early diagnosis of lung cancers, as prognostic markers and also for targeting specific therapies.

CHAPTER 59

Pathology of Lung Tumors

Amanjit Bal, Ashim Das

INTRODUCTION

The World Health Organization (WHO) 2004 classification of malignant epithelial lung tumors which is based purely on morphological features on hematoxylin and eosin (H&E) stained sections of resected specimens divides lung tumors into five major groups:
- Squamous cell carcinoma (SCC)
- Adenocarcinoma
- Small-cell carcinoma
- Large-cell carcinoma and
- Carcinoid tumors.

The other minor groups include *sarcomatoid carcinoma* and *salivary gland tumors*. A small group of *adenosquamous carcinoma* is also recognized. Recent updates recommend use of ancillary techniques for exact categorization of lung tumors. A standardized nomenclature and uniform criteria for diagnosis helps not only in consistency in diagnosis and treatment but also gives uniformity in epidemiologic and molecular studies.

PREINVASIVE LESIONS

Most of the malignant tumors develop through a phase of preinvasive component. The preinvasive lesions are:
- Squamous dysplasia/carcinoma in situ
- Atypical adenomatous hyperplasia (AAH) and adenocarcinoma in situ
- Diffuse idiopathic neuroendocrine cell hyperplasia.

Squamous cell carcinoma and many small-cell carcinomas may arise from these types of alterations. Basal cell hyperplasia, goblet cell hyperplasia, and squamous metaplasia are also identified as earlier changes of dysplasia/carcinoma in situ changes of squamous epithelium of central airways.

CLASSIFICATION OF LUNG CANCER

Traditionally, the epithelial tumors are divided into *non-small-cell and small-cell lung carcinoma* with a view that small-cell carcinoma has a different mode of treatment than non-small-cell carcinoma. The non-small-cell carcinoma includes squamous cell, adenocarcinoma, and large-cell carcinoma. It is now believed that non-small-cell carcinomas are heterogeneous both in molecular biology and also in treatment response.

One major change which has occurred in the 1999 WHO classification is the revision of the classification of neuroendocrine tumors and redefinition of bronchioloalveolar carcinoma. The introduction of preneoplastic process like AAH and diffuse neuroendocrine hyperplasia is also an important feature in this classification. The WHO classifications are predicated on the histological examination of the whole tumor on resected specimens. The lung adenocarcinoma is a heterogeneous form of lung cancer and most of them are histologically variable, both between cases and within individual tumor. Small biopsy samples which are routinely used may not be representative of the whole tumor and the tumor architecture cannot be appreciated in a small biopsy. The subtype accuracy for adenocarcinoma based on biopsy material is much lower than SCC. It has been found that most of the cases unclassifiable on small biopsy examination were adenocarcinoma in the surgically resected lung.

International Association for the Study of Lung Cancer, American Thoracic Society, and European Respiratory Society (IASLC/ATS/ERS) 2011, provided a new adenocarcinoma classification for uniformity in terminology and diagnostic criteria. This classification addresses the issues of both resected specimens and small nonresection cancer specimens (biopsies and cytology). The major recommendation of this classification was to discontinue the use of term "BAC" which was used for a broad spectrum of tumors like solitary small noninvasive peripheral lung tumors, invasive adenocarcinomas with minimal invasion, mixed subtype of invasive adenocarcinomas, and even for widespread advanced tumors with a low survival.

EPITHELIAL TUMORS

Squamous Cell Carcinoma

Squamous cell carcinoma typically occurs as a central mass but approximately 25% are located peripherally and 5% show central cavitation. Histologically, two features are important for diagnosis: (i) keratinization and (ii) intercellular bridges. The WHO classification recognizes four variants namely: (i) *papillary*, (ii) *clear cell*, (iii) *small cell*, and (iv) *basaloid*. The small cell variant of SCC, is a poorly differentiated variant which contains small tumor cells but retains cellular characteristics of a non-SCC, such as coarse chromatin, nucleoli, and distinct cell borders.

Adenocarcinoma

Minimally invasive adenocarcinoma: It is a small solitary adenocarcinomas with predominant lepidic growth and less than 5 mm invasion. The invasive component in minimally invasive adenocarcinoma (MIA) is defined as a histological subtype other than a lepidic pattern and the tumor cells infiltrating myofibroblastic stroma. MIAs are usually nonmucinous but rarely can be mucinous. These patients on complete resection will have 100% or near 100% disease-free survival.

Invasive adenocarcinoma: Most adenocarcinoma commonly presents as a peripheral nodule and only rarely shows cavitation. Occasional adenocarcinoma may present as a central or endobronchial tumor. Rare adenocarcinomas may produce a diffuse thickening of the visceral pleura, mimicking a mesothelioma. Histologically, a mixture of patterns is usually seen. These histological patterns may have different biological behavior with potential therapeutic applications for the patients. In fact, 80–90% of patients with adenocarcinoma show more than one histologic pattern.

Criteria for Diagnosis of Pulmonary Adenocarcinoma

- *Tumor architecture*: The form of patterns described above in an intact fragment of tumor is essential for the diagnosis of adenocarcinoma.
- *Mucin stains*: It is important to note that unequivocal SCC may also show occasional cells containing mucin and there are no unique, reliable individual cytological criteria that allow diagnosis of adenocarcinoma.
- *Immunohistochemistry*: Immunohistological approaches to refine the separation of squamous cell from adenocarcinoma are potentially valuable. Use of one adenocarcinoma marker and one squamous marker is suggested to preserve tissue for further molecular testing.

Small-cell Carcinoma

It constitutes approximately 25% of lung cancers and was also known as oat cell carcinoma or small-cell neuroendocrine carcinoma. Grossly these tumors are centrally located and show large areas of multifocal necrosis. Microscopically, in the majority of cases the bronchial or transthoracic core biopsy specimens, show an infiltrate of "small" cells with variable crush artifacts and nuclear smearing. The character of the cells should be seen in the better preserved areas. The cells have round or fusiform nuclei with stippled or ground glass chromatin and nuclear molding. Only small indistinct nuclei are seen. There can be some larger cells with large nuclei and occasional nucleoli. Abundant cytoplasm may be seen.

Large-cell Carcinoma

The WHO classifies large-cell carcinoma as a tumor of non-small cells with lack of light microscopic or histochemical evidence of glandular or squamous differentiation. These tumors are usually peripherally located with pleural and chest wall invasion. Microscopically, the tumor usually shows cohesive clusters of large or intermediate polygonal cells having abundant eosinophilic cytoplasm with large vesicular nuclei. There is always marked nuclear pleomorphism with numerous mitotic activity. The tumor cells are positive for pancytokeratin however do not show intercellular bridges or keratinization which are characteristic of SCC and are devoid of any gland formation as seen in adenocarcinoma.

Adenosquamous Carcinoma

The WHO defines a tumor as adenosquamous when both "adeno" and "squamous" components are present in a same tumor with each occupying at least 10% of total tumor areas. The origin of tumor is mostly due to its origin from a pluripotent cells with dual differentiation. The collision theory of adenocarcinoma and SCC, or squamous metaplasia of adenocarcinoma is unlikely.

NEUROENDOCRINE LESIONS OF THE LUNG

A spectrum of neuroendocrine lesions is seen in the lung. Among the pure neuroendocrine neoplasm, the recognized lesions are as follows: tumorlets, typical carcinoid, atypical carcinoid, large-cell neuroendocrine neoplasm, and small-cell carcinoma. A few non-small-cell carcinomas can show neuroendocrine differentiation. Many other tumors also have neuroendocrine properties, e.g. pulmonary blastoma, primitive neuroendocrine tumors, desmoplastic round cell tumors, etc.

- *Neuroendocrine hyperplasia*: Neuroendocrine cell hyperplasia is seen in association with fibrosis and inflammation. Diffuse hyperplasia can be noticed with or without airway fibrosis or obstruction.
- *Tumorlets* show localized proliferation of neuroendocrine cells in small airways in a background of pulmonary fibrosis or in association with bronchiectasis. This can be taken as large neuroepithelial bodies or a small typical carcinoid tumor.
- *Typical carcinoid tumor* is characterized by a large yellow tan lesion measuring 0.5 cm or more in the central bronchus immediately beneath the surface epithelium. It can occur more proximally in the trachea or in the peripheral airways. The histological features show organoid pattern with trabecular, insular, solid, and spindle cell morphology. Other histologic pattern like oncocytic, and melanocytic patterns are also seen.
- *Atypical carcinoid tumor*: These lesions are seen in the periphery of the lung in the majority of cases (60%) and are yellow-tan in color. Histologically, the tumor shows organoid pattern with prominent fibrous bands surrounding the groups of cells. The cells show more pleomorphism with increase mitotic figures and areas of necrosis.
- *Large-cell neuroendocrine carcinoma*: These tumors are located peripherally and show cytological features of non-small-cell carcinoma

having neuroendocrine features like organoid, palisading, rosettes or trabecular pattern. The cells are three times larger than the nuclear diameter of resting lymphocytes.
- *Small-cell carcinoma*: The previous WHO classification divided this tumor into three types: oat cell type, intermediate cell type and combined oat cell carcinoma. It has been observed that there were biological differences in the different subgroups. Small-cell carcinomas are centrally located and the tumors are soft and grey white with areas of multifocal necrosis. The tumors frequently metastasize to different organs.
- *Combined small cell-large cell carcinoma*: It is composed of small undifferentiated cells like small-cell carcinoma along with scattered large cells within the small cells. The large cells show variable eosinophilic cytoplasm with distinct cell border and having large vesicular nuclei and prominent nucleoli.
- *Combined small cell-non-small cell carcinoma*: It is characterized by a tumor with characteristic small cell morphology combined with a squamous carcinoma, adenocarcinoma or large cell undifferentiated carcinoma component.

STAGING OF LUNG TUMORS

An accurate staging of lung tumor is important for various reasons. It is extremely useful for treatment planning and evaluating the results of treatment; besides determination of prognosis.

Tumor Size (T Component)

It is an important prognostic indicator in the lung. The tumor diameters of 2 cm, 3 cm, 5 cm, and 7 cm are taken into account. T1a is less than or equal to 2 cm but T1b denotes greater than 2 cm but less than or equal to 3 cm. The T2 is subdivided into T2a which is greater than 3 cm but less than or equal to 5 cm whilst the T2b is designated as greater than 5 cm but less than or equal to 7 cm. The T3 tumor is greater than 7 cm.

Essential features which need discussion here are:
- *Measurement of tumor diameter*: The tumor should be measured before fixation. It is essential to subtract the adjacent region of pneumonia and atelectasis. Regions of central scarring and necrosis should be taken within the measurement of tumor.
- *Multinodularity of tumor*: In the 6th TNM staging system, the presence of additional nodules in the same lobe was classified as T4, and additional nodules in ipsilateral separate lobes were designated as M1 disease. The histology is important in two areas: the first is to distinguish synchronous primary tumors from intrapulmonary metastases and the second is changing the stage from stage IV to stage IIIA in node negative disease. This allows the clinician to consider surgery as a primary treatment option even when tumors are considered intrapulmonary metastases.

- *Differentiation of multiple primary tumors from metastases*: The multiple nodules are usually metastatic. However, if the tumor nodules are histologically different or show a totally different component in different nodules or have different cytological or stromal features or lack mediastinal lymph node metastasis or lymphatic emboli in common lymphatic drainage areas; then these nodules can be labeled as multiple synchronous primary tumors. In case of multiple primary nodules, the T status should be given maximum with the number of nodules to be mentioned either as M or actual number like T(m) or T(3).
- *Pleural invasion*: A definite pleural invasion is diagnosed when a tumor crosses the external elastic layer and can divided into (i) PL1 when it invades the elastic lamina, (ii) PL2 when it invades the mesothelial surface, and (iii) PL3 when it invades the parietal pleura/chest wall. An elastic stain is always indicated for accurate assessment of pleural invasion. When a tumor invades the pleura at the interlobar fissure and extends into the adjacent lobe, the staging remains T2.

Nodal (N) Component

N1 denotes when there is involvement of ipsilateral peribronchial, hilar, and intrapulmonary lymph nodes. N2 is designated when subcarinal and ipsilateral mediastinal lymph nodes are involved. Supraclavicular, scalene, and contralateral mediastinal lymph nodes are designated as N3.

Metastases (M) Component

When the tumor is confined to the lung, pleura, and pericardium, it is labeled as M1a but the discontinuous nodules in chest wall, diaphragm, or mediastinal structures, it is designated as M1b. The distant metastases (outside the lung or pleura) are also designated as M1b. The ipsilateral separate nodules are down staged to T4 but the contralateral nodules are to be designated as M1a.

CHAPTER 60

Lung Cancer: Clinical Manifestations

Javid Ahmad Malik

INTRODUCTION

Lung cancer produces more symptoms in adults, which include both respiratory and constitutional symptoms, than any other cancer. There are no distinct features between small cell lung cancer (SCLC) and non-small cell lung cancer (NSCLC). But the duration of symptoms of small cell cancer tends to be shorter due to its rapid dissemination to other organs.

The symptoms and signs of bronchogenic carcinoma may be caused by any of the following: the local tumor itself, invasion of the tumor into the adjacent structures, regional lymph node enlargement, growth at anatomically discontiguous sites after dissemination and effects of tumor products leading to various paraneoplastic syndromes. Accordingly, the spectrum of clinical presentation of lung cancer can be divided into: (1) local manifestations, (2) metastatic manifestations and (3) non-metastatic systemic manifestations (also called paraneoplastic syndromes). Most of the lung cancer patients in developing countries like India, compared to the patients in the developed countries, have lower mean age and advanced disease at diagnosis with 52% patients having evidence of metastases.

LOCAL MANIFESTATIONS

Hemoptysis

Although the cardinal symptom of lung cancer, particularly in an elderly smoker, hemoptysis is neither the most common feature nor diagnostic of cancer. Hemoptysis is one specific symptom that prompts rapid consultation from the physician. It is usually caused by bronchial mucosal ulceration, thus tends to be scanty. However, if the tumor erodes the bronchial artery or the pulmonary artery, hemoptysis may be massive resulting in potentially fatal hemodynamic or airway compromise. Chest radiographs are usually abnormal in patients with hemoptysis; but, in a small percentage of patients, it may be normal.

Cough

Development of new cough or a recent increase in the preexisting chronic productive cough in a middle-aged smoker raises suspicion of lung cancer. Appearance of new symptoms of cough that persist for more than 2 weeks should be considered as suspicious of malignancy in smokers of more than 35 years of age. Cough is the most common initial symptom present in more than 65% patients; productive cough is seen in about 25% patients. A change in the character of an established cough may actually point to the development of lung cancer.

Bronchorrhea, i.e. expectoration of large amounts of mucoid sputum, is present in 10% of patients who have some variants of invasive adenocarcinoma (formerly known as BAC or bronchioloalveolar carcinoma). Endobronchial tumors cause cough either by airway obstruction and its associated postobstructive pneumonia or by bronchial mucosal ulceration, whereas peripheral tumors cause cough primarily by pleural involvement.

Breathlessness

Dyspnea in patients with lung cancer can occur due to several causes as below:
- Direct lung involvement by the tumor (major airway obstruction, consolidation, carcinomatous lymphangitis)
- Indirect respiratory complications of the tumor (postobstructive pneumonia, pleural effusion, phrenic nerve paralysis)
- Treatment-related problems (anemia or radiation and chemotherapy-induced lung toxicity)
- Respiratory complications (pulmonary embolism and lung infections)
- Comorbid conditions (COPD, asthma, heart failure, prior lung resection, pericardial effusion and malnutrition).

Some patients of lung cancer have no obvious cause of breathlessness but may have significant respiratory muscle weakness, due to general weight loss and the muscle deconditioning of advanced illness.

Chest Pain

An ill-defined chest discomfort which is intermittent and aching in quality is common in bronchogenic carcinoma, occurs in up to 50% of patients at diagnosis. Direct spread of the tumor to the pleural surface causes pleuritic pain. This is commonly seen with peripheral neoplasms (adenocarcinoma or large-cell carcinoma) because of their tendency to seed pleura. The pain may be severe and continuous that also interferes with sleep once the malignancy spreads beyond the pleura into the chest wall. Local extension of the tumor from the apex of the lung (superior sulcus tumor) to eighth cervical, first and second thoracic nerves is responsible for shoulder pain that typically radiates along the ulnar distribution of arm may (Pancoast's syndrome).

METASTATIC MANIFESTATIONS

Intrathoracic Metastasis

Superior Vena Cava Syndrome

Symptoms of superior vena cava syndrome (SVCS) are often debilitating, tend to get exacerbated in supine position, include progressive swelling of neck, face, eyelids, arms and upper chest, conjunctival congestion, epistaxis, tinnitus, headache, disturbances in vision and sensorium. Neck veins are distended and nonpulsatile, well-developed collaterals are usually obvious on neck and anterior chest wall. SVC obstruction may get complicated with jugular venous and cerebrovascular thrombosis.

Malignant Pleural Effusion

Pleural effusions that occur due to direct pleural involvement occur in 7–15% of lung cancer patients. In addition, there may be paramalignant effusions that are not the direct result of malignant involvement of the pleura. Paramalignant pleural effusions occur due to various other complications of lung cancer such as postobstructive pneumonia, pulmonary embolism and infarction, chylothorax due to obstruction of the thoracic duct, radiation therapy and chemotherapy. Pleural effusion in lung cancer can sometimes develop due to concurrent nonmalignant disorders like congestive heart failure, renal disease or hypoproteinemia.

Recurrent Laryngeal Nerve Palsy

Recurrent laryngeal nerve, most commonly the left, is involved in 2–18% of lung cancer patients. Left recurrent laryngeal nerve is commonly involved due to entrapment by the tumor or by the metastatic mediastinal lymph nodes, as it passes over the left main bronchus and loops around the aortic arch. It results in paralysis of vocal cord which produces hoarseness of voice and cough. The cough lacks explosive quality of normal cough (bovine cough) and is associated with poor expectoration of tracheobronchial secretions and an increased risk of aspiration.

Phrenic Nerve Paralysis

Diaphragmatic paralysis may complicate lung cancer due to phrenic nerve entrapment by the tumor in the mediastinum. In unilateral phrenic nerve dysfunction, the patient may not have any specific symptom except for the elevated hemidiaphragm incidentally discovered on the chest radiograph.

In bilateral phrenic nerve paralysis, patients are severely symptomatic, have orthopnea and a downhill disease course.

Pancoast's Syndrome

Pancoast's syndrome results due to involvement of lower part of brachial plexus due to local extension of an apical lung cancer tumor. Pancoast tumor is also known as thoracic inlet or superior sulcus tumor. Typically, the syndrome is characterized by pain in the lower part of shoulder and inner aspect of arm along C8, T1 and T2 distribution. There is associated sensory loss, weakness and wasting of the small muscles of hand. Incomplete forms of the Pancoast's syndrome are also seen in clinical practice. Radiologically, in addition to the apical lung mass, Pancoast tumor is often characterized by the destruction of first and second ribs posteriorly and sometimes of transverse process or vertebral body. In anterior superior sulcus tumor, the predominant complaint is chest pain; the imaging studies reveal destruction of anterior ends of first and second ribs and invasion of subclavian vessels.

Horner's Syndrome

Horner's syndrome is a classical presentation of an apical (superior sulcus) tumor which invades the stellate ganglion formed by the fusion of lower cervical and first thoracic ganglia. Horner's syndrome comprises the following clinical components: ipsilateral ptosis, miosis, enophthalmos and lack of facial sweating (anhidrosis). Application of topical cocaine to the miotic eye fails to cause pupillary dilatation, while appropriate dilatation is noted in the unaffected eye. Horner's syndrome is usually a complication of superior sulcus lung tumor, but may very rarely complicate spontaneous pneumothorax that produces mediastinal shift and consequent mechanical traction of the sympathetic ganglion.

Involvement of Heart and Pericardium

Cardiac and pericardial metastases from bronchogenic carcinoma usually occur by direct lymphatic spread. In lung cancer, cardiac involvement with pericardium as the most common site is reported in 15% of the cases at autopsy.

Involvement of Esophagus

Dysphagia due to esophageal compression by massively enlarged metastatic hilar and mediastinal nodes is an unusual clinical feature of lung cancer and is generally a late symptom.

Extrathoracic Metastasis

Metastases from lung cancer may occur in virtually every organ system but are more common in brain, bones, liver, adrenal glands and lymph nodes. Extrathoracic spread of bronchogenic carcinoma makes a patient clearly inoperable. Metastatic spread is more common with small cell than with non-small cell lung cancer.

Brain Metastases

Lung cancer is the most common primary site for brain metastases. Squamous cell lung cancer metastasizes to brain less often than adenocarcinoma and large cell carcinomas. Sometimes, brain metastases form the only extrathoracic site of spread of lung cancer. Intracranial metastatic lung cancer usually presents with headache, nausea and vomiting, rarely with impaired intellectual function or personality changes. Seizures and motor or sensory neurological deficits may occur. Progressive neurological symptoms in cerebral metastases usually complicate the widespread disease. Rarely, brain metastases are detected when primary bronchogenic carcinoma is asymptomatic and radiological examination of the chest is normal.

Skeletal Metastases

Bronchogenic carcinoma frequently metastasizes to vertebrae and ribs; however, any bone in the body may be involved. Bony metastases usually produce pain which is invariably progressive. If the ribs are involved, pain gets aggravated by coughing and body movement. Skeletal metastases may also lead to pathological fractures. When bone marrow is invaded by metastatic lung cancer, it leads to cytopenias or leukoerythroblastosis.

Spinal Cord Compression

Epidural or vertebral metastases are rare but may complicate lung cancer producing an oncologic emergency. Such patients need immediate assessment by a neurologist. When present, spinal cord metastases are usually associated with cerebral metastases.

Adrenal Metastases

Involvement of adrenal glands by metastatic lung cancer, usually by small cell carcinoma, is common but rarely produces adrenal insufficiency. Solitary adrenal metastasis if resected along with primary lung tumor has a better prognosis with a 3-year survival rate of 38%.

Lymph Node Metastases

Enlarged metastatic lymph nodes are quite helpful in making diagnosis and facilitate staging of lung cancer. Supraclavicular lymph nodes are the most common sites seen in 15–20% of patients during the course of the illness.

Hepatic Metastases

Liver metastases occur commonly with lung cancer and their presence carries a very poor prognosis. Patient usually complains of fatigue and weight loss; on physical examination the liver is hard and irregularly enlarged. However, liver function tests are impaired only when the metastases are numerous and large. Both ultrasonography and CT scan are equally good in picking up hepatic metastases, a finding that makes the patient inoperable.

Paraneoplastic Syndromes

A number of clinical syndromes are known to be associated with malignant diseases but are not directly related to the primary or metastatic tumors. These paraneoplastic syndromes occur in 10% of patients with lung cancer. The mechanisms for paraneoplastic syndromes are not fully understood. It is likely that there is production of biologically active substances (e.g. polypeptide hormones or cytokines) by the tumor. There is impact of the size of the primary tumor with the severity of paraneoplastic symptoms. Sometimes, the paraneoplastic syndromes precede the diagnosis of malignant disease by months, or even years. More commonly, they occur late in the course of the illness or herald the first sign of recurrence of lung cancer. Paraneoplastic syndromes are more commonly seen with small cell cancers but can be present with any histological type. Paraneoplastic syndromes may simulate metastatic cancer thereby leading to inappropriate palliation rather than curative treatment of the underlying tumor. With successful treatment of lung cancer, the paraneoplastic phenomena usually resolve.

ENDOCRINE SYNDROMES

Cushing's Syndrome

Cushing syndrome present in 1–5% of patients with SCLC may be caused by ectopic production of corticotropin releasing hormone which leads to excessive ACTH secretion from the pituitary gland. Patients with small cell lung cancer usually do not develop the classical features because of a shorter lifespan. Diagnosis is usually suggested by features of acute hypercortisolism such as hypertension, hyperglycemia and hypokalemic alkalosis. Muscle weakness associated with hypokalemia, may be profound. Proximal myopathy and edema are commonly found on physical examination.

Hypercalcemia

Overall, 10% patients of lung cancer have hypercalcemia, which usually complicates squamous cell carcinoma that secretes parathyroid hormone-related peptide (PTH-rP). The diagnosis of PTH-rP associated paraneoplastic syndrome is considered if serum calcium level exceeds 10.5 mg/dL. Hypercalcemia initially produces nausea, vomiting, constipation, polyuria and nocturia resulting in hypovolemia and renal failure. As serum calcium goes up, the patient may become confused, and drowsy and ultimately, coma may supervene misleading the physician toward intracranial metastases. The clinical behavior of PTH-rP associated paraneoplastic syndrome is highly unpredictable, the patient may present with subtle symptoms or as medical emergency.

Syndrome of Inappropriate Antidiuretic Hormone

Syndrome of inappropriate antidiuretic hormone (SIADH) is more commonly associated with small cell lung cancer and occasionally present in other malignant tumors. ADH excess causes abnormal water retention, hyponatremia and low plasma osmolality. Urinary loss of sodium continues at a level inappropriate for plasma sodium concentration which results in urinary osmolality twice as high as concomitant plasma osmolality. In a patient of lung carcinoma with euvolemic hypo-osmolar hyponatremia, diagnosis of SIADH is made by the measurement of plasma and urinary osmolality.

Like for any other paraneoplastic phenomenon, the treatment of SIADH consists that of the underlying tumor. Other measures which may be effective to counter hyponatremia while awaiting the effects of chemotherapy include strict fluid restriction (i.e. 500 mL/day), which alone may be sufficient to maintain serum sodium above 128 mEq/L. If patient does not comply with fluid restriction or if it does not prove effective, demeclocycline, which blocks the action of vasopressin in the renal tubule, is used in a daily oral dose of 600–1,200 mg. Severe symptomatic hyponatremia is treated with hypertonic saline (3%) along with intravenous loop diuretic that enhance net free-water clearance. Sodium level should not be raised by more than 2 mEq/hour because it may lead to central pontine myelinolysis, an acute neurologic catastrophe. Unlike ectopic ACTH production, SIADH does not worsen the prognosis of small cell cancer.

Acromegaly

These patients develop thick leathery skin, prominent skin folds, hypertrophy of face and extremities and sometimes diabetes and hypertension. Increased plasma levels of GHRH and insulin like growth factor-1 (IGF-1) in the presence of a lung tumor, virtually establish the diagnosis. Lung cancer-related acromegaly promptly responds to surgical resection as well as to radiotherapy. Patients, who are not eligible for resection or irradiation, should receive octreotide, which inhibits GHRH secretion from the tumor and decreases GH and IGF-1 levels in the serum.

NEUROLOGICAL SYNDROMES

A number of poorly understood neurological syndromes have been described in about 5% of lung cancer patients, almost exclusively in small cell carcinoma. Some of the reported syndromes include Lambert–Eaton myasthenic syndrome (LEMS) and limbic encephalopathy. A number of other neurodegenerative diseases such as polyneuropathy, cerebellar degeneration, retinopathy, opsoclonus–myoclonus and autonomic neuropathy have also been described. There is no relationship of the tumor size with the severity of neurologic symptoms. They are more often seen in patients with limited disease. The primary malignant disease in some patients may remain undetected before death despite the presence of disabling neurological symptoms.

The diagnosis of a neurologic syndrome should, however, be made only after other possible causes are carefully excluded. Some of these manifestations may occur due to concurrent metabolic abnormalities such as electrolyte imbalance or other complications, like cerebral and spinal vascular disease, infections and drug toxicity. Presence of metastatic disease may also cause symptoms mimicking the neurological syndromes. These neurological symptoms often progress. The response of the neurologic syndrome to an effective chemotherapy is highly variable.

Eaton–Lambert Syndrome

These patients usually present with fatigue, dysphagia, dysarthria, visual blurring, muscle aches and weakness of pelvic girdle muscles. Unlike in myasthenia gravis, muscle weakness in LEMS is worse in the morning and improves during the day with exercise. Usually, there is no improvement with anticholinestrases. Extraocular muscle involvement is uncommon but ptosis may be often seen. There is increased muscle action potential with repeated nerve stimulation on electromyography. Demonstration of IgG autoantibodies in the serum of patients with small cell lung cancer confirms the diagnosis of Eaton–Lambert syndrome.

Eaton–Lambert syndrome usually resolves with chemotherapy of small cell carcinoma. If treatment of lung tumor does not improve neuromuscular weakness, remission may be induced with azathioprine, intravenous gamma globulin, diaminopyridine or plasma exchange.

Encephalomyelitis and Sensory Neuropathy

These patients may present with progressive sensory loss in hands and feet, myelopathy, brainstem involvement or features of limbic encephalopathy including behavioral changes, memory loss or convulsions. Autonomic neuropathy resulting in postural hypotension or gastrointestinal motility disturbances may also occur.

Paraneoplastic Cerebellar Degeneration

Some patients of small cell lung cancer develop cerebellar degeneration leading to nystagmus, impaired coordination and ataxia. These patients have anti-Hu antibodies in serum and frequently tend to develop encephalitis or sensory neuropathy.

Cancer-associated Retinopathy

It is a rare paraneoplastic syndrome that occurs as the first sign of occult small cell carcinoma of lung. Clinically, these patients have photosensitivity, rapid loss of vision, night blindness, visual field defects and arteriolar narrowing. In a given clinical setting, demonstration of anti-recoverin antibody establishes the diagnosis of cancer-associated retinopathy.

Opsoclonus and Myoclonus

This rare paraneoplastic syndrome is associated with both small cell and non-small cell lung cancers. The patient shows rapid involuntary conjugate eye movements in both the horizontal and the vertical directions. Some SCLC patients with this syndrome have anti-Hu antibody in serum.

HEMATOLOGICAL SYNDROMES

Granulocytosis

Granulocytosis with absolute white cell count of 10,000–25,000 occurs in 20% patients of non-small cell lung cancer. The increase in total white cell count may also be associated with neutrophilia and eosinophilia. Bone marrow biopsy is usually normal. Diagnosis is made on exclusion, granulocytosis per se does not produce any symptom in these patients.

Thrombocytosis

Paraneoplastic thrombocytosis is a common phenomenon observed in 40% patients of both small cell and non-small cell carcinomas. Like granulocytosis, lung cancer-associated thrombocytosis is asymptomatic, diagnosed if bone marrow biopsy is normal and platelet count exceeds 500,000/mm.

Thromboembolism

The pathogenetic basis of lung cancer-associated venous thromboembolism is not known, no proteins or cytokines have been linked to it. It can complicate both non-small cell and small cell cancers of lung. Trousseau's syndrome or recurrent migratory venous thrombophlebitis is more commonly associated with bronchogenic carcinoma than pancreatic or other gastrointestinal cancers. Isolated venous thrombosis is treated with oral warfarin, but long-term heparin is more effective than warfarin in recurrent thrombosis (Trousseau's syndrome).

SKELETAL

Digital Clubbing and Hypertrophic Osteoarthropathy

Digital clubbing is reported in about a third of patients more commonly among women. Hypertrophic pulmonary osteoarthropathy (HPOA) that is generally seen in stage IV clubbing is seen in 10% patients of NSCLC. Overexpression of vascular endothelial growth factor (VEGF) is one of the mechanisms postulated to be responsible for the development of clubbing and HPOA. Active deposition of new bone can be seen along the inner aspect of periosteum on bone scans. Usually, HPOA responds well to surgical resection of the primary lung tumor. In unresectable tumors, corticosteroids and nonsteroidal anti-inflammatory drugs are used for symptomatic relief. For symptom relief, vagotomy can also be done, if thoracotomy is undertaken with an attempt to cure.

MISCELLANEOUS SYNDROMES

There are various other unusual paraneoplastic syndromes known to be associated with bronchogenic carcinoma: renal (glomerulonephritis, nephrotic syndrome), vasculitic (systemic lupus erythematosus), systemic (fever, anorexia, cachexia) and metabolic (hypouricemia, lactic acidosis). Rarely, cutaneous manifestations such as dermatomyositis-polymyositis, scleroderma, acanthosis nigricans, papillary dermatosis, erythema gyratum repens, erythema multiforme, exfoliative dermatitis, Sweet syndrome, pruritus and urticaria can be present. Adenocarcinoma and large cell bronchogenic carcinoma are known to be associated with gynecomastia due to tumor cell production of human chorionic gonadotropin, which results in overproduction of testicular estrogen.

CHAPTER 61

Diagnosis and Staging of Lung Cancer

Nagarjuna V Maturu, Ajmal Khan, Navneet Singh

INTRODUCTION

The concept of staging in malignant disease originated from the historical observation that survival rates were better for patients with a localized tumor as compared to those with advanced disease. The lung cancer staging system is aimed at providing a common basis for categorization of the extent of disease, plan of treatment, estimation of prognosis, and ultimately for comparison of results of different treatment modalities on overall survival. Delay in the initial diagnostic workup can affect the stage, therefore, reducing this delay could increase the detection of potentially resectable tumors and, ultimately, patient survival.

DIAGNOSIS OF LUNG CANCER

Clinical Assessment

Clinical evaluation consists of a good history and physical examination. It should also be followed by tissue diagnosis and the information obtained on initial clinical evaluation is utilized to guide further testing.

Most patients complain of symptoms related to the primary tumor or its intrathoracic spread. Additionally, symptoms related to distant metastasis, paraneoplastic syndromes (Box 61.1) and/or nonspecific systemic symptoms, such as fatigue, weight loss, and generalized weakness may be present. Less than 10% of lung cancer patients are asymptomatic at presentation. Paraneoplastic syndromes are not directly related to the size or physical effects of primary or metastatic tumors. These occur in up to 10% of patients with

> **BOX 61.1:** Partial list of paraneoplastic syndromes associated with lung cancer.
>
> *Endocrine disorder:*
> - Syndrome of inappropriate secretion of antidiuretic hormone (SIADH)
> - Nonmetastatic hypercalcemia
> - Cushing syndrome
> - Gynecomastia
> - Hypercalcitonemia
> - Hypoglycemia
> - Hyperthyroidism
> - Carcinoid syndrome
>
> *Neurological syndromes:*
> - Subacute sensory neuropathy
> - Mononeuritis multiplex
> - Intestinal pseudo-obstruction
> - LEMS
> - Encephalomyelitis
> - Necrotizing myelopathy
> - Cancer-associated retinopathy
>
> *Skeletal disorders:*
> - Hypertrophic osteoarthropathy
> - Clubbing
>
> *Systemic syndromes:*
> - Anorexia and cachexia
> - Fever
>
> *Cutaneous:*
> - Acquired hypertrichosis lanuginosa
> - Erythema gyratum repens
> - Erythema multiforme
> - Tylosis
> - Erythroderma
> - Exfoliative dermatitis
> - Acanthosis nigricans
> - Pruritus and urticaria
>
> (LEMS, Lambert–Eaton myasthenic syndrome)

lung cancer due to the production of biologically active substances, such as polypeptide hormones, antibodies, or cytokines. Occasionally, one or more of these may precede the diagnosis of malignant disease, and at other times, may occur later during the course of illness or may even herald the first sign of recurrence.

Radiological Assessment

Initial chest radiograph plays a pivotal role in the recognition of lung cancer that may present as a straightforward spiculated mass, but its presence may also be inferred from other appearances, such as an unresolved pneumonia or lobar collapse. However, the radiographic appearance may be quite variable.

About 40% of chest radiographic appearances of lung cancer are related to the central tumors causing airway obstruction with secondary atelectasis and consolidation.

It is of great help compare the radiological lesions with old X-ray films, if these are available. Typically, the benign lesions have a longer doubling time of growth. Malignant nodules have a doubling time between 40 days and 360 days, while the benign have a prolonged period of more than 16 months. A 2-year stability of size is highly suggestive of a benign lesion. Nodule characteristics such as the presence of speculated margins may also favor malignant etiology.

Establishing a Diagnosis

Tissue diagnosis can be pursued best with sputum cytology or bronchoscopy, if the lesion is located centrally, and a transthoracic needle aspiration (TTNA), if the lesion is peripheral. A positive result from sputum cytology, bronchoscopy, or TTNA should be considered reliable because false-positive results typically have been reported to be less than 2%. Although these modalities are useful in confirming the diagnosis, the false-negative rate for all three has not been well defined, or remains too high to rule out the diagnosis effectively. Therefore, if the clinical suspicion for lung cancer diagnosis remains high, additional evaluation is usually required after a negative test result. In such cases for early diagnosis, special attention may be given to modern techniques like autofluorescence bronchoscopy (AFB) and electromagnetic navigation.

In patients with simultaneous pleural effusion, diagnostic thoracentesis should be considered. The sensitivity of pleural fluid cytology is only 60%, which increases to 80% with three separate fluid specimens and, therefore, a minimum of three samples should be evaluated by an experienced cytologist.

Once the tissue diagnosis has been achieved, the final component of the diagnostic assessment is a functional evaluation of the patient, including overall evaluation using performance status scales and evaluation for specific pulmonary status.

STAGING OF NONSMALL-CELL LUNG CANCER

Staging is done with TNM system in suspected nonsmall-cell lung cancer (NSCLC). The overall survival is the major determinant of T, N, and M descriptors. Clinical staging helps determine the next appropriate step in therapy, such as the decision to proceed with pathologic staging.

Primary Tumor Staging (T Staging)

The T stage of a tumor is defined by the local spread of the primary tumor. A computed tomography (CT) scan of the chest is the primary imaging modality for the assessment of T stage of tumor. The main disadvantages of CT chest include inability to differentiate the tumor mass from surrounding atelectasis, difficulty in defining the invasion of pleura, chest wall, and the mediastinum. In patients being considered for surgical resection, flexible bronchoscopy, if performed, will determine the proximal bronchial extent of the tumor. A distance of at least 2 cm from carina is necessary for pneumonectomy to be considered. A fused positron emission tomography (PET)/CT scan is more accurate than a CT chest for determining the T stage of the tumor. PET scan, if performed to determine the spread of disease outside the thorax, may be used to determine the T stage of the tumor. Similarly, magnetic resonance imaging (MRI) may be used in specific situations like superior sulcus tumors.

Mediastinal Staging (N Staging)

Mediastinal involvement is the threshold at which curative therapy may be implemented (IIIA is potentially curable while IIIB is generally not). Mediastinal lymph nodes are already present in 30–40% of patients at the time of diagnosis. Mediastinal lymph node staging can be achieved by noninvasive (imaging) and invasive (sampling) procedures.

Noninvasive Methods

Noninvasive imaging with the help of *chest radiography and CT of the chest* is the usual modality for clinical staging to know about the metastases in the regional lymph nodes. CT scan tends to both understage and overstage status of mediastinal lymph nodes. Even if the CT criteria are met for malignant nodes, there is still a need to prove by biopsy or resection that the nodes are truly malignant. *PET scanning* with [18F]-fluoro-2-deoxy-D-glucose (FDG) is most helpful to stage the disease, assess the treatment response and prognosis. Integrated PET/CT is better than either investigation done individually.

Invasive Mediastinal Staging

In many clinical situations, confirmation of the status of these nodes by an invasive test is necessary (especially when a curative treatment like surgical resection or concurrent chemoradiotherapy is being considered). These can be broadly classified into two groups:
- Mediastinoscopy
- Endosonographic procedures.

Invasive staging is helpful for both diagnosis of malignancy and its staging. The decision to use different investigations, however, depends upon several factors such as the following:
- Availability and expertise of different procedures at a given center/institution
- Location of lymph nodes to be assessed for histopathological/cytological examination
- Patient's general medical condition including performance status and comorbidities
- Morbidity and mortality of invasive procedures.

TABLE 61.1: Clinical pointers of metastatic malignancy.

History, examination, and investigations	Site of metastasis	Radiological investigation needed
Focal bony pain, bone tenderness, elevated serum calcium, ALP	Bone	Radioisotope (Tc99) bone scan; PET scan
Headache, focal neurological deficit, seizures, syncope, altered sensorium, projectile vomiting, focal neurological signs, papilledema	Brain	Contrast-enhanced MRI brain; contrast-enhanced CT head
Abdominal pain, hepatomegaly, elevated ALP, GGT	Liver	Ultrasound abdomen; CT abdomen; PET scan
Weakness, anorexia, vomiting, hyponatremia, hyperkalemia	Adrenal	Ultrasound abdomen; CT abdomen; PET scan
Soft-tissue mass	Muscles/skin	None

(CT, computed tomography; PET, positron emission tomography; MRI, magnetic resonance imaging; ALP, alkaline phosphatase; GGT, gamma-glutamyl transpeptidase)

Metastases (M) Staging

Approximately 30% of NSCLC patients have metastatic disease at presentation. The common sites for metastases in NSCLC are the brain, bone, liver, and the adrenals. The search for metastatic disease in a patient with NSCLC begins with accurate history and clinical examination (Table 61.1). The negative-predictive value of the clinical evaluation is high (>95%) to forego further diagnostic workup, if the clinical evaluation is negative. Radiological evaluation of metastasis is limited by the fact that it can only pick up macrometastases and not the micrometastases. The conventional workup for metastatic disease included CT of the upper abdomen, radionuclide bone scan, and MRI brain. PET/CT is most helpful to detect both intra- and extrathoracic metastases with a single test. It does not, however, diagnose brain metastases.

STAGING OF SMALL-CELL LUNG CANCER

Staging for small-cell lung cancer (SCLC) was traditionally done as limited disease (LD) or extensive disease (ED). LD implies disease restricted to one hemithorax (with or without regional lymph nodes and pleural effusion on the same side) therefore amenable to radiation with a single radiation port. Lately, it has been shown that use of the 7th and 8th editions of the TNM staging can prognosticate patients more accurately than the traditional system. For management purposes, the role of surgical resection is limited to patients with T1-T2 N0 M0 disease in case of SCLC. Invasive procedures of the mediastinum are meant for diagnostic purposes more than for staging. It is recommended to do CT scan of the thorax and upper abdomen, MRI of brain, and bone scan for complete workup of SCLC. Because of financial and logistic issues, MRI brain is used in select cases where the clinical evaluation is suggestive of brain involvement. There is only limited data on the role of PET scan in the management of SCLC patients. A whole body PET scan when performed in LD patients can help in radiation planning and also upstage the disease in up to 10% of the patients. Further studies are needed before the routine use of PET can be recommended in patients with SCLC.

CHAPTER 62

Approach to Management of Lung Cancer in India

Navneet Singh, Nagarjuna V Maturu, Digambar Behera

INTRODUCTION

Despite the various advances in the treatment options, overall prognosis of lung cancer is highly disappointing. The 5-year survival is seen in less than 15% cases with best of treatment. With the advent of targeted agents, it is equally important to confirm the exact histological subtype of lung cancer as well as its molecular profile.

In addition to staging the tumor, it is of paramount importance to also evaluate the patient for his/her ability to tolerate the treatment being planned. In patients being planned for surgical resection, a detailed workup should also be undertaken to evaluate their cardiopulmonary fitness. Spirometry, and if needed, diffusion capacity of the lung and, sometimes, cardiopulmonary exercise testing may be required to assess the pulmonary reserve of the patient. Similarly, a detailed cardiac evaluation would be needed prior to the surgery. Prior to initiating chemotherapy or radiotherapy, a baseline complete blood count and a biochemical profile (including renal and liver function tests, and blood sugars) are needed to decide on the optimal chemotherapy regimen and also to pick up asymptomatic abnormalities which may need to be corrected/monitored prior to initiating the treatment.

TREATMENT OF LUNG CANCER

A general outline for the management of NSCLC and SCLC is provided in Flowcharts 62.1 to 62.3. Management of patients with lung cancer involves

Flowchart 62.1: Surgical resection: The treatment of choice for stages I and II non-small cell lung cancer (NSCLC).

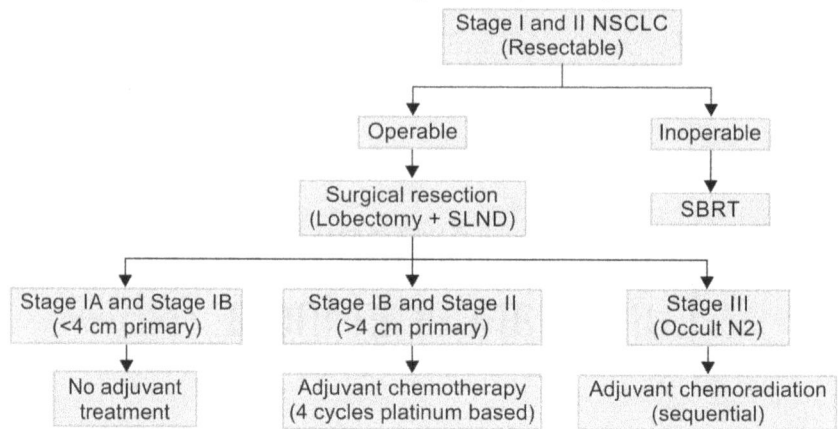

Note: Any patient with positive resection margins (R1-R2) needs adjuvant radiation therapy
SLND, systematic lymph node dissection; SBRT, stereotactic body radiation therapy

Flowchart 62.2: Approach to a patient with non-small cell lung cancer (NSCLC).

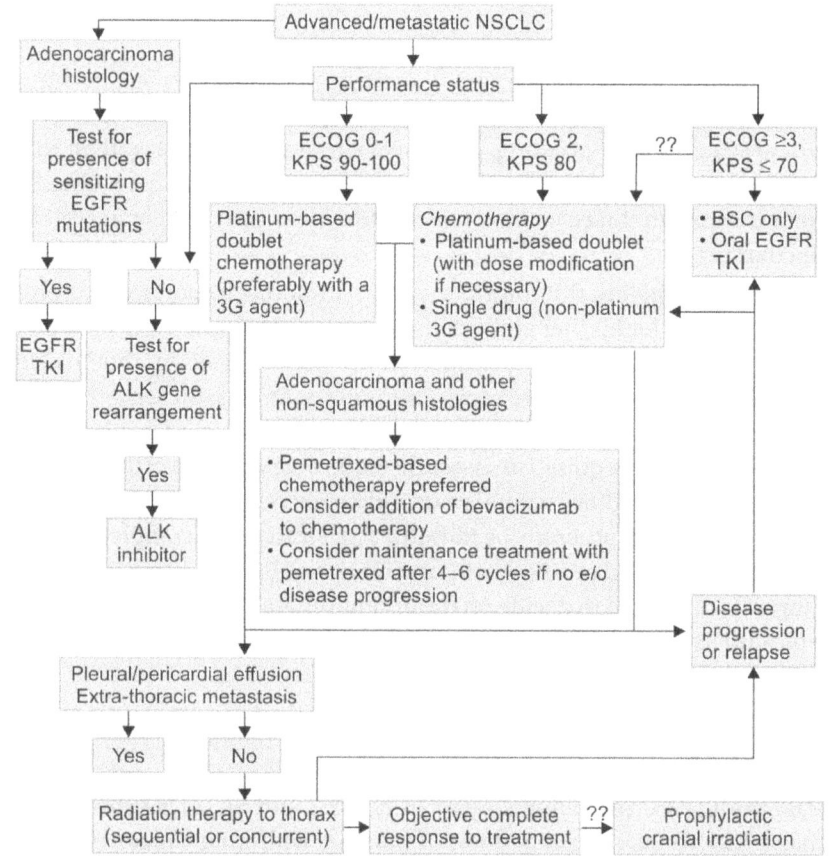

Flowchart 62.3: Approach to a patient with small cell lung cancer.

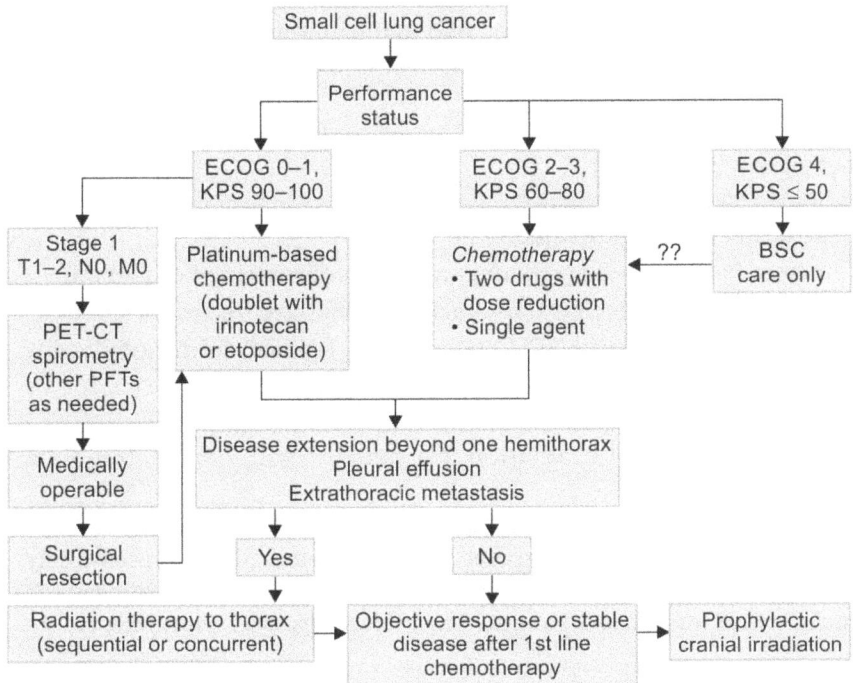

a multimodality approach. The various modalities available for treatment of lung cancer include the following:
- Surgical resection
- Radiotherapy
- Chemotherapy
- Molecular-targeted agents
- Immunotherapy.

Depending on the stage of the cancer and the performance status of the patient, these modalities are used either alone or in combination with either curative or palliative intent. In addition to these primary modalities, it is equally important to focus on palliation of patients' symptoms.

Surgical Resection (Flowchart 62.1)

Surgical resection is the treatment of choice for stage I and II NSCLC (T1–3 and N0–1) in patients with no preoperative mediastinal involvement. Surgery may be considered in a select subgroup of patients with stage IIIA disease, those with T3N1M0 disease or those with discrete and non-bulky single station N2 disease. In patients with preoperatively detected discrete and non-bulky N2 disease, adjuvant chemotherapy to downstage the tumor may be tried prior to surgical resection. Similarly, in a very select subset of patients with stage IV disease, i.e. those with resectable primary tumor and a solitary resectable metastasis, resection of both the primary and the metastatic site may be considered.

Radiotherapy

Radiation therapy (RT) is an integral part in the multimodality management of patients with lung cancers, both NSCLC as well as SCLC. The indication of RT in treatment of NSCLC includes:
- Curative intent RT in early stage lung cancer (when tumor is resectable but patient inoperable)
- Adjuvant RT (in tumors with R1–R2 resection margins or patients with N2 disease detected during surgery)
- Chemoradiation (for stage III lung cancer)—concurrent or sequential
- Palliative RT (thoracic or extrathoracic) in metastatic/recurrent NSCLC.

Similarly, for patients with SCLC, radiotherapy is beneficial in the following settings:
- Concurrent chemoradiation (for limited disease SCLC)
- Prophylactic cranial irradiation (for patients with partial/complete response LD-SCLC)
- *Palliative RT (thoracic or extrathoracic) in ED or recurrent SCLC*: Patients with metastatic/recurrent lung cancers with symptomatic focal disease may be considered for palliative radiation. Some of the common indications include CNS metastases, painful bony metastases, SVC syndrome, etc.

Chemotherapy

Almost all types of NSCLC are treated with platinum-based chemotherapy usually along with a third generation chemotherapy agent. For advanced/metastatic NSCLC without any driver (targetable) mutations/rearrangements, the current standard of care is chemotherapy. The greatest evidence is for the use of a platinum-based doublet. Chemotherapy for lung cancer is given in the following clinical scenarios:
- As adjuvant therapy following surgical resection (Stages IB and II)
- As neoadjuvant therapy to down stage the tumors before surgical resection (Stage IIIA)
- Along with radiotherapy (concurrent or sequential) in locally advanced lung cancer (Stage IIIA and IIIB)
- Palliative chemotherapy in metastatic lung cancer (Stage IV)

Chemotherapy when given for locally advanced and metastatic lung cancer can be further classified as first-line, maintenance and second-line chemotherapy.
- *First-line chemotherapy*: Chemotherapy given in a treatment of naïve patient is called the first-line chemotherapy. It is usually given for 4–6 cycles.
- *Maintenance chemotherapy*: Continuation of chemotherapy beyond 4–6 cycles at a lower intensity (usually single agent) in patients with stable or responsive disease. Maintenance therapy is given either as a continuation therapy (one or more drugs of the first-line regimen at a lower dose) or

switch maintenance, i.e. introduction of a new drug not included in the first-line regimen.
- *Second-line chemotherapy*: Second-line chemotherapy consists of an alternative treatment in patients with disease-progression on first-line therapy.
- *Adjuvant chemotherapy*: Because of the high risk of relapse (up to 70%), even in patients with completely resected tumors, adjuvant chemotherapy (ACT) is used to control the systemic micrometastases and decrease this systemic relapse and improve overall survival (OS). Most of the guidelines now recommend the use of any cisplatin-based regimen for adjuvant chemotherapy in stages II and IIIA. When given in the adjuvant setting, chemotherapy is started 4–6 weeks after the surgery and is generally given for up to four cycles.

    An oral chemotherapy drug, tegafur-uracil (the prodrug of fluorouracil) has been extensively studied as an adjuvant chemotherapeutic agent in Japanese patients. Two meta-analyses have shown that this drug improves the survival even in patients with stage I tumors though the benefit is mainly restricted to patients with adenocarcinoma.
- *Neoadjuvant chemotherapy:* Neoadjuvant chemotherapy (NACT) also has been studied in early as well as locally advanced lung cancers. Adjuvant therapy has become the standard of care in early stage lung cancer (stages I and II) because of the concern of disease progression while on NACT and the possibility of patient becoming inoperable due to the side effects of the chemotherapy regimens. The role of NACT followed by surgery in stage IIIA NSCLC patients is subject to debate since stage IIIA disease reflects a heterogeneous group. The gold standard in such patients remains definitive chemoradiation.

Chemoradiation for Locally Advanced Lung Cancer (Stage III)

Combined chemotherapy and radiation therapy (chemoradiation) is the current standard of care for patients with stage III lung cancer whose tumor is not fit for resection. This includes most patients of stage IIIB and also those with IIIA whose disease is deemed to be unsuitable for surgical resection. A meta-analysis of trials has shown chemoradiation to be superior to radiotherapy alone. Chemoradiation can either be given concurrently or sequentially. As radiation to the lung is delivered in fractions over 50–60 days, concurrent chemoradiation usually lasts 2 months and patients usually receive two cycles of chemotherapy. When given sequentially, standard 4–6 cycles of chemotherapy are given followed by thoracic radiation.

Chemotherapy for Metastatic Lung Cancer (Stage IV)

Chemotherapy with best supportive care (BSC) improves survival as well as the quality of life.

First-line Chemotherapy

There are several considerations which the treating physician has to look into while deciding the optimal first-line chemotherapy regimen for a given patient. The important ones are listed below:

- *Choice of platinum agent:* Platinum compound-based chemotherapeutic doublet regimens have become the standard of care. Cisplatin is usually the drug of choice in view of its superior response rates. Carboplatin is used only in the presence of relative contraindications to cisplatin.
- *Choice of third-generation agent to be used with platinum compound:* There are several factors which need to be considered while deciding the second agent to be combined with cisplatin/carboplatin.
    - *Cost of the regimen*
    - *Number of healthcare visits needed*
    - *Number of cycles*
    - *Dose intensity.*

Maintenance Chemotherapy

Maintenance chemotherapy (switch or continuation) is increasingly being used in patients who are stable/responsive after 4–6 cycles of chemotherapy if they have a good PS. Pemetrexed has been shown to improve OS when used as either continuous or switch maintenance following initial doublet platinum based chemotherapy.

Second-line Chemotherapy

Tolerance to second-line therapy is lesser than the first-line therapy but the considerations are similar. Usually, a single drug (non-platinum agent) is chosen which has not been used in the first-line therapy. The two chemotherapeutic drugs approved for use as second-line agents include docetaxel and pemetrexed (for non-squamous NSCLC). However, any of the other agents approved for first-line therapy may also be considered for use in second-/third-line therapy depending upon the treatment and toxicity profile for a given patient.

Chemotherapy for Small Cell Lung Cancer

Small cell lung cancer is also treated with chemotherapy with or without radiotherapy. Response is good even in patients with poor performance, therefore, a trial with doublet chemotherapy is generally given. Presently, a platinum-based regimen along with either etoposide or irinotecan remains the preferred choice.

Because of the aggressiveness of the tumor, most patients have a poor PS at the time of relapse and are not deemed candidates for chemotherapy. The only drug which has been approved for use in the second-line setting is topotecan. However, a number of drugs include irinotecan, etoposide, amrubicin can be used in the second-line setting. Unlike in NSCLC, the treatment options for

SCLC are limited for both first-line and second-line chemotherapy. None of the targeted agents has shown any benefit in SCLC treatment.

Immunotherapy

There have been exciting developments in the field of immunotherapy for advanced NSCLC in the last few months. Publication of large randomized trials involving use of PD-1/PDL-1 immune checkpoint inhibitors in the last 1 year or so has revolutionized the management algorithm for advanced NSCLC patients. Immunotherapy now represents a new frontier for treatment of patients with advanced NSCLC who have refractory disease during or relapsed disease following first-line chemotherapy. Nivolumab (a humanized IgG4 monoclonal antibody against PD-1) has been shown to be superior to standard single agent chemotherapy (docetaxel) in second-line therapy of advanced NSCLC for both squamous (CHECKMATE 017 trial) and nonsquamous trial (CHECKMATE 057 trial). Pembrolizumab (another anti-PD-1 monoclonal antibody) has also shown similar results in the KEYNOTE 010 trial but its usage is restricted to patients with PDL-1 expression more than or equal to 50 by immunochemistry in tumor tissue. Atezolizumab, on the other hand, is a monoclonal antibody against the PDL-1 and was superior to docetaxel for all histological subtypes of NSCLC (POPLAR trial). Patients with higher PDL-1 expression, in general, derive greater benefit from this class of drugs as opposed to those with lower expression. However, there is no consensus yet on the optimal method of testing for PDL-1 expression or on the optimal cutoff of PDL-1 expression to be used for selecting patients.

Trials are underway to address:
- Assess if combinations of two (PD-1/PDL-1 and/or CLTA-4) immune-check point inhibitors are more effective than single agents
- Role of PD-1/PDL-1 and/or CLTA-4 immune-check point inhibitors in small cell lung cancer
- Integration of PD-1/PDL-1 and/or CLTA-4 immune-check point inhibitors with other conventional treatment modalities (surgery, chemotherapy, radiation therapy) and with molecular targeted therapy.

The future is likely to witness emergence of a strategy wherein in addition to a standalone role, these agents may be incorporated in routine clinical practice in combination with other treatment modalities.

PALLIATION

Symptom control is the primary objective of treatment, especially in patients with locally advanced and metastatic disease (Stages IIIB and IV). These patients remain candidates for palliative treatment which is not only necessary but also justifiable.
- Treatment of locally advanced (especially endobronchial) disease is an important part of palliative care of lung cancer. Symptoms attributable to this include cough, dyspnea and hemoptysis. Interventional bronchoscopy,

wherever available, is helpful in alleviation of these symptoms since several procedures to relieve endobronchial obstruction can be performed. Wherever available, intra-lesion brachytherapy is another useful option for this purpose.
- Treatment of advanced mediastinal disease depends upon the structure that is being involved by the disease process.
- Treatment of metastatic disease:
  - Malignant pleural and pericardial effusion
  - Bone—Bisphosphonates are recommended for use in patients with proven osteoskeletal metastasis. Zoledronate is the most widely used drug for this purpose.
  - Brain and spinal cord—Here again, radiation therapy has an important role in providing symptomatic relief. Corticosteroids are used for the same purpose although there is a ceiling to both the dose used and the duration for which they provide clinical benefit.
- Treatment of nonmetastatic disease
  - Anemia
  - Cachexia
  - Deep venous thrombosis (DVT) and pulmonary thromboembolism (PTE)
- Treatment of complications of chemotherapy:
  - *Infection*: Infections, both pulmonary and extrapulmonary, may occur among patients with lung tumors. Postobstructive pneumonia is a frequent occurrence among patients with central tumors namely tumors arising from and occluding a major or lobar bronchus.
  - *Peripheral neuropathy*: This can be a complication of chemotherapy with taxanes and platinum agents. It can also occur as a paraneoplastic manifestation. Anticonvulsants and tricyclic antidepressants are used for the treatment of neuropathic pain.
- Treatment of comorbid illnesses
  - Chronic obstructive pulmonary disease (COPD)
  - Depression

CHAPTER 63

Targeted Agents for Nonsmall Cell Lung Cancer

Nagarjuna V Maturu, Navneet Singh

INTRODUCTION

Targeted therapy refers to treatment with pharmaceutical agents that affect a known molecular target in the cancer cell or tumor microenvironment. With the identification of oncogenic driver mutations, such molecularly directed agents have taken a key role in the management of lung cancer. The most important targets for specific drugs for lung cancer include the epidermal growth factor receptor (EGFR), the anaplastic lymphoma kinase (ALK) and the vascular endothelial growth factor (VEGF) pathways.

EPIDERMAL GROWTH FACTOR RECEPTOR–TYROSINE KINASE INHIBITORS

The discovery of EGFR mutations and specific EGFR–tyrosine kinase inhibitors (TKI) has forms the basis of treatment for advanced NSCLC with targeted agents. Various EGFR TKIs have been developed and subsequently approved for use in NSCLC patients (Table 63.1). The various drugs are now recommended for use as first-line agents, maintenance therapy as well as second-/third-line agents.

Clinical Indications

- *As first-line therapy in advanced NSCLC*: Epidermal growth factor receptor-Tyrosine kinase inhibitors have consistently shown improved progression-free survival (PFS), overall response rates (ORRs), lesser hematologic toxicity and better patient tolerability as compared to chemotherapy in

TABLE 63.1: Epidermal growth factor receptor–Tyrosine kinase inhibitors (EGFR–TKIs) agents for treatment of lung cancer.

Drug	Dose to be used	Approval for clinical use
First-generation EGFR-TKI		
Erlotinib	150 mg OD	Yes
Gefitinib	250 mg OD	Yes
Icotinib	125–150 mg TDS	Yes (In China only)
Second-generation EGFR-TKI		
Afatinib	50 mg OD	Yes
Dacomitinib	45 mg OD	No
Third-generation EGFR-TKI		
CO-1868	Still in phase I trials	No
AP-26113	Still in phase I/II trials	No

different studies. It is therefore recommended by all the international societies to start treatment with EGFR TKIs in EGFR mutated advanced/metastatic NSCLC patients. There is however no demonstrable difference in overall survival (OS) which is possibly due to significant crossover from the standard (chemotherapy) arm into the experimental (EGFR-TKI) arm at the time of disease progression in different trials.

The use of first-line EGFR-TKIs should be limited to patients with activating EGFR mutations. However, in patients with poor performance status, who cannot tolerate the standard doublet chemotherapy, EGFR-TKIs (especially erlotinib) may be considered irrespective of the mutation status as they have been shown to be non-inferior to single agent chemotherapy with better tolerability and superior to placebo/best supportive care.

- *As second-/third-line therapy in advanced NSCLC*: In pretreated and unselected NSCLC patients who progressed on or after chemotherapy (second/third line), the results of the RCTs show that EGFR-TKIs are either noninferior or superior to chemotherapy (for PFS) despite inherent limitations in the design of some of the trials. In patients who are known to be EGFR mutation negative, EGFR-TKIs even as second/third line therapy are best given only if patient has poor performance status (PS) and cannot tolerate chemotherapy.
- *As switch maintenance therapy in advanced NSCLC*: A pooled analysis of the three trials of erlotinib concluded that erlotinib as switch maintenance therapy improved both PFS and OS irrespective of the mutation status. Based upon the above data related to OS benefit, erlotinib but not gefitinib, has been approved for use as switch maintenance agent.
- *As adjuvant therapy (following surgery) in early NSCLC*: Use of erlotinib/gefitinib as adjuvant therapy after adjuvant chemotherapy is also being assessed. In patients unselected for EGFR mutations, there was no benefit seen with the use of these agents.

Practical Considerations

- *Dosing and drug interactions*: Both erlotinib (150 mg/day) and gefitinib (250 mg/day) are administered in once daily dosage. Bioavailability of erlotinib when taken orally is 60% on empty stomach and 100% when taken with food. This increases the adverse effects of the therapy and hence erlotinib is usually taken 1 hour before meals or 2 hours after food intake. The oral bioavailability of gefitinib (60%) is not affected by food intake and can be taken any time. The bioavailability of afatinib also increases when taken with food and hence is to be taken like erlotinib. The solubility of both erlotinib and gefitinib, but not afatinib, is pH dependent and their absorption is significantly decreased in the presence of H_2 blockers or proton pump inhibitors. Hence, the concomitant use of such agents is preferably avoided.

    When dose reduction is needed for erlotinib, changes are made in 50 mg decrements. Though therapeutic responses have been observed at doses as low as 25–50 mg/day, the main concern at such low doses is the low CSF penetration which would result in subtherapeutic levels in the central nervous system.

- *Resistance to EGFR-TKI therapy:* Epidermal growth factor receptor-tyrosine kinase inhibitors are to be continued as long as there is clinical response or stable disease and patient has an acceptable performance status. There is data to support continuation of EGFR-TKI use even after disease progression as the clinical deterioration occurs more rapidly once the agent is discontinued. Most of the patients, even those with initial good response, eventually have disease progression when continued on EGFR-TKIs. This is due to the development of acquired drug resistance. The median time to progression while on TKIs is approximately 12–14 months.

Clinical criteria have been proposed to identify acquired drug resistance to EGFR-TKIs as follows:
  - Patient should have been treated with an EGFR-TKI
  - The tumor shows an EGFR-activating mutation or shows objective clinical benefit from treatment with EGFR-TKI (defined by objective response or durable stable disease for 6 months as per RECIST or WHO criteria)
  - Systemic progression while on continuous treatment with EGFR-TKI in the last 30 days; and
  - No intervening systemic therapy between cessation of EGFR-TKI and the initiation of new therapy.

Adverse Drug Reactions and Monitoring

When the patient is on EGFR-TKIs, clinical monitoring for disease response is to be undertaken every 6–8 weeks, whereas monitoring for adverse reactions needs to be undertaken more frequently (once a month for the initial few months followed by less frequent monitoring later on). All EGFR-TKIs have group specific adverse drug reactions (ADR). The common side effects in decreasing order of frequency are skin rash, diarrhea, liver dysfunction and interstitial lung disease. They usually do not cause typical side effects associated with chemotherapy like myelosuppression, neuropathy, cardiac dysfunction and less commonly, mucositis, nausea, vomiting and alopecia.

The incidence of side effects (overall and grade 3/4) is most common with afatinib followed by erlotinib and gefitinib. Skin rash (acneiform/papulopustular) occurring on the face, scalp, chest and back is the most common ADR due to EGFR-TKI therapy (afatinib ~90%, erlotinib ~80% and gefitinib ~50%). This rash usually occurs in the first 2–4 weeks of initiation of treatment and is more common in non-smokers, elderly and in people with fair skin. Other mucocutaneous reactions include the development of stomatitis and paronychia.

The various modalities used are topical steroids, moisturizers, sunscreen agents and systemic agents like doxycycline and minocycline. Acne preparation such as benzoyl peroxide must be avoided as they can exacerbate the rash. If the rash is mild and controlled with topical therapies, the EGFR-TKI can be continued. In cases of severe rash, the agent needs dose modification or has to be discontinued and reintroduced at a lower dose.

Diarrhea is the next most common side effect occurring in up to 95%, 60% and 50% of the patients treated with afatinib, erlotinib and gefitinib respectively. Treatment usually is supportive care, discontinuation of the agent (if severe) till the diarrhea settles and use of loperamide. It is also recommended to periodically monitor liver function tests while on EGFR-TKI therapy as there have been instances of fulminant hepatic failure. Dose modification or interruption is suggested if the bilirubin exceeds three times the upper limit of the normal or the transaminase levels exceed five times the upper limit of the normal. Patients who develop hepatic toxicity usually tolerate gradual reintroduction of the agent once the liver function tests normalize.

Another life-threatening side effect of the EGFR-TKIs is the development of interstitial lung disease. The incidence of ILD is increased by previous chemotherapy, radiotherapy and preexisting interstitial lung disease. The onset of unexplained respiratory symptoms, when on these agents, should prompt drug interruption and once the diagnosis of ILD is established, the therapy should be permanently discontinued.

ANAPLASTIC LYMPHOMA KINASE INHIBITORS

Crizotinib is the first drug approved for use in patients with anaplastic lymphoma kinase (ALK) re-arrangement positive NSCLC. Crizotinib, an ATP-competitive inhibitor of anaplastic lymphoma kinase (ALK), is given at a dose of 250 mg twice a day. In the event of drug toxicity, dose reduction to 200 mg bd or 250 mg od may be considered. Similar to EGFR-TKIs, the plasma drug levels of crizotinib will vary with the use of CYP3A4 inducers and inhibitors. The CSF drug penetration of crizotinib is poor.

VASCULAR ENDOTHELIAL GROWTH FACTOR INHIBITORS

As an intact, functioning and expanding vascular network is a prerequisite for the growth of solid tumors, tumor vasculature has become an attractive target for antineoplastic therapies. Such agents can be divided as (a) vascular targeting agents (VTA), those which prevent angiogenesis (anti-VEGF therapies), i.e. formation of new vessels, and (b) vascular disrupting agents (VDA), those which cause the existing vessels to collapse thereby depriving the tumor of blood and oxygen. So far, anti-VEGF therapies are the only drugs which have shown some clinical promise. These agents include anti-VEGF monoclonal antibodies and anti-VEGF receptor small molecule tyrosine kinase inhibitors. None of the vascular targeting agents tested (e.g. ASA404) have shown any survival benefit.

Bevacizumab, a humanized monoclonal antibody against VEGF, is the only approved VTA for use in advanced nonsquamous NSCLC. This prevents new vessel formation and deprives the growing tumor of its vascular support. Several small molecule TKIs against VEGF receptor (nintedanib, vandetanib, sunitinib, sorafenib, axitinib, and vatalanib) have been tested in lung cancer. They compete with adenosine triphosphate (ATP) for the active site of the tyrosine kinase domain. Because of the conserved ATP binding site amongst various receptors, most of these small molecule TKIs inhibit multiple tyrosine kinase receptors.

CHAPTER 64

Hematopoietic and Lymphoid Neoplasm of Lungs

Gaurav Prakash, Pankaj Malhotra

INTRODUCTION

Hematolymphoid neoplasm of lungs can have two kinds of presentation: one, primary lung neoplasms, when the tumor originates from the lung or tracheobronchial tree and the other, secondary lung involvement by a hematolymphoid neoplasm located elsewhere in the body. Primary lung involvement by hematolymphoid neoplasms is an uncommon phenomenon; in such scenarios, the diagnosis is usually not suspected at the time of presentation. It is the cytology or biopsy of the tissue that gives first clue to the diagnosis. Secondary lung involvement by hematolymphoid neoplasms is not uncommon; the proof comes from bronchoalveolar lavage (BAL) fluid analysis, pleural fluid analysis, fine-needle aspiration or histopathology of the mass, the differential diagnosis includes infections that are far more common than the lung involvement by neoplasms. The lungs can also suffer, because of side effects of the systemic chemotherapy or radiotherapy used to treat lymphomas.

LYMPHOMAS

Lymphomas are diverse groups of neoplastic disorders which arise from lymphoid tissue. In most cases the lymphoid tissue is lymph nodal in origin. Extranodal lymphoid tissue present in normal individuals in various organs is a common site for development of extranodal lymphoma. In case of lungs, bronchial mucosa associated lymphoid tissue (MALT) is the main site of lymphoid tissue in the lung, this is often involved in the primary pulmonary lymphomas of the lung. Lymphomas are generally classified as Hodgkin's lymphoma (HL) and non-Hodgkin's lymphoma (NHL) based on the histopathology and immunohistochemistry. Involvement of the mediastinal group of lymph nodes is quite common in NHL but it is not included in pulmonary neoplasms.

General Considerations

In a case of lymphoma, the duration of symptoms can vary from weeks, months and sometimes years depending upon the rate of progress of the disease. Younger age is generally associated with more aggressive disease while both low-grade and high-grade presentations of lymphomas are common as the age advances. The systemic symptoms, such as fever, weight loss and night sweats, if present, connote aggressive behavior and high tumor burden which classify the patient into category B, while their absence is denoted as category A.

WHO classification of lymphomas is based on the morphology of lymphoma, cell of origin (B, T or NK cell lineage), immunophenotyping, chromosomal and molecular characteristics. Once the diagnosis of lymphoma is made, proper staging is required. Staging of both HL and NHL is done by Ann Arbor staging system (Box 64.1). Detailed investigations are required for proper work-up of patient with lymphoma (Box 64.2). The staging helps in prognostication as well as making therapeutic decisions whether only chemotherapy, only radiotherapy or both chemotherapy and radiotherapy, is required. Rarely, the surgery may be curative in localized lymphoma of the lung parenchyma when complete resection of the lesion is possible.

Overview of Primary Lung Involvement by Lymphomas

Patients can usually present with persistent cough, hemoptysis, dyspnea, wheezing, chest pain, discomfort or stridor. Patient may have fever, weight loss and night sweats (B symptoms). Chest skiagram is usually the first investigation that is required in these patients. This may show the presence of

---

BOX 64.1: Ann Arbor staging of lymphomas.

- *Stage I*: Involvement of a single lymph node or of a single extranodal organ or site (IE)
- *Stage II*: Involvement of two or more lymph node regions on the same side of the diaphragm, or localized involvement of an extranodal site or organ (IIE) and one or more lymph node regions on the same side of the diaphragm.
- *Stage III*: Involvement of lymph node regions on both sides of the diaphragm, which may be accompanied by localized involvement of an extranodal organ or site (III E) or spleen* (III S) or both (III SE).
- *Stage IV*: Diffuse or disseminated involvement of one or more distant extranodal organs with or without associated lymph node involvement.

Notes:
Fever more than 38°C, night sweats and weight loss more than 10% of body weight in the last 6 months of diagnosis are defined as systemic symptoms. Spleen involvement is considered as nodal.

> **BOX 64.2:** Workup of a lymphoma patient.
>
> - Lymph node biopsy (excisional or core) with immunohistochemistry
> - CECT neck/chest/abdomen including pelvis
> - Complete blood counts, ESR and bone marrow examination (aspiration and trephine biopsy)
> - Biochemical (urea, creatinine, uric acid, calcium, phosphorus, bilirubin, SGOT, SGPT, alk phos, blood sugar)
> - EKG, echocardiography or MUGA scan
> - Urine examination
> - Serum LDH, serum B_2 microglobulin
> - HbsAg, Anti-HCV, HIV
> - PET-CT scan
>
> *Workup in resource-constraints settings*
> - Get chest X-ray and ultrasound abdomen instead of CT or PET-CT scan.
>
> (CECT, contrast-enhanced computed tomography; ESR, erythrocyte sedimentation rate; SGOT, serum glutamic oxaloacetic transaminase; SGPT, serum glutamate-pyruvate transaminase; EKG, electrocardiogram; MUGA, multigated acquisition scan; LDH, lactate dehydrogenase; HbsAg, hepatitis B surface antigen; HCV, hepatitis C virus; HIV, human immunodeficiency virus; PET-CT, positron emission tomography-computed tomography)

nodule, mass, atelectasis, cavitation or other shadow. The differential diagnosis consists of infectious diseases (tuberculosis, histoplasmosis) or noninfectious diseases (lung carcinoma, bronchial carcinoid, sarcoidosis, and Wegener's granulomatosis). Sometimes, both lymphoma and infection may coexist in the lung and hence a biopsy is a must in these cases.

Diagnosis

Sputum examination for malignant cytology sometimes can give a clue to the diagnosis. The usual investigations that are carried out are bronchoscopy, endobronchoscopic ultrasound and transbronchial lung biopsy, or if needed, open lung biopsy. An adequate tissue specimen is the first and foremost requirement. Morphology along with immunochemical stains and rarely molecular analysis from the tissue specimen will clinch the diagnosis. If adequate tissue specimen is not possible, cytology with immunocytochemistry can suggest and confirm the diagnosis.

Treatment and Outcome

Patients who present with obstructive endobronchial lesions require rigid bronchoscopy and stenting. Sometimes, laser therapy with neodymium: yttrium-aluminum garnet laser (Nd:YAG) or photodynamic laser therapy (PDT) has been used in these life-threatening obstructive lesions. Lately, chemotherapy is used more frequently in primary lymphomas of the lungs because of the adverse long-term side effects of radiotherapy given to lung parenchyma. The principle of treatment varies according to the histology as well as to the burden/staging of the lymphoma.

Secondary Lung Involvement in Hodgkin's Lymphoma

The mediastinal lymph nodes are involved in almost two-thirds patients with HL, while the lung parenchymal involvement occurs in 10% of patients, which is usually the extension from the involved lymph nodes. The most common histological type of HL is the nodular sclerosis variety. If the mediastinal lymphadenopathy is more than one-third the size of the internal thoracic diameter or the transverse diameter is more than 10 cm, it is defined as bulky disease; these patients are candidates for mediastinal radiation after the chemotherapy. In order of decreasing frequency, the nodes involved are in the anterior mediastinum, aratracheal, hilar, subcarinal, peridiaphragmatic, paraesophageal and internal mammary nodes. The extension into the lung parenchyma occurs in the form of interstitial linear infiltrates or small nodules.

Hodgkin's lymphoma is considered as one of the curable malignancy depending upon the stage of the disease. Hence, it is important to know the stage of the disease before administration of chemotherapy. HL is also very sensitive to radiation therapy. The treatment of HL has evolved from only radiotherapy to chemotherapy alone or combination of both chemotherapy and radiotherapy. As a general rule, in the stage I and II disease, 2–4 cycles of chemotherapy (ABVD) followed by radiotherapy are used. Stage III and IV HL is usually treated by chemotherapy alone. However, at any stage if the bulky disease is present at baseline (defined as tumor size more than 10 cm), radiotherapy is always combined with chemotherapy.

Hodgkin's lymphoma with secondary lung involvement is treated initially with chemotherapy to reduce the size of tumor. Bleomycin, included in the treatment protocol (ABVD), is also toxic to lung and thus these patients should be monitored closely with pulmonary function tests. Female patients who receive mediastinal radiation for treatment of mediastinal mass are at risk of developing secondary breast and thyroid cancer. These patients should be kept on close follow-up for many years. In this subgroup, it is advisable to start screening for breast cancer by mammography at least 5 years before the recommended age of breast cancer screening.

Primary Lung Involvement in Non-Hodgkin's Lymphoma

The involvement of lymph nodes in NHL is generally noncontiguous (as opposed to contiguous spread in HL). The involvement of lungs can occur in up to 40% patients of NHL. NHLs are usually graded into indolent and aggressive subtypes. The most common variety of indolent lymphoma is MALT while aggressive lymphoma subtypes with predilection toward lung are diffuse large B-cell and lymphoblastic lymphoma and anaplastic large cell lymphoma. The treatment and prognosis are different for aggressive and indolent NHL, hence they are separately discussed.

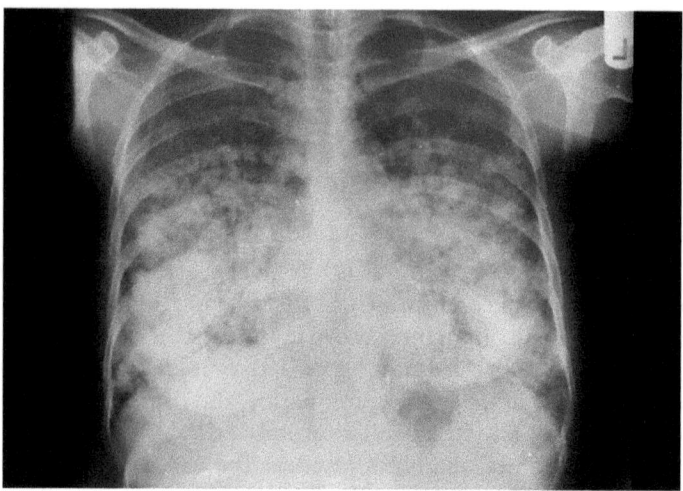

Fig. 64.1: Mucosa-associated lymphoid tissue lymphoma presentation in a 40-year-old lady.

Mucosa-associated Lymphoid Tissue Lymphoma

The most common type of primary pulmonary lymphoma is related to bronchus-associated lymphoid tissue clonal proliferation and is grouped under the category of mucosa associated lymphoid tissue lymphoma. Patients may be asymptomatic and lesions are detected on routine chest skiagram or they may have nonspecific chest symptoms that may occur due to other causes (Fig. 64.1). Due to rarity of these lymphomas, it is mostly on histology and immunohistochemistry of resected tissue that the diagnosis is made. In approximately 25% of patients, MALT lymphoma can present simultaneously at other sites such as the orbit, the salivary glands and the bone marrow. The differential diagnosis consists of other lung conditions in which lymphocyte proliferation occurs, such as follicular hyperplasia, lymphocytic interstitial pneumonia (usually bilateral) or hypersensitivity pneumonitis. Sometimes, the molecular techniques are required to accurately make the diagnosis of MALT lymphoma. These lymphomas when present for a very long period of time, can transform into a high-grade variety with systemic symptoms.

Low-grade lymphomas are considered incurable; hence, treatment is instituted only when the disease is symptomatic or progressive. Mostly, these lymphomas get treated either with single agent chemotherapy like chlorambucil, cyclophosphamide, deaminase inhibitors, monoclonal CD20 positive antibody or combination of these. The final treatment decision is based on the stage of the disease, age and performance status of the patient. Rarely, surgery alone or combined with radiotherapy is considered in these cases. The responses are excellent, but the disease tends to come back after some time.

Secondary Involvement of Lungs by High-grade Non-Hodgkin's Lymphoma

High-grade NHL generally presents with large mediastinal masses. The most common types are precursor T-cell lymphoblastic lymphoma/leukemia and primary mediastinal large B-cell lymphoma.

Primary Mediastinal Large Cell Lymphoma

Most of the presenting symptoms occur because of a rapidly enlarging mediastinal mass compressing various mediastinal structures. The presenting symptoms can be cough, hoarseness of voice, chest pain and dyspnea. Systemic B symptoms are present in one-fifth of patients. The work-up of these patients is the same as for other high-grade NHL. Mediastinal lymph node core biopsy either ultrasound guided, endoscopic guided or by thoracoscopy is required to accurately classify this condition. The treatment is similar to that for other diffuse large B-cell lymphoma [RCHOP (R: rituximab; C: cyclophosphamide; H: doxorubicin (hydroxydaunomycin); O: vincristine (Oncovin®); P: prednisolone (a steroid)] though many physicians treat with third generation chemotherapy regimens. Most patients require radiotherapy following chemotherapy since the mediastinal mass is usually more than 10 cm at presentation. If the treatment is initiated early, the response rates are similar to those seen with diffuse large B-cell lymphoma at other sites (60–70% depending upon the IPI).

Precursor T-cell Leukemia/Lymphoma

The presenting symptoms occur because of rapidly enlarging mediastinal mass compressing on the adjacent structures. In most cases, the disease is associated with HTLV-1 infection. The treatment is done with intensive chemotherapy, during which combination of various chemotherapeutic agents is given over few months as intensive phase. This is followed by maintenance chemotherapy for total duration of 2–3 years to prevent recurrence of the disease.

LYMPHOMATOID GRANULOMATOSIS

The disease is characterized by lung nodules or masses mostly in the lower lobes or periphery of the lung fields. In a substantial number of patients, central nervous system abnormalities in form of seizures or focal deficit and dermatological involvement in form of erythematous skin rashes, skin nodules or ulcers can occur. The disorder has been described as akin to post-transplant lymphoproliferative disorder. The disease usually presents in the middle to elderly age population; the usual symptoms are cough, hemoptysis and dyspnea.

The diagnosis is always made from surgical biopsy of the resected nodule or mass. Wegener's granulomatosis (WG) and T-cell lymphoma constitute the close differential diagnoses. Similar to WG, there is a granuloma formation but the cells are atypical, immature, and most B-cell show infectivity with Epstein-Barr Virus (EBV). Histological grade one and sometimes two can be observed without any treatment whereas grade three LYG always require treatment, usually akin to that for patients with diffuse large B-cell lymphoma.

SECONDARY INVOLVEMENT OF LUNG BY OTHER SYSTEMIC HEMATOPOIETIC AND LYMPHOID DISORDERS

Castleman Disease

Castleman disease (CD) (angiofollicular lymph node hyperplasia) presents like a single mass lesion that can present in the mediastinum, pleura, chest wall and rarely in the lungs. Mostly, young adults and middle-aged individuals are affected. The disease is mostly asymptomatic unless it presses on some of the important nerves or vessels. Resection of the mass is curable in these patients. No treatment is required, if the disease is asymptomatic. Prevalence of unicentric plasma cell variant is rare than the multicentric plasma cell variant.

Multicentric plasma cell variant usually presents in the middle age to elderly age group. The disease has become more common in the presence of HIV infection. The lesions can occur in the mediastinum, lungs and various extrathoracic and retroperitoneal regions. Systemic symptoms, such as fever, weight loss and fatigue are usually present in most of the patients. In many instances, the disease has been linked to the presence of human herpes virus 8 infection that can be demonstrated in the resected tissue specimen. Patients with multicentric Castleman disease require treatment in the form of systemic chemotherapy. If it is associated with HIV infection, antiretroviral therapy should be instituted as soon as possible.

Plasma Cell Dyscrasias

Plasma cell dyscrasias comprise a variety of disorders, such as, multiple myeloma, solitary or multiple plasmacytomas, Waldenström's macroglobulinemia and primary amyloidosis. All these disorders are characterized by neoplastic proliferation of immunoglobulin producing plasma cells. Lungs are secondarily involved in the disease process. The most common thoracic manifestation of multiple myeloma is in the form of plasmacytoma of ribs of adjoining vertebral column. Intraparenchymal nodules as well as interstitial infiltrates are less common but known manifestations. Although upper aerodigestive tract is one of the common sites of extramedullary plasmacytomas, primary pulmonary plasmacytoma is quite rare. Lung biopsy is often required to rule out involvement by an infectious disease. The treatment is directed toward the systemic disease. Major lung involvement is associated with poor prognosis.

Posttransplant Lymphoproliferative Disorders

Their spectrum ranges from benign polyclonal lymphoproliferation to malignant lymphomas. Most disorders occur during the first year after transplantation. Epstein-Barr virus infection acquired posttransplant is one of the important risk factors besides the degree of immunosuppression. There is some variation in the prevalence of PTLDs following different organ transplantation. The risk is probably greater among postlung and heart transplantation because the degree of immunosuppression is higher.

Intrathoracic presentation is mostly in form of lung nodules; patchy airspace disease and mediastinal lymphadenopathy. The differential diagnosis revolves around infectious diseases that can occur in patients on immunosuppression; hence a surgical biopsy of the lesion or image-guided biopsy from the intrathoracic lymph node is mandatory. More than 90% of lesions show positivity with EBV infection. Initial treatment consists of reduction in immunosuppression that probably works only in early lesions. In advanced lesions combination chemotherapy is the treatment of choice. The prognosis depends upon multiple factors, such as the stage and the grade of lesion, transplanted organ function and performance status of the patient. The mortality is usually high reaching up to 50% in some of the series.

Chemotherapeutic Drugs Lung Toxicity

Use of antineoplastic drugs can result in lung toxicity which is very difficult to distinguish from infectious diseases that occur in patients with hematological malignancies. Lung toxicity of anticancer drugs is a known complication. Lung involvement can present with nonspecific interstitial pneumonitis, organizing pneumonia, desquamative interstitial pneumonia, eosinophilic pneumonia, granulomatous pneumonitis, diffuse alveolar hemorrhage, retinoic acid syndrome, noncardiogenic pulmonary edema and acute respiratory distress syndrome. The classes of drugs involved in causation of these symptoms are anthracyclines, purine analogs, antiangiogenesis drugs, monoclonal antibodies, proteasome inhibitor, alkylating agents, antibiotics, arsenic trioxide and all transretinoic acid. The respiratory symptoms usually appear 2–14 days after the start of the offending drug. The index of suspicion should be kept high in patients where no infectious agents are identified and temporal correlation of symptoms is related to the administration of the drugs. Administration of corticosteroids in drug-induced toxicity is generally associated with gratifying results.

CHAPTER
65

Solitary Pulmonary Nodule

Alladi Mohan, B Vijayalakshmi Devi, Abha Chandra

INTRODUCTION

A solitary pulmonary nodule (SPN) is a small, focal, radiographic opacity of variable etiology. It may be caused by a variety of benign and malignant disorders including an early stage lung cancer. Advances in CT technology and ^{18}F-labeled 2-deoxy-D-glucose positron emission tomography (FDG-PET) have markedly improved the differential diagnosis of SPN. Comprehensive evaluation of an SPN requires detailed clinical work-up of the patient, imaging findings and appropriate use of invasive investigations.

TERMINOLOGY

Solitary pulmonary nodule is defined as a single, spherical, well-circumscribed, radiographic opacity that measures less than or equal to 3 cm in diameter, completely surrounded by the aerated lung and not associated with atelectasis, other parenchymal infiltrates, hilar or mediastinal lymphadenopathy, or pleural effusion. Localized pulmonary lesions that are greater than 3 cm in diameter are called *lung masses,* commonly the bronchogenic carcinoma. Smaller lung nodules (*subcentimeter* nodules) of less than 8–10 mm in diameter are much less likely to be malignant; they are difficult to accurately characterize by imaging modalities, and are often difficult to approach by needle biopsy. For practical purposes, the term SPN is used in the context of lung nodules that are at least 8–10 mm, but less than or equal to 3 cm in diameter.

The SPN has to be distinguished from multiple pulmonary nodules, the diagnostic significance and the algorithm for work-up are different. Furthermore, up to 20% of SPNs observed on chest radiographs may, in fact, be nonpulmonary in origin, may represent nipple shadow, skin lesions, rib fracture, end-on view of blood vessels, composite shadows, or monitor leads.

ETIOLOGY

Various etiological causes that manifest as an SPN are listed in Box 65.1. The etiological spectrum varies depending on the age group, geographical location of the patient and prevalence of risk factors for lung cancer.

BOX 65.1: Etiological causes of a solitary pulmonary nodule.

- Developmental
  - Bronchogenic cyst
  - Bronchial atresia with mucoid impaction
  - Sequestration
- Infections
  - Tuberculosis
  - Fungal infections (e.g. coccidioidomycosis, histoplasmosis, cryptococcosis, and aspergillosis)
  - Organizing pneumonia
  - Lung abscess
  - Septic embolus
  - Round pneumonia
  - Fungal infection (aspergillus)
- Neoplastic
  - Benign
    - Hamartoma
    - Chondroma
    - Teratoma
    - Lieomyoma
    - Endometriosis
  - Malignant
    - Carcinoma
    - Metastasis
    - Carcinoid tumor
- Vascular
  - Arteriovenous malformation
- Pulmonary infarction
- Hematoma
- Pulmonary artery aneurysm
- Lymphatic
  - Intrapulmonary lymph node
  - Lymphoma
- Inflammatory
  - Rheumatoid nodule
  - Wegener's granulomatosis
  - Sarcoidosis
- Airway
  - Mucous impaction (e.g. bronchiectasis)
- Others
  - Rounded atelectasis
  - Amyloidosis

CLINICAL EVALUATION

Majority of patients presenting with SPN are asymptomatic with the lesion being picked up incidentally in a chest radiograph or CT carried out for some other purpose. Clinical evaluation of a patient with SPN begins with a detailed history, and thorough physical examination. This is followed by appropriate imaging investigations and interventions for procuring tissue for cytopathological or histopathological diagnosis. Malignancy is rarely a cause of SPN in patients under 30 years of age; older the patient, higher is the likelihood that the SPN is caused by malignancy. History of tobacco smoking and other established exposures associated with an increased risk of lung cancer, such as, silica, air pollution, arsenic, cadmium, chromium and radiation (e.g. radon, X-rays, and gamma rays) should be obtained.

Some workers have developed models for predicting malignant etiology in a patient with SPN using multiple logistic regression analysis described older age, current or past tobacco smoking history, and history of extrathoracic cancer more than 5 years before nodule detection as independent predictors of malignancy. Others using multivariate analysis found current or former smoking status, increasing age, increasing nodule diameter, and decreasing interval since smoking cessation to be predictors of a malignant SPN. There have also been other attempts at predicting malignancy using the likelihood ratio form of Bayes theorem and neural networks.

IMAGING STUDIES

There are a number of characteristics which may point to the nature of SPN—benign or malignant (Table 65.1).

Chest Radiograph

The evaluation of an SPN usually begins with a review of the chest radiograph. Use of nipple markers or apical lordotic projections may help to distinguish

TABLE 65.1: Radiologic features suggestive of benign and malignant solitary pulmonary nodules.

Radiologic feature	Benign	Malignant
Size of the lesion	Smaller the size of a lesion, lesser is the risk of malignancy	Larger the size of a lesion, greater is the risk of malignancy
Border	Smooth	Irregular or spiculated (corona radiata)
Density	Dense, solid	Nonsolid, ground-glass
Calcification	Concentric, central, popcorn-like, or homogeneous patterns common	Usually noncalcified, or eccentric calcification
Satellite lesions	Common in granulomatous lesions	Rare
Wall thickness in a cavity	<5 mm	>15 mm
Doubling time	<1 month; >1 year	1 month to 1 year

normal anatomic structures from lesions causing an SPN. SPNs are often missed on chest radiographs especially if they are located below the diaphragm or behind the clavicles, ribs, or heart. Availability of dual-energy subtraction digital chest radiograph systems is expected to improve the pick-up rate of SPNs on chest radiographs. Presence of diffuse, central, laminated, and popcorn patterns of calcification are considered to be benign. But, stippled and eccentric patterns of calcification should prompt further work-up to rule out malignant etiology. When available, the current chest radiograph should be compared with a previous chest film. This will also facilitate the estimation of the growth rate (doubling time) of the SPN.

Computed Tomography

Computed tomography is the primary imaging modality in the evaluation of a patient with an SPN. The CT, by identifying whether the lesion is single or multiple, and by detecting atelectasis, other parenchymal infiltrates, hilar or mediastinal lymphadenopathy, or pleural effusion helps in characterizing the lesion as a true SPN. Following characteristics may help in the diagnosis of a malignant lesion:

- *Location of the nodule*: While malignant lesions are more likely to be located in the right lung and in the upper lobes, benign lesions are equally distributed throughout the lung fields.
- *Size*: Larger the SPN, higher is likelihood of malignancy; lesions greater than 3 cm in diameter should be considered malignant until proven otherwise.
- *Shape and margins:* Malignant SPNs rarely present with smooth margins. Presence of irregular spiculated margins (*corona radiata*) is highly suggestive of malignancy. Rarely, irregular margins can be observed even in benign lesions, such as lipoid pneumonia, focal atelectasis, tuberculoma, and progressive massive fibrosis. A lobulated margin is most often seen in hamartomas, but can be observed in malignant conditions, like peripheral carcinoid tumors, and adenocarcinomas. Presence of satellite lesions surrounding a larger central nodule is suggestive of granulomatous disease (e.g. tuberculosis).
- The *comet tail sign* is typically seen in rounded atelectasis and indicates a bundle of curvilinear bronchi and vessels extending into the hilar aspect of a peripherally located SPN that lies adjacent to pleural thickening.
- *Fat*: Presence of fat (attenuation value of between -40 and -120 Hounsfield units) within an SPN with smooth or rounded margins is suggestive of pulmonary hamartoma. Rarely, lipoid pneumonia, pulmonary metastases from renal cell carcinoma or liposarcoma presenting as an SPN may show fat.
- *Ground-glass attenuation*: The use of MDCT has facilitated the detection of "subsolid" nodules that contain a component of ground-glass attenuation. Atypical adenomatous hyperplasia, bronchioloalveolar carcinoma and invasive adenocarcinoma can present as subsolid nodules.
- The *halo sign* has been described in invasive aspergillus infection and bronchioloalveolar carcinoma and refers to a poorly defined rim of ground-glass attenuation around the SPN, the halo may represent hemorrhage,

tumor infiltration, or perinodular inflammation. The *reverse halo sign* (a focal round area of ground-glass attenuation surrounded by a ring of consolidation) has been described in cryptogenic organizing pneumonia and paracoccidioidomycosis.

- *Calcification*: Certain patterns of calcification within the SPN, such as central, laminated, diffuse, and calcification within a smooth or lobulated nodule are suggestive of a benign lesion, such as a granuloma; popcorn calcification is suggestive of hamartoma. Rarely, presence of eccentric calcification may be indicative of calcified granuloma engulfed by malignancy, amorphous calcification can be present due to dystrophic malignant calcification.
- *Cavitation*: Cavitation can be evident in necrotic malignant SPNs (e.g. squamous cell carcinoma) or conditions such as abscess, infectious granulomas (e.g. tuberculosis) vasculitides, early Langerhans cell histiocytosis and pulmonary infarction. Rarely, fluid-filled lesions from mucous impaction can present as a cavitating SPN.
- *Other internal characteristics:* Detection of cystic or "bubbly" lucencies within an SPN (Fig. 65.1) is highly suggestive of malignant etiology (e.g. lung cancer, especially adenocarcinomas with bronchioloalveolar cell features, and pulmonary lymphoma).
- *Contrast enhancement*: The SPNs that enhance less than 15 HU are almost certainly benign; malignant lesions, by virtue of increased vascularity tend to enhance avidly with the administration of intravenous contrast.
- *Growth*: An increase in nodule diameter by 26% corresponds approximately to one doubling in tumor volume. The doubling time for majority of malignant nodules is between 20 days and 300 days. A stable (no change in size) SPN for at least 2 years is likely to be benign and, usually, does not require further evaluation.

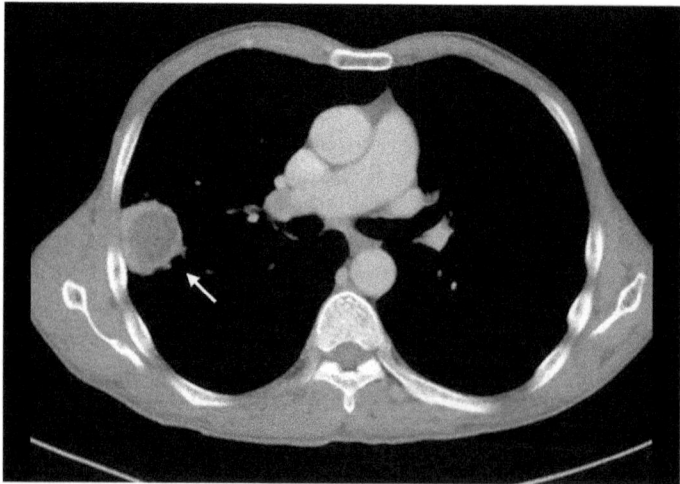

Fig. 65.1: Contrast-enhanced CT of the chest (mediastinal window) showing cystic lucency within the SPN (arrow). (SPN, solitary pulmonary nodule)

Magnetic Resonance Imaging

Magnetic resonance imaging (MRI), in spite of having the advantage of avoiding ionizing radiation, has been less frequently utilized than MDCT in evaluation of lung nodules because of its limited spatial resolution, effect of respiratory and cardiac motion on sequences with low temporal resolution. Half-fourier acquisition single-shot turbo spin-echo *(HASTE) imaging* facilitates identification of malignant tissues that manifest high signal intensity.

Positron Emission Tomography–Computed Tomography

Positron emission tomography–computed tomography (Figs. 65.2A to C) used to characterize an SPN typically shows increased metabolism of glucose in malignant SPNs; an SUVmax cut-off of 2.5 is used to differentiate benign from malignant SPNs. Currently, PET-CT is recommended only for nodules that are greater than 8–10 mm in diameter. Malignant causes of an SPN, such as a well-differentiated adenocarcinoma of lung (especially with a bronchioloalveolar cell carcinoma) and a peripheral carcinoid tumor can produce false-negative PET-CT results. The PET-CT has a low sensitivity for lesions of less than 1 cm in diameter.

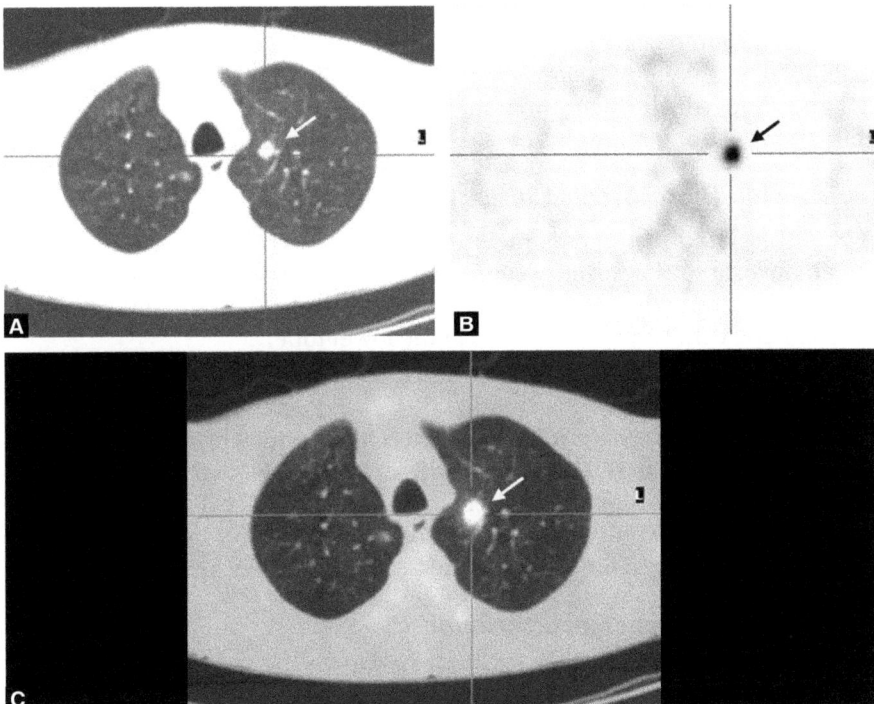

Figs. 65.2A to C: (A) CT of the chest (lung window); (B) F-18 fluorodeoxyglucose positron emission tomography (FDG–PET) showing an SPN (arrow); (C) PET–CT image of the same patient showing increased uptake in the nodule (arrow).
Source: Courtesy by Dr TC Kalawat, Department of Nuclear Medicine, Sri Venkateswara Institute of Medical Sciences, Tirupati.

Computer-aided Diagnosis

Computer-aided diagnosis (CAD) techniques, acting as a second interpreter, facilitate assessment of nodule size, volume, attenuation, and enhancement characteristics by performing global analysis of high-resolution MDCT data of the entire nodule. Further refinements in CAD, such as integration of multifunctional CAD platforms into *picture archiving and communication systems* (PACS) that provide easy accessibility during reader interpretation may facilitate more widespread use of these techniques.

Tissue Sampling Techniques

In spite of widespread use of various imaging techniques, characterization of some SPNs as benign or malignant is not possible, will warrant tissue sampling and histopathological or cytopathological diagnosis. Various methods, such as image-guided transthoracic fine-needle aspiration cytology (FNAC), needle biopsy, bronchoscopic biopsy with or without electromagnetic navigation systems, video-assisted thoracoscopic surgery (VATS), or open thoracotomy have been employed for procuring the tissue.

Image-guided Procedures

Image-guided transthoracic needle FNAC biopsy is frequently used for confirming the etiological diagnosis in patients with SPN in whom the pretest probability of a malignant lesion is high. Contraindications for transthoracic FNAC and biopsy include an uncooperative patient, presence of bleeding diathesis, severe bullous emphysema, and prior pneumonectomy.

Video-assisted Thoracoscopic Surgery

The video-assisted thoracoscopic surgery (VATS) technique facilitates procurement of tissue for frozen section examination to assist in decision about whether to proceed with a full lobectomy, especially from peripherally located SPNs and some centrally located SPNs in the lower lobe.

Fiberoptic Bronchoscopy

The sensitivity of fiberoptic bronchoscopy (FOB) for detecting a malignant SPN ranges from 10% for SPNs that are less than 1.5 cm diameter to 40–60% for SPNs that are 2–3 cm in diameter. Other factors that influence diagnostic yield of FOB include its proximity to bronchial tree. Several newer bronchoscopic modalities have emerged for evaluation of SPN in the recent years.

Radial Probe Endobronchial Ultrasound

Radial probe endobronchial ultrasound (R-EBUS) utilizes ultrasound to visualize structures within and adjacent to the airway wall. R-EBUS permits visualization of internal structure of PPN, this information may be helpful in predicting the histology of the lesion. Advances in R-EBUS technology have permitted visualization and performance of transbronchial biopsies of peripheral pulmonary nodules (PPN) without exposure to radiation.

Electromagnetic Navigation

Electromagnetic navigational bronchoscopy (ENB) is a novel image-guided localization technique. It is based on the principles of electromagnetism that facilitate placing endobronchial accessories in the target areas of lung. Combining ENB and R-EBUS has been found to increase the diagnostic yield close to 90%.

Ultrathin Bronchoscopy

Ultrathin bronchoscope by virtue of its smaller diameter (2.8–3.5 mm) has the advantage of facilitating insertion beyond the sixth-generation bronchi. For small peripheral lesions (<30 mm), this technique has a diagnostic yield ranging from 57% to 81%. CT fluoroscopy with ultrathin bronchoscopy has also been found to be useful for evaluation of SPNs.

Virtual Bronchoscopic Navigation

Virtual bronchoscopy (VB) facilitates simulation of actual bronchoscopy by application of three-dimensional (3D) display techniques to the airways. VB navigation (VBN) refers to use of virtual bronchoscopic images of bronchial path as a guide to navigate the bronchoscope. VBN coupled with ultrathin bronchoscopy, X-ray fluoroscopy, endobronchial ultrasound (EBUS) has been found to be useful in evaluation of SPNs.

MANAGEMENT

Initially, SPNs greater than 8 mm in size should be evaluated on past chest radiographs or CT (if available) to assess stability of the size. If the SPN has been stable for more than 2 years, such a patient may be followed-up without intervention unless morphological features are suggestive of malignancy. For SPNs 8 mm or larger, patients are categorized based on low, intermediate, and high pretest probability of cancer. Limited evaluation is recommended in case of patients who are not fit to undergo surgical excision. Biopsy should however be done to ascertain the etiological diagnosis in these patients to decide on appropriate therapy. Evaluation of patients who are fit to undergo lung resection is guided by their pretest probability of a malignant SPN. Patients with a low risk for malignancy require less frequent CT follow-up.

In summary, the approach to a patient is based on the pretest probability of cancer. This is decided on the basis of the size of the nodule, the presence or absence of risk factors for lung cancer (such as history of tobacco smoking), patient's age and imaging features of the SPN. The nodule should be monitored with serial high-resolution CT if the pretest probability of cancer is low. If the probability of cancer is high, aggressive diagnostic work-up should be undertaken to establish the histopathological or cytopathological diagnosis.

CHAPTER 66

Mediastinal Disorders

Arjun Srinivasan, SK Jindal

INTRODUCTION

Mediastinum consists of the thoracic cavity sans the lungs. Its boundaries include the parietal pleura laterally, the sternum anteriorly, the vertebral column and paravertebral gutters posteriorly, the thoracic inlet superiorly, and the diaphragm inferiorly. The lack of distinct anatomical planes between compartments, similar clinical manifestations due to spectrum of diseases and relative inaccessibility of the structures makes evaluation of mediastinal disorders a daunting task. The contents of the compartments are summarized in Table 66.1.

TABLE 66.1: Contents of mediastinal compartments.

Anterior	Middle	Posterior
Pericardial fat	Heart and pericardium	Azygos and hemiazygos veins
Thymus gland	Trachea, main bronchus and hila	Esophagus
Substernal extensions of thyroid and parathyroid glands	Innominate veins and superior vena cava	Azygos and hemiazygos veins
	Aortic arch and great vessels	Descending aorta
	Phrenic and vagus nerves	Sympathetic trunk
Lymph nodes	Lymph nodes	Intercostal nerves
		Thoracic duct
Connective tissue	Connective tissue	Connective tissue

IMAGING OF MEDIASTINUM

Conventional Chest Radiograph

Conventional chest radiograph is the first step in the evaluation of any chest symptom and mediastinal disease. Chest radiography can demonstrate site, size, density and the presence of calcifications, thereby narrowing the range of differential diagnoses. Additional views (oblique or lordotic) may be useful for distinguishing true images from composition images. Fluoroscopic examination and opacification of the esophagus will provide valuable complementary information.

Computed Tomography (CT)

Axial imaging avoids the problem of overlapping tissues with similar density. CT imaging helps demonstration of mediastinal spaces with their lymph nodes, relations with surrounding structures and blood vessels. CT is also indicated to characterize the lesions previously identified on standard X-ray as well as for assessment of the mediastinum in patients with a clinical suspicion of disease but negative X-ray. Improved resolution is required for better delineation of structures including point of origin, extension and relation to adjacent organs. This also helps to guide diagnostic procedures like fine needle aspiration or biopsy.

Magnetic Resonance Imaging (MRI)

MRI is used less frequently than the CT in the evaluation of mediastinal masses, mainly because of its lesser availability and higher cost; however, MRI has a capacity for multiplanar imaging and the ability to image vessels, and it can provide better tissue characterization than CT. Additionally, MRI is excellent in the evaluation of regions of complex anatomy such as the thoracic inlet, the perihilar, paracardiac, and peridiaphragmatic regions, and for the assessment of posterior mediastinal or paravertebral masses.

Ultrasonography

Traditional ultrasonography (US) has its role in evaluation of anterior mediastinal masses in children, especially thymic masses. Esophageal ultrasonography (eUS) and endobronchial ultrasonography (EBUS) are increasingly being used to detect mediastinal involvement in bronchogenic and esophageal carcinoma and guiding diagnostic aspiration of lymph nodes that would otherwise not be possible by conventional methods. EBUS-TBNA specimens are also found useful for rapid diagnosis of tubercular mediastinal lymphadenopathy.

Radionuclide Imaging

Positron emission tomography (PET) with or without CT has almost become a prerequisite in the preoperative evaluation of bronchogenic carcinoma to assess for resection. Radioactive iodine scans are useful in detecting mediastinal extension of suspected thyroid neoplasms. Technetium-99m (Tc-99) sestamibi can be used to detect parathyroid tissue.

DISEASES OF MEDIASTINUM

Pneumomediastinum

Free air in the mediastinum detected on a chest X-ray or chest computed tomography test (CT) is pneumomediastinum. It is "spontaneous" when occur, without surgical or medical procedures, chest trauma or mechanical ventilation, and in the absence of underlying lung disease. Secondary pneumomediastinum, though a rare entity, is far more common especially in recent times with mechanically ventilated patients. Anatomical continuity may lead to extensive subcutaneous emphysema over the head and neck area, interstitial emphysema, pneumoperitoneum or air may dissect the pleural layers/pericardium leading to associated pneumothorax/pneumopericardium. The source of air includes alveolar in spontaneous pneumomediastinum and that associated with mechanical ventilation. Other areas of origin include head and neck where it could be secondary to infection by gas-producing organisms or dental procedures requiring use of compressed gas at high pressures. Upper respiratory tract, tracheobronchial tree and extrathoracic gas are the source in trauma patients; uncommon sources include pneumoperitoneum and pneumoretroperitoneum in postsurgical patients.

Spontaneous Pneumomediastinum

The common presenting symptoms are chest pain and dyspnea. Pain typically radiates to the neck or back and is aggravated by bending forward, swallowing or deep inspiration. Other symptoms include cough and dysphonia. Differential diagnosis in any young person presenting with acute chest symptoms should include spontaneous pneumomediastinum (SPM). Severity of symptoms is usually moderate, patients tend to present within 24 hours of onset of symptoms. History regarding trigger events may help in clinching the diagnosis but no trigger can be identified in up to 40% of cases. Subcutaneous emphysema detected in up to 62% of reported cases is the most common physical finding and is usually restricted to the head and neck region. Hamman's crunch is reported in 30% of cases, careful auscultation with placement in left lateral position improves the chances.

Radiological findings: Some of the common findings in chest radiograph (PA view) include the following: air streaks in the superior mediastinum (sometimes up to the neck), the prominent silhouette of the heart (especially on the left) and subcutaneous emphysema of the shoulder and neck. The characteristic signs such as the double-bronchial-wall sign (bronchial wall sandwiched between inner and outer air) and the continuous diaphragm sign (the diaphragm of both sides appearing connected by leaked air between the inferior surface of heart and diaphragm) are relatively uncommon but highly useful for the diagnosis. Lateral views are more sensitive in detecting air and must be used when clinical suspicion is high and frontal radiographs are unrevealing. One must resort to computed tomography when strong clinical suspicion is present with normal chest radiograph. CT is also informative regarding additional lung disease and in complicated pneumomediastinum like Boerhaave's syndrome.

Differential diagnosis: Differential diagnosis includes pneumothorax, pulmonary thromboembolism, pericarditis and acute coronary syndrome. Whilst SPM is detected, one should be careful to rule out Boerhaave syndrome as it carries high mortality unlike SPM.

Treatment and clinical course: Symptoms tend to subside in 24–48 hours with complete radiological resolution. Symptomatic therapy with analgesics is all that is required in most cases. Antibiotics may be considered in the presence of signs of inflammation like fever after ruling out other differentials. Subcutaneous emphysema is drained using tunneled intravenous catheter if extensive. The most common complication is tension pneumothorax which needs prompt recognition and appropriate management. Recovery is total and recurrence uncommon (1.2%), unlike in spontaneous pneumothorax.

Pneumomediastinum in Mechanically Ventilated Patients

Mechanically ventilated patients especially those who are subjected to high tidal volumes, high peak inspiratory pressures, high positive end expiratory pressures (PEEP) and are fighting the ventilator are at high risk for developing pneumomediastinum. Air trapping (auto-PEEP) due to high frequency or underlying obstructive lung disease may also lead to an increase in peak inspiratory pressures. Unlike SPM, pneumomediastinum in mechanically ventilated patients can be life-threatening due to continuous positive pressure increasing the likelihood of associated tension pneumothorax. This may be incidentally detected on chest radiograph, but once detected, serial screening with chest radiograph is required to monitor pneumothorax. Chest tube drainage is needed if pneumothorax occurs regardless of how small it is if the patient continues to require positive pressure ventilation. In the presence of only pneumomediastinum, steps to curb increase in peak inspiratory pressures are taken if the patient cannot be safely taken off the ventilator. For respiratory support, it is preferable to use patient-triggered pressure-limited ventilation (e.g. inspiratory pressure support) or low-rate intermittent mandatory ventilation rather than mandatory volume-limited ventilation. Prophylactic bilateral chest tube insertion is not recommended in the absence of sudden deterioration.

Mediastinitis

Inflammation of the mediastinal structures is defined as mediastinitis. Based on the duration and severity of symptoms, it may be broadly classified into acute and chronic. Clinical presentation is dramatic and is often life-threatening in acute mediastinitis whereas the chronic tends to present as a mediastinal mass.

Acute Mediastinitis

Infection is the most common cause of acute mediastinitis but predominant inflammation could also occur with secondary infection as in esophageal rupture. With the advent of invasive endoscopic therapeutic procedures, esophageal perforation is the most common cause of acute mediastinitis. Other common causes include infection following sternotomy, descending necrotizing mediastinitis following neck infections, infection from tracheobronchial tree and, rarely, direct involvement as in anthrax mediastinitis.

Patients are usually gravely ill. High index of suspicion is the key to diagnosis especially in postprocedure patients as in esophageal manipulation or cardiac surgery. The patients may deteriorate rapidly developing multiorgan dysfunction within few hours. Computed tomography of the chest with contrast enhancement is the investigation of choice in these patients. Treatment of these patients requires appropriate antibiotics and surgical exploration.

Chronic Mediastinitis

The active form of chronic mediastinitis encompasses granulomatous disease, while mediastinal fibrosis represents the sequelae. The former tends to be asymptomatic whereas the latter presents as a mass. Symptoms depend upon the part of mediastinum which is involved. Histoplasmosis or tuberculosis is an important example of chronic mediastinitis. Either begins as an infection in the lung with mediastinal adenitis secondary to regional drainage. There can be associated perinodal inflammation in a subset of individuals with a residual breakdown of conglomerate of lymph nodes akin to matting seen in the periphery. This mass gets covered by a fibrous capsule and tends to calcify as it is usually seen on chest radiograph as a sequelae. In some individuals, the fibrous capsule tends to increase in thickness with compression and invasion of adjacent organs. In some patients with concomitant retroperitoneal fibrosis autoimmune phenomena might be responsible.

Clinical manifestations: Predominant symptoms are manifestations of mass effect on the adjacent organs. Primary symptoms include cough, chest pain, hemoptysis and dyspnea secondary to airway involvement. Trachea or any of the major bronchi can be involved. Compression or erosion of the right middle lobe is most common which may present as right middle lobe syndrome. Right paratracheal region involvement may lead to compression of superior vena cava, leading to superior vena cava (SVC) syndrome. Though malignancy accounts for up to 95% of SVC syndromes encountered in clinical practice, fibrosing mediastinitis is an important nonmalignant cause. Extrinsic esophageal compression presents as dysphagia and perforation as hematemesis or tracheoesophageal fistula. Mediastinal nerve compression leads to hoarseness of voice. Pulmonary vascular involvement can lead to pulmonary hypertension and cor pulmonale. Mediastinal fibrosis is occasionally reported to mimick sarcoidosis.

Management: Debulking of mediastinum should be attempted while being careful to avoid injury to surrounding structures. Antitubercular or antifungal can be given if specific infections are identified. Anti-inflammatory agents like steroids have been used with equivocal results but may be considered in an individual patient. Mechanical compression can be relieved by endovascular, esophageal or endobronchial stenting, where appropriate.

TUMORS AND CYSTS OF MEDIASTINUM

A mediastinal mass may be congenital or acquired in origin, the contents of the mediastinal compartments serve as points of origin. Hence localization of the mass in mediastinum gives a clue toward etiology but can be confirmed only by tissue sampling. Anterior mediastinal mass most commonly arises from thymus, lymph nodes, thyroid or primitive germ cells. The middle compartment which mostly comprises tracheobronchial tree, heart and esophagus is the site for duplication cysts. Posterior mediastinum abuts the vertebral body, enclosing the sympathetic trunk and vagal nerve; a mass arising from this region is likely to be of neural origin.

Plain chest radiograph in a suspected mediastinal mass provides information not only pertaining to the size and anatomic location but also about density and composition of the mass. CT scanning defines the characteristics of the mass and its relationship to the surrounding structures. It also identifies cystic, vascular, and soft-tissue structures. Multidetector-row CT scanning is also helpful to detect different characteristics of enlarged mediastinal lymph nodes. Magnetic resonance imaging (MRI) is primarily used to rule out or evaluate a neurogenic tumor. MRI is also helpful in the evaluation of the extent of vascular invasion or cardiac involvement.

Mediastinal sampling: Surgical methods such as thoracoscopy, cervical mediastinoscopy, extended cervical mediastinoscopy, and anterior mediastinostomy are employed for tissue diagnosis of mediastinal lesions. Needle biopsy may be done either through percutaneous (image-guided needle biopsy) or endoscopic routes. Endoscopic techniques include transbronchial needle biopsy, endobronchial ultrasound-guided transbronchial needle aspiration (EBUS-FNA), transesophageal endobronchial ultrasound-guided fine-needle aspiration (EUS-B-FNA) and transesophageal endoscopic ultrasound-guided fine-needle aspiration biopsy (EUS-FNA). Minimally invasive transcutaneous or transpulmonary image-guided fine-needle aspiration or biopsy is preferred over open surgical techniques as the diagnostic yield is comparable with a dramatic reduction in complication rates. Transbronchial needle aspiration (TBNA) through a flexible bronchoscope is the time-tested method for sampling enlarged subcarinal and hilar lymph nodes.

Cervical mediastinoscopy is the procedure of choice for sampling of multiple lymph node stations for accurate staging. It allows direct visualization and sampling of several groups of lymph nodes with high accuracy in patients with lung cancer. It is done under general anesthesia with 1–3% risk of major complications. Aortopulmonary, retrotracheal, posterior subcarinal, and inferior mediastinal lymph nodes are inaccessible. Alternative surgical techniques to access these groups include extended cervical mediastinoscopy, anterior mediastinotomy, and thoracoscopy.

Rapid on-site evaluation (ROSE) of EBUS-FNA samples is widely used for malignant lesions. Bioevaluator used to enhance the value of ROSE, is a device to know whether the tissues obtained by EBUS-TBNA are appropriate for pathological diagnosis. Image-guided percutaneous transthoracic needle biopsy using local anesthesia and conscious sedation allows access to virtually all mediastinal regions.

Anterior Mediastinal Masses

Thymoma

Thymomas constitute about 20% of anterior mediastinal neoplasms in adults. Systemic syndromes like myasthenia gravis (30–50%), hypogammaglobulinemia (10%) and pure red cell aplasia (PRCA) may present as primary manifestations and the mediastinal mass may be picked up incidentally during evaluation. There is a wide spectrum of histological diversity. Thymomas are classified based on cell type predominance as lymphocytic, epithelial, or spindle cell variants. The histological subtype is strongly related to the tumor invasiveness as well as prognosis. Thymomas may have cystic areas due to degeneration, necrosis or hemorrhage.

Most recently, thymic tumors are divided into thymomas, thymic carcinomas and neuroendocrine tumors. Diagnosis is easily established by percutaneous image-guided fine-needle aspiration but capsular invasion can only be made out on histopathologic examination of excision biopsy. Surgical excision is the only potentially curative option for both invasive and noninvasive thymomas. Adjunctive chemotherapy and radiation treatment may be needed for locally invasive or metastatic disease, or inoperable tumors.

Mediastinal Germ Cell Tumors

The germ cell tumors (GCTs) are either of true gonadal origin which represents spread from an occult or "burned out" primary tumor or of extragonadal origin with separate clinical and biological behaviors. It is currently believed that they arise from the primitive germ cells that fail to migrate during early embryonic development. They comprise about 15% of anterior mediastinal masses. GCTs are classified into the following three groups based on cell type:
- *Teratomas*: Teratomas are derived from at least two of the three primitive germs layers. They are subclassified into: mature and immature (malignant) teratomas based on the cell of origin. Mature teratomas are more common and are histologically well defined. Ectodermal tissues (skin, hair, sweat glands, and tooth-like structures) usually predominate. Mesodermal tissues (fat, cartilage, bone, and smooth muscle) and endodermal structures (respiratory and intestinal epithelium) are less common. Malignant

teratomas which may contain fetal or neuroendocrine tissue, have a favorable prognosis in children but can recur or metastasize. Mature teratomas tend to be silent or may present with cardinal mediastinal symptoms. Occasionally, the presentation may be dramatic with expectoration of hair or sebum due to endobronchial rupture of teratoma. Rarely malignant transformation may occur. Typical radiological picture is well-defined round or lobulated mass with up to 26% showing calcification due to presence of bone or teeth elements. CT or MRI may reveal sebaceous elements or fat, which may further support the diagnosis and help in assessing resectability. Complete surgical resection is the treatment of choice and adjuvant chemotherapy, if resection is incomplete.

- *Mediastinal seminoma*: Approximately, 40% of mediastinal GCTs are seminomas, occurring most commonly in males between second and the fourth decade. Gynecomastia and weight loss may occur as paraneoplastic manifestations besides the usual features of mediastinal tumors. Beta-human chorionic gonadotropin (β-hCG) is elevated in up to 10% of patients. Presence of an elevated alpha-fetoprotein (AFP) suggests an alternate diagnosis. Seminomas are bulky, lobulated, homogeneous masses on radiography. Local invasion is rare, but metastasis to lymph nodes and bones may occur. CT and gallium scanning are helpful to evaluate the extent of disease. Seminomas are highly radiosensitive. Radiotherapy alone or chemotherapy and radiotherapy are generally used. Neoadjuvant chemotherapy followed by surgery is offered in suitable cases.
- *Nonseminomatous GCTs*: The nonseminomatous malignant germ cell tumors which include embryonal cell carcinoma, endodermal sinus tumor, choriocarcinoma, or mixed germ cell tumors typically cause symptoms in young adult men. Unlike in seminomas, lactate dehydrogenase and serologic markers such as AFP and β-hCG are frequently positive. There is a unique association with hematologic malignancies with up to 20% of patients having Klinefelter's syndrome.

On chest radiography, these tumors are seen as large and irregular anterior mediastinal masses. Often there are extensive, central, heterogeneous areas of low attenuation due to necrosis, hemorrhage, and/or cyst formation. Pleural and pericardial effusions may commonly occur due to invasion of adjacent structures. Tumor may sometimes protrude through the chest wall causing a local bulge. Distal metastasis may also be present. The current standard of care chemotherapy consists of bleomycin, etoposide, and cisplatin. Complete response is rare, with most patients requiring resection of residual tumor. As compared to seminomas, nonseminomatous GCTs have a poor long-term survival with only 46% alive at 5 years in contrast to 86%.

Mediastinal Goiter

Clinically mediastinal extension of goiter is detected by inability to identify the lower border of thyroid during examination. Incidence is in the range of 1–15% among patients undergoing thyroidectomy. Most patients are euthyroid, appear as lobulated, encapsulated and heterogeneous tumors with classic cervicomediastinal continuity seen on CT. Radioiodine will show avid uptake if there is functional thyroid tissue. Due to retrosternal position, diagnostic sampling is difficult and exploratory thoracotomy with complete surgical excision is recommended as malignancy develops in a significant number of patients.

Mediastinal Lymphomas

Mediastinal involvement as a part of systemic disease is a common manifestation of lymphomas and figures among the top differentials while evaluating mediastinal lymphadenopathy. Primary mediastinal lymphomas are relatively a rare entity accounting for around 10% of all mediastinal lymphomas. Nodular sclerosing type of Hodgkin's lymphoma, large B-cell lymphoma and lymphoblastic lymphoma are the three most common lymphomas with mediastinal involvement. Presentation is similar to other mediastinal masses with constitutional symptoms (B symptoms) which predominate especially in Hodgkin's lymphoma. The treatment of mediastinal lymphomas is no different from lymphomas elsewhere, it primarily involves appropriate chemotherapy. Adjuvant radiotherapy may be justified in stage I or IIa disease or in the presence of superior vena cava syndrome. Relapsed disease is usually treated with high-dose chemotherapy followed by bone marrow transplantation.

Tumors of Middle Mediastinum

Mediastinal Cysts

These are congenital anomalies resulting from defects during embryonic development. They occur most commonly in the middle mediastinum, but neural-derived cysts are found in the posterior mediastinum. The presentation can be insidious due to compression of adjacent structures or acute due to infection or rupture.

Bronchogenic Cyst

Approximately, 40% of bronchogenic cysts are symptomatic with cough, dyspnea or chest pain whereas the rest are picked up during routine chest radiographs. They are seen as well-defined rounded masses on chest radiographs and on CT have similar Hounsfield unit as water. Air-fluid level signifies either bronchial communication or secondary infection. Diagnosis is confirmed by image-guided or endobronchial needle aspiration. Endobronchial needle aspiration of cyst with EBUS scope carries risk of infection and mediastinitis. Symptomatic cysts are managed by either surgical resection or therapeutic aspiration with or without instillation of sclerosing agent (ethanol or bleomycin) but controversy exists regarding management of asymptomatic cysts. Subjecting such patients to a major surgery must be weighed against potential long-term complications including malignancy when observation is planned.

Enterogenous Cyst

Radiological manifestations are similar to bronchogenic cysts, have slightly thicker walls and are nearer to esophagus. Barium meal study may show indentation along the posterior wall.

Pericardial Cysts

Unlike other cystic lesions of the middle mediastinum, pericardial cysts are often detected in the fourth to fifth decade. Therefore, the case for at least some of them being acquired cyst is strong but majority of them seem to be from the persistence of parietal recess during embryogenesis. Most are asymptomatic but can present with hemodynamic compromise secondary to cardiac compression or arrhythmia.

Lymphangiomas

Lymphangiomas classically present as cervical swelling and are clinically identified by the presence of fluctuation and transluminescence. In up to 10% of patients, there can be a mediastinal extension with associated chylothorax and hemangioma. They are congenital malformation of the lymphatics leading to saccular dilatation and cyst formation. Cervical lymphangiomas typically present in early childhood but isolated mediastinal lesions may present during adult life with symptoms of mediastinal compression.

Tumors of Posterior Mediastinum

Neuroenteric Cysts

Enterogenous cysts that are in continuation of or adjacent to vertebral anomalies are called neuroenteric cysts. Neuroenteric cysts are very rare congenital anomalies, result due to failure or incomplete separation of notochord from primitive foregut. Associated vertebral anomalies include butterfly vertebrae, hemivertebrae, and anterior spina bifida.

Neurogenic Tumors

Neurogenic tumors may arise from various neural elements: (i) peripheral nerve roots (neurofibroma, schwannoma, neurogenic sarcoma); (ii) the sympathetic ganglia (ganglioneuroma, ganglioneuroblastoma, and neuroblastoma); (iii) aorticosympathetic paraganglia (paravertebral paraganglioma), or rarely; (iv) the intrathoracic spinal canal (e.g. meningocele or meningomyelocele).

Nerve Sheath Tumors

They constitute about half to two-thirds of the neural tumors of posterior mediastinum. They are benign and extremely slow-growing tumors such as the neurilemmoma or schwannomas and neurofibromas. Schwannomas are generally encapsulated, firm masses consisting of Schwann cells whereas the neurofibromas are soft, friable, nonencapsulated and associated with neurofibromatosis. They generally complain of pain and nerve deficits. Treatment consists of surgical resection with or without adjuvant chemotherapy or radiotherapy.

Tumors of Autonomic Nervous System

These tumors arise from neuronal cells rather than the nerve sheath. They are either benign or encapsulated (ganglioneuroma) but can be fast growing, malignant and nonencapsulated (neuroblastoma).

Superior Vena Cava Syndrome

Superior vena cava syndrome (SVCS) is a common complication of lung cancer and non-Hodgkin's lymphoma (NHL). About 2–4% of lung cancer and NHL patients develop SVCS, together they constitute about 90% of cases of SVCS seen in modern practice. Benign causes constitute around 5–10% of cases, usually due to smoldering infections such as tuberculosis or fungus. Thrombosis of SVC due to iatrogenic procedures like central venous or Swan-Ganz catheter or insertion of pacemaker leads is another important cause of SVCs.

The severity of the complaints depends on the site of occlusion (site distal to azygos vein is more symptomatic than proximal) and the rate of onset of occlusion. If the occlusion is slowly progressive, the collaterals effectively decompress the system, hence the symptoms are minimal. The collateral channels include azygos, intercostal, mediastinal, paravertebral, hemiazygos, thoracoepigastric, internal mammary, thoracoacromioclavicular, and anterior chest wall veins. Collaterals often take several weeks to dilate and accommodate the diverted blood from SVC. Clinically, the site of obstruction at the level of SVC is identified by the direction of flow in the collaterals from above downwards both above and below the umbilicus. Patients present with symptoms of dyspnea, orthopnea, chest pain, hemoptysis, and swelling of neck, upper limbs and face, dilated veins in the upper chest wall, headaches, confusion and rarely seizures due to raised intracranial tension. Radiologic examination with a contrast-enhanced CT will identify the mass lesion and the presence of collaterals on CT is highly sensitive and specific for presence of SVCS. If suspected, CT angiography can detect the site and extent of the thrombus.

All patients should receive supportive care with oxygen supplementation, head-end elevation, restriction of fluids and diuretics. Use of steroids before the tissue diagnosis is established should be discouraged; it may lead to architectural distortion making subsequent biopsies difficult to interpret. Median life expectancy in patients with SVCS is approximately 6 months with a range of 1.5 to 9.5 months; estimates vary widely, depend on the underlying malignant condition.

CHAPTER 67

Diseases of the Chest Wall

Balamugesh T

The chest wall consists of the rib cage, rib cage muscles, and the diaphragm. Disorders involving the chest wall may affect ventilation and eventually lead to respiratory failure. Some of the important chest wall problems (Box 67.1) are discussed in this chapter.

KYPHOSCOLIOSIS

Kyphoscoliosis is a group of conditions in which patients have scoliosis (lateral curvature of the spine) and kyphosis (backward curvature of spine). Based on the etiology, the curvature abnormalities can be considered in three groups:
- *Congenital*—neurofibromatosis, Friedreich's ataxia, muscular dystrophy, Ehlers-Danlos syndrome, Marfan syndrome, etc.
- *Paralytic*: Poliomyelitis, muscular dystrophy, cerebral palsy, and Friedreich's ataxia
- Idiopathic.

BOX 67.1: Important nonmuscular diseases of the chest wall.
- Kyphoscoliosis
- Thoracoplasty
- Pectus excavatum
- Pectus carinatum
- Ankylosing spondylosis
- Obesity
- Flail chest
- Miscellaneous conditions

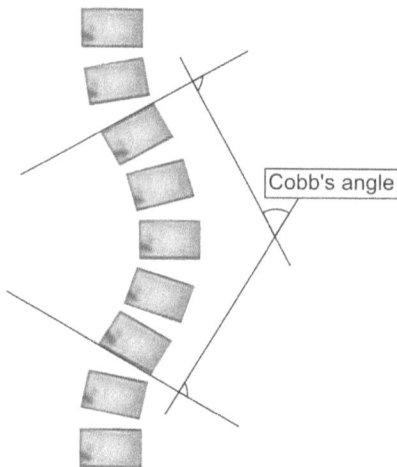

Fig. 67.1: Cobb's angle

Kyphoscoliosis is idiopathic in approximately 80%, with a female predominance (4:1).

The severity of kyphoscoliosis is determined radiologically using the Cobb's angle (Fig. 67.1). An angle of more than 10° defines scoliosis, and more than 100° is indicative of severe scoliosis with a higher risk of progression to respiratory failure.

Height cannot be used for predicted values for lung function in patients with kyphoscoliosis, because of the reduction in height due to spinal deformity; arm span should be used instead. Most commonly, one sees restrictive ventilatory pattern, i.e. reduction in vital capacity (VC) and total lung capacity in patients with severe kyphoscoliosis. Those with paralytic kyphoscoliosis have pronounced reduction in inspiratory muscle strength and have greater reduction in VC. Even in those with Cobb's angle more than 50°, there is significant reduction in inspiratory and expiratory muscle strength attributed to altered chest wall geometry and resultant mechanical disadvantage of the respiratory muscles.

Some patients have airway obstruction in addition to lung restriction; this is due to bronchial torsion and compression of central airways. These patients are at high risk of respiratory muscle fatigue and increased oxygen cost of breathing. There is reduced diffusing capacity for carbon monoxide in proportion to the reduction in lung volumes.

The most common abnormality in patients with kyphoscoliosis during sleep is hypoventilation. Since chest wall movement is compromised, any degree of diaphragmatic dysfunction can aggravate hypoventilation during sleep. Respiratory muscle function gets worsened due to untreated nocturnal desaturation leading to respiratory failure and cor pulmonale. The presence of obstructive sleep apnea can further worsen the nocturnal hypoventilation.

Prognosis is worse in those with a greater Cobb's angle and curvature at a higher level in the spine. In congenital and paralytic kyphoscoliosis, there can

> **BOX 67.2:** Indication of noninvasive ventilation (Consensus Conference Report, 1999).
>
> - Symptoms (e.g. fatigue, morning headaches, and dyspnea) or
> - Signs of cor pulmonale
>
> And one of the following:
> - Daytime arterial partial pressure of carbon dioxide ≥45 mm Hg
> - Nocturnal oxygen saturation ≤88% for 5 consecutive minutes
> - Progressive neuromuscular disease with maximal inspiratory pressure <60 cm H_2O or forced vital capacity <50% of predicted

be progressively worsening skeletal deformity leading to respiratory failure. Individuals with idiopathic kyphoscoliosis have a more benign course. Once cor pulmonale develops there is a rapid downhill course unless treatment is started. Death usually occurs as a result of respiratory failure or cardiac diseases and the risks are highest in juvenile and postpolio scoliosis. Pregnancy is poorly tolerated if the VC is less than 1 L.

Management

Mild kyphoscoliosis has a good prognosis, while more severe kyphoscoliosis can result in progressive respiratory failure and cor pulmonale. General measures include immunization against pneumococci and influenza, prompt treatment of respiratory infections, smoking cessation, avoidance of sedatives, maintenance of ideal body weight, and prevention of physical deconditioning by exercise. Supplemental oxygen may be required during activity or exercise. Specific treatment of nocturnal hypoventilation is by noninvasive positive pressure ventilation by a nasal or full-face mask (Box 67.2). The benefits of noninvasive nocturnal ventilation in patients with kyphoscoliosis include improvements in quality of life, gas exchange, sleep architecture, and reduction in pulmonary artery pressure. Long-term noninvasive ventilation also reduces the number of hospitalizations due to respiratory failure.

Surgery plays an important role in those with kyphoscoliosis secondary to neurological disorders among children and adolescents. Operative treatment traditionally consists of spinal fusion and/or insertion of Harrington rods, which may result in short-term improvement in lung function.

THORACOPLASTY

Thoracoplasty is a surgical technique that was used to collapse the lungs affected by tuberculosis, prior to the advent of antitubercular drugs. It consists of various combinations of rib removal, artificial pneumothorax, phrenic nerve resection, and compression of lung by foreign material. The patients who underwent thoracoplasty subsequently developed restrictive lung disease and chronic respiratory failure as they aged.

The severity of dysfunction was related to the number of ribs removed, presence of fibrothorax, degree of fibrosis of the underlying lung, phrenic nerve damage, and degree of scoliosis. The development of cardiorespiratory or respiratory failure depends upon the presence of preoperative contralateral artificial pneumothorax, older age at operation, and the presence of cavities. Currently thoracoplasty is used in rare situations like postpneumonectomy complications, persistent tubercular bronchopleural fistula, and sputum positive drug-resistant tuberculosis.

PECTUS EXCAVATUM

Pectus excavatum, also known as "funnel chest", is characterized by excessive depression of sternum. It is more common among boys than girls. The etiology is not clear but a defect in connective tissue surrounding sternum and imbalance of forces counteracting the inward pull of diaphragm on xiphisternum during development has been implicated. Upper airway obstruction due to enlarged tonsils and adenoids predisposes to pectus excavatum. Marfan syndrome has a higher incidence of pectus excavatum. Incidence of congenital heart disease is also higher among those with pectus excavatum.

Most individuals with pectus excavatum remain asymptomatic. The most common complaint is cosmesis. Dyspnea out of proportion to the mild restrictive ventilatory defect is seen. Majority of them have cardiac murmurs mimicking pulmonary stenosis caused by cardiac displacement. Chest radiograph frequently shows right paracardiac opacity due to parasternal soft tissues and should not be mistaken for middle lobe infiltrate. Electrocardiographic abnormalities include the presence of T inversion in right chest leads, right axis deviation, P wave inversion in V1, and a QR pattern.

The benefit from a structured program of physical therapy to improve posture and the appearance of the chest may benefit the patients with minimal deformity. Surgery is indicated only in severe situations or for cosmetic purposes in patients with pectus index of above 3.25 (measured on CT scan), cardiac compression, displacement, mitral valve prolapse, murmurs, or conduction abnormalities.

PECTUS CARINATUM

There is excessive anterior protrusion of sternum (pigeon breast) which may also be associated with other congenital anomalies such as a cardiac lesions and coarctation of aorta. Pectus carinatum may occur due to premature obliteration of the sternal sutures or due to inadequate segmentation during fetal life or due to malattachment of diaphragm. There is no functional defect with pectus carinatum and surgery is indicated only for cosmetic reasons.

ANKYLOSING SPONDYLOSIS

Ankylosing spondylosis (AS) belongs to a group of conditions with strong association with Human Leukocyte Antigen-B27 in which there is inflammation of axial skeleton. There is inflammation and bony ankylosis of vertebral structures, costovertebral, and sternoclavicular joints. This leads to reduction in chest expansion. Chest expansion at the level of 4th intercostal space less than 2.5 cm in an young adult with back pain should raise the suspicion of AS. Exercise intolerance and dyspnea are uncommon, unless there is associated underlying lung fibrosis, diaphragmatic dysfunction or cardiac disease.

Fibrobullous upper lobe disease may develop in about 1–4% of patients, especially men with chronic disease. Apical fibrosis can be detected on high-resolution computed tomography (CT) scan in about 9%. The cause of apical fibrobullous changes is unknown. Some of the possible mechanisms may include diminished upper lobe ventilation due to chest wall rigidity, altered apical mechanical stress due to rigid thoracic spine, recurrent pulmonary infection due to impaired cough, and respiratory mechanics. Occasionally, there is formation of fungal ball (mycetoma or aspergillomas) in the cavities or the bullae. Other rare complications include pleural effusion, pneumothorax, airway obstruction by cricoarytenoid joint ankylosis, and amyloidosis of the lung. About 20% of patients who were on sulfasalazine have been found to have asymptomatic interstitial lung disease detected by high-resolution CT scanning.

Treatment is focused on symptom relief and maintenance of posture and mobility. Physiotherapy to improve chest wall movements and breathing exercises are important. Tumor necrosis factor antagonists have recently revolutionized the management of patients with AS.

OBESITY

The body mass index (BMI) is positively associated with morbidity and mortality. An individual with a BMI between 18.5 kg/m^2 and 24.9 kg/m^2 is normal; a BMI between 25 kg/m^2 and 29.9 kg/m^2 is overweight, and a BMI greater than 30 kg/m^2 is obese. Those with a BMI greater than 40 kg/m^2 (morbid obesity) are especially predisposed to develop restrictive lung disease. The respiratory morbidity due to obesity can be considered under three categories: (i) Simple obesity (SO) with minimal effects on respiration; (ii) Morbid obesity eucapnic individuals with compromised pulmonary function; and (iii) Obesity hypoventilation syndrome (OHS) with hypercapnia during awake state. Obstructive sleep apnea can coexist with any of these.

Pulmonary Function Tests

Both the thoracoabdominal pattern and lung function tests are altered during spontaneous respiration. The fat in the chest wall and abdomen causes reduction in functional reserve capacity with near normal residual volume and a marked reduction in expiratory reserve volume (ERV). Airway resistance is increased in obesity due to abnormalities in lung tissue and small airways rather than in the large airways. This leads to expiratory flow limitation and orthopnea. The work of breathing and oxygen cost of breathing are markedly increased in OHS. Respiratory muscle strength is preserved in SO, but reduced in OHS due to deconditioning and fatty infiltration of muscle. This along with disordered respiratory control and blunted respiratory drive contributes to hypercapnia in OHS.

Treatment

Weight loss induced by either diet or surgery helps in improvement of ERV and improvement of hypoxia in patients with OHS. In patients with OHS noninvasive ventilation helps improving gas exchange and daytime symptoms.

FLAIL CHEST

Flail chest is characterized by the presence of paradoxical movements of a segment of rib cage during respiration due to fractures of ribs most commonly of lateral chest wall, posteriorly. Generally this happens when there are double fractures of three or more contiguous ribs or a combination of sternal and rib fractures. Trauma due to fall or automobile accidents is the most common cause of flail chest. Rarely, a flail segment is caused by pathological fractures of ribs. The negative intrapleural pressure during inspiration causes the flail segment to move inward instead of expanding outward.

Treatment

Treatment consists of adequate pain relief to prevent atelectasis and improve tidal volume. It can be achieved with medications, intercostal nerve blocks, and epidural anesthesia. Stabilizing the flail segment by external strappings is not very successful. Positive pressure ventilation can provide effective stabilization by eliminating the negative intrapleural pressure. Earlier mechanical ventilation was used to provide the ventilation. But recently noninvasive continuous positive airway ventilation together with regional anesthesia has been found to reduce morbidity and avoid complications. In severe injuries, a variety of surgical procedures are described for fracture fixation and improvement of respiratory mechanics.

MISCELLANEOUS CONDITIONS

Cervical Ribs

Cervical ribs occur in about 0.5% of the population. They are usually asymptomatic. But rarely can cause thoracic outlet syndrome due to compression of subclavian vessels or cervical nerve roots. The presence of symptoms is not dependent on the size of the rib, since the fibrous attachment itself may cause compression. While the neurological complications can be managed by shoulder muscle strengthening exercises, rib resection may be needed to address the vascular complications.

Tietze Syndrome or Costochondritis

The etiology of this condition is unknown. It presents with pain and swelling of one or more of the upper six costal cartilages. It is more common in young adults with no sex predisposition and affects predominately second costal cartilage. Coughing or deep breathing may exacerbate the pain. The condition may persist for long periods of weeks, months or years. There are no X-ray changes, biopsy also shows normal cartilage. Thickened cartilage with in homogeneously increased echogenicity and hypoechoic halo may be seen on ultrasonography.

Rib Notching

Coarctation of aorta is the most common cause of rib-notching, i.e. erosion of the inferior border of ribs (inferior rib notching) due to the enlarged intercostal arteries. The first two and the last three ribs are never involved. Other causes include subclavian artery obstruction, Takayasu's arteritis, pulmonary arteriovenous fistula, and intercostal neuroma. Superior notching of third to sixth ribs is sometimes reported in poliomyelitis and in patients with connective tissue disorders.

Chest Wall Hernias

Lung herniation through chest wall can occur after thoracotomy, trauma, violent coughing, and sneezing. Prosthetic herniorrhaphy was successfully performed in these patients without any complications.

Tumors of the Chest Wall

Metastatic tumors of the chest wall are more common than the primary tumors. Breast is the most site of primary malignancy. Lipoma and fibrosarcoma are the most common benign and malignant soft tissue tumors of the chest wall while osteochondroma and chondrosarcoma are the most common benign and malignant tumors of the bony thoracic skeleton.

Tuberculosis of the Thoracic Cage

Tuberculosis can sometimes involve the costal cartilages, sternoclavicular, and acromioclavicular joints. Tuberculosis of the spine with paravertebral abscess can also cause multiple lesions of the costovertebral portions of the ribs. Cold abscess of the chest wall, due to tuberculosis of the intercostal lymph glands, can be seen commonly at three sites: (i) near the erector spinae muscles when pus tracks along the posterior primary division of the intercostal nerve; (ii) lateral chest wall, when pus tracks along the anterior division; and (iii) near costal cartilages. It manifests with painless fluctuant swelling. Diagnosis is made by aspiration and investigations of pus. Tuberculosis responds fairly well to conventional antitubercular chemotherapy.

CHAPTER 68

Diffuse Alveolar Hemorrhage

Stagaki E, Karakontaki F, Polychronopoulos V

DIFFUSE ALVEOLAR HEMORRHAGE SYNDROMES

Alveolar hemorrhage (AH) is a potentially life-threatening clinicopathological syndrome characterized by diffuse intraalveolar bleeding which originates from the pulmonary microcirculation (pulmonary arterioles, alveolar capillaries and pulmonary venules). Localized pulmonary hemorrhage originating from the bronchial circulation in airway disorders such as bronchiectasis, infection and tumors should not be confused with diffuse alveolar hemorrhage (DAH).

The characteristic clinical trial of DAH includes hemoptysis, diffuse alveolar infiltrates and a drop in hematocrit. Hemoptysis may be absent in up to one-third of patients even in severe AH. DAH generally occurs acutely but sometimes can be subacute as well as recurrent. DAH should be distinguished from other diseases causing hemoptysis (Box 68.1).

Diagnostic Evaluation

Causes of AH can be broadly divided into immune and nonimmune.

Clinical Evaluation

The history should be directed to exclude conditions that can cause hemoptysis: coagulopathy, mitral stenosis, recent bone marrow transplantation and preexisting autoimmune disorders. Smoking history, use of different medication and illicit drugs as well as history of exposures to inhaled agents, infected animals or their urine, immersion in contaminated water (swimming, fishing, and floods), bites and recent stay in tropical areas should be also

BOX 68.1: Histology and causes of diffuse alveolar hemorrhage.

Pulmonary capillaritis:
- Antineutrophil cytoplasmic antibody (ANCA)-associated granulomatous vasculitis
- Microscopic polyangiitis
- Isolated pulmonary capillaritis (ANCA positive and negative)
- Systemic lupus erythematosus (SLE)
- Rheumatoid arthritis
- Mixed connective tissue disorder
- Scleroderma
- Polymyositis
- Primary antiphospholipid antibody syndrome
- Henoch–Schönlein purpura
- Behçet syndrome
- IgA nephropathy
- Goodpasture syndrome
- Idiopathic glomerulonephritis (pauci-immune or immune complex related)
- Acute lung transplant rejection
- Idiopathic pulmonary fibrosis
- Diphenylhydantoin
- Retinoic acid toxicity
- Autologous bone marrow transplantation
- Myasthenia gravis
- Cryoglobulinemia
- Ulcerative colitis
- Propylthiouracil

Bland pulmonary hemorrhage:
- Idiopathic pulmonary hemorrhage
- Mitral stenosis
- Left heart failure
- Subacute bacterial endocarditis
- Goodpasture syndrome
- SLE and rarely other connective tissue diseases
- Coagulation disorders
- Drugs: Trimellitic anhydride, Isocyanate exposure, penicillamine, amiodarone, nitrofurantoin
- Polyglandular autoimmune syndrome
- Multiple myeloma

Diffuse alveolar hemorrhage
- Bone marrow transplantation
- Crack cocaine inhalation
- Cytotoxic drug therapy
- SLE
- Radiation therapy
- Acute respiratory distress syndrome

inquired. Following symptomatic inquiry should be helpful for different systemic disorders:
- General symptoms (fever, asthenia, and weight loss)
- Nasal symptoms (crusty rhinitis, septal erosions, and sinusitis)
- Ocular symptoms (episcleritis, retinal vasculitis, and iridocyclitis)
- Skin changes (palpable purpura, subcutaneous nodules, erythema, and livedo)
- Musculoskeletal symptoms (arthralgias, myalgias, and synovitis)
- Neurological symptoms (mono- or multineuritis)
- Signs of glomerulonephritis.

Chest Imaging

Findings of air space disease on chest radiograph (CXR) or high-resolution computed tomography (HRCT) are generally nonspecific. There can be ground-glass alveolar opacities which are either patchy or diffuse, consolidation with air bronchogram, or multiple nodules reflecting acinar filling. Pulmonary apices and costodiaphragmatic angles are relatively spared. Chest radiograph may be almost normal in mild AH.

Laboratory Investigations

Initial blood testing consists of hemogram, routine biochemistry, coagulation status and baseline markers of inflammation [erythrocyte sedimentation rate (ESR) and C-reactive protein]. A urinalysis should always be ordered, because renal involvement is very often associated with pulmonary capillary disease even if symptoms from renal disease may be subtle. The underlying pathology may be either a segmental necrotizing glomerulonephritis rapidly progressing to renal failure, Wegener's granulomatosis (WG), and microscopic polyangiitis (MPA) or other systemic vasculitides, e.g. systemic lupus erythematosus (SLE) or even may be pauci-immune idiopathic glomerulonephritis (Goodpasture's syndrome). Laboratory investigation should also include auto antibodies in order to determine the underlying antineutrophil cytoplasmic antibody (ANCA) with determination of cytoplasmic (c-ANCA) or perinuclear (p-ANCA) fluorescence and anti-PR3 or anti-myeloperoxidase (MPO) specificity [ANCA-associated vasculitis (AAV)]. Also, the following should be ordered:
- Anti-glomerular basement membrane (GBM) (Goodpasture disease)
- Antibodies associated with connective tissue diseases including antinuclear antibody (ANA) antibodies, anti-ds DNA antibodies, rheumatoid factor (RF), anti-cyclic citrullinated peptide, anti-nucleoproteins, and anti-phospholipids (SLE, RA), creatinine kinase and complement levels (myositis).

There are three main patterns of staining on indirect immunofluorescence: (1) c-ANCA, a coarse granular staining of the cytoplasm; (2) p-ANCA, with staining chiefly around the nucleus, leaving the cytoplasm unstained; and (iii) atypical ANCA. Only the PR3-ANCA with c-ANCA combination and the MPO-ANCA with p-ANCA combination are sensitive and specific for AAV. Positive and negative predictive values of ANCA for WG and MPA depend on the pretest probability of the disease as well as on its analytical accuracy.

Bronchoscopy: Bronchoalveolar Lavage

Bronchoscopy with bronchoalveolar lavage (BAL), serves two purposes: documentation of AH and exclusion of infection. Serial samples of BAL showing increasing hemorrhagic appearances are diagnostic of DAH. Presence of hemosiderin-laden macrophages in BAL represents 20–30% of the total macrophage count, suggests subacute DAH. These may be absent in DAH of less than 72 h duration, as it takes 48–72 h for macrophages to accumulate.

Histopathology

Although diagnostic biopsy remains the gold standard, a confident diagnosis can be made without tissue biopsy in a sufficient number of patients. So, the decision to obtain biopsy specimen (renal, lung, other sites—skin, upper airway, etc.) should be made taking into consideration the risk of the procedure and the likelihood of biopsy findings to alter the therapeutic approach.

CAUSES

Granulomatosis with Polyangiitis (Wegener Granulomatosis)

Granulomatosis with polyangiitis (GPA) is a necrotizing granulomatous inflammation, usually involving the upper and lower respiratory tract histologically characterized by necrotizing vasculitis predominantly involving the small to medium vessels. Pulmonary capillaritis with hemorrhage are frequent. Extravascular inflammation of granulomatous or nongranulomatous origin is also common. Necrotizing glomerulonephritis and ocular vasculitis are often present. About 90% of GPA patients present upper or lower airway involvement or both. In many patients, ear and nose or sinus symptoms are usually the predominant features. Persistent ear, nose, and throat (ENT) symptoms, accompanied by fever, malaise, anemia, should warn the clinician for the possibility of GPA.

Ear, nose, and throat involvement: Serous otitis, chronic or subacute otitis and/or mastoiditis are the main manifestations of ear involvement. Hearing loss is the result of either serous otitis or nerve involvement. Nose involvement is characterized by epistaxis, necrotizing inflammation with crusting, chondritis, septum perforation and saddle-nose deformity. Oropharynx may present ulcerations; "strawberry" gingival hyperplasia due to petechiae caused from interdental papillae is a rare, but almost pathognomonic manifestation of GPA.

Tracheal involvement: The most frequent location of tracheobronchial involvement is the subglottic area. The result of subglottic stenosis is wheezing which mimics asthma; subglottic involvement is more often (for unknown reason) in young ladies, and in many cases the disease is diagnosed and treated unsuccessfully as asthma.

Airway involvement is found in 15–55% of patients with GPA. Bronchoscopy may reveal nonspecific findings as: mucosal edema and erythema, ulceration, cobblestone mucosa, polypoid lesions. Occasionally, one may find necrotic mass (pseudotumor), submucosal tunnels, membrane formation, localized or multiple stenoses, cartilaginous deformities (tracheobronchomalacia).

Lung involvement: The lungs may be involved by GPA in two ways: (1) pulmonary nodules/masses or (2) diffuse consolidations (due to AH/pulmonary capillaritis). Nodules are usually multiple, may cavitate. Nodules represent granulomatous lesions of the lung; as they heal, the cavities become thin walled before disappearing. Relapses of disease as reappearance of nodules occur at the area of first location. Usually the nodules are asymptomatic, in contrast to alveolar consolidations, but when they appear in a patient with ENT and/or general symptoms (fever, malaise, and anemia), physicians should think of the possibility of GPA.

Alveolar hemorrhage is the result of pulmonary capillaritis, it is considered as severe disease as it may rapidly lead to respiratory failure. In the emergency department (ED) or ICU, patients presenting with acute respiratory failure and acute respiratory distress syndrome (ARDS)-like picture should always be evaluated for the possibility of DAH, provided that cardiogenic pulmonary edema is excluded. Such patients with AH usually have coexisting hematuria due to the presence of glomerular erythrocytes in urine. Coexisting severe desaturation and dramatic fall of hemoglobin are very common. Mortality is very high (50%) in this situation and renal failure occurs in a very short time (few days or even hours). Early treatment with high doses of steroids and immunosuppression has to be started immediately, even if the diagnosis has not be confirmed with ANCA tests.

Other thoracic manifestations of GPA: Pleural effusions—10% of GPA patients usually present with small pleural effusions, which are exudative in nature. Mediastinal adenopathy revealed only in CT scans, occurs rarely (10% of cases).

Heart involvement is often asymptomatic and underdiagnosed. Granulomatous infiltration of the myocardium is common; wall motion abnormalities and conduction abnormalities are well described, complete heart block may represent the first disease manifestation.

Skin manifestations: About 20–50% of GPA patients may develop skin involvement over the course of the disease. Leukocytoclastic vasculitis (palpable purpura with or without petechial lesions) is the most common manifestation, may represent an indicator of generalized form of the disease.

Nervous system: The most common abnormality is multiple peripheral mononeuropathy, which is thought to be caused by vasculitis of vasa nervorum. Granulomatous infiltrations of the pituitary gland can cause diabetes insipidus; rare manifestations are meningeal involvement.

Renal involvement is the most serious manifestation of the disease, along with alveolar capillaritis. The histological pattern does not differ at all from the pattern of MPA. Immunofluorescence shows no or only scant immune deposits in GPA and MPA, in contrast to the linear distribution of immune deposits along the basement membranes in Goodpasture's syndrome or the granular immune complex deposits in SLE.

Ocular disease occurs in 50% usually as keratitis, conjunctivitis, scleritis, episcleritis, retro-orbital pseudotumor or optic neuritis.

Musculoskeletal symptoms are common, with most patients experiencing arthralgias and myalgias.

Chest Imaging

Chest imaging may reveal nodule (s) or masses, with or without cavitation. The presence of patchy or diffuse alveolar infiltrations is indicative of AH and may appear as pneumonia. CT findings are more specific of AH.

Laboratory Testing

Every patient with prolonged fever, anemia, malaise and nodular mass or alveolar infiltrations, should be evaluated for the possibility of GPA. It is important to emphasize that asymptomatic proteinuria may be present for weeks or even months before renal failure; so patients with prolonged ENT disease and general or specific symptoms should have a simple urine examination. c-ANCA presents very high specificity for GPA (PR3 positive) but in limited disease, the sensitivity of method is below 70%. c-ANCA PR3 positivity is also indicative of relapse of the disease; ANCA disappearance after the treatment is a good marker for response to treatment.

Treatment of Granulomatosis with Polyangiitis

The limited disease may be treated with methotrexate (MTX) alone or with the combination of oral cyclophosphamide (CYC) plus corticosteroids. The results are excellent, achieving remission 6 months after initiation of treatment in 90-94% of patients. Treatment with the combination of trimethoprim-sulfamethoxazole (T/S) could suffice, in patients with limited ENT or nodular lung disease, provided there is no evidence of capillaritis. If drug allergy to the drug exists, desensitization using oral pediatric T/S solution has to be tried.

Patients with the severe form of the disease, where the symptomatology is caused primarily by inflammation of the small vessels and capillaries (AH, focal necrotizing glomerulonephritis, scleritis, sensorineural hearing loss, mononeuritis multiplex, CNS involvement, leukocytoclastic vasculitis of the skin), have to be immediately treated with the combination of prednisone (1 mg/kg/day) and oral CYC (2 mg/kg/day).

Cyclophosphamide may also be given intravenously (intermittent, high dose: pulse therapy) with the advantages of more effectiveness of inducing remission and lower overall side effects (hemorrhagic cystitis, bladder cancer, myelodysplasia, infections). After 6 months of treatment with oral or IV CYC, the drug is substituted (after remission has been achieved) by oral azathioprine (AZA), which seems to be as effective as CYC in maintaining remission of the disease for 18 months. Patients who do not tolerate the drug well, may receive MTX or mycophenolate mofetil and leflunomide.

Rituximab seems to be as effective as CYC for induction of remission. It can also be used with success in patients with relapsing disease who have been treated with CYC.

Disease Sequelae

The saddle nose deformity, large airway obstruction, subglottic stenosis, and end-stage renal disease are important disease sequelae and they deserve special therapeutic attention. Intratracheal and bronchial dilation may be used for airway obstruction in order to avoid, if possible, tracheostomy. Patency of trachea or mainstem bronchi may be restored by placement of silastic airway stents. Renal transplantation improves quality of life and prognosis for patients on continued dialysis.

Microscopic Polyangiitis

There are several common features between MPA with GPA patients; distinction may be difficult in early disease. MPA is also different from polyarteritis nodosa (PAN). The typical histology consists of pauci-immune focal or segmental necrotizing glomerulonephritis, similar to that seen in GPA. The majority of MPA patients have p-ANCA with specificity for MPO. Renal involvement is the most frequent organ manifestation occurring in 79% of patients, followed by skin (63%), peripheral nerve (58%), and gastrointestinal involvement (30%), whilst lung is involved in only 25% of patients (half of these present with AH). Occasionally, MPA may be associated with pulmonary fibrosis, either in the form of acute interstitial pneumonia or more commonly, resembling idiopathic pulmonary fibrosis. Treatment of MPA includes prednisone and CYC, remission occurs in up to 93% of patients, whilst the relapse rate varies between 8% and 30%. The overall 5-year survival is about 75%. The overall mortality is about 50%.

Eosinophilic Granulomatosis with Polyangiitis (Churg–Strauss–EGPA)

Eosinophilic granulomatosis with polyangiitis (EGPA) is an eosinophilic-rich and necrotizing granulomatous inflammation which predominantly affects the small to medium vessels. EGPA is always associated with asthma and eosinophilia which distinguish the disease from GPA and MPA. Asthma with or without allergic rhinitis and nasal polyps usually precedes vasculitis by a mean of several years and is usually refractory to standard therapy; its onset is late in life and becomes more severe when the vasculitis starts. Chest X-ray reveals transient peripheral alveolar-type infiltrates in more than 70% of the cases. Nodular lesions or eosinophilic pleural effusion can be seen occasionally. DAH is extremely rare, in contrast to GPA and MPA.

Cardiac disease is common and is an important cause of mortality due to congestive heart failure, pericardial effusion and restrictive cardiomyopathy. Peripheral nervous system may also be involved. Renal involvement is less common than in GPA and MPA.

Patients with EGPA respond very well to high dose of systemic corticosteroids. In patients with life-threatening manifestation of the disease, such as nervous system involvement, glomerulonephritis, heart involvement or DAH, CYC should be added to corticosteroids. For remission maintenance other less toxic immunosuppressive drugs could be used, i.e. AZA or MTX in combination with tapering dose of corticosteroids. RTX has also been successfully used in EGPA.

Besides the ANCA-associated small vessel diseases, there are several other diverse vasculitides known to affect the lung although these entities are better associated with extrapulmonary disease. For example, giant cell arteritis (GCA), Takayasu's arteritis (TA), polyarteritis nodosa, Behçet syndrome, and IgA vasculitis may also involve pulmonary vessels.

Giant Cell Arteritis

Giant cell arteritis is a granulomatous arteritis which predominantly affects the aorta and/or its major branches (carotid, vertebral and temporal arteries). GCA is often associated with polymyalgia rheumatica. The most typical features include new onset severe headache, a palpably tender or nodular temporal artery and visual symptoms. Constitutional symptoms of low-grade fever, malaise and weight loss are common. Pulmonary complications reported in up to 25% of patients include cough, sore throat, and hoarseness. Therapy consists of corticosteroids which usually lead to the resolution of pulmonary symptoms.

Takayasu's Arteritis

Takayasu's arteritis is a large vessel vasculitis affecting predominantly the aorta and its major branches in young patients, especially women. It is characterized by stenosis, occlusion and sometimes aneurysms of the large arteries. Initial symptoms in patients with TA often consist of malaise, weight loss and arthralgias. After weeks or months, vascular lesions appear and ischemic disease of the involved organs develops. Typically, there is variability of pulses of the upper and lower extremities and intermittent claudication of the affected vascular territories. Progressive and relapsing disease may cause aortic insufficiency, renovascular hypertension, and ischemia of the affected organs. Mild-to-moderate pulmonary hypertension has been reported in up to 70% in series from Japan and Mexico. The diagnosis is established by demonstration of aneurysms and occluded vessels on classic or magnetic resonance angiography. Corticosteroids constitute the mainstay of the therapy, MTX, may be used for severe cases. Surgical bypass procedures may be considered for severe disease in individual cases.

Polyarteritis Nodosa

Polyarteritis nodosa is a necrotizing vasculitis of medium-sized arteries and does not affect capillaries. It rarely affects the lung, more commonly the bronchial than the pulmonary arteries. It does not cause AH or glomerulonephritis. An association with hepatitis-B virus has been documented in a minority of patients. Immunosuppression with antiviral agents is the treatment of choice in such cases.

Behçet Disease

Behçet disease (BD) is characterized by recurrent aphthous oral ulcerations, and two or more of the following: genital ulcers, uveitis, skin involvement with cutaneous nodules or pustules, meningoencephalitis. The vasculitis in BD may affect both arteries and veins, so that arterial aneurysms and major venous occlusion can occur accordingly. The most common pulmonary manifestation is pulmonary artery aneurysms, typically presenting as hemoptysis. The aneurysm may be single or multiple, unilateral or bilateral. Thrombi within the aneurysms are common. Other manifestations include lung infiltrates, recurrent pneumonias and bronchial occlusion. Fever, elevated ESR, and anemia are common. Treatment of choice consists of combination of prednisone with another drugs, such as colchicine, MTX, AZA or cyclosporine. Anticoagulation should be avoided in case of arteritis. Prognosis is poor in patients with pulmonary involvement, since 30% die within 2 years due to fatal pulmonary hemorrhage.

IgA Vasculitis (Henoch–Schönlein)

Henoch-Schönlein is a vasculitis with IgA1-dominant immune deposits, affecting small vessels. IgA vasculitis (IgAV) usually affects the skin, joints, and gastrointestinal tract. Glomerulonephritis may commonly occur which is similar to IgA nephropathy. Pulmonary capillaritis and DAH are often reported in patients with IgA immune complexes which are present in the serum, lungs, and kidney. Treatment comprises corticosteroids and immunosuppressive drugs.

Cryoglobulinemic Vasculitis

Cryoglobulinemic vasculitis, vasculitis associated with serum cryoglobulins and vascular deposition of immune complexes and complement pulmonary lesions are not uncommon with small vessel leukocytoclastic vasculitis or medium-sized artery involvement. Interstitial lung disease is the most common lung manifestation. DAH is uncommon.

Isolated Pulmonary Capillaritis

Isolated pulmonary capillaritis is confined to the lung without any clinical or serologic features of an associated systemic disease. Most cases are pauci-immune but some may show serum p-ANCA positivity. Prognosis is better when compared with DAH occurring in the presence of systemic vasculitis or a collagen vascular disease. Treatment approach is similar to that of MPA and GPA.

Vasculitis Associated with Systemic Disease

Systemic Lupus Erythematosus

Diffuse alveolar hemorrhage due to pulmonary capillaritis with prominent immune complex deposits or due to bland hemorrhage in systemic lupus erythematosus (SLE) occurs in approximately 4% of patients. In 80%, the DAH occurs in patients with known SLE, it must be distinguished from acute lupus pneumonitis and infectious pneumonia. Almost always the onset is abrupt with pulmonary infiltrates, fever, dyspnea, and hemoptysis (although the latter may be absent in 50%). Glomerulonephritis is usually present. For cases with not known SLE, prolonged fever with malaise and anemia, which is not obviously attributed to other causes especially if accompanied by hematuria, should be considered highly suspicious for SLE. Therapy consists of corticosteroids, CYC and plasmapheresis. Mortality from DAH in SLE (36–62%), mostly occurs due to respiratory failure or superimposed infection. It is important to search for infection and administer broad-spectrum antibiotics. Relapses are often reported.

Diffuse alveolar hemorrhage is also reported in other connective tissue diseases such as rheumatoid arthritis, mixed connective tissue disease, systemic sclerosis, polymyositis, and anti-phospholipid antibody syndrome.

Other Vasculitis Associated with Systemic Diseases

Granulomatous vasculitis of systemic and pulmonary arteries is sometimes reported in sarcoidosis, inflammatory bowel diseases, such as ulcerative colitis. Infiltration of pulmonary vessels by the lymphoid cells which may even be necrotic may be seen in lymphoproliferative disorders affecting the lung.

Drug-associated Vasculitis

Alveolar hemorrhage due to capillaritis attributable to immune mechanism can occur due to drugs: D-penicillamine, propylthiouracil, phenytoin, and transretinoic acid. D-penicillamine can cause both AH and glomerulonephritis with granular deposits of immune complexes in the glomerular capillaries. Other drugs (amiodarone and less frequently, nitrofurantoin) may cause DAH associated with underlying bland hemorrhage or DAD (without evidence of capillaritis).

Antiglomerular Basement Membrane Disease

Antiglomerular basement membrane (anti-GBM) disease is a rare autoimmune disorder (one case per 1,000,000 population per year) characterized by rapidly progressive glomerulonephritis and AH. It is caused by autoantibodies directed against the NC1 domain of the α3 chain of the basement membrane collagen type 4 located on alveolar and glomerular basement membranes. Both pulmonary and renal involvement is seen in about half of cases while there is only renal impairment in the other half. The disease is limited to the lungs in fewer than 10% of patients. Active cigarette smoking is reported to increase the risk of DAH.

The diagnosis is established by the detection of anti-basement membrane antibodies either in serum (in 80% of cases) or in the renal glomeruli. The antibody deposits in the kidneys are seen on immunofluorescence staining of renal biopsy present in a linear fashion along glomerular basement membranes. Antibody deposits are sometimes present in the lungs in about 20% of patients. Such patients may demonstrate p-ANCA (MPO) positivity and more likely to develop DAH. The standard treatment consists of a combination of plasmapheresis, corticosteroids and CYC. Plasmapheresis is aimed at rapid removal of circulating antibodies while immunosuppressive therapy aims at stopping antibody synthesis.

OTHER CAUSES OF DIFFUSE ALVEOLAR HEMORRHAGE

More than half the cases of AH are of nonimmune origin due to heart diseases (especially mitral stenosis and left ventricular failure), infections, drugs (not causing vasculitis), and coagulation disorders. Such causes should not be overlooked.

Hemodynamic Causes

Alveolar hemorrhage in mitral stenosis and left heart disease may be chronic and occult or less frequently, acute and massive. It occurs due to elevated pulmonary venous pressure. The raised hydrostatic pressure in pulmonary capillaries and/or bronchial veins at the surface of bronchial mucosa may lead to capillary rupture in the alveolar spaces and/or airway lumen. Nonvalvular systolic or diastolic left heart disease, mitral regurgitation and pulmonary veno-occlusive disease may also cause AH.

Infections

Opportunistic pulmonary infections such as cytomegalovirus, adenovirus, invasive aspergillosis, mycoplasma, legionella and strongyloides in immunocompromised patients may sometimes cause DAH. Infectious diseases that most frequently cause DAH in immunocompetent patients are leptospirosis, influenza A (H1N1), dengue, malaria, and *Staphylococcus aureus* infection [especially strains producing Panton–Valentine leukocidin (PVL)]. Hanta viruses, CMV, and TB may also cause AH, although such cases are rare. Certain angioinvasive bacteria and fungi may cause vasculitis, vascular necrosis and vascular occlusion with pulmonary infarcts. Diffuse alveolar damage (DAD) and immune mechanisms may play a role in the manifestation of DAH due to pulmonary infections.

Coagulation Disorders

Coagulation disorders may cause DAH without inflammatory capillaritis. Thrombocytopenia, either drug induced or secondary to idiopathic thrombocytopenic purpura or hemolytic uremic syndrome is well-recognized cause of DAH. All drugs acting on hemostasis, including oral anticoagulants, heparin, thrombolytic agents and antiplatelet agents including anti-glycoprotein IIb/IIIa have also been incriminated in the occurrence of AH.

Diffuse Alveolar Damage

Diffuse alveolar damage which occurs in acute interstitial pneumonia, either idiopathic or associated with collagen vascular disease, can sometimes be responsible for DAH. DAD causing DAH may also complicate bone marrow and stem cell transplantation, cytotoxic drug therapy, sirolimus, nitrofurantoin, crack cocaine inhalation, severe viral infections, and radiation therapy.

Idiopathic Pulmonary Hemosiderosis

Idiopathic pulmonary hemosiderosis (IPH) characterized by recurrent episodes of AH, chronic anemia and pulmonary fibrosis, is a rare disease. Around 80% of cases occur in childhood in the first decade of life while the remaining occur in adults usually before the age of 30 years. There is no capillaritis in these patients, the alveolar basement membranes are thickened but remain intact. There is abundant amount of hemosiderin-laden macrophages and red blood cells in the airspaces. The diagnosis of IPH is primarily made by exclusion. The cause and pathogenesis of IPH are not known. Immune mechanisms have been suspected since it appears to respond to immunosuppressant therapy. Corticosteroids are beneficial to control the acute phase as well as to prevent recurrences.

CHAPTER
69

Pulmonary Hypertension: A Third World Perspective

Lakshmi Mudambi, Zeenat Safdar

INTRODUCTION

Pulmonary hypertension (PH) is defined hemodynamically by the presence of elevated mean pulmonary artery pressure (PAP) more than or equal to 25 mmHg that may further lead to right ventricular (RV) failure and premature death. Pulmonary hypertension is classified into groups based on similar pathological and hemodynamic characteristics and treatment approaches (Box 69.1): Group 1 is defined by a mean PAP more than or equal to 25 mm Hg with a pulmonary artery wedge pressure (PAWP) or left ventricular end-diastolic pressure (LVEDP) less than or equal to 15 mm Hg, and pulmonary vascular resistance (PVR) more than 3 wood unit. These criteria account for PH associated with multiple other diseases including chronic obstructive pulmonary disease (COPD). On the other hand, pulmonary venous hypertension [(PVH) diagnostic group 2] is defined by a mean PAP more than or equal to 25 mm Hg with PAWP or LVEDP more than 15 mm Hg.

In group 3, PH and RV enlargement occurring secondarily to chronic lung or chest wall disease, recognized as chronic cor pulmonale has been long considered as an independent disease, especially in the developing countries. The problem continues to pose a challenge in differential diagnosis and management of PH. The disorders of respiratory regulation and chronic central hypoventilation with hypoxemia and carbon dioxide retention are also included in this group. Chronic hypoxia in these conditions is responsible for the development of PH leading to RV failure.

BOX 69.1: Updated classification of pulmonary hypertension (PH) (5th World symposium on PH).

Group 1: Pulmonary arterial hypertension (PAH)
- Idiopathic PAH
- Heritable: BMPR2, Alk1, ENG, SMAD9, CAV1, KCNK3, unknown
- Drug- and toxin-induced
- PAH assoicated with
  - Connective tissue disease
  - Nongenital heart disease
  - HIV
  - Schistosomiasis
  - Portal hypertension
- 1' pulmonary veno-occlusive disease amd/or pulmonary capillary hemangiomatosis
- 1" persistent pulmonary hypertension of newborn (PPHN)

Group 2: Pulmonary hypertension due to left heart disease
- Left ventricle systolic dysfunction
- Left ventricle diastolic dysfunction
- Valvular disease
- Congenital/acquired left heart inflow/outflow tract obstruction and congenital cardiomyopathies

Group 3: Pulmonary hypertension owing to lung disease and/or hypoxemia
- Chronic obstructive pulmonary disease
- Interstitial lung disease
- Other pulmonary disease with mixed restrictive and obstructive pattern
- Sleep-disordered breathing
- Alveolar hypoventilation disorders
- Chronic exposure to high altitude
- Developmental abnormalities

Group 4: Chronic thromboembolic pulmonary hypertension (CTEPH)

Group 5: Pulmonary hypertension with unclear multifactorial mechanisms
- Hematological disorders: Chronic hemolytic anemia, myeloproliferative disorders, splenectomy
- Systemic disorders: Sarcoidosis, pulmonary histiocytosis, and lymphangioleiomyomatosis
- Metabolic disorders: Glycogen storage disease, Gaucher disease, thyroid disorders
- Others: Tumoral obstruction, fibrosing mediastinitis, chronic renal failure, and segmental PH

CLINICAL FEATURES

The symptoms of PH are mostly nonspecific: fatigue, dyspnea, worsening exercise tolerance, sporadic chest pains, abdominal distension, and pedal edema. With disease progression, the RV gets overburdened, leading to right heart failure. There is worsening of symptoms due to fall in the cardiac output causing presyncope or even syncope.

PHYSICAL EXAMINATION

Physical examination is nonspecific in the early and compensated phase. Specific physical signs may include prominent jugular "a" wave and left parasternal heave. On cardiac auscultation, there will be an accentuated second heart sound (P2), presence of midsystolic murmur (caused by turbulent flow across the pulmonary artery) and right sided S4 gallop. Signs of right heart failure (pulsatile liver, marked distention of jugular veins, ascites, and peripheral edema) develop with further disease progression. Other signs, such as hepatojugular reflux and inspiratory augmented tricuspid murmur (Carvallo's sign) may also be present. Cold extremities and systemic hypotension may be present when cardiovascular collapse ensures.

Signs of chronic lung disease, such as those of emphysema, interstitial lung disease (ILD) or chest wall abnormalities (e.g. kyphoscoliosis) are present in cases of chronic cor pulmonale. Stigmata of collagen vascular disease (CVD) include skin changes of scleroderma (skin thickening/tightening, nail fold changes, and telangiectasis), butterfly rash of lupus and heliotrope rash of dermatomyositis/polymyositis. The incidence of pulmonary arterial hypertension (PAH) is higher in patients with mixed connective tissue disease and reported as high as 38%. HIV infection has been associated with an increase prevalence of PAH up to 0.5%.

DIAGNOSTIC EVALUATION

Diagnostic evaluation is aimed at two components: (i) diagnosis of the presence and severity of PH, and (ii) etiological diagnosis.

When clinical history and examination suggest PH, the first diagnostic screening tool is the echocardiogram. If the echocardiogram reveals elevated right ventricular systolic pressures or evidence of RV dysfunction and the suspicion for PH is high, a right heart catheterization should be undertaken as it is the gold standard for establishing the diagnosis (Flowchart 69.1).
The following tests are used in the evaluation of PH:

Electrocardiogram

Suggestive electrocardiogram (ECG) findings include: right-axis deviation, "rSR" pattern in lead V1, tall R wave and small S wave with R/S ratio more than 1 in lead V1, qR complex in lead V1, large S wave and small R wave with R/S ratio less than 1 in lead V5 or V6; or S1, S2, S3 pattern. Right precordial leads may show ST-T segment wave depression. Right atrial enlargement manifests with tall P wave (>2.5 mm) in leads II, III, and aVF and frontal P-axis of 75°.

Chest Radiography

Plain chest radiography (CXR) shows enlarged main and hilar pulmonary arterial shadows with attenuated peripheral pulmonary vascular markings (pruning) and RV enlargement. Right ventricular enlargement is better seen

Flowchart 69.1: Evaluation of pulmonary hypertension.

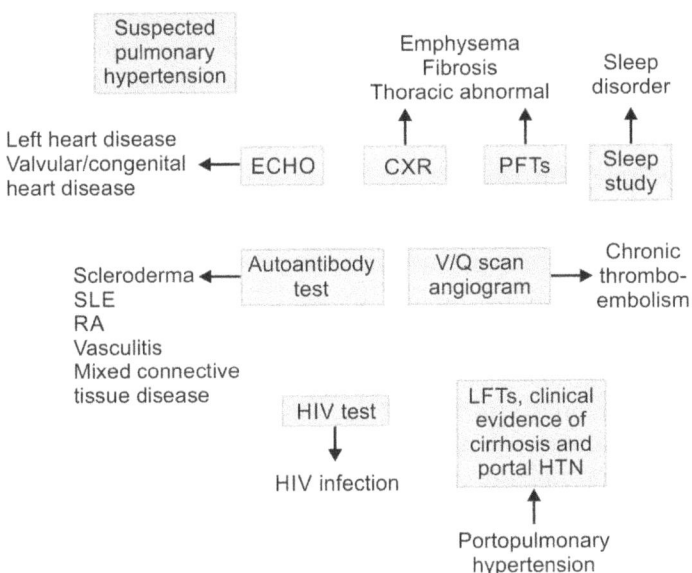

on the lateral films as impingement of the anteriorly situated RV silhouette into the retrosternal clear space. In a case of chronic cor pulmonale, CXR may also show evidence of emphysema, presence of other lung parenchymal diseases or of chest wall deformity.

Echocardiogram

Echocardiogram (ECHO) is a commonly used, simple and noninvasive screening tool for evaluation of PH. ECHO provides detailed assessment of biventricular function and anatomy. Doppler ECHO can be employed to assess the right ventricle systolic pressure (RVSP) in the presence of tricuspid regurgitation jet. In the absence of pulmonary artery outflow obstruction or stenosis, the PAP approximately equals the RVSP.

Ventilation–perfusion Scan

This is an important test to determine the presence of chronic thromboembolic hypertension (CTEPH) disease. CTEPH is a potentially curable by patients undergoing pulmonary endarterectomy. Ventilation–perfusion (V/Q) scan is also useful to look for the presence of an underlying lung disease that will be evident as ventilation defects.

Computerized Tomography of the Chest

Pulmonary vein anatomy in the thorax can be better appreciated on multidetector row CT with three-dimensional volume rendering. Presence of abnormalities in the pulmonary venous drainage points to the need of prompt evaluation for structural anomalies causing PH. The helical CT chest is helpful to define RV dysfunction after acute pulmonary embolism if it shows right ventricular dilation and deviation of interventricular septum toward LV. High-resolution CT chest is of particular help diagnose a chronic lung disease, such as the bronchiectasis, COPD or ILD.

Pulmonary Function Tests

Isolated reduction in DLCO in the absence of other lung pathology may be the only abnormal finding on lung function testing.

Serological Evaluation

A complete evaluation for serological markers of systemic lupus erythematosus, scleroderma, rheumatoid arthritis, polymyositis/dermatomyositis and mixed connective tissue diseases should be undertaken early in patients with PAH. Elevated antinuclear antibodies may be seen in up to 40% of patients with PAH.

Right Heart Catheterization

This remains the gold standard to determine the presence of pulmonary arterial versus PVH by providing true measurements of mean PAP, right atrial pressure and cardiac output, and pulmonary capillary wedge pressure.

Pulmonary vasoreactivity is most commonly seen in idiopathic PAH, hereditary PAH or anorexigen-associated PAH. Unfortunately, less than 10% of patients elicit a positive vasodilator response and 50% of initial responders remain responsive on repeat vasodilator testing. Still, patients who show vasoreactivity appear to have a better prognosis when treated with long-term calcium channel blocker therapy than those who do not have a positive response.

Six-minute Walk Test

Exercise capacity in a PH patient is assessed by a six-minute walk distance (6MWD). Several randomized clinical trials have demonstrated the prognostic ability of a 6MWD and used 6MWD as the primary end point.

PATHOPHYSIOLOGY

Pulmonary arterial hypertension involves pulmonary arteries of less 500 μm. It is characterized by intimal proliferation, medial hypertrophy, and adventitial hyperplasia. The muscularization of the small pulmonary arteries leads to decreased vascular lumen. Endothelial dysfunction has a main role in PH. There is increased production of endothelin-1, the most potent vasoconstrictor known to mankind, in the diseased pulmonary vasculature. There is increased production of vasoconstrictor endothelin-1 as well as thromboxane and decreased production of vasodilator, such as prostacyclin and nitric oxide (NO).

Nitric oxide is recognized as an important endothelium derived vasodilator playing a major role in maintaining vascular tone in normoxemic pulmonary vasculature. Increased shear may contribute to the increase in vascular tone in the presence of reduced NO production. In addition to excessive vasoconstriction, both endothelin and thromboxane has vascular remodeling effects that lead to muscularized pulmonary arterioles.

In addition to medial hypertrophy, and intimal fibrosis, PH is associated with thrombi in situ in small muscular pulmonary arteries. The increased platelet aggregation may be due to abnormal arachidonic acid metabolism as shown by an elevated urinary metabolite of thromboxane A2 (TXA2) and reduced urinary metabolite of prostacyclin (PGI_2) in PH.

MANAGEMENT

Treatment of the etiological cause constitutes the cornerstone of management of PH associated with chronic lung or heart disease. The role of pulmonary pressure lowering drugs is neither established nor recommended in PH associated with left heart failure or lung disease.

Oxygen Therapy

Hypoxic vasoconstriction plays an important role in the pathophysiology of PH. Oxygen therapy is a cornerstone in management of hypoxemia in these patients.

Anticoagulation

Improved survival has been demonstrated in patients with idiopathic PAH who were treated with oral anticoagulation. Therefore, anticoagulation is recommended in idiopathic PAH patients with no contraindication for anticoagulation.

Diuretics

In the presence of signs of right heart failure (peripheral edema, ascites, hepatomegaly) use of diuretics is strongly encouraged. Patients should be advised to maintain near-normal intravascular volume and monitor salt and water intake. Diuretics commonly used are furosemide (loop diuretic) and spironolactone (aldosterone receptor antagonist). Aggressive diuresis should be avoided to prevent systemic hypotension, acute renal failure, and hemodynamic compromise.

Digoxin

Digoxin has not been extensively studied in PAH. Digoxin may be useful in refractory right heart failure to augment RV function and increase cardiac output in PAH.

Vasodilator Therapy

Multiple pharmacological agents modulate vascular remodeling in addition to their pulmonary vasodilatory effects. Several drugs are now available to treat PAH associated with group 1 diseases. Specific drug therapies for the three major pathways [(i) endothelin pathway, (ii) prostacyclin pathway and (iii) NO pathway] implicated in the pathogenesis of PAH include: (i) prostanoids—epoprostenol, treprostinil, inhaled treprostinil, iloprost, oral treprostinil; (ii) Endothelin receptor antagonists—bosentan, ambrisentan, and macitentan; (iii) Phosphodiesterase 5 inhibitors—sildenafil, tadalafil and soluble guanylate cyclase stimulator—riociguat.

These agents are not indicated to treat PH related to left heart disease (group 2 PH) or lung disease (group 3 PH).

In summary, PH is a serious disease that carries a high mortality. Although echocardiogram is a good screening tool, the diagnosis is confirmed on right heart catheterization. Determining the etiology of PH is important since current pharmacological agents are approved only for specific diagnostic groups of PAH. Since use of PH-specific therapy is not recommended in management of PH in diagnostic groups 2, 3, and 5 is targeted at treatment of the underlying cause (left-sided heart disease/valvular disease, sleep apnea, lung disease, obesity hypoventilation syndrome, etc.).

CHAPTER 70

Pulmonary Thromboembolism

Devasahayam J Christopher, Richa Gupta

INTRODUCTION

Pulmonary thromboembolism (PTE) generally includes syndromic manifestations of both pulmonary embolism (PE) and deep vein thrombosis (DVT). In most cases PE takes its origin from DVT. About 50% of patients with proximal DVT are likely to have an associated, clinically asymptomatic PE on lung scan. DVT can be found in the lower limbs in about 70% of patients with PE, if sensitive diagnostic methods are used. Patients who present with PE have greater risk of death related to the initial acute episode or to recurrent PE. Two-thirds of cases are unsuspected and unconfirmed antemortem. Furthermore, it is well known that only one-third of cases suspected to be PE on the basis of clinical symptoms turn out to have other conditions after investigations (Fig. 70.1).

PATHOPHYSIOLOGY

There are three important factors related to clot formation (Virchow's triad): (i) venous stasis, (ii) increased blood coagulability, and (iii) injury to the vein wall. Thrombosis in the deep veins of the lower limbs, particularly between the knee and the inguinal ligament, is the most common source of pulmonary emboli. PE is infrequently due to thrombosis of the pelvic veins, veins of the upper extremities or other organ systems (e.g. hepatic and renal veins). The thrombus dislodges and travels through the venous circulation and lodges in one of the pulmonary arteries. The embolism initially results in an area of the lung that is ventilated but underperfused, resulting in an alveolar dead space. Release of vasoactive substances like serotonin from the platelets and the

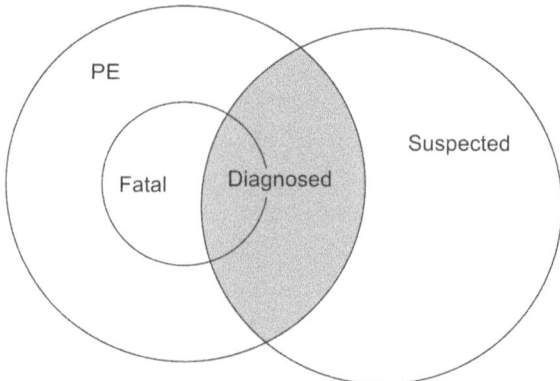

Fig. 70.1: Relationship between suspected and diagnosed pulmonary embolism (PE).

Flowchart 70.1: Pathophysiology of pulmonary embolism—formation of deep vein thrombosis (DVT) and embolization into pulmonary arteries leads to acute increase in pulmonary vascular resistance, which increases the demand on the right ventricle and may decrease the cardiac output. This combination of effects can lead to right ventricular dysfunction, infarction, and even cardiac arrest.

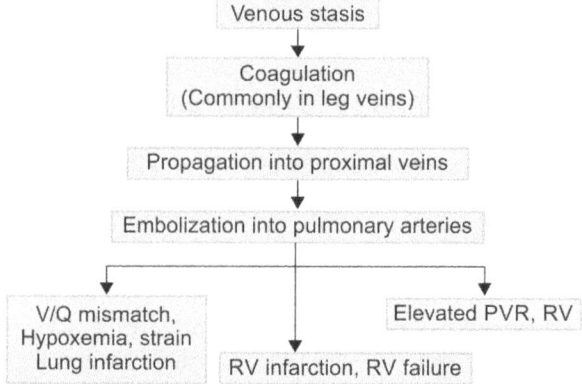

blockade of the pulmonary artery by the clot cause an elevation of pulmonary vascular resistance. This results in an increase in right ventricular work load, leading to a redistribution of blood flow and increase in right ventricular work load, which if excessive may result in right ventricular failure (Flowchart 70.1). Once this occurs there is a fall in the pulmonary blood flow and reduction of left ventricular filling, causing systemic hypotension.

Airway obstruction resulting from the reflex bronchoconstriction further contributes to the ventilation–perfusion (V/Q) mismatch. After about 24 hours, there is depletion of surfactant; this may result in atelectasis and edema in the affected area. Pulmonary embolism causes infarction in only about 10% of cases. Pulmonary parenchyma has three potential sources of oxygen—the pulmonary arteries, the bronchial arteries and the alveoli of which at least two need to be compromised for infarction to develop; this usually happens only in patients with coexisting cardiopulmonary disease. Moreover, complete occlusion of the pulmonary artery is not common.

RISK FACTORS

There are several important risk factors for venous thromboembolism (VTE) to develop (Table 70.1). But the predictive values of these factors are different; VTE can also occur in patients in the absence of identifiable predisposing factors.

CLINICAL FEATURES

The clinical features vary widely from one patient to another. In most patients, suspicion of PE arises by clinical symptoms, such as dyspnea, chest pain and syncope, either alone or in combination.

The initial presentation usually falls into one of the following three categories:
- *Pulmonary infarction syndrome*: The patients who fall in this category, which is generally mild, present with dyspnea and pleuritic chest pain.
- *Isolated dyspnea*: In these patients, the only symptom is acute shortness of breath. These patients are often hypoxic and PE is deemed to be moderate.
- *Circulatory collapse*: Patients in this category present with circulatory collapse, characterized by shock or syncope. PE is deemed to be severe.

Further, pleuritic chest pain, with or without dyspnea, is one of the most frequent presentations of PE. Retrosternal angina-like chest pain, (which

TABLE 70.1: Risk factors for pulmonary embolism.

Conditions for PE	Major risk factors	Minor risk factors
Surgery and fractures	• Abdominal/pelvic surgery • Hip/knee replacement • Postoperative ICU care • Bone fractures especially of tibia and femur	• Oral contraceptive pills • Hormone replacement therapy • Myocardial infarction • Congestive cardiac failure • Congenital heart disease • Superficial venous thrombosis • Indwelling central vein catheter • Chronic obstructive airways disease • Increasing age • Occult malignancy • Thrombotic disorders • Long distance sedentary travel • Obesity
Malignancy	• Pancreatic • Bronchial • Genitourinary • Stomach and colon • Breast • Advanced/metastatic	
Obstetrics	• Pregnancy—late • Puerperium • Cesarean section	
Immobilization (especially lower limb)	• Plaster of Paris cast • Paralysis • Hospitalization • Institutional care	
Others	Previous proven VTE	

(PE, pulmonary embolism; VTE, venous thromboembolism)

may reflect right ventricular ischemia) is seen with moderate to large sized embolism. Dyspnea may be insidious in onset and progressive over several weeks. Diagnosis of PE is considered by exclusion of other causes of dyspnea. Syncope which indicates a severely reduced hemodynamic reserve is a rare presentation of PTE.

Tachypnea is the most common sign. Other general physical signs include tachycardia, fever, diaphoresis, and cyanosis. Crackles, wheezes and pleural friction rub may be heard on chest auscultation. Cardiac examination may reveal parasternal heave, loud pulmonary component of the second heart sound, third or fourth heart sound. Hepatomegaly and hepatojugular reflux may also be present. But these findings are common to several cardiopulmonary disorders and so have low specificity.

Since lower limb DVT is the cause of PE in the majority of cases, it is prudent to look for features of DVT, namely, local pain, tenderness, redness, and warmth.

DIAGNOSIS

The diagnosis of PE requires the integration of a careful history and physical examination with laboratory testing and appropriate imaging modalities.

Routine and Ancillary Investigations

Routine investigations like chest X-ray, electrocardiography (ECG) and 2D-echo are of limited value in the diagnosis of PE. More importantly they contribute in excluding many common conditions with similar clinical presentation like; acute myocardial infarction, acute aortic dissection, pneumonia, pneumothorax, cardiac failure, etc. Chest radiographic abnormalities are commonly seen in patients with PE; however, they are not helpful diagnostically, because they are nonspecific. Electrocardiogram abnormalities are also nonspecific, may show sinus tachycardia and atrial arrhythmia. In particular, new-onset atrial flutter should increase suspicion of acute PE.

Echocardiography is best used to assess the impact of acute PE on right ventricular function in suspected or proven case. The findings may include a regional pattern of right ventricular dysfunction, akinesia of the mid free wall, and right ventricular free wall but normal apical contractility (McConnell's sign). Acute right ventricular infarction may also cause a similar appearance. Rarely, echocardiogram may identify emboli in-transit in the right atrium.

Arterial blood gas analysis may show hypoxemia and hypocapnia. Blood gases may be normal, especially in younger patients in the absence of any cardiopulmonary disease. Pulmonary embolism should be considered in any patient with significant unexplained hypoxemia even when the chest radiograph is normal or near normal.

The levels of D-dimers in plasma are raised in PTE as a result of fibrin degradation and intravascular coagulation. The levels reflect the fibrinolytic activity on preexisting thrombi and not necessarily the rate of thrombus formation. But D-dimer levels are also elevated in various conditions like cancer, inflammation, peripheral vascular disease, and hospitalized patients, including obstetrics cases.

Serum troponin may be elevated in acute PE, indicating right ventricular ischemia or microinfarction. Brain natriuretic peptide (BNP) levels may also be elevated in acute PE, because of right ventricular dilation. This may serve as a clue to the diagnosis, but are also nonspecific.

Diagnostic Imaging for Suspected Pulmonary Embolism

Deep Venous Thrombosis Testing

Compression ultrasonography (CUS) is used to look for DVT which is seen in 30–50% of patients with PE and helps as an indirect method for diagnosing PE. Finding a proximal DVT in patients suspected of PE is sufficient to warrant anticoagulant treatment. Incomplete compressibility of the vein, which indicates the presence of a clot is the only validated diagnostic criterion for DVT; the flow criteria are unreliable. CT can be avoided in patients with contraindications to contrast dye and/or irradiation in the presence of positive proximal CUS.

Radioisotope Ventilation–Perfusion Scan

Ventilation–perfusion scintigraphy (V/Q scan) is a helpful test for diagnosis of suspected PE. Diagnostic accuracy of the V/Q scan is greatest when the test is combined with clinical probability:
- Likelihood of PE is 95% in patients with high clinical probability of PE and a high-probability V/Q scan.
- Likelihood of PE is only 4% in patients with low clinical probability of PE and a low-probability V/Q scan.
- A normal V/Q scan virtually excludes PE.
- Strong clinical suspicion of PE in the presence of a nondiagnostic VQ scan should lead to further evaluation [computed tomography angiography (CTA), pulmonary angiography or lower limb DVT studies]. Although rare, the radioisotopes may cause an allergic reaction.

Computer Tomography Pulmonary Arteriography

Computed tomography pulmonary arteriography (CTPA) has become the most commonly used diagnostic modality for patients with suspected PE. One of the most commonly cited benefits of CTPA is its ability to detect alternative pulmonary abnormalities that may explain the patient's clinical presentation. With spiral CT, the location and the magnitude of the thrombus is demonstrated and both mediastinal and parenchymal structures are evaluated, which may provide important alternate or additional diagnoses.

The advent of the multidetector CT (MDCT) angiography largely overcame the limitations with regards to the accuracy of spiral CT. MDCT angiography has several distinct advantages: reduced scanning time, thin sections and markedly improved visualization of segmental and subsegmental vessels.

Pulmonary Angiography

Pulmonary angiography remains the gold standard for the confirmation of the diagnosis. It is indicated if other investigations are inconclusive or there is cardiovascular collapse and hypotension. It requires placement of a catheter into the pulmonary artery for injection of the dye. The catheter is inserted through the femoral, internal jugular or the subclavian vein. The features indicating the presence of an embolus include intraluminal filling defect and abrupt vascular cutoff in pulmonary arteries. Fatal complications occur in 0.5–1.3% of the procedures and minor complications in 2% of patients.

MANAGEMENT

General Management

It is often recommended to hospitalize the patient for 24–48 hours for initial bed rest. Analgesics are administered for treatment of severe pleuritic pain. Opiates should be avoided in patients with incipient cardiovascular collapse, because of the fear of vasodilatation. High percentage inspired oxygen is required for management of hypoxemia but severe hypoxia may require assisted ventilation. Colloids are administered for treatment of hypotension with monitoring of central venous pressure; high right atrial pressure (15–20 mm Hg) should be maintained to ensure maximal right ventricular filling. Inotropic agents should be used to provide circulatory support. Diuretics and vasodilators which lower the blood pressure are not indicated.

Specific Treatment

From point of view of therapy patients suffering from PE can be classified into one of the following subsets:
- *Stable pulmonary embolism*: Normotensive patients (when SBP ≥90 mm Hg) and no evidence of right ventricular dysfunction.
- *Submassive pulmonary embolism*: Normotensive patients (SBP ≥90 mm Hg) with evidence of right ventricular dysfunction.
- *Massive pulmonary embolism*: Patient is hypotensive in cardiogenic shock (SBP <90 mm Hg) or cardiac arrest or there is fall in systolic BP by more than 40 mm Hg for at least 15 min.

Anticoagulation is the mainstay of treatment for acute PE. The main objectives of anticoagulant therapy in the initial treatment of PE are to prevent thrombus extension while allowing endogenous fibrinolysis to proceed and to prevent early and late recurrences of VTE.

Stable PE can be managed in hospital or on an outpatient basis with anticoagulation either with unfractionated heparin (UFH) or low molecular weight heparin (LMWH) or factor Xa inhibitor—fondaparinux. Massive and submassive PE carries high mortality; modalities to achieve early reperfusion of the pulmonary arteries may be lifesaving by reversing the right ventricular dysfunction. The various options available are—thrombolysis, surgical embolectomy and percutaneous catheter embolectomy.

Anticoagulant Therapy

Anticoagulant treatment plays a critical role in the management of patients with PE and is required universally regardless of whether they have undergone reperfusion therapy for massive and submassive PE. Anticoagulants help in preventing formation of new thrombus, death and recurrent events with an acceptable rate of bleeding complications. The agents that are used for anticoagulation are as follows.

Unfractionated Heparin

Unfractionated heparin acts by binding to antithrombin and catalyzing the inactivation of thrombin factor Xa and other clotting factors. Besides, it also binds with other plasma proteins which can lead to nonhemorrhagic side effects, such as heparin-induced thrombocytopenia (HIT) and osteoporosis. Since the anticoagulant effect of UFH which can be rapidly reversed, it is the agent of choice for patients with PE who are at high risk of bleeding (Table 70.2).

The important complications associated with heparin are bleeding, immune mediated platelet activation leading to HIT and osteoporosis. Sometimes dermatological side effects, such as necrosis, alopecia, and hypersensitivity are encountered.

Low-molecular Weight Heparin

Low molecular weight heparins (LMWH), derived from UFH by chemical or enzymatic depolymerization have more predictable pharmacokinetic and pharmacodynamic properties. LMWH have a longer half-life and a lower risk of nonhemorrhagic side effects than heparin; moreover, they can be administered through simple subcutaneous route without the need for laboratory monitoring. LMWH should be given with care in patients with renal failure. Initial anticoagulation for patients with severe renal impairment (creatinine clearance <30 mL/min) should be provided preferably with intravenous UFH.

TABLE 70.2: Regimens of heparin therapy.

Intravenous route	Subcutaneous route
• 80 U/kg bolus followed by 18 U/kg/h infusion, 70 U/kg bolus followed by 15 U/kg/h for cardiac or stroke patients OR • 5,000 U bolus followed by 1,000 U/h infusion	• Initial dose of 333 U/kg subcutaneously followed by 250 U/kg twice daily, OR • I/V bolus of 5,000 U followed by 250 U/kg twice daily

Fondaparinux

Fondaparinux is a synthetic polysaccharide with anti-Xa activity. It has been shown to be as effective as heparin and is not associated with HIT. Dosage is required once daily and is weight related. It is contraindicated in severe renal failure (creatinine clearance <30 mL/min).

Long-term Anticoagulation

Long-term anticoagulation to prevent clot recurrence is usually achieved by oral vitamin K antagonists (VKA) like warfarin or acenocoumarol). However, it should be initiated once PE has been reliably confirmed. Oral anticoagulation with warfarin is initiated with dose between 5 mg and 10 mg, preferably on the first treatment day, along with parenteral anticoagulants with subsequent dosing based on the international normalized ratio (INR) response. A starting dose of 5 mg or 7.5 mg warfarin is preferred over higher doses.

Monitoring of Oral Anticoagulants

Anticoagulation therapy should be monitored with measurement of INR after the initial two or three doses of oral VKA therapy. Monitoring should be done at regular intervals of no longer than every 4 weeks for patients on a stable dose of oral anticoagulants.

Newer Oral Anticoagulants

Dabigatran etexilate (direct thrombin inhibitor, IIa), rivaroxaban, and apixaban (direct coagulation factor Xa inhibitor) are FDA approved newer oral anticoagulants for clinical use. Newer oral anticoagulants have the potential to overcome the short comings of VKAs. These can be administered in fixed doses without need for close laboratory monitoring with no significant food-drug interactions. However, they are costly and lack specific antidotes as well as long-term safety data. Newer studies on these aspects will help in deciding more widespread use of newer oral anticoagulants in clinical practice.

Duration of Anticoagulation Therapy

Duration of anticoagulant treatment depends on the risk benefit assessment by weighing the estimated risk of recurrence after treatment discontinuation and the risk of bleeding complications while on treatment. Recurrences during and after treatment are quite unusual when the risk factors for VTE are temporary. Long-term anticoagulation is required for recurrent embolism. In patients with persisting underlying risk factors (such as deficiency of antithrombin III, protein C or protein S), the anticoagulation is usually prolonged to several years, possibly lifelong.

Thrombolytic Therapy

Thrombolytic therapy is recommended as the first-line treatment for patients with massive PE (hemodynamic compromise/imminent cardiac arrest).

The therapy not only helps in achieving rapid resolution of PE; but also rapid hemodynamic improvement. It has no role in the management of hemodynamically stable patients, except perhaps in the subgroup of patients with submassive PE (right ventricular dysfunction but normal systemic arterial pressure), in which there is some evidence for its efficacy. Thrombolytic treatment is most effective when administered soon after the onset of PE, but benefit may extend for up to 14 days from the onset of symptoms. While thrombolysis may be lifesaving in massive and submassive PE, the extent of long-term survival and reduction in mortality at 90 days remains unclear.

Drawbacks of thrombolytic therapy are—high cost, risk of severe and often fatal bleeding and allergic reactions (specifically to streptokinase).

Inferior Vena Caval Filters

Inferior vena caval (IVC) filter devices in the inferior vena cava prevent the emboli from distal drainage areas traveling to the pulmonary circulation. In view of the associated complications, the routine use of IVC filters is not recommended. IVC filters are also associated with late sequelae, including the recurrent DVT episodes and development of the postthrombotic syndrome. The two main indications for the use of filters are absolute contraindications to anticoagulation and high risk of VTE recurrence.

Surgical Management

Surgical Embolectomy

Surgical embolectomy has been reserved for a selective group of patients who have massive PE with hemodynamic instability requiring cardiopulmonary resuscitation or who have failed thrombolytic therapy or have contraindications to its use. It may also be performed in patients with patent foramen ovale and intracardiac thrombi.

Catheter Embolectomy

As alternatives to surgical embolectomy, other methods, such as catheter-based mechanical pulmonary embolectomy, local intraembolic thrombolytic therapy, or both may be considered. Indications for these procedures are similar to those for surgical embolectomy.

Various biomarkers have been used for risk stratification. There is a greater risk of death in patients with PE with high levels of BNP, pro-BNP, and cardiac troponins (both T and I). Similarly, elevated troponin level is associated with a fivefold increase in short-term mortality. Troponin levels may predict outcomes not only in patients with shock, but also in those who are hemodynamically stable at presentation.

CHAPTER
71

Pulmonary Vascular Malformations

Gautam Ahluwalia

INTRODUCTION

The diagnosis of pulmonary vascular malformations (Box 71.1) has revolutionized with the advent of multidetector computed tomography (MDCT). Though pulmonary arteriovenous malformations (PAVMs) are not very common, they constitute an important differential diagnosis in patients presenting with hypoxemia, paradoxical embolism, and nodules on chest radiographs. PAVMs are also known as pulmonary telangiectasias, cavernous angiomas of the lung, pulmonary arteriovenous fistulae or aneurysms. Most PAVMs are congenital in nature. However, these abnormalities can also develop later in life as acquired conditions (Box 71.2). PAVMs occur more frequently in

---

BOX 71.1: Pulmonary vascular malformations.

Congenital:
- Congenital pulmonary artery stenosis
- Congenital pulmonary artery aneurysms
- Pulmonary arteriovenous malformations (PAVMs)
- Bronchopulmonary sequestration (BPS)
- Congenital pulmonary airway malformation (CPAM)
- Hybrid lesions of BPS and CPAM
- Anomalous pulmonary venous return
- Pulmonary venous varices

Acquired:
- Pulmonary artery pseudoaneurysm
- Pulmonary emboli

> **BOX 71.2:** Acquired conditions presenting with pulmonary arteriovenous malformation (PAVM).
>
> - *Hepatic:* Cirrhosis
> - *Cardiovascular:* Mitral stenosis
> - *Infections:* Actinomycosis, schistosomiasis
> - *Malignancy:* Metastatic thyroid carcinoma
> - Postoperative congenital cyanotic heart disease patients
> - Trauma

women as compared to men. The male:female ratio is 1:2. In neonates, there is male preponderance.

HEREDITARY HEMORRHAGIC TELANGIECTASIAS OR RENDU–OSLER–WEBER SYNDROME

Hereditary hemorrhagic telangiectasias (HHT) is a syndrome encompassing arteriovenous malformations (AVMs) in nose (>95%), skin (>80%), lungs (>30%), gastrointestinal tract (>30%), liver (>30%), and brain (>10%). HHT has an autosomal dominant inheritance with an age-related penetrance; all patients manifest the disease by the age of 40 years. It is important to appreciate that AVMs in HHT (though present from birth) manifest clinically only in adult life after the AVM vessels have been exposed to pressure in the initial decades of life. The early clinical features include the appearance of cutaneous telangiectasia or epistaxis. Later on, the patients may present with dyspnea, pulmonary hemorrhage or obscure gastrointestinal bleeding.

PATHOGENESIS

By definition, telangiectasia is a localized tortuous enlargement of the postcapillary venule with perivascular lymphocytic infiltration and smooth muscle proliferation. AVM is a direct communication between the pulmonary artery and the pulmonary vein with aneurysmal enlargement of the feeding artery. It is hypothesized that there is incomplete resorption of vascular septae, between arterial and venous plexuses during fetal development. Other postulation supports a defect in the terminal arterial loop, which results in dilatation of thin-walled capillary sacs.

Anatomically, there are three characteristic appearances of PAVMs: (i) large single sac; and (ii) plexiform mass of dilated vascular channels; or (iii) direct tortuous communication between artery and vein. Pathologically, they consist of two elements—vascular channels lined with endothelium form the first element and the connective tissue stroma with no connection with lung parenchyma form the second element. Most PAVMs have paper thin walls, similar to the AVMs occurring in other parts of the body. Occasionally, PAVM may become calcified or contain a thrombus.

CLINICAL FEATURES

In early life, patients with PAVM are asymptomatic or may present with cyanosis, cardiac failure or respiratory failure. Most patients become symptomatic in the fourth or the fifth decade. Symptoms occur more frequently in patients with PAVM and HHT than in patients with PAVM alone. Moreover, symptoms correlate with the size and number of PAVM. Single and less than 2 cm PAVM are asymptomatic. Patients with multiple PAVMs have a higher probability of presence of symptoms.

Epistaxis is the most common symptom in PAVM. Epistaxis may precede the development of external telangiectasia by 10–30 years in HHT. Epistaxis may occur spontaneously or result from minor trauma to the nasal telangiectasia present. One in two patients with HHT develops epistaxis in the first two decades of life with almost all the patients developing it by the fifth decade. The presence of lung nodules (PAVM) and the history of recurrent epistaxis should raise the suspicion of HHT.

Dyspnea is the next common symptom after epistaxis. It is most frequently observed with large or multiple PAVM. Platypnea is another characteristic pulmonary symptom, although it is also observed in other conditions. Hemoptysis is the third most common symptom after epistaxis and dyspnea. Gastrointestinal hemorrhage occurs in 20–30% patients. This symptom manifests in later life with 50% patients developing between 30 years and 58 years and the remaining after the age of 58 years. Infrequently, occult bleeding from extrapulmonary sources, including from superficial telangiectasias over skin and mucosa may result in iron-deficiency anemia. Many nonspecific symptoms may occur from complications, such as hypoxemia, polycythemia or cerebrovascular accidents due to the presence of AVM in the brain.

On general physical examination, superficial telangiectasia present on face, oral cavity, chest and upper extremities are the sole findings in these patients. The predominant skin lesions are found on the lower lip, tongue, nose, and skin. The HHT lesions of 1–3 mm size are slightly rounded with dendrite-like projections, ruby-colored and sharply demarcated from adjacent skin and mucosa. Unlike the flat and readily blanchable spider nevi in chronic liver disease, the telangiectasia of HHT are papular and do not completely blanch with pressure. PAVM patients with significant hypoxemia develop cyanosis and clubbing, almost all patients with PAVM and dyspnea manifest clubbing.

On chest examination, murmurs or bruits increasing on inspiration are heard in almost one out of two patients with PAVM. The murmurs also increase when the PAVM assumes a gravitationally dependent position. Though the triad of dyspnea, clubbing, and cyanosis is considered specific for PAVM, it is observed in only 10% cases.

INVESTIGATIONS

On arterial blood gas analysis, hypoxemia especially orthodeoxia (decrease in saturation from supine to sitting position) are observed in PAVM. Pulmonary function tests have no role in the diagnosis.

Chest radiography is the initial investigation raising the suspicion of PAVM in a patient. It may reveal a lobulated and sharply defined pulmonary nodule in the lower lobe. The size of the nodule which is usually single, varies from 1 cm to 5 cm. Smaller PAVM may reveal only a nonspecific increase in pulmonary vascular markings, which may wax and wane over a period of time. On fluoroscopy, PAVM lesions in the lung reveal pulsations during Valsalva maneuver. Intrapulmonary shunts can be best demonstrated on contrast echocardiography. With normal anatomy, the contrast bubbles injected in the peripheral vein are visualized in the left atrium after a delay of three to eight cardiac cycles (2–5 seconds). On the other hand, they are visualized in the left atrium within one cardiac cycle of appearing in the right atrium in the presence of an intracardiac shunt.

Multidetector computed tomography has become the investigation of choice. The high-resolution volumetric images can be attained with a single breath hold. Moreover, three-dimensional reconstruction of the lesion on MDCT assists in the characterization of the vascular lesions. Smaller lesions missed on the chest radiograph can be diagnosed by MDCT. This modality also helps in the differentiation of PAVM from other vascular lesions of the lung (Box 71.1). The use of contrast as a timed bolus can help to delineate the arterial and venous phases to further characterize the feeding arterial supply and venous drainage.

MANAGEMENT

One in four PAVM slowly enlarge in size, whereas the remaining lesions are unchanged over years. The growth rate varies from 5 mm to 10 mm every 5–15 years. It has also been observed that enlargement is more common in patients with HHT compared to patients without HHT. The main modalities of therapy include surgery and embolotherapy. The various procedures included local excision, segment resection, lobectomy or pneumonectomy. In patients unfit for surgery, the transection of pulmonary artery was also used as a treatment modality. Video-assisted thoracoscopic surgery is a preferred choice.

Embolization of the feeding artery was first used in the year 1977. The embolic material includes vascular plugs, coils, balloons, and alcohol. Currently, embolotherapy is the modality of choice. It avoids general anesthesia and there is no loss of pulmonary parenchyma. It is also the procedure of choice in multiple and/or bilateral PAVM. As compared to surgery, periprocedural mortality and morbidity with embolization is almost negligible. There is no role of hormonal therapy, unlike anecdotal reports in patient with AVM of other regions. The role of antibiotic prophylaxis to avoid the chances of cerebral abscess needs emphasis before dental and surgical procedures in these patients.

OTHER PULMONARY VASCULAR MALFORMATIONS

Rarely there is congenital stenosis of pulmonary arteries (proximal interruption, anomalous origin of the left pulmonary artery or pulmonary artery sling) detected incidentally on chest radiography or MDCT. Sometimes, acquired anomalies, such as the diffuse or focal enlargement of pulmonary arteries may be seen. The acquired abnormalities commonly result from causes, such as pulmonary hypertension, pulmonary artery aneurysm, and intravascular pulmonary metastasis.

Congenital Pulmonary Artery, Aneurysm, and Pseudoaneurysm

Most pulmonary artery aneurysms and pseudoaneurysms are caused by trauma (including the iatrogenic causes, such as the malpositioned Swan-Ganz catheters, and chest tube insertion), infection (fungal, tuberculosis, and pyogenic), and vasculitis (Behçet's syndrome). The pulmonary artery aneurysms due to tuberculosis known as Rasmussen aneurysms generally occur in the upper lobe. Pulmonary artery aneurysm and pseudoaneurysm may sometimes occur in the presence of pulmonary hypertension, congenital pulmonary stenosis, neoplasm (bronchogenic carcinoma), and connective tissue disease (Marfan syndrome). It is important to detect pulmonary artery aneurysms and pseudoaneurysms since they carry a high risk of rupture-related morbidity and mortality.

Anomalous Pulmonary Venous Return

Anomalous pulmonary venous return (APVR) is a congenital disorder which can be either total or partial. Total APVR is characterized by total mixing of systemic venous and pulmonary venous blood within the heart and causes cyanosis. In contrast, cyanosis is not present in partial anomalous pulmonary venous return (PAPVR). Anatomically, these are vascular malformations of the pulmonary circuit. However, as a matter of convention both these entities are considered as congenital heart diseases.

Bronchopulmonary Sequestration

Bronchopulmonary sequestration (BPS) is a condition characterized by sequestration of mass of nonfunctioning lung tissue with an anomalous systemic blood supply but tracheobronchial connection. The sequestrated lobe/segment can be either solid or cystic in nature. Both the intrapulmonary (more common) and extrapulmonary forms are commonly seen on the left side (intrapulmonary occurring more frequently in left lower lobe). In fact, a high index of suspicion is required to suspect these conditions to enable an early diagnosis on MDCT.

Congenital Pulmonary Airway Malformation

Congenital pulmonary airway malformation (CPAM), earlier known as congenital cystic adenomatoid malformation (CCAM), is a developmental abnormality of the lower respiratory tract. It is an uncommon condition which may present with respiratory distress in the neonatal period or remain asymptomatic until later in life. Incidental cases are now detected on routine prenatal ultrasound examination, more recently by fetal magnetic resonance imaging. During embryogenesis, CPAM results from abnormalities of branching morphogenesis of the lung. The different types of CPAMs are postulated to originate at different levels of the tracheobronchial tree. They may develop at different stages of lung development, possibly influenced by in utero airway obstruction and/or atresia. Surgical excision is the only definitive treatment.

CHAPTER 72

Approach to Respiratory Sleep Disorders

Ruchi Bansal

INTRODUCTION

Disorders of respiration during sleep are common in the general adult population of sleep-related breathing disorders includes obstructive sleep apnea (OSA), central sleep apnea, nocturnal hypoventilation and hypoxemia, and nocturnal manifestations of general pulmonary diseases, such as asthma and chronic obstructive pulmonary disease. The evaluation of an individual suspected of a respiratory sleep disorder includes an extensive sleep history, physical examination, and diagnostic testing. Controversy exists regarding the utilization of in-laboratory versus home nocturnal polysomnography (PSG); however, in-laboratory sleep studies remain the diagnostic "gold standard." Despite this, the use of out-of-center sleep testing (OCST) has now been included in the diagnostic criteria for OSA in the newest iteration of the International Classification of Sleep Disorders, (ICSD-3) with the caveat that OCST may underestimate the severity of sleep apnea.

SLEEP HISTORY

Sleep complaints are varied and can often be attributed to respiratory sleep disorders. Although insomnia is often related to comorbid psychiatric disease, medical disease, or an idiopathic etiology, patients with respiratory sleep disorders often perceive their inability to sleep as insomnia and do not make the connection between their complaints and breathing abnormalities during sleep. Poor sleep quality, excessive daytime sleepiness, frequent nocturnal arousals and poorly consolidated sleep, changes in cognition and disruption of a bed partner's sleep due to the nocturnal activities of the patient are common

TABLE 72.1: Common sleep complaints of patients and bed partners.

Patient's complaints	Bed partner complaints
Snoring	Disruptive/crescendo snoring
Excessive daytime sleepiness	Restlessness
Poor sleep quality	Choking/gasping
Frequent nocturnal arousals	Limb movements/kicking bed partner
Insomnia	Concern of breathing cessation
Morning dry mouth	
Morning headache	
Nocturia	
Palpitations	
Cognitive deficits	

reasons for individuals to undergo sleep evaluation; loud snoring, restlessness, choking sounds, and limb movements/kicking are all common complaints of bed partners of individuals with respiratory sleep disorders (Table 72.1).

Although snoring is present primarily during sleep, patients can often perceive snoring resulting in a respiratory effort-related arousal (RERA) and also complain of loud breathing and snoring while awake. Choking and gasping during nocturnal arousal is caused by frank obstructive events; the patient increases respiratory effort against a subtotally or totally occluded glottis, with subsequent opening of the glottis on arousal resulting in a loud snort. Morning dry mouth is attributed to increased airflow through the oropharynx. Morning headache is often a manifestation of sleep-related hypercapnia in individuals whose respiratory sleep disorder is associated with nocturnal alveolar hypoventilation. Nocturia has been associated with OSA and is felt to be due to intrathoracic pressure changes and consequent release of natriuretic hormones during obstructive events. Finally, limb movements during sleep are a common physical manifestation of the arousal response associated with respiratory events.

A complete medication history is essential in evaluating the patient with sleep complaints. Respiratory suppressants, such as narcotics and benzodiazepines, may increase the risk of OSA in individuals who are at risk for this disorder. Narcotic medication is additionally associated with opioid-induced central sleep apnea syndrome. The use of REM-suppressant medication may decrease the severity of an individual's sleep-disordered breathing.

PHYSICAL EXAMINATION

Examination of the upper airway is an essential component of the evaluation for respiratory sleep disorders. Although complete evaluation of the upper airway requires endoscopic visualization of structures and radiologic imaging (X-ray cephalometry, computed tomography, and magnetic resonance imaging), a general physical examination in the pulmonologist or sleep specialist's office often provides important clues to the diagnosis of respiratory sleep disorders and will guide future diagnostic modalities. The Mallampati classification system was initially developed in the anesthesia literature to predict the difficulty of direct laryngoscopy; this scoring system has been shown to be an independent predictor of the presence and severity of OSA in patients with suspected respiratory sleep disorders. Finally, neurologic evaluation is important to determine the risk of nocturnal hypoventilation from neuromuscular disease and central sleep apnea from cerebrovascular disease (as manifested by focal neurologic deficits). Although the findings on physical examination are nonspecific, they are essential for complete evaluation of the patient presenting to sleep clinic.

NOCTURNAL POLYSOMNOGRAPHY

Although clinical prediction models used to estimate the presence of OSA in various populations have been evaluated, in-laboratory nocturnal PSG remains the "gold standard" diagnostic method in determining the presence of a sleep-related breathing disorder. In-laboratory PSG is a complex medical procedure that enables recording and analysis of a wide spectrum of physiologic processes during sleep. The complexity of this test provides important cardiopulmonary and electromyographic information in the context of electroencephalographically derived sleep stages and body position. Although PSG is considered the "gold standard" for diagnosing sleep-related breathing disorders, it is not infallible. Data loss, artifact, and measurement error may affect the analysis of the raw data. Scoring of sleep studies is performed by sleep technicians; intra- and interrater event recognition errors and differences in respiratory event definitions among different sleep laboratories (discussed below) can result in over- or underestimation of respiratory events

On the basis of objective findings, we are able to classify respiratory events into apnea (obstructive, central, or mixed), hypopnea, RERA, hypoventilation, and Cheyne–Stokes breathing. An apnea is defined as a reduction in the amplitude of the nasal thermistor by more than or equal to 90% for 10 seconds; if the event is associated with respiratory effort, it is classified as obstructive, if no respiratory effort is present, it is a central event, and if it starts out without respiratory effort but respiratory effort resumes in the latter portion of the event, a mixed apnea. In the current version, a hypopnea is defined as a reduction in the nasal pressure transducer amplitude by more than or equal to 30% lasting more than or equal to 10 seconds with a concomitant more than or equal to 3% drop in oxygen desaturation or an EEG arousal. The number of apneas and hypopneas that occur per hour of sleep are combined to provide an apnea-hypopnea index (AHI), which is utilized as a measure of severity of disease.

OUT-OF-CENTER SLEEP TESTING

Out-of-center sleep testing encompasses a wide spectrum of diagnostic technology utilized to determine the presence or absence of sleep-disordered breathing outside of a formal in-laboratory study. Advantages of using portable monitoring include decreased time to diagnosis of sleep-disordered breathing, improved comfort due to the patient being able to be studied in a comfortable and familiar environment, and decreased costs associated with diagnostic testing.

SLEEP QUESTIONNAIRES

Sleep questionnaires, which quantify the severity of symptomatic daytime somnolence and/or screen for the presence of OSA, assist the sleep physician in determining an individual's risk for primary sleep disorders. The Epworth Sleepiness Scale (ESS), a self-administered tool to measure subjective daytime sleepiness, is one of the most commonly utilized questionnaires in sleep medicine due to its simplicity and brevity. Although screening tests in general are most useful when they demonstrate high sensitivity, the tests described above are not perfectly discriminating tools; the specificities of the above questionnaires are 64% and 43%, respectively. Caution when interpreting the results of screening questionnaires for OSA should be employed.

RESPIRATORY DISORDERS DURING SLEEP

Asthma

Although sleep apnea syndromes are the most commonly diagnosed and treated disorders in a sleep medicine practice, many disease entities seen in a general pulmonary practice manifest with significant nocturnal symptoms. Nocturnal asthma, which is defined by a drop in forced expiratory volume in 1 second (FEV_1) of at least 15% between sleep and awake states associated with increased airway hyperresponsiveness and inflammation, has gained increasing awareness and is likely underreported. Prior to focusing on the specific treatment of nocturnal symptoms of asthma, it is imperative that the patient has adhered to standard asthma therapy which ideally manages asthma symptoms throughout the course of a 24-hour period.

Chronic Obstructive Pulmonary Disease

The presence of both COPD and OSA has been termed the "overlap syndrome" and denotes worsened nocturnal gas exchange parameters as compared with either disease entity alone. Oxygen saturation of hemoglobin is significantly affected by the presence of OSA, airways obstruction, and the "overlap syndrome". Potential pathophysiologic mechanisms for the degree of oxyhemoglobin desaturation in the overlap syndrome include altered respiratory mechanics due to lung disease, ventilation/perfusion abnormality, and pulmonary parenchymal abnormalities due to underlying lung disease. Management of the overlap syndrome includes positive airway pressure (continuous or bilevel mode), pharmacologic management of airways obstruction, and oxygen supplementation when indicated.

Hypoventilation/Hypoxemia Syndromes

While gas exchange parameters are important for the diagnosis of hypoventilation/hypoxemia syndromes, the causes of these gas exchange abnormalities is comprised of a heterogeneous group of disorders that affect the ability of the respiratory system to compensate for sleep-related changes in ventilatory control mechanisms and respiratory mechanics. Disorders included in this group include neuromuscular and chest wall disorders, various pulmonary disorders, and idiopathic disorders (congenital central alveolar hypoventilation). The primary pathophysiology of nocturnal hypoxemia relates to the inability of the respiratory system to maintain adequate ventilation, resulting in an elevation of alveolar partial pressure of carbon dioxide and a subsequent reduction of alveolar oxygen, consistent with the alveolar gas equation; an alternate cause of hypoxemia likely relates to increasing ventilation and perfusion mismatch in poorly ventilated lung regions. Clinical features of alveolar hypoventilation include poor sleep quality, nocturnal and/or morning headache, daytime sleepiness and loss of energy, decreased intellectual performance, loss of appetite and weight loss, and features of progressive right heart failure/cor pulmonale. Treatment for sleep-related hypoventilation/hypoxemia syndromes is disorder-specific, although noninvasive ventilation in the bilevel mode is often a necessary adjunctive measure utilized in all of these disorders; short-term improvement in clinical symptoms and the suggestion of a mortality benefit, particularly in individuals with neuromuscular disease, is present when noninvasive ventilatory support is utilized.

Neuromuscular disorders that may result in nocturnal hypoventilation/hypoxemia include amyotrophic lateral sclerosis (ALS), spinal cord injury, diaphragmatic paralysis, myasthenia gravis, Eaton–Lambert syndrome, post-polio syndrome, myopathic disorders, and Charcot–Marie–Tooth syndrome. Individuals with ALS, a neurodegenerative disorder characterized by loss of motor neurons and resultant progressive weakness and atrophy of skeletal muscles including accessory muscles of respiration, are at risk for both diurnal and nocturnal hypoventilation/hypoxemia.

Although the diminished function of respiratory muscles is the primary defect in neuromuscular disorders during sleep, individuals with chest wall disorders (kyphoscoliosis, ankylosing spondylitis, trauma, pleural disease, history of thoracoplasty, and obesity) and pulmonary disease (COPD, asthma, IPF, and CF) are at risk for nocturnal hypoventilation/hypoxemia due to several additional mechanisms. During REM sleep, bursts of rapid eye movements are associated with inhibition of accessory muscles of respiration; ventilation and gas exchange thus depend solely on the diaphragm. During wake, individuals with chest wall and/or pulmonary disease may already have gas exchange abnormalities due to their underlying disease; normal increases in $PaCO_2$ associated with sleep onset compounds the underlying gas exchange problems, resulting in worsening hypoxemia. Obesity results in reduced chest wall compliance due to the mass load placed on the thoracic cage; the reduction in compliance is further exacerbated in the supine position, worsening ventilatory function during sleep by increasing the work of breathing.

CHAPTER
73

Respiratory Sleep Disorders

Aditya Jindal

INTRODUCTION

Respiratory sleep disorders are among the most common diseases affecting humans and encompass a wide spectrum of diseases. These range from obstructive sleep apnea/hypopnea syndrome (OSAHS) where the pathology is peripheral to central sleep apnea (CSA) where the respiratory center is involved. The field of sleep medicine is heavily dominated by OSAHS, which is the most common sleep disorder. The introduction of positive airway pressure (PAP) therapy led to a revolution in the field, with newer devices and treatments announced on a regular basis.

CLASSIFICATION

Sleep disorders involving the respiratory system can be classified as given in Box 73.1.

This classification is based on the basic underlying pathophysiology of disease. Disorders like OSAHS are rooted in peripheral airway obstruction while central sleep disorders arise out of a complex interaction between respiratory center dysfunction and feedback mechanisms. It should be noted that this is not an exhaustive classification and is only meant to serve as a guide for the proper approach to respiratory sleep disorders.

Obstructive Sleep Apnea/Hypopnea Syndrome

Obstructive sleep apnea/hypopnea syndrome is most common respiratory sleep disorder worldwide, with an estimated prevalence of at least 2-4% of

> **BOX 73.1: Classification of respiratory sleep disorders.**
> - Peripheral
>   - Obstructive sleep apnea/hypopnea syndrome
> - Central
>   - Central sleep apnea
>   - Congenital
>   - Drug induced, e.g. opioids
>   - Medical disease induced, e.g. stroke, high altitude, etc.
>   - Complex sleep apnea (treatment emergent)
>   - Obesity hypoventilation syndrome
> - Miscellaneous
>   - Overlap syndrome
>   - Chest wall neuromuscular diseases

the middle-aged population and, in some estimates, up to 10% of the total population. OSAHS is diagnosed in the presence of cessation of airflow—partially or completely—due to upper airway obstruction. The main symptoms of OSAHS occur secondary to recurrent airway obstruction during sleep and excessive daytime sleepiness because of disturbed sleep during the nighttime. Other than direct symptoms of OSAHS, the disorder is also associated with early onset cardiovascular disease, diabetes mellitus and cerebrovascular disease, with significant morbidity and mortality.

Pathophysiology

Obstructive sleep apnea/hypopnea syndrome is a syndrome characterized by repetitive, intermittent collapse of the upper airway during sleep, leading to obstruction to airflow, either complete (apnea) or partial (hypopnea). Airway patency depends on a balance of factors promoting or reducing airway tone. The pressure below which airway collapse occurs is called Pcrit or the critical closing pressure. Factors which promote airway closing include anatomical factors (retrognathia, age, gender, race) and disease processes (obesity, lack of physical activity, enlarged tonsils, adenoids). Over a period of time, the pharyngeal muscles undergo changes leading onto the development of cricopharyngeal myopathy, which further exacerbates the process.

Intermittent and repetitive airway collapse is responsible for the consequences of OSAHS. Collapse leads to hypoxia with disturbed sleep and daytime sleepiness. Hypoxia also causes repeated sympathetic stimulation with the subsequent deleterious cardiovascular and cerebrovascular side effects. The hypoxia also leads to metabolic derangements and the predisposition to diabetes mellitus and hypertension.

Symptoms

The typical patient of OSAHS is a middle-aged, obese individual who complains of disturbed sleep, snoring, and daytime sleepiness, and may have hypertension and diabetes. In general, symptoms can be divided as nocturnal, diurnal or remote. Nocturnal symptoms include disturbed sleep, snoring, choking or gasping during the night, witnessed pauses during sleep and nocturia. Less common symptoms are leg cramps, nightmares and syndromes such as restless leg syndrome and paroxysmal limb movements of sleep.

Diurnal symptoms are due to both sleep deprivation and excessive daytime sleepiness. These are early morning headaches, feeling of inadequate sleep, lack of concentration, irritability and a tendency to fall asleep at any time, including while driving. This has been associated with an increased frequency of vehicular accidents.

Remote symptoms are those caused due to the pathophysiological consequences of OSAHS and include weight gain, obesity and the development of the metabolic syndrome. Hypertension may develop at a younger age than usual and may be more difficult to control, requiring the use of extra medication. Diabetes mellitus may also develop at an earlier age. Both cardiovascular and cerebrovascular diseases are more prevalent in these patients.

Diagnosis

The diagnosis of OSAHS requires the demonstration of the presence of repeated airway collapse causing apneas/hypopneas. This is done by the means of a full night polysomnography (PSG) or sleep study. The PSG measures multiple bodily parameters like electroencephalogram, electrooculogram, muscle tone, nasal and oral airflow, respiratory and limb movements, oxygen saturation, etc. Based on the analysis of the recordings, an apnea-hypopnea index (AHI) is calculated. The AHI is the number of times the patient develops apneas or hypopneas per hour of sleep. The diagnosis of OSAHS is made when the AHI is greater than 5. The severity of OSAHS can also be calculated based on the AHI:
- 5–15 → mild OSAHS
- 16–30 → moderate OSAHS
- More than 30 → severe OSAHS.

In addition to the sleep study, patients may also require a directed screening to check for associated diseases like diabetes, hypertension and cardiac disease. Thyroid levels should also be checked to rule out hypothyroidism as it can mimic many of the symptoms.

Treatment

Treatment in OSAHS consists of the following:
- *General measures*: Patients should avoid the use of nicotine, alcohol and caffeine as these agents precipitate OSAHS. Obese patients should be advised to lose weight; a physically active lifestyle should be adopted. Comorbid conditions, which may also lead to sleep disturbances, should be controlled. Positional therapy may be tried in less severe cases or in cases of documented positional OSAHS. Sleep hygiene should be promoted; the components of sleep hygiene are given in Box 73.2.
- *Positive airway pressure therapy:* The main therapy of OSAHS is PAP therapy. The basic principle involves the application of positive pressure to the airway during sleep. The airway is a distensible tube—the positive pressure

> **BOX 73.2:** Components of sleep hygiene.
>
> - Avoid nicotine, alcohol and caffeine, especially 3–4 hours before bedtime.
> - Avoid the use of electronic screens like TV, mobile phones, tablets, etc. before bedtime.
> - Have regular physical activity 4–5 hours before bedtime.
> - The room used for sleep should be dark and maintained at a comfortable temperature.
> - Use the bedroom only for sleep.
> - Have regular time to go to sleep and to wake.

acts as a pneumatic splint, keeping the airway open. The obstruction is relieved and the symptoms of OSAHS resolve thereafter.

Positive airway pressure therapy has been found to be safe and effective. The AHI can be brought down significantly and all symptoms of OSAHS relieved somewhat. Excessive daytime sleepiness may disappear and significant weight loss may occur. One may notice a reduction in the dose and number of antihypertensive and antidiabetic medications. The one main drawback is that PAP therapy has to be used daily.

There are many modes of PAP therapy. These include the following:
- Continuous positive airway pressure (CPAP): The PAP is applied only during the expiratory phase of respiration.
- Bilevel positive airway therapy (BiPAP): PAP is applied both during inspiration and expiration and the pressures can be different during both the phases.
- Automatic PAP: The airway pressure or resistance is calculated automatically and the pressure delivered is varied from breath to breath based on this calculation. Both CPAP and BiPAP can be given by this method.
- Other modes: These include average volume assured pressure support (AVAPS), adaptive support ventilation (ASV) and others.

Positive airway pressure therapy is delivered by means of a small portable ventilator; the patient interface is an oronasal or nasal mask. Other types of interfaces such as nasal pillows, full-face masks, etc. are also available. There is also the option of giving humidified air to prevent airway from drying. Patients who are prone to jaw opening during sleep can be advised to use a chinstrap.

- *Oxygen therapy:* Oxygen is not the primary treatment of OSAHS and should only be used when there is documented hypoxia in the absence of respiratory events or as an add-on therapy after proper titration. Care should be taken to prevent depression of the respiratory center due to excess oxygen, especially in patients with type 2 respiratory failure.
- *Pharmacotherapy:* Pharmacotherapy generally has no role in the treatment of OSAHS. The only indication is that of modafinil and armodafinil for treatment of excessive daytime sleepiness, which is refractory to treatment or in patients who do not tolerate or want PAP.

- *Other therapies*: These include the use of oral devices for mandibular repositioning and for prevention of tongue displacement. Surgical procedures to widen the airway have also been tried. These therapies are indicated for persons with specific anatomical abnormalities or for those who are intolerant or do not want PAP therapy.

Prognosis and Follow-up

As mentioned earlier, untreated OSAHS is a disease with considerable morbidity and mortality. The use of proper therapy leads to a significant difference in the quality of life, symptoms and complications. Patients on PAP therapy should follow up regularly; repeat polysomnography may be indicated in case of complications. Otherwise, a repeat procedure is generally not indicated before 2 years. The treatment of OSAHS is continually evolving and with better understanding of the pathophysiology and disease mechanisms, even better treatments are expected.

Central Sleep Apnea

Central sleep apnea syndrome (CSAS) is a constellation of multiple disorders which present similarly and have a similar mechanism of generation. These causes of CSAS include congestive heart failure, brain strokes, opoid overuse, high altitude, etc. CSAS may occur in addition to the underlying disease and may not be the presenting manifestation. All these disorders are either hyperventilation or hypoventilation associated and arise due to a malfunction of the central and peripheral respiratory control mechanisms coupled with feedback dysfunction.

The symptomatology of CSAS is similar to that of OSAHS with the caveat that the symptoms of the underlying disease may predominate. The diagnosis requires the demonstration of central apneas on a full night polysomnography. Cheyne–Stokes respiration is a special type of CSAS in which there is crescendo–decrescendo pattern of respiration; this is seen in 30–40% of patients with congestive heart failure.

The treatment of CSAS is controversial with the efficacy of PAP therapy not clearly established. However, a trial of treatment is definitely warranted in all patients, who should be titrated with a full night polysomnography. The use of ASV in patients of congestive heart failure with a low ejection fraction has been shown to be associated with higher mortality in a major trial conducted recently and its use has been withdrawn for this indication. Otherwise, treatment of the underlying cause is of primary importance and may help in resolving symptoms in some cases.

Complex Sleep Apnea

Complex sleep apnea is a type of CSA which emerges during treatment of OSAHS. Specifically, patients of OSAHS who are started on PAP therapy, may develop central apneas while on PAP. This has been proposed to be due to the use of higher pressures and over-titration, which leads to hyperventilation and an enhanced negative peripheral feedback. However, the exact mechanism is yet to be clearly elucidated. The treatment consists of prevention by proper titration and sometimes use of ASV.

Obesity Hypoventilation Syndrome

Obesity hypoventilation syndrome (OHS) is another sleep-related respiratory disorder which is characterized by the triad of obesity, hypoventilation and hypersomnolence. The diagnostic criteria include all of the following:
- *Obesity*: Body mass index more than 30 or 35 kg/m²
- *Hypoventilation*: PO_2 less than 70 mm Hg and PCO_2 more than 45 mm Hg
- OSAHS
- Absence of any other cause.

The diagnosis requires a high index of suspicion, especially in patients suspected to have OSAHS. These patients are obese and have all the symptoms characteristic of OSAHS. In addition, symptoms suggestive of chronic hypercapnia and right heart failure may predominate, e.g. morning headaches, peripheral edema, plethora, etc. A full night polysomnography is required along with demonstration of arterial hypercapnia.

The treatment is similar to that of OSAHS, with an additional stress on weight loss. Bariatric surgery may be required; however, there is an increased mortality in this setting. Also, treatment of right heart failure is required.

CONCLUSION

Sleep-related respiratory disorder is among the most common, underrecognized and underdiagnosed diseases. A high index of suspicion is needed for diagnosis. Treatment is definitely required as these disorders are associated with high morbidity and mortality burdens. In the Indian context, significant challenges remain to the initiation of therapy. New research is constantly shedding light on pathophysiology and treatment.

CHAPTER 74

Respiratory Failure

Abinash Singh Paul, Ritesh Agarwal

INTRODUCTION

Respiratory failure is defined by the presence of failure of gas exchange functions—oxygenation and carbon dioxide elimination. In clinical practice, respiratory failure is said to be present if while breathing room air, the PaO_2 values are less than 60 mm Hg. It is further classified as *type I* (or hypoxemic respiratory failure), if the $PaCO_2$ levels are less than 45 mm Hg, or *type II* (or hypercapnic respiratory failure), if the $PaCO_2$ levels are more than or equal to 45 mm Hg.

CLASSIFICATION

Respiratory failure may be further classified as acute or chronic depending on the rapidity of its onset (Table 74.1). Acute respiratory failure (ARF) refers to disorders of recent onset (hours to days). In these situations, respiratory failure has developed before physiologic compensation can occur. On the other hand, chronic respiratory failure (CRF) develops over months to years, allowing compensatory mechanisms to improve oxygen transport and to buffer respiratory acidosis. ARF can also be superimposed on CRF, as in acute exacerbations of chronic obstructive pulmonary disease (COPD). There is life-threatening derangements in arterial blood gases and acid-base status in ARF. The manifestations of CRF, on the other hand, may not be clinically apparent. Acute type 1 respiratory failure commonly occurs in lung parenchymal, cardiovascular system and lower airway diseases. The causes are due to various physiological processes primarily due to ventilation-perfusion (V/Q) mismatch but also include other mechanisms, such as low inspired concentration of oxygen, impairment of diffusion, intrapulmonary shunting, and low mixed venous oxygen content (Table 74.1).

TABLE 74.1: Causes of respiratory failure.

Acute	Chronic
Type 1 Acute pulmonary edema Pneumonia Acute lung injury/acute respiratory distress syndrome Pneumothorax Severe acute asthma	*Type 1* Interstitial lung diseases—idiopathic pulmonary fibrosis, sarcoidosis and others Lymphangitis carcinomatosis Chronic pulmonary embolism Chronic heart failure
Type 2 Acute exacerbations of chronic obstructive pulmonary disease Tension pneumothorax Guillain–Barré syndrome Myasthenia gravis Laryngeal edema Inhaled foreign body	*Type 2* Chronic obstructive pulmonary disease Obesity hypoventilation syndrome Motor neuron disease and other neuromuscular disorders

MECHANISMS

Hypoxemic (Type 1) Respiratory Failure

A low PaO_2 and a normal or low $PaCO_2$ characterizes hypoxemic respiratory failure (also called type 1, nonventilatory or normocapnic respiratory failure). Although there are four pathophysiological mechanisms that can cause hypoxemia namely low partial pressure of O_2 (FiO_2), diffusion impairment, right-to-left shunt and V/Q mismatch, the underlying physiologic aberration causing hypoxemia is predominantly V/Q mismatch. Acute respiratory distress syndrome (ARDS) is a classic example of acute hypoxemic respiratory failure.

In most pulmonary diseases, hypoxemia is finally the result of V/Q mismatch (Fig. 74.1). An area of lung that is well perfused but not ventilated acts as a right to left shunt ("physiological shunt") whereas an area that is well ventilated but not perfused acts like a dead space ("physiological dead space"). The spectrum of V/Q ratios in a healthy lung would vary between zero (perfused but not ventilated) to infinity (ventilated but not perfused). Physiologic dead space, is rarely, if ever the cause of hypoxemia. In an alveolar–capillary unit with a V/Q ratio of zero (physiologic shunt), the blood leaving the unit has the composition of mixed venous blood entering the pulmonary capillaries, i.e. PO_2 of 40 mm Hg and PCO_2 of 46 mm Hg whereas in an alveolar–capillary unit with a high V/Q ratio (physiologic dead space), the small amount of blood leaving the unit has partial pressures of O_2 and CO_2 as 150 mm Hg and 0 mm Hg approaching the composition of inspired gas.

The efficiency of gas exchange can be evaluated clinically by measuring the PaO_2, $PaCO_2$ and the alveolar-arterial (A–a) DO_2 gradient. Thus, patients with hypoxemia may be divided into those with a normal gradient and those with an increased gradient (Flowchart 74.1). The alveolar PO_2 can be calculated from the alveolar air equation: $PaO_2 = (P_B - P_{H2O}) FiO_2 - (PaCO_2/R)$, where

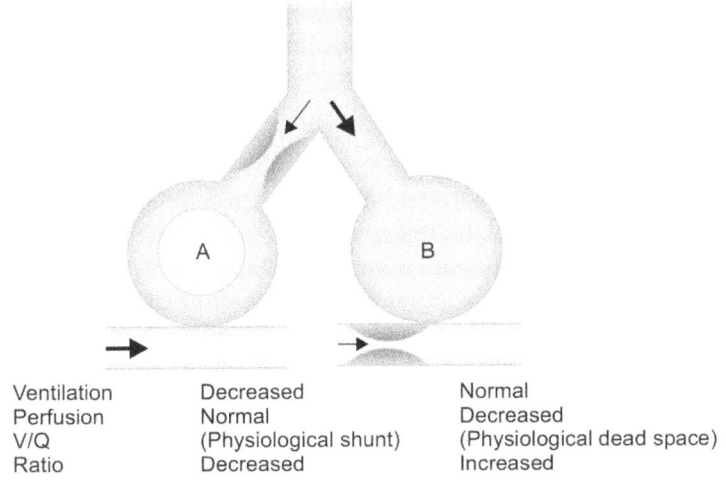

Fig. 74.1: Primary mechanism of hypoxemic respiratory failure—shunt physiology. (A) Diminished ventilation; (B) Decreased perfusion.

Flowchart 74.1: Importance of calculating alveolar–arterial gradient in patients with acute respiratory failure.

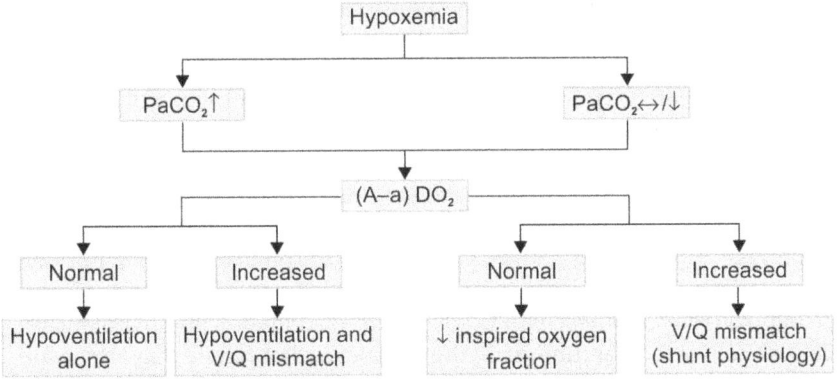

(V/Q, ventilation-perfusion; PaCO₂, partial pressure of carbon dioxide in arterial blood; (A-a) DO₂, alveolar-arterial oxygen difference)

PaO_2 is the alveolar PO_2, FiO_2 is the fraction of inspired O_2, P_B is barometric pressure (760 mm Hg at sea level), P_{H2O} is the water vapor pressure (47 mm Hg at sea level) and R is the respiratory exchange ratio (assumed to be 0.8). The alveolar–arterial gradient is then derived by subtracting PaO_2 from PaO_2. On room air, the (A-a) DO_2 is normally less than 15 mm Hg. In a healthy individual, it increases by 3 mm Hg every decade and can be as high as 30 mm Hg in elderly patients. Hypoxemic respiratory failure most often occurs due to conditions that increase the (A-a) DO_2.

Hypercapnic (Type 2) Respiratory Failure

The normal respiratory rate is about 12-16 times per minute with the tidal volume of each breath being around 500 mL. About 30% of the air inspired with each breath remains in the conducting airways of the lung and does not reach the alveoli. This *anatomic dead space* comprises of the component of inspired air that does not participate in gas exchange. The component of the anatomic dead space is increased in diseases where some alveoli are ventilated but not perfused. Alveolar ventilation falls if total dead space ventilation is increased but total minute ventilation is unchanged. Gas exchange is determined by alveolar ventilation rather than total minute ventilation.

The $PaCO_2$ is directly proportional to the amount of CO_2 produced per minute and inversely proportional to alveolar ventilation (V_A), according to the relationship—$PaCO_2 = 0.863 \times VCO_2/V_A$, where CO_2 is expressed in mL/min, V_A in L/min, and $PaCO_2$ in mm Hg. $PaCO_2$ falls when alveolar ventilation increases, and $PaCO_2$ rises when alveolar ventilation decreases. Maintaining a normal level of O_2 in the alveoli (and consequently in arterial blood) also depends on provision of adequate alveolar ventilation to replenish alveolar O_2. Thus, hypercapnic respiratory failure results from any cause that leads to decrease in alveolar ventilation.

CLINICAL MANIFESTATIONS

A combination of arterial hypoxemia and tissue hypoxia leads to the typical manifestations of hypoxemic failure. Hypoxemia causes hyperventilation due to stimulation of carotid body chemoreceptors with resultant tachypnea. There may be cyanosis; the degree depends on the concentration of the hemoglobin and the patient's perfusion. Hypoxia stimulates anaerobic metabolism with generation of lactic acid that further stimulates ventilation. Mild hypoxia may also lead to impaired mental performance. With progression of hypoxia, alteration in the sensorium, somnolence, coma and seizures, can occur leading to permanent brain damage. Hypoxemia causes stimulation of the sympathetic nervous system resulting in tachycardia, diaphoresis and systemic vasoconstriction. Severe hypoxia may manifest with bradycardia, vasodilation and hypotension. Myocardial ischemia, infarction, arrhythmias and cardiac failure may also result.

Symptoms and signs of ARF include those due to presence of acute hypoxemia as well those due to the underlying cause of respiratory failure. Acute hypercapnic respiratory failure which usually occurs due to central nervous system disturbances present with central nervous system depression resulting in lethargy, somnolence, asterixis and restlessness. It may also cause tremors, slurred speech, headache, papilledema and coma. Symptoms of hypercapnia and hypoxemia frequently overlap.

DIAGNOSIS

Arterial Blood Gas Analysis

The arterial blood gas analysis includes the measurement of pH, PaO_2, $PaCO_2$ and HCO_3. While the O_2 content in the blood depends on the solubility of O_2 in

plasma and the quantity of hemoglobin, the PaO_2 determines the percentage of hemoglobin saturated with O_2, based on the position on the oxyhemoglobin dissociation curve. Oxygen content in blood can be determined by the equation—
O_2 content = $1.34 \times$ [hemoglobin] $\times O_2$ saturation $+ 0.0031 \times PaO_2$, i.e. the sum of O_2 dissolved in plasma and the amount of oxygen bound to hemoglobin.

In arterial blood, the amount of O_2 dissolved in plasma (approximately 0.3 mL O_2 per deciliter of blood) is trivial compared to the amount bound to hemoglobin (approximately 20 mL O_2 per deciliter of blood). PaO_2 is the important measurement to assess the effect of respiratory disease on the oxygenation status. The PaO_2 gives an assessment of the hypoxemia whereas the oxygen content denotes the level of hypoxia.

Pulse Oximetry

Pulse oximetry is a noninvasive assessment of the oxygenation status as measurement of PaO_2 requires arterial puncture. The pulse oximeter calculates SaO_2 based on measurements of absorption of two wavelengths of light by hemoglobin in pulsatile, cutaneous arterial blood. The oximeter is relatively insensitive to changes in PaO_2 above PaO_2 of 60 mm Hg (corresponding to SaO_2 of 90%), since the oxyhemoglobin dissociation curve becomes relatively flat above this level. Oximetry is insensitive in conditions where cutaneous perfusion is decreased (such as hypotension); other forms of hemoglobin, such as carboxyhemoglobin and methemoglobin, cannot be distinguished from oxyhemoglobin when only two wavelengths are used making the SaO_2 values as unreliable in the presence of significant amounts of either of them. The pulse oximeter does not provide any information about CO_2 elimination.

Chest Radiograph

Chest radiography frequently reveals the cause of respiratory failure. It may not however distinguish between cardiogenic and noncardiogenic pulmonary edema which may require additional clinical assessment and echocardiography.

Pulmonary Function Tests

Pulmonary Function Tests (PFTs) are not generally indicated in patients with ARF, though these are valuable in the evaluation of CRF.

A decrease in forced expiratory volume to forced vital capacity (FEV_1/FVC) ratio indicates airflow obstruction, whereas a reduction in both the FEV_1 and FVC in the presence of a normal FEV_1/FVC ratio suggests restrictive lung disease. Respiratory failure generally occurs only when the FEV_1 is less than 1 L in obstructive diseases and when the FVC is less than 1 L in restrictive diseases.

TREATMENT

Most patients of ARF are critically ill making it important that the management is undertaken in a high dependency unit or intensive care unit (ICU) setting.

Oxygen Therapy

Hypoxemia is a grave and immediate threat to organ function. Oxygen therapy is started immediately on admission after an arterial blood sample is obtained for assessment of blood gas tensions. The goal of supplemental oxygen is to maintain a PaO_2 of 55–60 mm Hg corresponding to SpO_2 of 89–92%. Administration of excess amounts of oxygen can blunt this ventilatory drive with resultant hypercapnia and acute respiratory acidosis superimposed on type 2 respiratory failure that could be potentially life threatening. Excess oxygen therapy has been shown to prolong hospital stay probably because it can lead to generation of harmful reactive oxygen species, which can exacerbate tissue injury. Excess oxygen can also lead to hypercapnia by ventilation perfusion disturbances, Haldane effect and by causing numerous areas of microatelectasis. Another reason why PaO_2 is not increased more than 60 mm Hg is because it corresponds to oxygen saturation (SaO_2) of around 90%; from the oxygen content equation, we can conclude that there is no benefit of increasing PaO_2 above 60 mm Hg except in situations of hyperbaric oxygen delivery.

The type of oxygen delivery device that is used is an important consideration in acutely ill patients. Low-flow oxygen delivery systems provide oxygen at flow rates that are lower than patient's inspiratory demands; thus these systems allow entrainment by room air when the total ventilation exceeds the capacity of the oxygen reservoir. The final concentration of oxygen delivered depends on several factors, such as the ventilatory demands of the patient, the size of the oxygen reservoir and the rate at which the reservoir is filled. At a constant flow, the larger the tidal volume of the patient, the lower the FiO_2; similarly, the smaller the tidal volume, the higher the FiO_2. On the other hand, the high-flow systems which also use devices that entrain fixed proportion of room air, provide a constant FiO_2 by delivering the gas at flow rates exceeding the patient's peak inspiratory flow. In acute situations, it is always better to use high-flow devices as one can, to a reasonable extent, guarantee the oxygen delivered. On the other hand, with the use of a low flow device, oxygen delivery would not be dependent on the patient's minute ventilation. Once the patient has been stabilized, one can shift to nasal prongs, as it proves more comfortable for the patient.

The high-flow nasal cannula has been used in adults with respiratory failure. It delivers high-flow heated humidified oxygen through nasal prongs and supplies much higher flow rates (up to 40 L/minute) than the traditional nasal cannula. Such types of high-flow cannulae may help for short-term management of severe hypoxemia.

Noninvasive Ventilation

Noninvasive ventilation (NIV) is defined as provision of inspiratory pressure support plus continuous positive airway pressure (CPAP) via a nasal or facemask, i.e. without an endotracheal airway. CPAP is not traditionally a ventilatory mode since it does not actively assist inspiration. CPAP is considered a form of NIV only when used for management of respiratory failure.

> **BOX 74.1:** Protocol for application of noninvasive ventilation in acute respiratory failure.
>
> - Full face mask better tolerated in the acute setting
> - Start with an inspiratory pressure support of 6–8 cm H_2O and continuous positive airway pressure (CPAP) of 3–4 cm H_2O
> - Adjustments
>   - Increase inspiratory pressure and CPAP by 2 cm H_2O and 1 cm H_2O, respectively
>   - Titrate to tidal volume (>5 mL/kg), respiratory rate (<35 breaths/minute) and blood gases
>   - Maximum inspiratory pressure and CPAP generally used is 15–16 cm H_2O and 7–8 cm H_2O, respectively
> - Air leaks should be minimized.
> - CPAP is rarely used in acute respiratory failure.

Noninvasive ventilation success depends upon proper fit and comfortable interface (mask) and ventilator settings. Full-face masks are used for ARF whereas nasal masks are preferred for the chronic setting. The optimal ventilator settings are determined by the ability to reduce the work of breathing against the discomfort imposed by high pressures (Box 74.1). This is assessed clinically by reduction in respiratory rate to less than 30-35 breaths per minute by providing an adequate level of pressure support (usually more than 8-10 cm H_2O).

It is difficult to set the optimal duration of the initial NIV trial but one should expect a response within 1-4 hours of initiation. Any patient who fails an NIV trial should be promptly intubated and mechanically ventilated. Delays in endotracheal are shown to be associated with decreased survival.

With the remarkable success of NIV in COPD, it has been tempting to try and use this in the setting of asthma, which seems similar. However, most trials do not show unequivocal benefit in asthma. NIV must be used cautiously, if at all in asthma. The mask should not be allowed to delay or interfere with inhaled therapy in any case. There are constant efforts to try and expand the role of NIV beyond the currently accepted four settings mentioned above. In these, benefit has been proven beyond doubt.

Endotracheal Intubation and Invasive Ventilation

Patients who are in severe respiratory distress and those who fail treatment with oxygen and NIV generally require endotracheal intubation and invasive ventilation. Another indication for intubation is airway protection in patients with altered mental status. The aim of invasive ventilation is to correct hypoxemia and maintain alveolar ventilation appropriate to patient's metabolic requirements.

An important consideration is the ventilator that should be used for mechanically ventilating these patients. No ventilator is clearly better than any other. The machine is selected on the basis of the spectrum of patients, the financial resources of the ICU and the available expertise in handling the equipment. Clearly, the people operating the ventilator are more important than the machine. Other important issue is the mode to be used for mechanical ventilation. No mode is clearly superior. The choice of a particular mode is often guided by institutional policy or personal preference. One controversial area is the choice of a volume controlled or pressure controlled strategy. There is no strong evidence base for the pressure controlled ventilation although logically it is likely to be equivalent to the volume-controlled mode because it is the settings rather than the mode that is the important issue. It is best to initiate ventilation with a volume assist-controlled mode ventilation and once the patient improves, shift the patient to pressure support ventilation. Newer modes of ventilation are increasingly being promoted to decrease the hazards of conventional ventilation and improve patient–ventilator interactions. However, none of the newer mode of ventilation has been shown superior to conventional modes. Also, the indications, efficacy and safety are still clinically uncertain and are not being widely utilized. Much controversy has been witnessed over lung protective ventilation with all the adjunctive maneuvers versus high frequency ventilation and finally extracorporeal membrane oxygenation (ECMO).

Extracorporeal Membrane Oxygenation

The use of ECMO for severe ARF in adults continues to expand, in spite of the lack of evidence justifying its use. ECMO should be utilized in centers with availability of sufficient expertise to ensure its safety—it is a complex, high-risk, and costly modality. It is the most useful intervention in ARDS not responding to other measures. Significant benefit is seen if analysis is restricted to better quality studies of venovenous ECMO and the subgroup with H_1N_1. Benefits in reversing hypoxemia may not necessarily translate into mortality benefit. Almost 50% of patients on ECMO survive up to discharge even with conditions usually associated with a high chance of death. Complications such as renal failure, pneumonia or sepsis, and bleeding are frequent.

In conclusion, the management of respiratory failure hinges on two basic principles, i.e. oxygen therapy for alleviation of hypoxemia and aggressive treatment of basic disease. Oxygen should be administered through high-flow (Venturi mask) system. NIV should be judiciously used in ARF as inappropriate use of NIV may lead to delayed intubation in some patients. Eventually, mechanical ventilation is required in patients who fail NIV or develop respiratory arrest. ECMO is useful in patients who remain hypoxemic despite 100% oxygen.

CHAPTER
75

Acute Respiratory Distress Syndrome

Jean I Keddissi, D Robert McCaffree

The acute respiratory distress syndrome (ARDS) is a serious and frequently encountered entity in modern intensive care units. For decades, attempts to define ARDS lacked specific criteria, causing uncertainty in terms of its true incidence, natural history and appropriate management. The term "acute respiratory distress syndrome" has now replaced the initial terminology of adult respiratory distress syndrome since it does occur in children as well. An international expert panel, convened by the European Society of Intensive Care Medicine, with endorsement from the American Thoracic Society and the Society of Critical Care Medicine, proposed a revised definition in 2012. Known as the Berlin definition, it drops the term acute lung injury. The Berlin definition of ARDS includes the following characteristics:
- Development within 1 week of a known clinical insult
- Bilateral radiographic opacities
- Pulmonary edema that cannot be fully explained by cardiac failure or fluid overload
- The new definition uses the degree of gas exchange abnormality to classify the syndrome as mild (200 <PaO_2/FiO_2 ≤300), moderate (100 <PaO_2/FiO_2 ≤200) or severe (PaO_2/FiO_2 ≤100). The arterial oxygen partial pressure to fractional inspired oxygen (PaO_2/FiO_2) should be measured at a positive end-expiratory pressure (PEEP) more than or equal to 5 cm H_2O, with noninvasive ventilation (NIV) possible in the mild group. These groups correlated with mortality and duration of mechanical ventilation.

ETIOLOGY

Sepsis is the most common cause of ARDS. Sepsis with ARDS carries the worst prognosis of 40%. Other frequently encountered etiologies include

> **BOX 75.1:** Clinical entities associated with acute respiratory distress syndrome (ARDS) or acute lung injury.
>
> - Acute pancreatitis
> - Acute upper airway obstruction
> - Aspiration (gastric acid, near drowning)
> - Drugs (amiodarone, tocolytics, salicylates, opiates, etc.)
> - Iatrogenic ARDS
> - Inhalation injury
> - Neurogenic pulmonary edema
> - Nonthrombotic embolic events (amniotic, tumor, etc.)
> - Pneumonia
> - Pulmonary embolism
> - Reperfusion injury (postlung transplant, lung reexpansion)
> - Sepsis (most common)
> - Shock
> - Transfusion-related acute lung injury (TRALI)
> - Trauma

pneumonia (bacteria, virus, fungal), aspiration, shock and trauma (Box 75.1). The presence of multiple predisposing factors increases the risk significantly. Additionally, observational data suggest that inappropriate ventilatory settings in mechanically ventilated patients may contribute to the development of ARDS (i.e. iatrogenic ARDS).

CLINICAL PICTURE

Clinically, the picture is characterized by the rapid onset of hypoxemic respiratory failure in a patient with a predisposing underlying condition. The hypoxemia is typically refractory to oxygen replacement, frequently requiring the institution of invasive mechanical ventilation. Radiographically, bilateral patchy or asymmetric infiltrates are present, frequently indistinguishable from those seen in cardiogenic pulmonary edema. Computed tomography (CT) typically reveals areas of consolidation, alveolar filling with atelectasis, predominantly in the dependent zones. In later stages, the CT may reveal diffuse interstitial opacities, with bullae formation. Pulmonary compliance is decreased, and evidence of pulmonary hypertension and right ventricular failure may be seen. Pneumothorax may develop in 10–13% of the cases, but is not clearly related to the airway pressures, nor is it associated with a significantly increased mortality rate.

PATHOPHYSIOLOGY

Acute respiratory distress syndrome is a progressive syndrome, characterized by distinct histopathological stages. Initially, an acute, exudative stage is characterized by the presence of alveolar edema in the absence of an elevated hydrostatic pressure. This edema is secondary to capillary injury, with increased alveolar-capillary membrane permeability, a feature considered to be the hallmark of ARDS. As a result, massive amount of edema fluid and plasma proteins leak into the alveolar space, with subsequent formation of hyaline membranes. These membranes appear in the first 24–48 hours, reach a maximum around day 4, and start to decrease after 6–7 days. Maximal alveolar fluid clearance, when present, is associated with better clinical outcomes.

There is accumulation of activated inflammatory cells, primarily macrophages and neutrophils, in the interstitium. It is not clearly known if the inflammatory cells are the cause or the result of the lung injury. Proinflammatory cytokines are released into the lungs, including interleukin (IL)-1β, IL-8, and tumor necrosis factor (TNF)-α. These cytokines play a major role in the lung response to infection or injury, but have a potential role in the cellular response, microvascular injury, and the extrapulmonary organ failures seen in ARDS. In addition, neutrophil matrix metalloproteinase (MMP)-9 level is significantly increased.

Surfactant activity and composition is altered, resulting in elevated surface tension, leading to alveolar collapse. Furthermore, the presence of excess protein in the alveolar space leads to the disintegration of the large phospholipids macroaggregates into smaller aggregates, which are less active and dysfunctional. In addition to the decreased lung compliance, this results in impaired gas exchange and increased pulmonary arterial pressures.

Although the above injury may resolve completely after the acute phase, some patients progress and develop evidence of pulmonary fibrosis, with persistent hypoxemia. In addition to new blood vessel formation, there is filling of alveolar space with mesenchymal cells and their products. Fibrosis starts on around day 3, and becomes dominant at day 7. Therefore, day 7 is considered as the cutoff between the early stage (exudative phase) and late stage (proliferative phase) of ARDS. Finally, it appears that the presence of pulmonary fibrosis diagnosed on the basis of fiberscopic transbronchial lung biopsy closely correlates with mortality in established ARDS.

MANAGEMENT

General Measures

Careful search of the underlying etiology is crucial in the management of patients with ARDS. Treatable infections should be addressed, and the need for surgical drainage evaluated. The patients should be monitored for the development of nosocomial infections. Adequate nutrition should be provided with the enteral route always preferred when feasible. In addition, patients should be placed on prophylaxis against gastrointestinal bleeding and thromboembolic events.

Invasive Mechanical Ventilation

Endotracheal intubation and mechanical ventilation are almost always needed in patients with ARDS. Mechanical ventilation aims to correct the severe hypoxemia encountered in this setting. Historically, normalizing the partial pressure of carbon dioxide was also considered a primary goal. Although lifesaving, it became gradually evident that mechanical ventilation can have major negative consequences in terms of exacerbating lung injury, through a process termed as ventilator-induced lung injury (VILI).

- *Tidal volume:* High tidal volume and high airway pressures were thought to be beneficial in opening collapse alveoli (i.e. recruitment). However, if one considers the fact that collapsed alveoli have low compliance, and do not adequately participate in tidal ventilation, the potential for injury with the use of high pressure or volume becomes evident. Hyperinflation and overdistension lead to the development of VILI. At this point, one can ascertain that a tidal volume of 6 mL/kg is better than 12 mL/kg in ARDS. However, it is important to use the ideal body weight, and not the actual weight, to calculate the tidal volume.

    One also has to remember that the use of low tidal volume can result in CO_2 retention, i.e. permissive hypercapnia with respiratory acidosis. This could be treated with a higher respiratory rate, and with the administration of sodium bicarbonate. The latter remains controversial, and likely unnecessary, except in the presence of severe acidosis. The pH at which the use of bicarbonate is necessary (if at all) is controversial. There is some experimental data to suggest that permissive hypercapnia is not only safe, but potentially beneficial. Nevertheless, hypercapnic strategy should be used with caution in patients with heart disease. Hypercapnia is contraindicated in patients with raised intracranial pressure.

- *Positive end-expiratory pressure:* The primary target is about 90% arterial oxyhemoglobin saturation in patients with ARDS. This may be difficult to achieve, even in the presence of high FiO_2. This constitutes the main indication for PEEP in ARDS. Used primarily as a means of supporting oxygenation, PEEP increases the functional residual capacity, and prevents small airways and alveoli from collapsing, leading to improvement in the ventilation–perfusion (V/Q) matching. It also prevents the repetitive opening and closing of alveoli, referred to as atelectrauma.

    Clinicians have to be aware of the potential for side effect associated with PEEP, primarily circulatory depression and barotrauma. Consequently, the concept of best PEEP in ARDS remains elusive, with some advocating the use of the pressure–volume curve as a means to determine the best PEEP, as one component of an overall safe ventilatory strategy (Fig. 75.1). Based on several trials, it appears that high levels of PEEP do not improve survival in patients with ARDS. Since side effects may occur with these high levels, the lowest PEEP that keeps acceptable levels of oxygenation and airway pressure may be used.

- *Mode of ventilation:* Traditional volume-assist-control mode remains widely used in patients with ARDS, whether in daily clinical practice, or in most recent large clinical trials. It has the advantage of being relatively simple and easy to monitor compared to the newer modalities. No studies have shown an outcome benefit when using newer modes of ventilation.

    Airway pressure release ventilation (APRV) is a relatively new modality that has been advocated to be used in ARDS. It is a pressure-targeted,

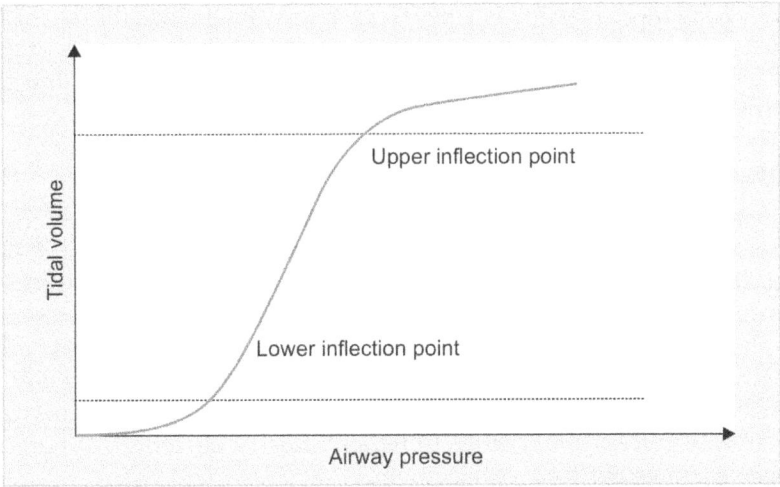

Fig. 75.1: Pressure–volume relationship curve. Positive end expiratory pressure above the lower inflection point prevents the cyclic opening and collapse of alveolar units, while ventilation above the upper inflection point leads to alveolar overdistension and lung injury. Ventilation within these two points can potentially reduce the risk of iatrogenic alveolar injury.

time-cycled mode that shares some similarities with pressure-controlled ventilation, allowing the ability for spontaneous breathing. High frequency oscillatory ventilation (HFOV) is another mode that aims to optimize alveolar recruitment while avoiding overdistension. It delivers a very low tidal volume (1–2 mL/kg) at very high frequency (3–15 breaths/s). Gas exchange occurs through nonconventional mechanisms such as diffusion. Two large multicenter studies showed no improvement in, or potentially worsening, outcome. Therefore, it cannot be recommended in patient with ARDS. Other ventilatory modalities include the use of partial liquid ventilation. Perfluorocarbon is a liquid with characteristics that make it appealing to use in ARDS, but it should be considered experimental until more definitive studies are done.

- *Recruitment maneuvers in acute respiratory distress syndrome:* Recruitment maneuvers involve the application of a high and sustained airway pressure, enough to open collapsed alveoli. This is done in the presence of sufficient PEEP application that will maintain these units open. The goal is to reverse the atelectasis and improve oxygenation. However, the effect on oxygenation has been variable, and the potential for adverse hemodynamic effects is concerning.

Noninvasive Ventilation

The use of noninvasive ventilation (NIV) in hypercapnic respiratory failure has been shown to decrease the need for intubation, the length of stay, as well as the mortality rate. Its effect on patients with hypoxemic respiratory failure, including ARDS, is less clear. Based on these studies, it appears that careful patients' selection is a key to success when using NIV in ARDS. One must consider the patients' comorbidities as well as the severity of the respiratory failure when deciding whether to institute NIV, or proceed directly to endotracheal intubation with invasive mechanical ventilation.

Fluid Management or Pulmonary Artery Catheter

On one hand, many patients with ARDS have underlying sepsis, may have intravascular fluid deficit, and/or are hypotensive. On the other hand, the fact that ARDS is a normal pressure pulmonary edema means that any fluid administration has the potential to worsen the pulmonary edema, increase the alveolar flooding, and decrease the PaO_2/FiO_2. Trials have suggested those ARDS patients who achieve negative fluid balance have improved outcome. In addition, excessive fluid administration in trauma-related ARDS patients was associated with increased mortality. Generally, most of the reports support a conservative strategy of fluid management.

Prone Position

The use of prone position in ARDS consistently results in oxygenation improvement. Several mechanisms have been suggested, including atelectasis reversal, alveolar recruitment, with increased lung volume, decreased shunt fraction and improved V/Q mismatch. Prone position may also release the effect of the heart weight on the left lung, as well as better drainage and clearing of respiratory secretions. It appears that prone position improves oxygenation, and likely affects the outcome of patient with severe ARDS. Current evidence does not support its routine use in patients with less severe ARDS, especially that a survival benefit has not been demonstrated in this population.

Other Supportive Therapies

- *Inhaled nitric oxide (iNO)* is a powerful vasodilator. When used in patients with ARDS, it has the potential to improve the V/Q mismatching, with reduction in the pulmonary vasoconstriction and hypertension seen in those patients. iNO has practically no systemic effects since it is rapidly deactivated by the hemoglobin. The effect on oxygenation is dose dependent—maximal improvement is seen with 1 and 10 parts per million (ppm). In clinical practice, as with any salvage therapy in ARDS, iNO may be utilized in patients with refractory hypoxemia, keeping in mind that the beneficial effect is likely to be time limited.
- *Surfactant therapy:* Replacement therapy is an appealing modality, with animal models showing improvement in gas exchange. In addition, survival of neonates with ARDS was improved with the use of surfactant. Surfactant replacement may have the potential to improve oxygenation in ARDS, but no effect on mortality is yet demonstrated. However, more studies are needed to control for several variables, including the type of surfactant used, the route of administration (nebulized vs bronchoscopic), and the duration of therapy.

- *Steroids*: The use of steroids in ARDS has been one of the most controversial issues over the last several decades. As powerful anti-inflammatory agents, it is reasonable to expect some beneficial effect in such an intense inflammatory milieu. Favorable outcomes and survival benefits with prolonged administration of systemic steroids are seen only when given before day 14 of ARDS. Any possible benefit should be weighed against the potential for adverse effects, including infections and neuromuscular weakness.
- *Extracorporeal membrane oxygenation (ECMO)* uses an extracorporeal circuit that directly oxygenates and removes CO_2 from the blood. In ARDS, it may be used as salvage therapy in patients with severe gas exchange abnormalities despite maximal ventilatory support. It can also be used to supplement positive-pressure ventilation, in order to limit inspiratory airway pressures, thus allowing the use of lung protective ventilation. Considering the potential for adverse events (including intracranial bleeding), its use in ARDS remains controversial, and well-designed controlled trials showing clear survival benefit are needed.

PROGNOSIS AND OUTCOME

The outcome depends primarily on the underlying cause of lung injury. Survival to discharge from hospital is lowest in ARDS patients with sepsis, and highest in patients with trauma. Presence of chronic liver disease, nonpulmonary organ dysfunction, advanced age and sepsis are some of the predictors of death. Initial indices of oxygenation and ventilation do not predict outcome.

In conclusion, except for the low tidal volume strategy, and more recently, the use of prone position in severe ARDS, no intervention was shown to be unequivocally effective in reducing mortality. Nevertheless, salvage therapies are available (e.g. iNO), with relatively good impact on oxygenation. One should use them only in patients with refractory hypoxemia. And, even though the quality of clinical trials has improved over the last decade, further studies are still needed to advance our understanding of this syndrome, and to translate that understanding into reduced morbidity and mortality.

CHAPTER
76

Sepsis

Sean E Hesselbacher, Walter G Shakespeare, Kalpalatha K Guntupalli

INTRODUCTION

The term sepsis is used to describe the systemic inflammatory response syndrome (SIRS) that is due to an infection. Noninfectious SIRS can progress similarly to sepsis, but is treated differently, so will not be discussed here. When sepsis progresses to cause organ dysfunction, hypoperfusion or hypotension, it is severe sepsis. The final stage in the progression of sepsis is septic shock which is sepsis-induced hypotension despite adequate fluid resuscitation along with the presence of perfusion abnormalities. The natural progression of severe sepsis and septic shock lead to irreversible organ failure and death. These definitions remain widely used in both clinical and research settings, though the sponsoring organizations have abandoned them as obsolete.

The new definition of sepsis does not require an infection to be confirmed if it is strongly suspected clinically. The definitions of severe sepsis and septic shock remain essentially unchanged. A staging system, intended to be used to stratify patients, is based on their baseline risk for adverse outcomes and their potential to respond to therapy. It is known as the PIRO system, which stands for *P*redisposition, *I*nsult or *I*nfection, *R*esponse, and *O*rgan dysfunction.

PATHOGENESIS

By definition, sepsis is the result of one or more pathogens invading the body and causing infection. The most common causes of sepsis worldwide are bacterial agents (93%). Sepsis can also result from viruses, fungi, and protozoa; in fact, almost any pathogen that causes infection can result in sepsis. When considering the likely etiology of sepsis in an individual patient, it is important to consider the prevalent pathogens in the region, the setting in which the infection was acquired [outpatient, hospital or intensive care unit (ICU)], and host factors including immunosuppression, comorbidities, medications, lifestyle and travel. There are clearly host abnormalities which lead to sepsis that do not depend entirely on the invading organism.

Early sepsis is characterized by the activation of CD4+ Th1 cells and the release of proinflammatory mediators, leading to systemic inflammation and SIRS. The propagation of sepsis is complicated, involving multiple systems and pathways, with resulting end-organ damage. Innate immune cells also activate complement C5a, with the resulting activation of the complement cascade. The complement cascade not only augments the inflammatory response, but is also involved in a complex feedback loop with both the intrinsic and extrinsic coagulation pathways. The coagulation cascades themselves are activated by the damaged tissues that triggered the sepsis in the first place, and uncontrolled activation results in microvascular thrombosis, inhibited fibrinolysis, and disseminated intravascular coagulation (DIC).

The result of the combination of systemic inflammation, cytokine storm, arterial hypotension, and DIC is often multiple organ dysfunction and failure. The late phase of sepsis is characterized by immunosuppression. Previously activated Th1 cells evolve into CD4+ Th2 cells, with the production of anti-inflammatory cytokines. Persistent inflammation and activation of the complement cascade results in apoptosis of immune cells, neutrophil dysfunction, hypothermia and anergy. As the sepsis resolves, the immunosuppressed state will eventually recover. In patients with severe baseline comorbidities, however, the immunosuppression may progress, with resulting death.

CLINICAL FEATURES AND EVALUATION

The patient with sepsis will often present with symptoms of SIRS. In general, these patients may complain of fever or chills, fatigue, malaise, anorexia, and sometimes complaints specific to the source of infection. Whether or not there are complaints reflecting organ dysfunction, such as confusion or decreased urine output, the clinician must always be aware of these signs, which can reflect progressing sepsis. Physical examination findings should always begin with vital signs and a general impression of the patient. Septic patients will show vital signs reflective of SIRS, including fever or hypothermia, tachycardia, tachypnea and possibly hypotension.

It is important to recognize that the rapid evolution of the septic patient's condition can change rapidly and serial evaluation is important to recognize decompensation. Basic laboratory data can help in the diagnosis of sepsis and organ dysfunction. These basic investigations should include complete and differential blood counts, chemistry panel, including glucose, liver function tests and coagulation tests. The Surviving Sepsis guidelines have consistently recommended early evaluation of serum lactate, while data on procalcitonin and C-reactive protein have not shown significant benefit. Any organ system can show the effects of sepsis, mortality increases with the number of organ systems affected. Table 76.1 provides a summary of some of the findings that can be seen in organ system dysfunction.

Cultures will ideally be drawn prior to the initiation of antibiotics, but only if it will not delay the dosing of antibiotics. Cultures should be taken from the blood and from the presumed site of infection. If the site of infection is unknown, cultures from multiple sites may be taken, which may eventually reveal the source. More invasive monitoring may be indicated in case of severe sepsis or septic shock to guide the therapies. Arterial blood gas assessment is required in patients with acid-base disorders and more frequently in mechanically ventilated patients. Patients with hypotension will most likely need invasive blood pressure monitoring, which may require arterial catheterization. To date, there has been no evidence that pulmonary arterial catheterization has been beneficial in patients with sepsis, severe sepsis or septic shock and should not be routinely placed.

PROGNOSIS

Sepsis not resulting in organ dysfunction or septic shock, carries good prognosis. Progression of sepsis to severe sepsis and septic shock portends escalating mortality. The severity of a septic episode is often graded by the number and type of organ dysfunction or failure. There is a mortality risk associated with most individual organ failures (Table 76.1), which may or may not improve with specific treatment. Additionally, studies have consistently shown an escalating mortality rate associated with a higher number of concurrent organ system failures suggesting that multisystems organ failure (MSOF) may represent a final common pathway leading to death. Younger age has been consistently shown to be a positive prognostic factor; patients less than 44 years of age and with absence of comorbidities have a mortality of less than 10%.

Multiple ICU scoring systems have been developed to assist the clinician in medical evaluation and treatment decisions in critically ill patients (Table 76.2). The Acute Physiology and Chronic Health Evaluation (APACHE II) remains perhaps the most widely used scoring system, mostly due to the vast literature based on this system and the availability in the public domain free of cost. The scoring system assigns points for 12 acute physical examination or laboratory findings, as well as age and chronic health; the higher the sum of the points, the higher the predicted mortality. The APACHE II score is currently recommended to determine the suitability of potentially harmful treatments in septic patients. Other scoring systems, such as the Multiple Organ Dysfunction Score (MODS) and Sequential Organ Failure Assessment (SOFA) systems, each assigns points (0–4) based on the degree of acute dysfunction in six systems. Again, higher sums predict higher mortality. Other scoring systems also exist for use in septic patients, each with advantages and disadvantages.

TABLE 76.1: Organ systems affected in severe sepsis and septic shock.

Organ system	Clinical manifestations	Associated mortality	Management (in addition to supportive care)
Nervous system	Encephalopathy	24%	Sedation, stimulus control
	Critical illness neuromyopathy	21–55%	Avoid aggravating medications (neuromuscular blockade, corticosteroids)
Respiratory	ARDS, hypoxemic respiratory failure	21–47%	Oxygen, mechanical ventilator support
Cardiovascular	Hypotension, tachycardia	28–43%	Vasopressors, inotropes, mechanical CV support
	Myocardial injury and dysfunction	29–48%	
Kidneys	Oliguric or anuric acute kidney injury	15–46%	Electrolyte management, renal replacement therapy
Hematologic	Cytopenias	23–53%	Blood product transfusions
	Coagulopathy	17–51%	
	Microvascular thrombosis/ disseminated intravascular coagulation (DIC)	43–50%	
Gastrointestinal	Shock liver, acute hepatic failure, hyperbilirubinemia, Ileus	14–54% Not defined	Avoidance of hepatotoxic agents Bowel rest, parenteral nutrition
Endocrine	Hyperglycemia	22–53%	Insulin
	Adrenal insufficiency	25–80%	Glucocorticoids
	Thyroid hormone abnormalities	44–62%	Generally none (in sick euthyroid), other abnormalities may require specific treatment
Skin	Rash, wounds	Varies by cause	Wound care, prevent superinfection

MANAGEMENT

The ideal treatment would target a common pathway or several pathways at once. More practical is the use of several agents at the same time, in a strategic manner, to stop or slow the progression at several key points. To simplify the

TABLE 76.2: Scoring systems applicable to sepsis.

Scoring system	Description	Advantages	Disadvantages
GCS (Glasgow Coma Score)	Neurologic scale (3–15) to assess level of consciousness	Simple; applicable to all trauma and medical patients; used in other scoring systems	Single organ system
APACHE II (Acute Physiology and Chronic Health Evaluation)	Calculated (0–71) within 24 hours of admission using common physiologic and demographic data, and prior health status	Widely used; online scoring systems; can assist in treatment decisions	Imprecise in predicting the mortality of a single patient; revised (APACHE III) in 1991
SOFA (Sepsis-related/Sequential Organ Failure Assessment)	Calculated (0–24) based on degree of organ failure in 6 systems	Can be calculated sequentially in the same patient	Multiple possible comparisons (admission, maximum, change in maximum), not one standard
MOD (Multiple Organ Dysfunction) score	Calculated (0–24) based on degree of organ failure in 6 systems	Can be calculated sequentially in the same patient	Complicated CV measures; similar to but less prevalent than SOFA
SAPS II (Simplified Acute Physiology Score)	Calculated on 17 variables after 24 hours, using common physiologic and demographic data and prior health status	Can be used in a variety of diseases; compare the morbidity of a patient/group with others	Imprecise in predicting the mortality of a single patient; revised (SAPS III) in 2005

complex care, several elements of care are combined together to implement as a group, i.e. sepsis "bundles". The effect on outcomes of the use of a bundle is significantly more than implementing the individual elements alone.

Antibiotics and Infection Source Control

The effective use of proper antibiotics is the only therapy that can truly stop sepsis before it gets going. Antibiotics, if given early, will either destroy or halt the replication of the pathogen and, in some cases, will also absorb the toxins released. The antibiotic selection must be appropriate for the clinical situation.

In the septic population, the appropriate initial antibiotic is any antibiotic that will target the causative pathogen. There are few cases where the microbiologic answer is available immediately. A suggested strategy is to administer a regimen of antibiotics that will broadly cover most, if not all, of the microbes to which the individual patient is at risk. Once the organism has been isolated, the antibiotics can be titrated as appropriate. In some cases, antibiotics alone will not be enough to clear infection without additional intervention. Some examples of this scenario include abscess formation, deep-seated skin or soft tissue infections, and infected mechanical devices. Abscesses may be present in a septic patient with no identifiable source of infection. Drainage of the abscess may be needed to clear the infection completely.

Interventions for source control should be undertaken with the lowest potential risk for the patient for example choosing to perform a percutaneous cholecystostomy drainage versus laparoscopic cholecystectomy. Indwelling mechanical devices such as pacemakers or artificial joints present a therapeutic dilemma. Every attempt should be made to remove the infected foreign body from the patient, allowing the antibiotics to clear infection, though that approach is not always practical.

Hemodynamic Support and Monitoring

Sepsis-induced hypotension is caused by a number of factors, which result in intravascular hypovolemia and arterial vasodilation. The goal of correcting hypotension is to maintain adequate tissue perfusion which is determined by the surrogate marker of lactate and the SvO_2. Aggressive hydration is the backbone of management in sepsis. Crystalloids are the fluid of choice in resuscitation of sepsis due to an abundance of data demonstrating no significant benefit when compared to colloid.

It is important to remember that adequate volume resuscitation be attempted prior to initiation of vasopressors. Arterial catheterization should be placed when patients require vasopressor or inotropic therapy. Norepinephrine is the initial choice of vasopressor in patients with septic shock, adjunct vasopressors can be added as dictated by the clinical scenario. Epinephrine is now the second-line agent of choice for the majority of patients with septic shock. Data has shown dopamine to be an inferior vasopressor in sepsis and is now only recommended in certain patients (low risk of tachyarrhythmias or relative bradycardia). Patients with severe sepsis and septic shock can develop cardiac dysfunction and show signs of low cardiac output (cool clammy skin, worsening $ScvO_2$) which could require inotropic therapy. Dobutamine or epinephrine remains the agent of choice.

Ventilatory Support

Respiratory failure is common in sepsis and is often multifactorial in nature. It may be due to the inability to maintain supraphysiologic ventilation, which is a result of high metabolic requirement or as a compensation mechanism for metabolic acidosis. Alternatively, hypoxemic respiratory failure may develop due to acute lung injury, as a direct result of infection, or as a consequence of change in mentation often seen during the sepsis syndrome. These patients often require invasive mechanical ventilation which should target low tidal volumes (6 mL/Kg) and higher positive end expiratory pressure (PEEP) to maintain low plateau pressures (<30 cm H_2O) similar to ARDS management. In general, patients with sepsis can be tried on noninvasive positive pressure ventilation (NIPPV) but clinicians should have a low threshold for intubation. Patients with multiorgan failure may require prolonged periods of mechanical ventilation and discontinuation may require resolution of acid-base disturbances, organ recovery and weaning of vasopressors.

Glucose Control

Hyperglycemia alone portrays increased mortality in critically ill patients, and intensive insulin therapy has been shown to improve mortality in a surgical ICU population. Proposed benefits of glucose control include prevention of immune dysfunction, reduction of systemic inflammation, endothelial protection, and preservation of mitochondrial structure and function, all of which are important in sepsis.

Corticosteroids

The use of corticosteroids in the treatment of sepsis has had a long and complex history, yet its use remains controversial. Understanding the history of corticosteroids in sepsis is important and review of all the literature compelled the Surviving Sepsis Campaign to recommend not to routinely use hydrocortisone in patients if their hemodynamics is stable with fluids and vasopressors. The ACTH stimulation test has no role in identifying patients who will benefit from hydrocortisone and should not be done routinely. If patients meet acceptability criteria for corticosteroids, they should be given hydrocortisone 200 mg separated over 4 different doses per day.

Standardized Protocols

Perhaps the most important development over the past decade is the refinement of protocols, or quantitative resuscitation strategies, regarding the evaluation and management of sepsis. An "early goal-directed therapy" protocol was created for a single center for severe sepsis and septic shock. In this protocol, patients meeting set criteria for severe sepsis and septic shock were monitored closely in the emergency room for 6 hours, undergoing a sequence of measures (volume resuscitation, vasopressors, red blood cell transfusion, and dobutamine) aimed at improving tissue perfusion, as defined by the $ScvO_2$ of 70%. The protocol resulted in absolute reduction in 28-day mortality of 16%; similar results and reduction in ICU usage were noted when the protocol was translated into clinical practice.

GOALS OF CARE

As described earlier, severe sepsis often affects debilitated individuals, with numerous comorbidities that increase expected mortality from sepsis episode. It is vital to have open discussions with the patient (if possible) and caregivers regarding the severity of the illness, likely outcomes and treatment recommendations. Goals of care discussion should be undertaken as soon as is reasonable but not longer than 72 hours after admission to the ICU. Frank discussions with the patient and caregiver may minimize suffering for the patient and reduce stress on the caregiver.

SPECIAL CONSIDERATIONS

Nutrition remains an important aspect in the management of the critically ill patient with severe sepsis or septic shock. Low-dose feeds started within 48 hours of diagnosis even in patients with severe sepsis and septic shock, with recommendations to attempt avoidance of total parenteral nutrition, if possible, within the first 7 days. There is increasing evidence that episodes of delirium can have longstanding deleterious effects on neurocognition. All care should be taken to avoid delirium altogether and if that is not possible, shorten its duration. Many practitioners have gone toward an analgesic (presumably opiate)-based sedation with avoidance of benzodiazepines to avoid delirium.

Despite much hope and good preliminary data, statin therapy has not been shown to improve clinical outcomes of patients with sepsis-associated ARDS.

In summary, considerable progress has been made in the understanding and management of sepsis. The Surviving Sepsis Campaign and implementation of sepsis bundles have significantly lowered the mortality from sepsis. Yet, severe sepsis and septic shock continue to remain life-threatening conditions stressing the need for further improvement in management strategies.

CHAPTER 77

Nonpulmonary Critical Care

Liziamma George, Mark Astiz

INTRODUCTION

Patients are admitted to critical care units with several disease processes other than respiratory failure. In addition, patients admitted with respiratory failure often develop further organ dysfunctions that require aggressive management.

GASTROINTESTINAL DISEASE IN CRITICAL CARE

Gastrointestinal Bleeding

Upper gastrointestinal (GI) bleed is defined as bleeding above the level of the ligament of Treitz while lower GI bleed is bleeding below the level of the ligament of Treitz. Recurrent acute or chronic bleed from the digestive tract without an obvious etiology after a normal esophagogastroduodenoscopy (EGD) and colonoscopy is known as obscure GI bleed.

Upper Gastrointestinal Bleeding

Clinical manifestations depend on the rate and amount of bleeding. A pulse more than or equal to 100 beats/minute, systolic blood pressure less than 100 mm Hg, postural changes, an increase in the pulse of more than or equal to 20 beats/minute or a drop in systolic blood pressure of more than or equal to 20 mm Hg on standing are significant. Airway protection is needed for patients with altered mental status or massive hematemesis. History of alcohol abuse, nonsteroidal anti-inflammatory drug (NSAID) usage, liver disease, and family history of GI or other malignancies, recent retching, prior surgery, and other medication usage may point to the etiology of GI bleed. Elderly patients, who potentially have an age-related compromised cardiac reserve, may present with symptoms of chest pain and shortness of breath rather than GI bleed, suggestive of myocardial ischemia. Other symptoms, such as fatigue and dyspnea tend to occur with chronic blood loss. Signs specific for upper GI bleed include hematemesis, bloody gastric lavage, melena and hematochezia.

Irrespective of the bleeding site, the management of acute GI bleeding should include hemodynamic stabilization, localization of the bleeding site, and specific therapeutic intervention. Supplemental oxygen should be provided to ensure adequate tissue oxygenation and all patients should also be placed on cardiac monitors. Intravascular volume repletion with crystalloid infusion through two large bore (16 or 18 gauges) intravenous lines should begin immediately. Patients with unstable vital signs even after initial stabilization should be transfused with packed red cells.

In cases with exsanguinating blood loss, attempts at localization and control of bleeding through endoscopic or surgical procedures should be done simultaneously. The threshold for transfusion must be individualized. Most hemodynamically stable patients do not require a transfusion for a hemoglobin level is greater than 7 g/dL, while hypotensive actively bleeding patients will require more aggressive transfusions.

Medical therapy should be used as an adjunct to endoscopic therapy. Pre-endoscopic continuous infusion of proton pump inhibitors (PPIs) decreases the need for endoscopic intervention. Administration of a PPI has also been shown to decrease rebleeding, surgical intervention and mortality. Continuous PPI infusion is given for 72 hours for acute GI bleed.

Angiography and embolization is recommended for patients in whom acute bleeding is not controlled by endoscopic treatment.

Lower Gastrointestinal Bleeding

These patients tend to present with hematochezia or maroon colored stools.

The initial stabilization of lower GI bleed is not different from that of upper GI bleed. The localization of bleeding is done by colonoscopy which identifies the bleeding in 60–80% of cases. The other options are nuclear scanning using technetium-99m-labeled red blood cell (Tc-99m RBC) scan and arteriography. A multidetector computed tomography (CT) scan was used to localize massive GI bleeding in some reports. Arteriography of both superior and inferior mesenteric arteries can be used to identify the source of bleeding. Some studies recommend radionuclide scanning before angiography so as to decrease the incidence of negative tests.

Management of GI bleed in patients with anticoagulation and antiplatelet therapy. It is recommend to stop antiplatelet agents and anticoagulation until hemostasis is achieved in consultation with the cardiologists or vascular physicians. The decision to use platelets, fresh frozen plasma (FFP), prothrombin complex concentrate (PCC) and vitamin K should be individualized.

Acute Variceal Hemorrhage

Acute variceal hemorrhage is one of the complications of portal hypertension requiring critical care unit admission. Patients with Child-Pugh classification of B or C have a higher incidence of variceal bleed and are associated with a mortality of 15-20%. The specific treatment strategies include the use of medications, endoscopy, surgical interventions, transjugular intrahepatic shunt, balloon tamponade and the prevention of recurrent bleeding. After initial stabilization of the patient, medications directed toward splanchnic vasoconstriction should be utilized to decrease portal pressure. The commonly used agents are vasopressin, terlipressin, somatostatin and its analogs. Vasopressin causes direct vasoconstriction of splanchnic arterioles leading to decreased portal pressure. The major side effects include systemic vasoconstriction, particularly coronary vessels. The use of nitrates in addition to vasopressin is recommended to decrease these side effects with added therapeutic benefit. Notably, vasopressin has minimal effects on rebleeding. Terlipressin, a vasopressin analog can be used as an alternative to vasopressin, which has less side effects than vasopressin. Somatostatin, an indirect vasoconstrictor of splanchnic circulation, rapidly decreases the portal pressure with minimal side effects. It is superior to vasopressin in patients with variceal hemorrhage. The infusion is continued for 2-5 days and has no significant effect on mortality.

Endoscopic banding or sclerotherapy is the definitive treatment for acute variceal bleed. However, combination of both medical and endoscopic therapies is most beneficial to control bleeding. Endoscopic therapies are associated with complications, such as ulceration, mediastinitis, esophageal perforation as well as sepsis. Balloon tamponade is considered when medical and endoscopic approaches fail to achieve hemostasis or when there is a lack of expertise to perform endoscopic interventions.

Acute Liver Failure

Acute liver failure is defined as the onset of hepatic encephalopathy and coagulopathy within 26 weeks of jaundice in a patient with preexisting liver disease. Patients should be managed in a critical care unit at the onset of encephalopathy. Fulminant hepatic failure can occur within 8 weeks of jaundice. While acetaminophen toxicity is the major cause of liver failure in western world, infections are the predominant etiology in developing countries. Most common causes of hepatic failure in India include hepatitis E virus (44%), hepatitis B virus (15%), hepatitis A virus (2%), and unknown (31%).

Management of Complications

Hepatic encephalopathy is a reversible neurological dysfunction, occurring in patients with liver failure. Neurotoxins like ammonia, oxidative stress, production of false neurotransmitters, and alteration in blood-brain barrier are implicated for its development. In addition to correction of precipitating factors, ammonia production in the gut is reduced with the use of lactulose and nonabsorbable antibiotics, such as neomycin and rifaximin. Infections contribute significantly to the mortality of these patients and should be treated aggressively. For patients developing hypotension intravascular volume repletion if they are hypovolemic, vasopressors and inotropic support for vasodilatation and low cardiac state should be instituted.

Spontaneous Bacterial Peritonitis

Spontaneous bacterial peritonitis (SBP) is an infection of ascitic fluid in the absence of an intra-abdominal source of infection. It is a common and life-threatening complication of cirrhosis. SBP occurrence is rare in noncirrhotic patients as opposed to cirrhotic ones. Bacterial translocation into ascitic fluid is commonly believed to be a causative factor for the development of SBP, however current research shows that SBP is the result of the interplay of several factors, such as prolonged bacteremia resulting from defective local and humoral immunity, intrahepatic shunting of blood, defective bactericidal action of ascitic fluid, and transabdominal introduction of infection. SBP should be suspected in all cirrhotic patients with ascites, as the clinical manifestations can be very subtle as well as nonspecific, with a broad range of clinical expression.

Severe Acute Pancreatitis

Acute pancreatitis is an inflammatory condition of the pancreas resulting in abdominal pain and elevation of the serum levels of the pancreatic enzymes. It is a self-limiting disease in most cases. About 20% of patients develop acute necrotizing pancreatitis, leading to multiorgan failure and death. The common etiologies include gallstones, alcohol consumption, hypertriglyceridemia, smoking, hypercalcemia, drugs, trauma, pancreatic divisum, and infections.

Pancreatic enzymes are activated within the acini causing damage to the pancreatic tissues and vasculature. In necrotizing pancreatitis the inflammation extends into the adjacent tissues. Patients present to the intensive care unit (ICU) with fever, tachycardia, shock, and multiorgan dysfunction.

A contrast-enhanced abdominal CT-scan should be performed for patients with acute pancreatitis who require admission to the ICU. Fluid resuscitation at a rate of 5–10 mL/kg/hour of isotonic solution is required to prevent acute renal tubular necrosis. In addition to the vital signs, monitoring hematocrit for hemoconcentration can guide the adequacy of fluid resuscitation. Pain is managed with meperidine, morphine, or fentanyl. Infections caused by enteric gram-negative organisms increase the morbidity and mortality of these patients. CT-guided aspiration and drainage of collections should be performed in patients in whom infection is suspected. Open necrosectomy is not favored. Early enteral feeding via a nasojejunostomy or nasogastric tube is associated with decreased infectious complications and early recovery compared to parenteral nutrition.

HEMATOLOGY IN CRITICAL CARE

Anemia

Anemia, acute or chronic is a frequent problem in critically ill patients admitted into ICUs. The proinflammatory state seen in critically ill patients results in a blunted erythropoietic response to anemia in addition to abnormalities in iron metabolism, further complicating the clinical course.

The clinical consequences of anemia will depend on the degree of anemia, the rate at which it has developed, the oxygen demands of the patient which tends to be high in the critically ill, as well as the ability of the patient to compensate for these changes. High-risk groups in which anemia is considered to be less tolerated and more vulnerable to adverse outcomes include the elderly, critically ill patients and patients with respiratory, coronary or cerebrovascular disease. The symptoms and signs are nonspecific.

Anemia of acute onset, such as in GI bleed is typically treated with the administration of physiologic crystalloids, colloidal fluids or red cell transfusions. However, in patients with a more chronic evolution of anemia, treatment will depend on the underlying etiology. Iatrogenic causes such as phlebotomy are common in the ICU and range from 40 mL/day to 70 mL/day. Blood conservation techniques, such as use of small volume phlebotomy tubes, point-of-care analysis and closed, no-waste sampling systems may contribute to the reduction in anemia.

Approximately 70% of critically ill patients are transfused and receive their initial transfusion within the first 48 hours in the ICU. For those patients staying greater than a week in the ICU about 73–85% of them will receive red cell transfusions. Higher transfusion rates have been reported to be associated with increased hospital acquired infections, increased ICU length of stay, higher rates of coagulation abnormalities, more severe organ failure as well as increased mortality rates. Erythropoietin is associated with more thrombotic events.

Indications for Red Blood Cell Transfusion in the Intensive Care Unit

In patients with hemorrhagic shock, initial resuscitation should be done using crystalloids. If the shock is not corrected after 2 L of crystalloids, packed red blood cell (PRBC) transfusion is indicated to improve oxygen delivery to the tissues and should be guided by hemodynamic parameters rather than hemoglobin measurement. Aggressive measures to control bleeding should accompany resuscitation. Blood lactate levels can be used to guide the adequacy of resuscitation. In patients with hemodynamically stable anemia, transfusion is indicated if the hemoglobin level drops below 7 g/dL and should be guided by the patient's condition rather than the absolute number.

Massive transfusions, defined as the transfusion of 10 or more units of red cells in 24 hours, are necessary in patients with hemorrhagic shock; however, such transfusions are associated with hypothermia, metabolic acidosis and coagulopathy. Hypothermia occurs due to transfusion of stored cold blood and impairment of metabolism leading to delayed clearing of toxins and cytokines. Dilutional coagulopathy along with consumption coagulopathy occurs in these patients and this is further exacerbated by hypothermia that can occur with massive transfusions. Massive transfusions are also associated with hyperkalemia, hypocalcemia, hypomagnesemia, metabolic alkalosis and acidosis. Transfusion-related acute lung injury (TRALI) occurs within 6 hours of transfusion with signs and symptoms of acute respiratory failure. The proposed mechanisms are reaction of donor antibodies against the recipient white blood cells (WBCs) and pulmonary vascular endothelial activation leading to WBC sequestration and endothelial damage.

Thrombocytopenia

Thrombocytopenia occurs frequently in critically ill patients and is the most common coagulation problem in this group of patients. Depending on the cut-off level utilized to define thrombocytopenia (i.e. $<150 \times 10^9$/L vs $<100 \times 10^9$/L), the type of population being assessed (e.g. medical vs surgical/trauma) and the period of the ICU course (e.g. <4 days vs ≥4 days) being studied, the incidence of thrombocytopenia has been reported to range from 15 to 60%. The decreased risk of bleeding with platelet counts between 100 and 150×10^9/L has resulted in a cutoff level of less than 100×10^9/L being proposed as the definition of thrombocytopenia in the critically ill.

Platelet concentrates are made by centrifugation of either whole blood or plasma and by apheresis of blood. Simply transfusing patients with platelets to raise levels may be unwarranted, ineffective and even contraindicated in some critically ill thrombocytopenic patients. It is essential to determine the typically multifactorial etiology of thrombocytopenia in these patients and subsequently correct the underlying cause. Prophylactic platelet transfusion is given to patients who are actively bleeding with thrombocytopenia or when platelet counts fall below 10×10^9/L.

Coagulopathy in the Intensive Care Unit

Coagulopathy occurs in critically ill patients due to the underlying illness or medications. Fresh frozen plasma is indicated for the replacement of single coagulation factor deficiency, multiple factor deficiencies, for patients with DIC associated with bleeding, during plasma exchange in patients with thrombotic thrombocytopenic purpura and for severe bleeding associated with warfarin-induced coagulopathy. Prothrombin complex concentrates can be used as an alternative to FFP for reversal of anticoagulation due to warfarin. They achieve more rapid reversal with significantly less fluid administration. Cryoprecipitate is given to patients when plasma fibrinogen levels are less than 1.5–2.0 g/L. Tranexamic acid, an inhibitor of fibrinolysis, should be considered for trauma patients at risk for significant bleeding in whom it is demonstrated to improve survival and decrease the need for transfusions.

RENAL DISEASE IN CRITICAL CARE

Acute Kidney Injury

Acute kidney injury (AKI), formerly referred to as acute renal failure, is said to occur when renal dysfunction takes place suddenly and/or rapidly. The etiology of AKI has typically been separated into three categories, namely, prerenal, intrinsic renal and postrenal azotemia thereby guiding the mode of therapeutic intervention. However, in ICU patients, etiology of AKI is usually a result of multiple factors which could easily fall into any, or more commonly, a combination of the aforementioned categories, thus complicating the manner in which such patients can be treated successfully.

Clinical Presentation

The reduction in GFR and urine output can result in fluid overload which may further progress into congestive heart failure and hypotension, raised intra-abdominal pressure from retroperitoneal tissue edema and ascites, hypertension from intravascular volume overload as well as pulmonary compromise from congestion and pleural effusions. Electrolyte abnormalities such as metabolic acidosis and hyperkalemia commonly occur predisposing to cardiac arrhythmias. Critically ill patients with AKI can also develop a compromised inflammatory and immune response which increases the risk for infection, pneumonia, shock or other multiorgan failure. The uremic state in these patients can contribute to the development of anorexia, vomiting, encephalopathy, pericarditis, bleeding diathesis, polyneuropathy, and anemia from increased erythrocyte destruction which can be further complicated by weakness and easy fatigability.

Management

Treatment strategies are initially targeted at correcting the suspected underlying cause. Such treatment may include but is not limited to fluid resuscitation with or without inotropic or vasopressor support to maintain hemodynamic stability and renal perfusion, correction of metabolic abnormalities, discontinuation of nephrotoxic agents or dosage adjustments of medications eliminated through the kidney, as well as the provision of adequate nutrition.

With regards to fluid resuscitation, there is no difference in survival when comparing crystalloids with colloids (albumin). Furthermore, though fluid resuscitation can be crucial in these patients, a positive fluid balance is also associated with an increased mortality.

The role of diuretic agents in the treatment of AKI remains controversial. Diuretics did not improve overall mortality, need for renal replacement therapy (RRT) or shorten the duration of AKI. At the present time, there is no evidence supporting the routine use of diuretics in patients with AKI or to convert oliguric renal failure to nonoliguric renal failure. In addition, there is no consensus regarding the most appropriate time to start RRT for AKI. However, severe hyperkalemia, severe metabolic acidosis, uremic complications such as encephalopathy, pericarditis, pleuritis or bleeding diathesis, and volume overload are generally considered to be absolute indications for RRT, which could either be continuous or intermittent.

Similarly, there is also no consensus regarding the dose of hemofiltration or the renal replacement modality, i.e. continuous versus intermittent. A detailed description of modes of RRT is beyond the scope of this chapter.

Prevention

Early recognition of underlying risk factors and prevention of additional injuries in high-risk patients are particularly important. Maintaining adequate renal perfusion, prevention of hyperglycemia and avoidance of nephrotoxins are some of the strategies used for this purpose.

Radioiodine contrast-induced nephropathy can be prevented by using a low volume nonionic low osmolar or iso-osmolar agent in a well-hydrated patient. There is no significant advantage in using sodium bicarbonate over sodium chloride solution. Prophylactic administration of N-acetylcysteine to prevent renal failure is also controversial. In patients, who must undergo radiological studies utilizing contrast, adequate hydration, use of prophylactic N-acetylcysteine, avoidance of other nephrotoxic agents, and use of low volume nonionic low or iso-osmolar agents are recommended.

ENDOCRINE EMERGENCIES IN CRITICAL CARE

Thyroid Storm

Hyperthyroid patients present with palpitations, unexplained weight loss, diarrhea, and intolerance to heat and muscle weakness. Thyroid storm is a hyperthyroid state where the symptoms are exaggerated and associated with 20-50% mortality. The common causes are Graves' disease, chronic and subacute thyroiditis, postpartum thyroiditis, and excessive iodine intake. It can also be precipitated by stress, surgery, sepsis or cardiovascular events in a preexisting hyperthyroid patient.

Patients can present with cardiac arrhythmias, widened pulse pressure, congestive heart failure, systemic inflammatory response syndrome, hypotension, psychosis, delirium and coma. The laboratory findings specific to the thyroid gland include a low or undetectable thyroid-stimulating hormone (TSH) level and a high thyroxine (T_4) level.

Management

Patient should be stabilized with fluids if hypotensive or with diuretics in case of congestive heart failure. Adequate oxygenation should be maintained and often these patients may need mechanical ventilatory support. Fever should be controlled by cooling and the use of acetaminophen. Specific treatment initially involves the prevention of thyroid hormone synthesis by using thioamides. Either propylthiouracil or methimazole can be used. Propylthiouracil has the advantage of decreasing peripheral conversion of T_4 to triiodothyronine (T_3).

Lugol's iodine (10 drops 3 times daily) or saturated solutions of potassium iodide [SSKI (5 drops every 6 hours)] is used for this purpose. It is important to give iodine only after giving hormone synthesis blocking agents. Lithium carbonate also decreases the release of thyroid hormone but is rarely used due to its toxicity. The third step is to give agents to prevent conversion of T_4 to T_3. These include glucocorticosteroids and iodinated contrast solutions. The administration of β-blockers will counteract the sympathetic stimulation and propranolol is the drug of choice. It is given intravenously 1 mg/minute. Alternative agents are nadolol or esmolol. Patients with contraindications to β-blockers can be given calcium channel blockers as an alternative.

Myxedema Coma

Myxedema coma is a rare but life-threatening complication that results from severe untreated hypothyroidism or long-standing hypothyroidism. It can be precipitated by trauma, surgery, severe infection, and cold stress especially with the usage of sedative, hypnotic and narcotic medications.

Clinical and Diagnostic Features

Myxedema is characterized by distinct clinical features rather than by laboratory findings suggestive of hypothyroidism. The role of laboratory findings is to confirm the diagnosis and delineate coexisting or precipitating conditions. Low TSH levels along with low total and free serum T_4 and T_3 levels are noted in primary hypothyroidism. High TSH levels with below normal levels of T_3 are seen in secondary hypothyroidism. Low sodium levels with elevated levels of lactate dehydrogenase (LDH) and creatinine are also seen.

Management

Supportive care, treatment of hypothermia, monitoring of the neurological and respiratory status should be emphasized along with the supplementation of thyroid hormones. The optimal dose of thyroid replacement remains controversial. Both thyroid storm and myxedema coma are associated with significant mortality and early recognition and treatment are important for a favorable outcome.

Acute Adrenal Insufficiency

Acute adrenal insufficiency is seen in patients with bilateral adrenal hemorrhage, undiagnosed adrenal insufficiency with stress, trauma, surgery, drugs especially etomidate and previous steroid therapy, and pituitary apoplexy. Diagnosis is difficult due to diurnal variation of cortisol secretion. Cortisol levels are higher in the morning and lower in the evening. A cortisol level of less than 3 µg/dL in the morning is diagnostic of adrenal insufficiency and a level less than 10 µg/dL is suggestive of the diagnosis. The supportive measures include volume administration with isotonic fluids with glucose in case of hypoglycemia. Precipitating causes must be sought and treated.

Diabetic Ketoacidosis and Hyperosmolar Hyperglycemic State

Diabetic ketoacidosis (DKA), hyperosmolar hyperglycemic state (HHS) and drug-induced hypoglycemia are the major complications of diabetes mellitus. Both DKA and HHS are due to insulin deficiency and excessive counter-regulatory hormones.

Diabetic ketoacidosis and HHS patients usually present with nausea, vomiting, abdominal pain, shortness of breath, polyuria, and polydipsia. As the condition worsens they develop neurological symptoms which may progress to coma. The initial evaluation should assess hemodynamic status and airways. Metabolic acidosis is the hallmark of DKA.

Management

If potassium is less than 3 mEq/L, replenish potassium to above 3.3 mEq/L before initiating insulin. Sodium bicarbonate is given only when the arterial pH is less than 7. The insulin infusion is typically continued until ketoacidosis is resolved. Blood glucose should be monitored every hour while on an insulin infusion while other laboratory tests, i.e. basic metabolic profile, are monitored every 3-4 hours. The complications of untreated DKA and HHS are cerebral edema particularly in children and noncardiogenic pulmonary edema. Patients must be monitored for hypoglycemia and hypokalemia. Almost all patients with DKA develop a nonanion gap metabolic acidosis with treatment and phosphate repletion is not recommended for patients with DKA. Hypoglycemia in diabetic patients occurs either due to insulin excess or as a result of failure of the counter regulatory hormones. Symptoms and signs are usually non-specific. Severe hypoglycemia causes seizure and coma and should be treated with glucagon 0.5-1 mg subcutaneous or intramuscularly as well as intravenous glucose (dextrose).

NEUROLOGICAL DISORDERS IN CRITICAL CARE

Acute Ischemic Stroke

A stroke is a focal neurological deficit that is typically of acute onset and results from a disruption of the cerebral blood flow. It usually occurs suddenly, but occasionally progresses in a more gradual fashion. The majority of stroke presentations result from cerebral ischemia, while hemorrhage (intracerebral or subarachnoid) causes the rest. The advent and widespread utilization of thrombolytic therapy within 3 hours of developing ischemic stroke, has revolutionized the management of what was once considered a condition with few treatment choices. Thrombotic strokes tend to present with clinical features that evolve over hours to days whereas embolic strokes have a sudden or rapid onset at maximum severity at the time or presentation.

Time is of the essence and initial management at time of presentation involves stabilizing the patient, performing a prompt clinical evaluation, as well as laboratory and imaging studies, and thereby assessing the need for resuscitation, oxygen supplementation or intubation, fever, blood sugar or blood pressure control, and thrombolysis. Fever, hyperglycemia and hypotension following an ischemic stroke have been associated with poorer outcomes and should be treated. Immediate treatment of hypertension is controversial and currently recommended for patients with systolic pressures greater than 220 mm Hg not undergoing fibrinolysis.

Subarachnoid Hemorrhage

Subarachnoid hemorrhage (SAH) accounts for 10% of cerebrovascular accidents (CVAs) and is associated with significant morbidity and mortality (50%). The risk factors for SAH include cigarette smoking, heavy alcohol consumption, uncontrolled hypertension, use of sympathomimetic drugs, cocaine abuse, estrogen deficiency and some hereditary conditions like polycystic kidney and Ehlers–Danlos syndrome. Patients present with unusual or severe sudden onset headaches. Warning bleeds and sentinel headaches are relatively uncommon.

The management of SAH is centered on three aspects namely: (i) general management; (ii) definitive treatment (identifying and treating the causative lesion and preventing rebleeding); and (iii) treatment of complications.

General management involves ICU monitoring, discontinuation of all antithrombotic medications and correction of any coagulopathy if present. Definitive treatment involves either surgical clipping or endovascular coiling. There is a decreased mortality and a nonsignificant increase in rebleeding in patients treated with endovascular coiling as opposed to surgical clipping. The timing of intervention should be as early as is feasible.

Maintenance of euvolemia is recommended to prevent vasospasm. Induced hypertension should be considered for patients with delayed cerebral ischemia due to vasospasm. Balloon angioplasty and the administration of intra-arterial vasodilators are indicated in patients with vasospasm that is refractory to medical therapy.

Intracerebral Hemorrhage

Intracerebral hemorrhage (ICH) (bleeding within the skull) occurs within the brain parenchyma or surrounding meningeal spaces. Brain hemorrhage can occur from defects in the vessel wall, such as aneurysms, arteriovenous malformations, small vessel microaneurysms, coagulopathy, and increased blood pressure or trauma. Intracerebral hemorrhage accounts for 10–30% of all stroke hospital admissions and is associated with high mortality. Intracerebral hemorrhage commonly occurs in the cerebral lobes, cerebellum, basal ganglia, thalamus, and brainstem with extension into ventricles with large hematomas. Cerebral edema and neuronal damage in the surrounding parenchyma also occurs.

Initial management of these patients includes evaluation of the airways, breathing, and circulation. Mechanical ventilatory support is usually recommended for patients with GCS of less than 8, but should be guided by the clinical presentation. The secondary effects of ICH include expansion of the hematoma, increased ICP, perihematomal edema, intraventricular hemorrhage, and hydrocephalus. Treatment involves a combination of both medical and surgical interventions. Elevated blood pressure is common in patients with ICH and is feared to contribute to the expansion of hematoma. Lowering blood pressure to less than 140 mm Hg systolic did not decrease hematoma volume or mortality but may in a subset of patients improve functional outcome. Hyperventilation has an immediate and transient effect on cerebral circulation. It lowers CPP by cerebral vasoconstriction and may be associated with exacerbations of ischemia in local regions of the brain. It is recommended to lower the $PaCO_2$ to 30-35 mm Hg in situations of an intractable rise in CPP. Hyperthermia worsens neurological damage by increasing the metabolism in ischemic brain tissues. Therapeutic cooling to a temperature of 30-32°C and gradual rewarming may improve outcomes. The role of ventriculostomy and CSF drainage has not been studied prospectively, but is an effective method of decreasing ICP, especially in the phase of hydrocephalus.

In addition to these specific treatments, patients should be treated adequately for pain. Sedation and neuromuscular blockade may be needed for patients who are intubated. Also, blood glucose should be lowered to less than 150 mg/dL, but hypoglycemia should be avoided. Since most of the seizures are nonconvulsive in nature, prophylactic seizure medications must be used initially.

Patients with ICH have a high incidence of venous thromboembolism and should receive prophylaxis initially with pneumatic compression stockings and later subcutaneous heparin 5,000 units every 8 hours after day 4 of ICH onset. Patients who developed venous thromboembolism should be treated with an inferior vena caval (IVC) filter. Warfarin treatment increases the incidence of ICH and the risk is proportional to the degree of anticoagulation and the presence of amyloid vasculopathy. The reinstitution of warfarin therapy should be carefully assessed on an individual basis. ICH associated with antifibrinolytic therapy carries a worse prognosis than warfarin associated ICH and is treated with platelets and cryoprecipitate.

Surgical treatment is not beneficial except in certain selected conditions. Recommendations for surgery are as follows: (i) cerebellar hematoma with neurological deterioration, brainstem compression or hydrocephalus should be removed as soon as possible; (ii) patient with large lobar clots within 1 cm of the surface of the brain, evacuation of supratentorial ICH by standard craniotomy may be considered; and (iii) the usefulness of urokinase infusion into the clot, or minimally invasive evacuation of the clot or routine decompressive craniotomy is currently unknown.

Status Epilepticus

Seizures are a common condition seen in 3.3–34% of ICU patients. They can result from either a primary neurological pathology, such as a stroke, brain tumor or central nervous system (CNS) infection, or develop as a neurological complication of critical illness as in patients with metabolic abnormalities, drug/substance toxicity or withdrawal, or hypoxemia. Status epilepticus is said to occur when seizures are recurrent or refractory lasting more than 5 minutes or repetitive in nature without regaining consciousness in between episodes. It is a life-threatening emergency that necessitates urgent diagnosis and treatment and is classified as either being convulsive or nonconvulsive. The convulsive form tends to be the more severe and common type and is characterized by repeated seizure episodes associated with a postictal state, while the nonconvulsive form is characterized typically by an altered mental status and a lack of obvious physical manifestations.

The EEG not only serves as a diagnostic tool, but also aids in monitoring response to treatment, as patients may still be actively seizing even though motor signs have subsided. Treatment involves eliminating seizure activity as well as preventing the development of further episodes. Benzodiazepines are the initial drug of choice. Intravenous lorazepam 1–2 mg, midazolam 2–5 mg or diazepam 10–20 mg can be given at first but these doses can be increased up to 5–10 mg, 5–20 mg or 20–40 mg over 5 minutes in cases of recurrent or refractory seizures. Intramuscular midazolam is an effective alternative if intravenous access is not available.

In patients not responding to the increased doses of benzodiazepines, second-line agents that have been used include phenytoin (loading dose 20 mg/kg at 50 mg/minute) or fosphenytoin (20 mg/minute at 150 mg/minute). Other alternative second-line agents that can be used include intravenous medications like levetiracetam and valproic acid. In patients, who still continue to have seizure episodes (>60 minutes), induction of a pharmacological coma may be necessary with infusions of phenobarbital, propofol or midazolam. Continuous EEG monitoring is also preferred, particularly in patients with nonconvulsive status epilepticus. Status epilepticus is a serious condition in critically ill patients and is associated with a mortality of approximately 20%. Early recognition and treatment is necessary to prevent the potentially severe neurological consequences.

CHAPTER

78

Critical Care in Nonpulmonary Conditions: Poisoning, Envenomation, and Environmental Injuries

Dhruva Chaudhry, Inderpaul Singh Sehgal

INTRODUCTION

A large number of patients admitted in the intensive care units (ICUs) include those admitted due to nonpulmonary causes like poisoning, snake envenomation, trauma, environmental injuries or tropical infections (malaria, leptospirosis, tetanus, etc.) where life may be threatened with or without involvement of lungs, respiratory muscles or both.

POISONING

Poisoning is defined as the exposure of an individual to a toxin through ingestion, inhalation or direct skin contact. It can be either accidental as is common in children or suicidal which is more common in adults. It is believed that majority of poisoning in critical care units occurs due to pesticides and fumicides used across the country as most of the cases of severe intoxication and deaths.

Toxic ingestion presents variably. Patients often arrive with known drug overdose or toxic exposure, such as in the setting of illicit drug use, suicidal attempt, or accidental exposure. In others, history is unclear, particularly when there is associated trauma or alterations in mental status. Clinical features may be specific for a toxic syndrome (or toxidrome) but just as often nonspecific and suggestive of other disorders.

The protean manifestations of intoxication mandate a higher index of suspicion to facilitate decision and immediate treatment, while the nature of the ingestion is confirmed. Following steps are important in the management:

Management

Resuscitation and Stabilization

Initial step is to identify and treat immediate life-threatening problems and revolves around pneumonic ABCD (airway; breathing; circulation; drugs, decontamination).

Airway: Airway patency and stabilization must be established.

Breathing: It includes oxygenation and ventilation. In case of doubts regarding the patient's ability to handle secretion or maintenance of spontaneous respirations, endotracheal intubation should be done immediately. Hypoxemia should be corrected immediately to avoid anoxic damage to brain, myocardial ischemia, and cardiac arrhythmias.

Circulation: Circulatory manifestations of poisoning can range from hypotension, hypertension, bradycardia, and tachycardia to cardiac arrest.

Drugs and decontamination: Give an antidote when there is reasonable certainty of a specific diagnosis. Decontamination includes facilitation for increased drug removal.

- *Decontamination of skin*: Rapid action is required for poisoning with organophosphates and organochlorines (OCLs) which are rapidly absorbed through the skin.
- *Gastrointestinal decontamination*: Oral activated charcoal alone may be enough for small amounts of ingested poisons while gastric emptying is recommended for large ingestions, especially of substances which delay gastric emptying. Gastric emptying is not done for corrosive poisons.

Increased Drug Removal

Urinary manipulation: Forced diuresis is fraught with risks of pulmonary edema and electrolyte imbalance. It is commonly used for toxicity of acidic drugs (e.g. salicylates and phenobarbital) as they are more rapidly excreted with alkaline urine. Electrolyte imbalance such as alkalemia, hypernatremia and hypokalemia may occur following this therapy.

Hemodialysis: Hemodialysis is helpful for the following indications: (a) Potentially lethal amounts of a dialyzable drug which is either known or suspected; (b) Presence of deep coma, apnea, severe hypotension, fluid and electrolyte or acid–base disturbance; (c) Extreme body temperature changes that cannot be corrected by conventional measures; (d) Poisoning in patients with severe kidney, cardiac, pulmonary, or hepatic disease. Continuous renal replacement therapy has been used successfully in management of lithium poisoning. The benefit in cases of most other poisons is not certain.

Repeat dose charcoal: Elimination of some drugs (phenytoin, carbamazepine, and dapsone) can be hastened by use of repeated doses of activated charcoal (20–30 g orally or via gastric tube every 3–4 hours). Activated charcoal may act by absorbing drugs excreted into the gut lumen (gut dialysis).

Diagnosis of Poisoning

The identity of the ingested substance or substances is usually unknown. History is the single most important indicator of toxic ingestion, but occasionally a comatose patient is found or the patient is unable or unwilling to give a coherent history.

Symptomatic Patient

In symptomatic patients, treatment of life-threatening complications takes precedence. Detailed diagnostic evaluation can be undertaken after stabilization.

Following complications may occur, depending upon the type of poisoning:

Coma: Coma commonly usually occurs following ingestion of large number of drugs and toxins. Respiratory failure is the most common cause of death in a comatose patient. Aspiration of gastric contents in the lungs may also occur in patients who are obtunded or having seizures. The initial emergency management of coma is on lines of ABC. Immediately after stabilizing the coma patient, a "coma cocktail" of thiamine, dextrose and naloxone should be administered. All comatose or convulsing patients should receive 50–100 mL of 50% dextrose.

Agitated or convulsing patient: Agitated, violent or acutely psychotic patients unresponsive to verbal feedback and reduction in environmental stimuli require pharmacological treatment or physical restraints to establish patient safety. Organic causes of agitation other than drug overdose should be considered like drug withdrawal, head trauma with subdural hematoma, intracerebral hemorrhage and hypoglycemia, etc. Seizures are a major cause of drug-related morbidity and mortality. They are caused by multiple drugs and toxins. Prolonged or repeated seizures may lead to hypoxia, metabolic acidosis, hyperthermia, and rhabdomyolysis.

Temperature alteration: Both hypothermia and hyperthermia are common with intoxication. Significantly abnormal temperature must be immediately identified and aggressively treated to prevent life-threatening complications. For hypothermic patient, gradual rewarming is preferred unless the patient is in cardiac arrest. Hyperthermia should be aggressively managed by removing all clothes, spraying the patient with tepid water, and fanning the patient.

Circulatory manifestations: Circulatory manifestations of drug overdose are common and varied, including cardiac arrest, atrial and ventricular arrhythmias, hypo- and hypertension. Hypertension requires treatment especially if there is no prior history, in case the patient is symptomatic or if the diastolic blood pressure is greater than 105–110 mm Hg. Hypotension is empirically treated with repeated 200 mL intravenous boluses of 0.9% saline or other isotonic crystalloid (up to a total of 1–2 liter). Most patients are likely to respond to fluid therapy. If this is not successful, dopamine at a dose of 5–15 µg/kg/min by intravenous infusion may be given. Pulmonary artery catheterization may be done if hypotension persists.

Pupil size: Pupil size can be of help in diagnosis of intoxications (Table 78.1).

Laboratory evaluation: Clinical laboratory data include assessment of three gaps of toxicology: (1) the anion gap, (2) the osmolal gap, and (3) the arterial oxygen saturation gap.

1. *Anion gap:* Metabolic acidosis associated with an elevated anion gap is usually due to accumulation of lactic acid or other acids. It is measured by:

   AG = [Na+] − [Cl− − HCO_3^-]

   The normal value is 12 ± 4 mEq/L. There are various causes of disturbed anion gap (Box 78.1).

2. *Osmolal gap:* Certain drugs and toxins of low molecular weight produce discrepancy between measured and calculated plasma osmolality. Osmolality is calculated by:

   Calculated osmolality = 2 [Na$^+$] + [BUN/2.8] + [Glucose/18] + [Ethanol/4.6]. Methanol and ethylene glycol are unique in producing both severe metabolic acidosis with elevated anion gap and an elevated osmolal gap.

3. *Oxygen saturation gap:* Carbon monoxide and methemoglobin interfere with oxygen binding to hemoglobin; thereby significantly decrease arterial

TABLE 78.1: Drugs causing pupillary alterations.

Miosis	Mydriasis	Nystagmus
Narcotics	Deep coma	Barbiturate
Phenothiazine	Alcohol	Phenytoin
Barbiturate	Atropine	Phencyclidine
Organophosphate	Anticholinergics	Alcohol
	Glutethimide	
	Diphenhydramine	
	Cocaine	

BOX 78.1: Drugs associated with anion gap disturbance.

Increased anion gap
- Carbon monoxide
- Cyanide
- Ethanol*
- Ethylene glycol*
- Formaldehyde
- Methanol*
- Salicylates

Decreased anion gap
- Hyperkalemia
- Hypercalcemia
- Acute lithium intoxication
- Bromide
- Hypermagnesemia

*Also have an increased osmolal gap.

oxygen content without lowering PaO$_2$. Oxygen saturation measured by pulse oximetry is falsely high in these setting causing an elevated arterial oxygen gap (>5% difference between calculated from arterial blood gas determination and saturation measured by co-oximetry).

4. *Toxicology screening*: Toxicology screening provides direct evidence of ingestion, but initial supportive measures should never await results of such analysis.

Treatment

After general supportive measures enumerated above, certain drugs or toxins can be managed by specific antidotes (Table 78.2).

Organochlorine Poisoning

Organochlorine compounds include dichlorodiphenyltrichloroethane (DDT), chlordane, hexachlorocyclohexane and eldrin. Organochlorines are well absorbed by ingestion, inhalation and minimally through skin. These agents are central nervous system (CNS) stimulants and work by inhibiting GABA and glycine pathways. This leads to inhibition of chloride channels preventing influx of Cl$^-$ resulting in neuroexcitation, i.e. inhibitory control is lost.

Organochlorines are highly lipid soluble resulting in slow redistribution, prolongation of elimination half-life and thus increased duration of toxicity. Clinical features include predominance of neurological symptoms ranging from hyperexcitability, irritability, delirium, myoclonus, and facial paresthesias in mild toxicity to seizures and status epilepticus in severe toxicity. In addition, these agents may produce myocardial irritability with ventricular fibrillation.

TABLE 78.2: Antidotes to various drugs and poisons.

Drug/poison	Antidote
Acetaminophen	N-acetylcysteine
Anticholinergics	Physostigmine
Anticholinesterases	Atropine
Benzodiazepines	Flumazenil
Beta-blockers	Glucagon
Calcium channel blocker	Calcium chloride, glucagon
Cyanide	Amyl nitrite, sodium nitrite, sodium thiosulfate
Digoxin	Digoxin-specific antibodies
Ethylene glycol	Ethanol
Heavy metals	Dimercaprol (BAL), EDTA, penicillamine
Opioids	Naloxone
Hypoglycemic agents	Dextrose, glucagon

Management

History is important for making the diagnosis. Laboratory evaluation is generally not helpful but these agents can be detected in serum and urine. Treatment includes oxygen administration, intubation to treat hypoxia secondary to seizures, aspiration, and respiratory failure. Seizures are treated with benzodiazepines (lorazepam 0.04 mg/kg, midazolam 0.05 mg/kg or diazepam 0.2 mg/kg). If they still persist, phenobarbitone or anesthesia with sodium thiopental may have to be used. EEG monitoring should be a routine in these cases to observe seizure activity.

Atropine and epinephrine should be avoided for the control of dysrhythmia in OCL-sensitized myocardium. Cholestyramine, a bile salt binding substance has been found to be helpful in reducing the absorption of these compounds (4 g 4 times/day for at least 2–3 days for ingestional poisoning).

Herbicide Poisoning

Herbicides are pesticides used to kill weeds. Herbicides may be classified as chlorophenoxy, bipyridyl, and urea-substituted compounds. Chlorophenoxy compounds dioxins and furans are the common chemicals in this group. Other agents are 2,4-dicholoro-phenoxyacetic acid (2,4-D), 4-chloro-2-methylphenoxyacetic acid (MPCA).

The metabolic pathway and mechanism related to toxicity are unknown. Skeletal muscle toxicity can result in respiratory failure or rhabdomyolysis. Toxicity can result from inhalation, or ingestion. Clinical features include eye and mucous membrane irritation. After ingestion, nausea, vomiting, and diarrhea follow. Cardiovascular findings include hypotension, tachycardia, and dysrhythmias. Muscle toxicity manifests by muscle tenderness, fasciculation, and myotonia with resulting rhabdomyolysis.

Treatment

Diagnosis is based on history of exposure. There is metabolic acidosis and hepatorenal dysfunction. Myoglobinuria and elevated creatinine levels indicate rhabdomyolysis. Treatment is supportive, including decontamination measures and respiratory support. Alkalinization is not of any proven benefit, but may be tried for severe toxicity.

Opioids

The term "opioids" is an all-inclusive term for antagonists, endogenous, and exogenous substances that possess morphine-like activity. The most commonly abused opioids are heroin and methadone. Mild intoxication with opioids is characterized by euphoria, drowsiness, and constriction of both pupils. Hypotension, bradycardia, hypothermia, pulmonary edema, coma, and respiratory arrest may occur with more severe intoxication. Death may usually occur due to apnea or pulmonary aspiration of gastric contents. Propoxyphene may cause seizure and prolongation of QRS interval. Methadone has been associated with QT interval prolongation and torsades de pointes.

Treatment

Naloxone, a specific opioid antagonist, can rapidly reverse the signs of narcotic intoxication. It is administered in an intravenous dose of 0.4–2 mg; repeat dose may be given to awaken the patient. Very large doses (10–20 mg) may be required for patients intoxicated by some other opioids (propoxyphene, codeine, fentanyl derivatives). The duration of effect of naloxone is only 2–3 hours; repeated doses are needed for intoxicated with long-acting drugs such as methadone. Continued observation is necessary for at least 3 hours after the last dose of naloxone. In severest forms associated with respiratory depression, intubation and ventilation may be required.

ENVENOMATION

Snake Envenomation

Snake envenomation is an occupational hazard of farmers as well as plantation and agriculture workers. In India, big four, i.e. (1) cobra (*Naja naja*), (2) common krait (*Bungarus caeruleus*), (3) Russell's viper (*Daboia russelii*) and (4) Saw-scaled viper (*Echis carinatus*) are responsible for nearly all the reported cases of severe envenomation and death due to snakebites.

Snake venom is a combination of procoagulant enzymes, hemorrhagins, cytolytic or necrotoxins, hemolytic and myolytic phospholipases A2 and pre/postsynaptic neurotoxins in isolation or in combinations. The result is myonecrosis, consumption coagulopathy, neuroparalysis leading to life-threatening respiratory paralysis, myocarditis, hypotension, and renal failure. This explains the diversity of clinical symptoms of snake envenomation. Certain patterns are species or genus specific thereby allowing clinical identification and treatment.

Cobra and common krait belong to family Elapidae and their bites are primarily responsible for neuroparalytic presentation. Cobra venom acts predominantly postsynaptically whereas krait venom presynaptically and dysautonomia is common. Viperine bites (Russell's viper and Saw-scaled viper) cause severe coagulopathy leading to hemorrhagic manifestations, cardiac toxicity, capillary leak and acute renal failure. There occurs significant local necrosis leading to compartment syndrome. In addition, it is not uncommon to see marked myonecrosis, but it is more common in sea snakebites. In South India and Sri Lanka, neuroparalysis may also be associated with Russell's viper. Cobra bites are associated with significant local necrosis like viperine bites and occasionally with hemolysis.

Clinical Features

Clinical presentation primarily depends on the type of snake and amount of venom injected. Majority of patients with clinically significant toxicity will have malaise, nausea, vomiting, abdominal pain, drowsiness, weakness, and prostration.

Local symptoms are minimal or nearly absent in krait bite. In cobra and viperine bite, there is a swelling at the site of bite, which may expand rather rapidly. It is not uncommon to have regional lymphadenopathy.

Systemic manifestations are usually preceded by significant nausea and abdominal pain. In Elapidae bites, patient complains of blurring of vision, double vision, and inability to keep eyes open, drooping of the eyelids followed by difficulty in swallowing, speech and complete bulbar paralysis. The progression leads to development of respiratory and flaccid areflexic paralysis. There occurs complete internal as well as external ophthalmoplegia. In its full-blown form, it can mimic brain death with wide dilated nonresponsive pupils. In Indian subcontinent, snakebite should always be considered as the cause of this presentation especially when it presents acutely even in the absence of history or fang marks, krait usually has little or no local reaction.

Bleeding from the site of the bite may be the first manifestation of coagulopathy. Patients can bleed from any site; the most dreaded is intracranial hemorrhage. Due to bleeding, a patient can have pituitary apoplexy or acute Addisonian crisis leading to refractory hypotension. Hematuria may be associated with loin pain. Hypotension, cardiac arrhythmias and pulmonary edema are also seen frequently because of associated toxic myocarditis.

Treatment

Snakebite is an emergency and usually happens in rural settings where medical facilities are minimal. Once in the hospital, if severe envenomation is present, the patient should be managed in intensive care (Box 78.2).

The limb should be immobilized preferably with a splint and bandage (pressure bandage if available). Do not apply the bandage if there is a swelling at the site of bite, do not raise the limb. Never ever open the bandage quickly, especially in the absence of life support equipment; it can lead to sudden deterioration in patient's condition.

The only specific treatment for snake envenomation is anti-snake venom (ASV) prepared from horses' sera. Indications for its use are: coagulopathy, neuroparalysis, hypotension/cardiovascular toxicity, acute renal failure, severe myonecrosis leading to myoglobinuria and local swelling more than half of the bitten limb (provided not related to ligature) or if local swelling is rapidly enlarging.

BOX 78.2: Potentially lethal conditions associated with snakebite and its treatment needing admission in intensive care unit (ICU).

- Circulatory shock, cardiac dysfunction, pulmonary edema
- Hemorrhage, hypovolemia
- Coagulopathy, disseminated intravascular coagulation (DIC)
- Coma, seizures, intracranial hemorrhage
- Cranial nerve dysfunction
- Rhabdomyolysis, renal failure, hyperkalemia
- Gastrointestinal bleeding
- Respiratory failure
- Anaphylaxis (to component of venom or antivenom)

Sensitivity must be checked prior to ASV infusion, preferably intradermally. Usually patients are given 50-100 mL of reconstituted ASV in serious envenomation as an infusion over 1 hour, after premedication with chlorpheniramine maleate (5 mg) and ranitidine (50 mg). It can also be given as a bolus especially when the patient is bleeding profusely with rate not more than 2 mL/min. Whole blood CT should be repeated every 4-6 hourly or till the bleeding stops. Recurrence of bleeding after initial improvement is not uncommon. ASV should be given till bleeding stops and clotting time normalizes.

Anti-snake venom will not have a dramatic effect in neuroparalysis. If patient develops bulbar palsy or has difficulty in swallowing or speaking, airway must be protected. Patient must be intubated before giving ASV and ventilated if respiration is shallow or tachypneic. ASV is a foreign protein; allergic reactions including anaphylaxis are not unknown. Patients developing renal failure need hemodialysis. Hyperkalemia should be looked for and managed aggressively. All patients should be given tetanus immunization. Antibiotics may be given to cover gram-negative and anaerobes (gentamicin and metronidazole or amoxicillin and others), whenever there is an intense local reaction and swelling.

Snake envenomation, usually has a good outcome if recognized early and treated aggressively.

Scorpion Sting and Envenomation

Scorpion bite is common in tropics and subtropics. It is commonly associated with outdoor activity. There are more than 90 species of scorpion whose venom is lethal; nearly 50% of them are found in India. Scorpion venom primarily acts on gated channels primarily sodium channels leaving them open thereby leading to constant stimulation. Similarly, they also have an effect on calcium-dependent K^+ channels in various cells and organs. Venom effects on presynaptic membranes lead to cholinergic as well as adrenergic hyperstimulation resulting in massive release of catecholamines and stimulation of angiotensin-renin axis. The autonomic storm is associated with intense vasoconstriction, cardiac stimulation with increased myocardial oxygen demand and marked metabolic abnormalities like pheochromocytoma crisis ending in myocardial necrosis and failure. In addition, activation of cholinergic stimulation takes place. Therefore, clinical syndrome is dominated by features of autonomic crisis including severe cardiovascular effects and cholinergic stimulation.

Clinical sign and symptoms depend primarily on the amount of venom released in the body. If venom gets injected in the veins, the presentation of envenomation can occur in as little as 5-10 minutes. There occurs intense severe pain at the site of the sting. It worsens on taping at the site of the bite (tap sign), may be associated with burning and paresthesiae. Systemic envenomation is characterized by tachycardia and hypertension in the initial stages. There may be sweating, lacrimation and fasciculations. In severe envenomation, patient develops pulmonary edema, dysrhythmias, hypotension which later become refractory. Muscle paralysis and priapism are not uncommon to see.

Treatment

Scorpion bite is an emergency and patients with systemic manifestation must preferably be managed in critical care units. Immobilize the affected part and keep it below the heart. Lymphatic venous compression may be applied an inch proximal, to prevent venoms absorption. Pain can be relieved by giving ice packs as well as analgesics. Ice packs are most effective when applied earlier, preferably within 2 hours of the sting.

One must follow the principles of resuscitation, i.e. establish airway, breathing, and circulation and shift the patient to intensive care for monitoring. Administer oxygen and maintain saturations to more than 90%. Fluids should be administered to prevent hypovolemia which is not uncommon in these seriously sick patients.

Antivenin is the treatment of choice, should be administered at the first opportunity after stabilization of the patient. Usual starting dose is 10 mL of the reconstituted ASV; can vary from 10 mL to 30 mL or more depending on the severity and evolution of toxicity. Antivenom neutralizes only free venom, therefore ongoing toxicity may continue. One has to use either more ASV or preferably prazosin (a postsynaptic α_{-2} blocker) which reverses most of the effects of the venom.

Combination of sympathetic α-blocker (prazosin) with β-blocker is most effective in reversing the effects of venom in patients who primarily have hyperdynamic cardiovascular changes manifested by tachycardia and hypertension. Beta-blockers must never be used alone. Golden rule is to treat it like pheochromocytoma crisis. Prazosin alone has decreased the mortality from 30–40% to less than 3%. If ASV is not available, the patient must preferably be treated with prazosin. Insulin-glucose-K^+ infusion as well as other antihypertensives like nifedipine and captopril have also been used. All patients must receive antitetanus prophylaxis.

ENVIRONMENTAL INJURIES

Environmental injuries are commonly seen in medical practice. If hypothermia is common during winters or at high altitude, hyperthermia is commonly seen during the summer and in humid tepid warm months when environmental temperature may go as high as 45°C. Increased outdoor activities like excursions including swimming, travel or accidents add to the growing number of people involved in near-drowning or traumatic injuries requiring life-supporting treatment.

Hypothermia

Definition

Primary or accidental hypothermia is defined by a fall in core body temperature to less than 35°C (95.0°F), mostly due to exposure to cold environment. Hypothermia is classified as mild (35–32°C), moderate (32–28°C) or severe (<28°C).

Epidemiology

The common predisposing factors are extremes of age, military combatants and winter sport participants. Dehydration, malnutrition and certain common drugs like β-blockers, calcium channel blockers; antibiotics can also contribute to cause hypothermia. It may also be seen in endocrinopathies like hypothyroidism, postoperative states and alcohol intoxication.

Pathophysiological Changes

Hypothermia is caused when normal heat-generating mechanism by posterior pituitary and heat conservation mechanism by anterior pituitary are disturbed by extreme cold exposure. Every organ shows changes due to effect of hypothermia. The initial response of cold stress on cardiovascular system is peripheral vasoconstriction with tachycardia and increased myocardial oxygen consumption. There is associated increase in blood pressure. As temperature goes down up to 28°C, myocardial depression ensues resulting into bradycardia, decrease in cardiac output and index with resultant QRS broadening, prolongation of QT segment, and hypotension. Atrial and ventricular arrhythmias occur with profound hypothermia. J wave or Osborn wave present at the junction of QRS and ST segment in lead II and V6 is diagnostic of hypothermia, when temperature goes down below 32°C.

Cerebral metabolic activity decreases linearly as hypothermia sets in. Cognitive functions are the first to be affected. EEG activity slows down as temperature goes down and is totally silent at 19-20°C. Triphasic waves are characteristic in electroencephalogram of hypothermia.

Initial hyperventilation is followed by hypoventilation, increased secretions, ventilation perfusion mismatch, noncardiogenic pulmonary edema, acute respiratory distress syndrome, and lastly respiratory arrest. Below 30°C, respiratory rate is generally 5-10/min. Renal system responds by cold diuresis probably due to inhibition of ADH release.

Coagulopathies are frequent during hypothermia. Prolongation of activated partial thromboplastin time with normal prothrombin time and normal international normalized ratio occur at up to temperatures of 30°C; below this temperature, picture of disseminated intravascular coagulopathy with thrombocytopenia sets in. Leukocytosis with hemoconcentration occurs secondary to volume contraction from diuresis.

Treatment

Principles of resuscitation should take precedence and be followed carefully. Method of rewarming depends on the severity of hypothermia and should be accompanied with adequate cardiac and hemodynamic monitoring. Passive external rewarming, active external rewarming, or active core rewarming are the accepted methods of rewarming.

Active external rewarming is done by creating heated environment around the patient by putting heating pads, warm blankets, infrared lights or immersion in warm water. It raises the body temperature by 0.5-0.6°C/h. This method is controversial as it results into a phenomenon called core temperature after drop, defined as decrease in core temperature due to sudden peripheral vasodilatation resulting at times into life-threatening arrhythmias.

Active core rewarming is the method of choice in severe hypothermia. It is done by infusing warm intravenous fluids (up to 42°C), body cavity warm lavages, and inhalation of heated air or by extracorporeal circuit. This method is best in increasing body temperature to the magnitude of 1–2°C/h.

Associated conditions must be identified and treated. In cases of myxedema coma leading to hypothermia, thyroxine with steroids should be given.
In spite of aggressive management, mortality with hypothermia continues to remain high.

Hyperthermia

Hyperthermia is defined as increased body temperature with abnormal thermoregulation. The spectrum of hyperthermia includes heat cramps or miliaria rubra at one end to life-threatening heat exhaustion and heat stroke at the other.

Heat exhaustion is generally present in individuals who sweat profusely during extreme environmental heat load and thus become hypovolemic. The symptoms are vague, can range from general irritability, fatigue, increased thirst, decreased urine output and light-headedness. Muscle cramps occur later in the course of the illness. Temperatures are generally elevated to up to 40°C. Rhabdomyolysis does not usually occur in heat exhaustion. Treatment consists of exposing the individual to cool environment and aggressive fluid resuscitation. Encourage oral intake in conscious patients, if patient has vomiting, intravenous fluids should be administered.

Heat stroke is a medical emergency. It can be differentiated from heat exhaustion by temperature elevation of more than 40.6°C, is associated with central nervous system symptoms. Another peculiar symptom is absence of sweating. This syndrome is also associated with multiorgan failure with rhabdomyolysis, disseminated intravascular coagulation (DIC) and renal failure. These patients have classical CNS symptoms like agitation, delirium, hallucinations, convulsions and finally coma. They have cerebral edema on autopsy. Tachycardia is a universal finding; low cardiac output with hypotension refractory to volume loading and vasopressors is generally present. High-grade fever stimulates respiratory center leading to hyperventilation respiratory alkalosis, hypocalcemia and tetany. Acute renal failure and elevation of hepatic enzymes are seen in approximately 25–30% of patients, probably due to thermal cell injury. Vomiting and diarrhea are common. Patches of gut ischemia can occur due to compensatory mesenteric vasoconstriction. Thrombocytopenia with DIC resulting into petechial hemorrhages, hematuria, and alveolar hemorrhage is a common feature of heat stroke.

Heat stroke is of two types—(1) classic heat stroke, which is due to environment exposure, and (2) exertional heat stroke that occurs after strenuous exercise mostly in hot humid environment. Exertional heat stroke is the severe form, has higher incidence of multiorgan dysfunction and mortality.

Management

After addressing to airway and breathing, fluid resuscitation should be done. Cold intravenous fluids can be used. Cooling of the patient should be undertaken once fluid resuscitation has been done. The aim of any cooling method is to bring down the temperature to 39°C. External cooling is the most common and easiest method. It is done by placing the patient in cool environment and by putting ice packs in groin, axilla and over the chest. Even pouring tap water over the body and then fanning the patient will decrease temperature by evaporative cooling. Cool water immersion is one of the most common methods of cooling. Internal cooling can be done by lavages of body cavities by cool water. Blood samples should be taken to check for multiorgan dysfunction.

Drowning and Near-drowning

The World Health Organization defines drowning as "the process of experiencing respiratory impairment from submersion or immersion in a liquid". The major reasons leading to drowning are: unattended children, alcohol abuse, restricted swimming capability, exacerbation of preexisting conditions (seizure, myocardial infarction), risky behavior, and exhaustion.

Drowning is a continuum of events that occur when the victim's airway lies below water. It starts with breath-holding leading to laryngospasm, and resultant respiratory acidosis and hypoxemia. This further leads to respiratory efforts and intake of large quantities of water in lungs causing severe acid-base changes and finally respiratory arrest. Drowning is associated with cerebral edema, raised intracranial pressure (ICP), acute respiratory distress syndrome, noncardiogenic pulmonary edema, myocardial dysfunction, cardiac arrhythmias, acute tubular necrosis, hepatocellular damage and hypothermia. These patients generally have hypoxic-ischemic injury.

Management

Basic cardiopulmonary resuscitation and treatment of pulmonary edema remain mainstay of the treatment.

Cardiopulmonary resuscitation should be started by the bystander till healthcare personnel arrive. Cold wet clothes should be removed from the victim's body. Airway and breathing should be addressed immediately. Cervical spine immobilization should be undertaken. Patient should be electively intubated and mechanically ventilated if the breathing pattern is poor. Once the patient reaches the hospital, controlled ventilation with low levels of PEEP should be used initially. Generally, these patients have pulmonary edema, so continuous positive airway pressure mode can also be used. Invasive monitoring is generally not required.

In summary, environmental hazards can manifest after natural or man-made disasters lead to extensive resource utilization. The presentation and management of each injury has a characteristic course, results are rewarding if timely protocolized management is followed.

CHAPTER 79

Pulmonary Hypertension in the Intensive Care Unit

Charles Peng, Roxana Sulica

INTRODUCTION

Pulmonary hypertension (PH) is a heterogeneous group of disorders characterized by elevated pulmonary pressures and associated right ventricular dysfunction. Pulmonary hypertension is defined hemodynamically as an increase in the mean pulmonary artery pressure (mPAP) above 25 mm Hg, measured at right heart catheterization. Pulmonary arterial hypertension (PAH) has the additional criteria of normal left-sided heart filling pressures, as shown by pulmonary artery wedge pressure (PAWP) or left ventricular end-diastolic pressure less than 15 mm Hg, and elevated pulmonary vascular resistance [pulmonary vascular resistance (PVR) >3 Wood units). Elevated pulmonary pressures in critical care settings may lead to acute right ventricular decompensation, with systemic hypotension and death.

RIGHT HEART IN HEALTH AND DISEASE

Abnormalities involving the pulmonary vasculature leading to an increase in PVR lead to right heart strain. The ability of the right ventricle (RV) to adapt and compensate for physiologic changes depends on the acuity of the change in PVR, preexisting RV hypertrophy, and its ability to extract and utilize oxygen in different disease states. RV failure is characterized by low cardiac output (CO) and systemic hypoperfusion, despite normal or high central venous pressure, and it is usually due to one of three possible mechanisms: increase in the RV afterload (most common), decreased RV contractility, and changes in the RV preload.

In situations with acutely elevated PVR the ability of the RV to compensate is quickly exceeded, with contractile failure and systemic hypotension if the RV systolic pressure is higher than 60 mm Hg. When PVR is chronically elevated, the RV hypertrophies and dilates, which increases the preload, thereby augmenting the RV stroke volume. RV dilatation and volume overload lead to RV geometrical changes, with increased tricuspid regurgitation and leftward shift of the interventricular septum, with reduction in the left ventricle (LV) diastolic filling, a phenomenon known as ventricular interdependency. Progressive RV dilatation ultimately results is RV pressure overload and RV myocardial ischemia with further decreases in RV contractility.

Patients in the intensive care setting are particularly susceptible to factors that can worsen pulmonary pressures. Hypoxia, leading to low alveolar FiO_2, causes hypoxic vasoconstriction that can lead to an increase in PVR. Other factors that exacerbate vasoconstriction include academia and hypothermia. Conditions that increase catecholamine release and sympathetic output, such as sepsis and pain or agitation, respectively, will also worsen PVR. Intensive care unit (ICU) patients have higher metabolic demand, and they are particularly sensitive to conditions leading to right heart ischemia. Inadequate LV filling leading to low CO exacerbates global hypoperfusion, and subsequent metabolic acidosis causes further worsening PVR and right heart ischemia.

PULMONARY HYPERTENSION IN THE CRITICALLY ILL PATIENT

Right ventricular failure complicates a number of commonly encountered conditions in the ICU, either as de novo development of RV dysfunction [e.g. acute pulmonary embolism (PE) or acute respiratory distress syndrome], or by further deterioration of the RV function in patients with preexisting PAH and intercurrent comorbidities (e.g. sepsis or arrhythmia in patients with PAH). It is currently recognized that the most common cause of PH is LV failure and presence of right ventricular dysfunction increase mortality in patients with LV congestive heart failure. RV ischemia, congenital abnormalities, intrinsic myocardial abnormalities and pericardial disease are all common causes of RV dysfunction. In all these circumstances, therapy is directed at the primary cause of decompensation.

In the mechanically ventilated patient, the positive pressure ventilation increases the intrathoracic pressure, which impedes the venous return, compromising the RV preload. Concomitantly, there is an increase in the RV afterload induced by the positive-end expiratory pressure (PEEP) application and alveolar distension. In patients with ARDS, mechanical ventilation is the primary supportive treatment modality. The current standard of care is to provide low tidal volume with accompanying optimal PEEP to achieve lung protection and provide adequate oxygenation. Due to poor compliance of the lung, the functional residual capacity (FRC) is reduced with alveolar collapse causing intrapulmonary shunting. Therefore, improvement in FRC by the application of PEEP counteracts the derecruitment of alveoli units and reduces intrapulmonary shunting, improving oxygenation, which in turn decreases the hypoxic vasoconstriction and PVR.

The prototype of acute RV dysfunction due to afterload increase in the ICU is the case of acute PE. RV dysfunction is prevalent in acute PE, but in approximately 5% of cases it results in cardiogenic shock due to massive clot burden. RV afterload increases, because of the mechanical obstruction by the thrombus and by hypoxic and cytokine-mediated pulmonary vasoconstriction. Resultant RV dilatation leads to increased myocardial oxygen demand and ischemia, and LV preload reduction, which ultimately may result in hypotension and cardiogenic shock. This group of patients requires initial fluid resuscitation and vasopressors, similar to circumstances with right ventricular infarction. Thrombolysis therapy should be considered in patients with refractory hypotension, and in dire conditions, surgical or catheter directed embolectomy may be required.

Diagnosis and monitoring of pulmonary hypertension and RV dysfunction in the ICU may be done by both invasive and noninvasive techniques (Table 79.1).

Echocardiography

For patients with suspected PH and RV decompensation, bedside transthoracic echocardiography (TTE) is an ideal diagnostic tool given its portability, noninvasive nature, as well as the ability to be repeated frequently. These attributes have positioned echocardiography as the first-line modality in the assessment of right ventricular structure and function, and to estimate pulmonary artery pressure.

TABLE 79.1: Diagnosis and monitoring of the patient with severe PH in the ICU.

	Test modality	Parameters and notes
PH and RV dysfunction	• Echocardiography • PA catheter • Biomarkers	• RA/RV size RV function • PA saturation, CO, mPAP • BNP, troponin
Systemic perfusion	• Blood pressure • Urinary output • Lactate	• Arterial line if unstable • Goal <2 mmol/L
Fluid status	• CVP • Urinary output • Echocardiography • Liver function tests	• Goal 10–15 mm Hg or less • Negative fluid balance • LV filling • Increased in liver congestion
Oxygenation Oxygen-carrying capacity	• Pulse oximetry • ABG • Hemoglobin (Hb)	• Goal O_2 saturation >90% • Goal PaO_2 >60 mm Hg • Goal Hb >10 g/dL
Heart rate and rhythm	Continuous cardiac monitor	• Avoid tachyarrhythmias

(PH, pulmonary hypertension; ICU, intensive care unit; RV, right ventricular; PA, pulmonary artery; CO, cardiac output; mPAP, mean pulmonary artery pressure; BNP, brain natriuretic peptide; CVP, central venous pressure; LV, left ventricular; ABG, arterial-blood gas)

Echocardiography allows clinicians to evaluate cardiac chamber dimensions, interventricular septal motion, and tricuspid regurgitant jet velocity. These are important parameters for estimation of pulmonary artery pressure. Additionally, echocardiography can help establish an etiology, such as left heart failure or valvular disease. Furthermore, Doppler echocardiography, incorporating bubble contrast via agitated saline can detect intra- and extracardiac shunts. A pulmonary artery systolic pressure more than 40 mm Hg by echocardiogram is generally regarded as abnormal although overestimation and underestimation of pulmonary artery pressure is frequent.

Pulmonary Artery Catheterization

Right heart catheterization is the gold standard for the diagnosis of pulmonary hypertension. This is accomplished in the ICU setting by using a pulmonary artery catheter that is inserted through either the right internal jugular (RIJ) vein, the left subclavian vein, or femoral veins (right preferred). Values measured include right atrial pressure [central venous pressure (CVP)], pulmonary artery systolic and diastolic pressure, and the PAWP. A PAWP more than or equal to 15 mm Hg suggests left-sided disease while a PAWP less than or equal to 15 mm Hg is consistent with pulmonary arterial hypertension. CO and cardiac index can be measured either by thermodilution or the Fick method.

An important calculation during right heart catheterization is PVR expressed in Wood units. Measurement of the oxygen saturation in the pulmonary artery is an important marker of the adequacy of the systemic oxygen delivery and it is a useful parameter to guide the use of inotropes in the ICU patient with PH.

Biochemical Markers

Serum troponin has been extensively studied as a marker of PH primarily in the disease prognosis. Troponin T release due to RV myocyte injury was found to be associated with higher heart rates and increased serum N-terminal-pro brain natriuretic peptide (NT-proBNP) levels, and reduced 6-minute walk distance and mixed venous oxygen saturation. Serum troponin I elevation was shown to be associated with RV pressure overload secondary to acute PE. BNP levels are inversely correlated to 6-minute walk distance and VO_2 maximum in patients with idiopathic PAH.

RIGHT VENTRICULAR FAILURE IN PATIENTS WITH PREEXISTING PULMONARY ARTERIAL HYPERTENSION

Patients with preexisting PAH are particularly susceptible to development of RV failure and numerous conditions and circumstances may lead to ICU admission. RV failure is the most common cause of death in PAH, both in outpatient and inpatient settings. Predictors of poor outcomes in PAH patients admitted with RV failure include hyponatremia, renal dysfunction, tachypnea, hypotension, need for inotropes, elevated levels of such biomarkers and BNP, and tricuspid regurgitation severity. Cause of PAH may be also a risk factor for postdischarge mortality, which is significantly higher in patients with connective tissue disease compared with idiopathic PAH patients.

MANAGEMENT OF THE PULMONARY ARTERIAL HYPERTENSION PATIENT WITH DECOMPENSATED RIGHT HEART FAILURE

General principles to follow for patients with PAH in RV failure are to identify and treat the triggering factor, to improve RV function (optimization of the RV preload, decrease the RV afterload, increase cardiac contractility), and to maintain systemic perfusion. A number of vasoactive and inotropic agents are used in the ICU management of the PH patient (Table 79.2). An algorithmic approach should be followed for the critical care management of the patient with PAH and decompensated RV failure (Fig. 79.1).

Identify and Treat the Triggering Factor

Most commonly encountered triggering factors for an acute episodes of right heart failure include infection, arrhythmias, pericardial effusion, trauma, anemia, acidosis, hypoxia, pregnancy, acute PE, discontinuation of specific PAH therapy or discontinuation of diuretics. Atrial tachyarrhythmias, such as atrial fibrillation and atrial flutter are commonly seen in PAH patients with decompensated RV failure and can further contribute to hemodynamic compromise, as poor atrial contractions impair RV filling and contractility.

Improvement of the Right Ventricular Function

After initially focusing on reversing triggering factors, management strategies shift toward improving RV function via modification of RV preload, contractility, and afterload.

TABLE 79.2: Agents used in PH management in the ICU (receptors, effects on inotropy, chronotropy, PVR, SVR, and dosing ranges).

Vasoactive agents and inotropes						
Medication	Receptors	Inotropy	$HR\uparrow^a$	Dose	PVR	SVR
Dopamine	Dopaminergic	±	±	≤5 µg/kg/min	–	
	α = β	Yes	Yes	5–10 µg/kg/min		↑
	α > β	Yes	Yes	>10 µg/kg/min		↑
Dobutamine	$β_1$ $β_2$	Yes	Yes	2–20 µg/kg/min[b]	↓	↓
Norepinephrine	α > β	Yes	Yes	0.03–1.5 µg/kg/min	↑	↑
Vasopressin	V_1/V_2	No	No	0.01–0.04 units/min	↓	↑
Phenylephrine	α	No	No	0.05–8 µg/kg/min	↑	↑
Milrinone[c]	PDE III	Yes	±	0.375 µg/kg/min	↓	↓↓

[a]Chronotropy and potential for arrhythmias.
[b]Doses of 2–5 µg/kg/min may be adequate for the inotropic effect, while minimizing the hypotension risk.
[c]Milrinone may be of benefit in PAH/PVH patients in whom more pronounced systemic hypotensive effect may benefit the LV afterload.
(PH, pulmonary hypertension; ICU, intensive care unit; PVR, pulmonary vascular resistance; SVR, systemetic vascular resistance; HR, heart rate; PDE, phosphodiesterase)

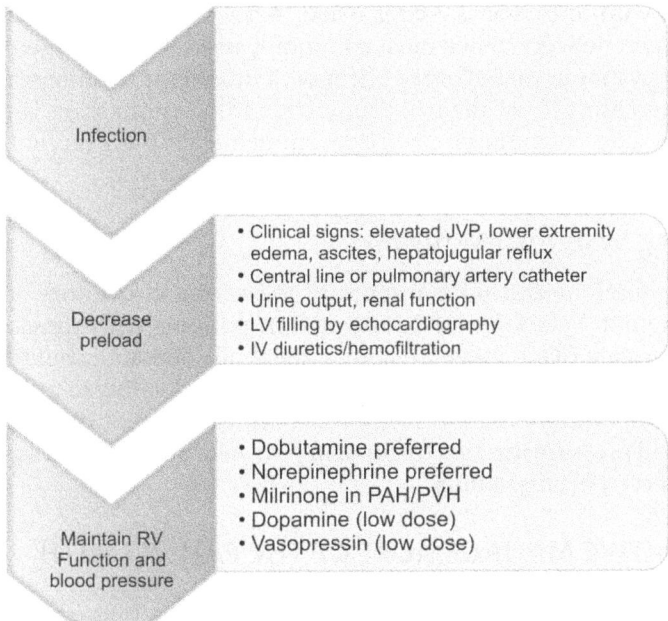

Fig. 79.1: ICU management of the PH patient with decompensated RV failure. (JVP, jugular venous pressure; LV, left ventricular; IV, intravenous; PAH/PVH, pulmonary arterial hypertension/pulmonary venous hypertension; ICU, intensive care unit; PH, pulmonary hypertension; RV, right ventricular)

Optimizing preload of the RV is a complex process because both over- and underfilling of the RV can lead to further decompensation. It should be noted that, as opposed to the ischemic RV which is preload dependent, the failing RV in advanced PAH is functioning of the descending portion of the Frank-Starling curve, in which case further volume expansion may lead to clinical deterioration by worsening the CO. Reducing the intravascular volume is the major goal of therapy in the treatment of both left and right heart failure. Patients with signs of right ventricular failure, i.e. peripheral edema, warrant the introduction of intravenous diuresis, along with sodium and fluid intake restriction, to maintain a negative fluid balance. Judicious administration of fluid or blood products should be carefully considered in certain settings, such as sepsis or significant anemia.

Optimizing RV afterload by using pulmonary vasodilators and targeted PAH therapies is critical in the management of decompensated RV failure. It should be noted that patients with an established diagnosis of PAH on appropriate therapy, in general, should not have their PH medication dose adjusted or stopped. This is especially important with continuous prostacyclin therapy, as a reduction or discontinuation of IV infusion may cause acute withdrawal of the inotropic support to the RV, leading to cardiovascular collapse.

Increase in the cardiac contractility may be achieved by the use of inotropic agents. In general, they are indicated when RV failure and fluid overload cannot be managed with diuretics alone, or when there is evidence of decreased systemic oxygen delivery. Since most commonly used inotropic agents have also a direct systemic vasodilatory effect with attendant hypotension, it is sometimes necessary to use them in conjunction with vasopressors. Given the proarrhythmic effect of the inotropes it is recommended to place on continuous heart monitor while receiving inotropes.

Maintaining Systemic Perfusion

Adequate systemic perfusion is important to prevent circulatory collapse and RV ischemia. Vasopressor is indicated in patients with shock, when there is inadequate CO to meet the body's metabolic demands, but they can have deleterious effect on the pulmonary vasculature, leading to pulmonary vasoconstriction and increased RV dysfunction. Norepinephrine increases systemic blood pressure through α_1-mediated vasoconstriction and a positive inotropic effect by β_1 stimulation.

PERIOPERATIVE MANAGEMENT OF THE PATIENT WITH PULMONARY ARTERIAL HYPERTENSION

Pulmonary hypertension is a known risk factor for perioperative complications, both for cardiac and noncardiac surgery. During the perioperative period, several factors can contribute to worsening of pulmonary hypertension and RV failure. These include and are not limited to hypoxia, fluid overload, left ventricular dysfunction, embolic events, increased sympathetic tone, effect of anesthesia on cardiac function and positive pressure ventilation. Mortality rates of cardiac surgery in patients with PH are up to 25% and most studied predictors of complications are increased mPAP, PVR and no response to vasodilatory agents.

In general, patients with mild-to-moderate PH can undergo low-risk and most of the intermediate-risk procedures without complication. Severe PH and presence of RV dysfunction require careful perioperative management. In cases of significant RV failure risk–benefit ratio of the proposed procedure may preclude surgery and alternatives have to be sought.

During the postoperative period, careful attention must be paid to analgesia as anesthetics begin to lose their effect and cause worsening PH and RV ischemia due to PVR increases secondary to pain. Rebound PH may also occur during mechanical ventilation or pulmonary vasodilator weaning.

Physicians working in the intensive care setting should be knowledgeable in the diagnosis and management of patients with PH. With the advent of advanced therapies, it is essential to understand the vascular physiology and pharmacotherapy, due to comorbid conditions often existing in this population. Similarly, conditions that can worsen pulmonary vascular resistance, such as increasing airway pressures from mechanical ventilation and metabolic derangements, should be recognized and managed promptly, as decompensation can occur abruptly.

CHAPTER
80

Mechanical Ventilation: General Principles and Modes

GC Khilnani, Vijay Hadda

INTRODUCTION

Conceptually, mechanical ventilation is the process to provide O_2 and CO_2 transport between the environment and the alveolar pulmonary capillary interface, with the help of a device. The target of this process is to maintain appropriate partial pressure of oxygen (PaO_2) and partial pressure of carbon dioxide ($PaCO_2$) in arterial blood along with reduction in work of breathing. The basic principles and application of different ventilators are similar.

INDICATIONS OF MECHANICAL VENTILATION

Mechanical ventilation is often used to manage ventilatory or oxygenation failure or an impending failure. Failure to ventilate or oxygenate adequately may be caused by several pulmonary or extrapulmonary conditions, belonging to three distinct groups:
- *Depressed respiratory drive*: Respiratory drive is depressed in conditions of drug overdose (narcotic, sedative, and alcohol), acute spinal cord injury and head trauma. Several neurologic disorders (coma, stroke), sleep disorders (e.g. sleep apnea), and metabolic alkalosis can also cause respiratory depression.
- *Excessive ventilatory workload*: Ventilatory work is commonly increased due to acute airflow obstruction in diseases, such as chronic obstructive pulmonary disease (COPD), asthma, and epiglottitis; dead space ventilation (pulmonary embolism and emphysema) and acute respiratory distress syndrome (ARDS). Other conditions like cardiovascular decompensation [decreased cardiac output, ventilation/perfusion (V/Q) mismatch], shock, increased metabolic rate (fever), drugs and decreased compliance

(atelectasis, pneumothorax, and obesity) also cause excessive ventilator work.
- *Ventilatory pump failure*: This includes chest trauma (flail chest, tension pneumothorax), premature birth (idiopathic respiratory distress syndrome), electrolyte imbalance (hyperkalemia or hypokalemia), and geriatric patients (muscle fatigue).

BASIC ASPECTS OF MECHANICAL VENTILATION

Phase Variables

The actual factors that provide the four components of a ventilator-delivered breath are called the phase variables. These factors or variables are responsible for changing one phase of respiratory cycle into the next and for controlling what occurs during that portion of breath. The four phases of a breath consists of:
- Inspiratory phase
- Change from inspiration to expiration
- Expiratory phase
- Change from expiration to inspiration.

In each of these four phases, a certain variable (time, pressure, volume or flow) is measured and used to initiate, maintain and end the phase. There are three terms required to describe phase variables:

Triggering of Breath

Triggering is the term applied to the variable that changes from expiration to inspiration.

When a variable, such as time, pressure, volume or flow reaches a preset value and causes the ventilator to change from expiration to inspiration, the ventilator is said to be triggered by that parameter. Ventilators can also be manually triggered in most cases. This is accomplished by activating the "manual breath" control.

Limiting a Breath

Limiting is a term used to describe the variables that have a limiting value during inspiration or expiration, which could be time, flow or pressure. The length of inspiration is the time from the beginning of inspiratory flow to the start of expiratory flow. Limiting in simple words means the variable can reach the preset value, but never goes higher than that.

Cycling of Breath

Cycling is defined by the preset variable, causing the ventilator to end the inspiration and switch to expiration. During this process, a preset variable (time, pressure, volume or flow) is actually measured by the ventilator; the information is used by the ventilator to determine when to end the inspiratory flow.

Time-cycled ventilation: Here, time-cycling terminates the inspiratory gas flow and changes to the expiratory phase, when a preselected time interval has lapsed after the start of inspiration.

Pressure-cycled ventilation: In this cycling, ventilation terminates the inspiratory phase when a preselected airway pressure has been achieved. They are used predominately for intermittent positive pressure breathing, ventilator support at home and while using inverse ratio ventilation.

Volume-cycled ventilation: The inspiration is terminated after delivery of a preselected volume of gas.

Flow-cycled ventilation: If a preset flow ends the inspiratory flow, the breath is flow-cycled. Flow-cycled ventilation is independent of airway pressure, tidal volume (VT) or duration of inspiration.

Patient–ventilator Interactions

Most of the modern mechanical ventilations (MVs) use piston or bellow systems of high pressure gas source to drive the gas flow. Newer MVs allow interaction of patients with ventilator that range from simple triggering of mechanical breaths to more complex processes (interactive modes). These interactions can affect the functions of tidal breath, such as the flow pattern and breath timing. The patient's interactions are based on three physiological variables:
- Ventilatory drive when inspiration starts
- Ventilatory requirement, i.e. how much flow and volume are required to satisfy the metabolic demand.
- Timing of the integrated circuits generating the respiratory rhythm, as measured by the duration and ratio of inspiratory time (TI) to total breath cycle duration.

Similarly, ventilator interacts with the patient on the basis of three technologic variables:
- The inspiratory trigger, i.e. the point at which the ventilator starts to deliver flow, volume, and pressure.
- The delivery of the gas, i.e. the algorithm used by the ventilator to assist ventilation through delivery of flow, volume or pressure.
- Cycling or when the ventilator stops, assisting the inspiratory effort and letting the patient exhale spontaneously.

Interactive modes prevent muscle atrophy and facilitate fatigue recovery by allowing muscle activity. The interactions are called synchronous when the ventilator is sensitive to initiation, modulation, and termination of a patient's ventilatory effort.

MODES OF MECHANICAL VENTILATION

A patient can be mechanically ventilated with a number of different modes. The primary targets are to improve gas exchange, provide patient comfort and speed up weaning from mechanical ventilation. All the ventilators are equipped to deliver either volume-set or pressure-set ventilation. In volume-set ventilation, a preset VT is delivered at whatever pressure it is required while in pressure-set modes, a fixed inspiratory pressure (P_{insp}) is applied to the respiratory system.

Irrespective of the VT, both pressure-set and volume-set ventilators usually achieve the same level of ventilation in fully paralyzed patients.

The pressure-set ventilation has the advantage of greater physician control over the peak airway pressure (P_{rw}) and the peak alveolar pressure (P_{alv}); the chances of ventilator-induced lung injury (VILI) are therefore less. This can be also achieved by using a low VT strategy (typically 5–8 mL/kg) in volume-set ventilation. Pressure-set modes also allow a greater control over inspiratory flow rate and therefore potentially increased comfort. But the pressure-set modes result in increased airflow resistance and lung stiffness thereby decreasing the minute ventilation. Volume-set modes provide ventilation, but require pressure alarms to detect new abnormalities in respiratory mechanics.

Controlled Mechanical Ventilation

The term controlled mechanical ventilation (CMV) has been used to describe a volume or pressure-controlled and time-triggered form of ventilation. The operator sets the desired VT (volume controlled) or peak airway pressure (pressure controlled), respiratory rate/frequency (f), TI and inspiratory:expiratory (I:E) ratio. The patient's ventilation is totally controlled by ventilator and patient cannot trigger the ventilator (Fig. 80.1). Controlled mechanical ventilation may be responsible for excessive ventilation, use of sedatives and muscle relaxants. Muscle atrophy frequently results from their disuse. Further, use of heavy sedation/neuromuscular blockade imposes a great risk of apnea/hypoxia in case of accidental ventilator disconnection.

Volume-controlled (Targeted) Ventilation

Volume-controlled (targeted) mode requires that the operator set a desired VT. Usually, the operator also sets the rate or TI and gas flow, including flow pattern. During this mode of ventilation, the peak pressure varies from breath-

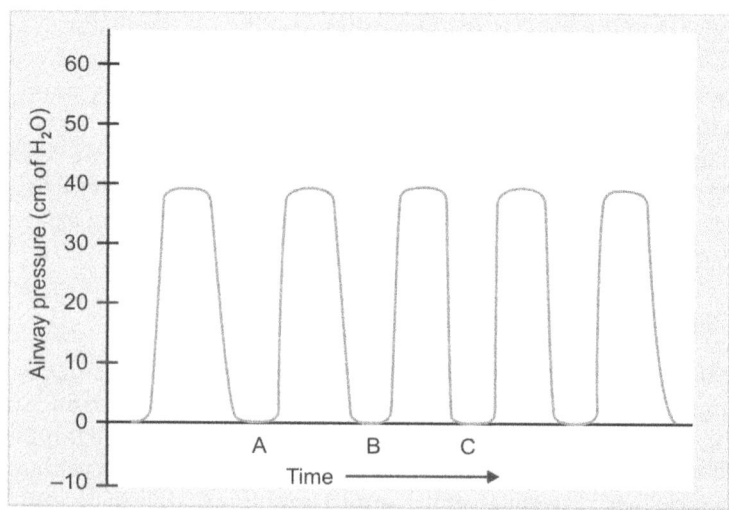

Fig. 80.1: A graphical presentation of controlled mechanical ventilation.

to-breath depending on several factors, primarily patient's lung compliance. However, volume delivered is usually constant.

Pressure-controlled (Targeted) Ventilation

Pressure-controlled ventilation (PCV), unlike volume targeted modes, is pressure and time cycled, generates VTs that vary with the impedance of the respiratory system. The ventilation is determined by f, the P_{insp} increment [P_{insp}-positive end-expiratory pressure (PEEP)], and I:E ratio. A working understanding of factors that determine volume delivery is necessary for proper implementation of this mode of ventilation.

Advantages: Pressure-controlled ventilation facilitates ventilation with a lung protective strategy. When one of the goals of ventilator management is to limit alveolar overdistention, PCV ensures that P_{alv} never exceeds prefixed threshold value (usually 30–35 cm H_2O). Pressure limits and decelerating flow profiles are thought to produce more uniform distribution of forces within the lung, possibly reducing the risk of barotrauma. PCV leads to improved oxygenation, higher static and dynamic compliance along with improved measures of work of breathing. PCV is increasingly used in ARDS patients to deliver inspiratory reserve volume (IRV), in which the TI exceeds the expiratory time (TE).

Disadvantage: Pressure-controlled ventilation, especially when done as IRV, generally requires sedation and sometimes paralysis, which may have adverse effects on weaning.

Assist-control Mode of Ventilation

This is the most commonly used mode of ventilation all over the world. It delivers controlled breaths as well as assists patient triggered breaths. During assist-control mode of ventilation (ACMV), operator can set the inspiratory flow rate (V•), f, and VT. In some ventilators, one must set the total minute ventilation and rate, thereby determining VT and indirectly determining V•. In fully paralyzed or sedated patients, ACMV behaves like CMV delivering tidal breaths per minute at an operator set rate.

On ACMV mode, patients continue to perform inspiratory work even on ventilator. Clues to patient effort are also often available from the airway pressure tracing (Fig. 80.2). On ACMV, the work of breathing can be increased, by either increasing the magnitude of the trigger or by lowering VT. Lowering of "f" alone at the same VT, generally has no effect on work of breathing.

Indications

The ACMV mode is most often used to provide full ventilatory support in the first place. Typically, these patients are having stable respiratory drive (an adequate inspiratory effort of at least 10–12 breaths/min) and therefore can trigger the ventilator into inspiration. The time-triggering control rate (back up rate) is generally considered as safety net, to provide adequate ventilation in case the patient stops triggering the ventilator. In general, the accepted

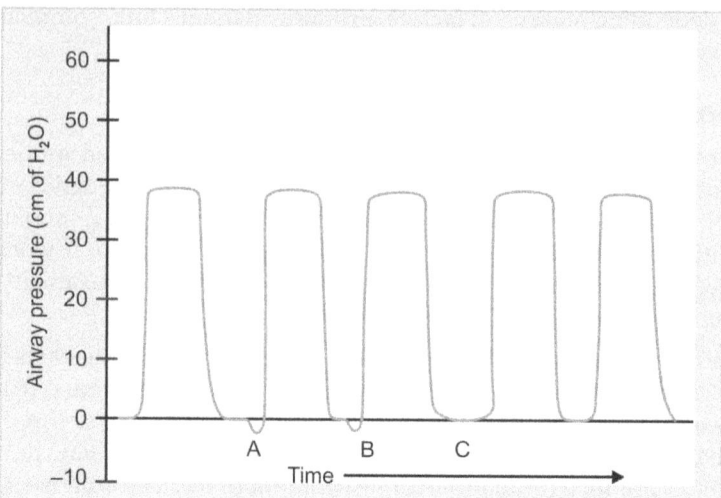

Fig. 80.2: A graphical presentation of assist-controlled mechanical ventilation. Each assisted as well as controlled-breath triggers a mechanical ventilator to deliver VT. The assisted breath is characterized by a negative deflection at the beginning of inspiration (breath A and B). While in controlled breathing, there is no negative deflection at the onset of inspiration (breath C).

minimum control rate for ACMV mode is 2–4 breaths/min, lower than the patient's assist rate or a minimum control rate of 12–15 breaths/min.

Advantages

There are two advantages of ACMV mode. First, the work of breathing, which is required in minimal when trigger sensitivity is set appropriately and when ventilator supplies adequate flow that meets or exceeds patient's inspiratory demand. Second, if the patient has an appropriate ventilatory drive, this mode allows the patient to control the respiratory rate, and hence the minute ventilation.

Complications

Alveolar hyperventilation or respiratory alkalosis is the most important complication associated with ACMV mode. Patients on ACMV have higher pH and lower $PaCO_2$, when compared to intermittent mandatory ventilation (IMV). This may be an important consideration in patients having inappropriately high respiratory drive/rate due to disease/injury to respiratory center.

Synchronized Intermittent Mandatory Ventilation

Synchronized intermittent mandatory ventilation (SIMV) works as CMV in fully paralyzed patients, where ventilation is determined by the mandatory f, VT, and V. But the patient exerts respiratory work during his own as well as some during the mandatory breaths. The patient can trigger additional breaths by lowering airway opening pressure (Pao) below the trigger threshold (Fig. 80.3).

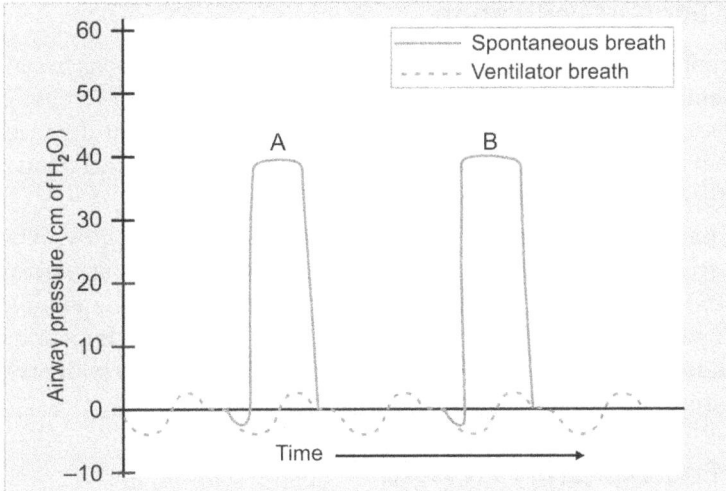

Fig. 80.3: A graphical presentation of synchronized intermittent mandatory ventilation (SIMV). Tracing is showing two mandatory breaths (A and B) and five triggered breaths. In SIMV, the mandatory breaths may be delivered slightly sooner or later (during a small window period) than the preset time, so that the anticipated breath during this is converted into mechanical breath.

In case, this triggering effort comes in a brief, defined interval (synchronization window) before the next mandatory breath is due; the ventilator will deliver the mandatory breath ahead of the scheduled breath, in order to synchronize with the patient's inspiratory effort.

The SIMV mode is often used to gradually augment the patient's work of breathing for weaning. This can be achieved by lowering either the mandatory breath or the VT. This approach prolongs the process of weaning.

Indications

The primary indication of SIMV is to provide partial ventilatory support to enable the patient to provide a part of minute volume. For practical purposes, full ventilatory support is provided usually for the first 24 hours. After this initial period of full ventilator support, the usual practice of partial ventilatory support, such as SIMV, is tried. SIMV promotes spontaneous breathing and use of respiratory muscles, which results in:
- Maintenance of respiratory muscle strength and avoid muscle atrophy
- Reduced ventilation-perfusion mismatch
- Decreased mean airway pressure
- Help in weaning.

Synchronized intermittent mandatory ventilation has inherent property to provide a spontaneous breathing work load that gradually increases patients' muscle strength and endurance. The primary disadvantage is breath wasting, which may occur when patient breathes outside the synchronization window.

Pressure Support Ventilation

Pressure support ventilation (PSV) is delivered during spontaneous breathing in a mechanically ventilated patient. The trigger signal consists of a change in airway pressure or flow. Ventilation is determined by P_{insp}, patient-determined f and patient effort. The ventilator delivers a breath that is flow cycled but time limited after detection of spontaneous patient effort.

Better patient comfort is the most important advantage of PSV. When a patient is well maintained (on clinical and ABG parameters) at a pressure support (PS) of 5–7 cm of H_2O, it indicates that patient can be extubated. Patients' own effort is essential for PSV. PSV can account for a large fraction of total minute ventilation, even when set at rather low levels in patients with normal respiratory system mechanics.

Positive End-expiratory Pressure

Positive end-expiratory pressure increases the end expiratory or baseline airway pressure to a value greater than atmospheric pressure (Fig. 80.4). Positive end-expiratory pressure is not a stand-alone mode, but applied in conjunction with other ventilatory modes. It helps recruit or stabilize lung units and improve oxygenation in patients with hypoxemic respiratory failure.

Advantages

Use of PEEP has positive effects on both the gas exchange and lung mechanics. Following are the advantages of PEEP:

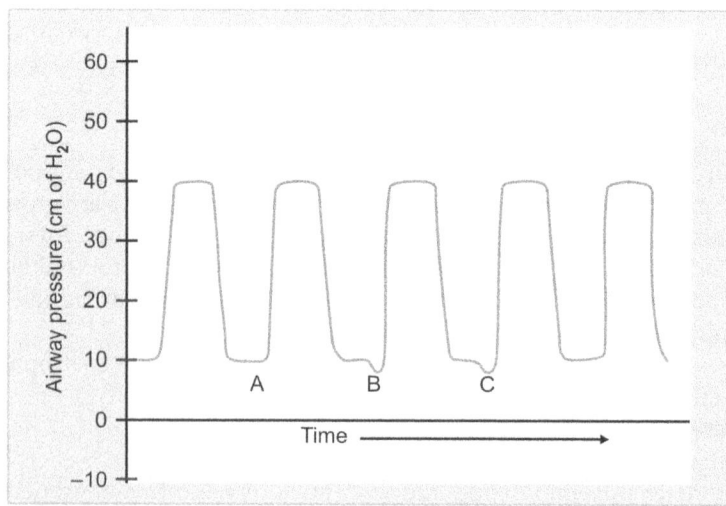

Fig. 80.4: Pressure tracing of assist-controlled mode with a positive end-expiratory pressure (PEEP) of 10 cm of H_2O. "A" is controlled breath, while "B" and "C" are assisted breath with PEEP.

- Gas exchange:
  - Redistribution of fluid within the alveoli and reduction of intrapulmonary shunting
  - Improved arterial oxygenation (PaO_2)
  - Reduced FiO_2 need with decreased risk of oxygen toxicity.
- Lung mechanics:
  - Avoidance of alveolar collapse
  - Stabilization and recruitment of lung units
  - Increased functional residual capacity
  - Improved lung compliance
  - Decreased risk of ventilator-induced lung injury (avoidance of repetitive collapse of lung units at end-expiration followed by reopening during inspiration).
  - Decreased inspiratory work of breathing due to auto-PEEP (in patients with obstructive airway disease).

Indications

Indications of PEEP include the respiratory failure due either to intrapulmonary shunting or decreased functional residual capacity, for example, acute lung injury and ARDS, cardiogenic pulmonary edema, diffuse pneumonia requiring mechanical ventilation, atelectasis associated with severe hypoxemia and other forms of severe hypoxemic respiratory failure. PEEP is also used in patients with COPD, where there is significant intrinsic PEEP. External PEEP is given approximately at the level of 80% of the intrinsic PEEP. It helps in the easy triggering of breath by counteracting intrinsic PEEP.

Complications

The hazards associated with use of PEEP include:
- Decreased venous return and cardiac output leading to hypotension
- Barotrauma
- Increased intracranial pressure
- Alteration in renal function and water metabolism.

Continuous Positive Airway Pressure

Conceptually, continuous positive airway pressure (CPAP) is not a mode of ventilation, but rather a means of raising functional residual capacity while patient is breathing spontaneously. In this mode, ventilatory support is pressure-limited and pressure or flow-triggered, i.e. the spontaneous breath has a pressure limit that remains nearly the same, (within few centimeters of water) during both inspiration and expiration (Figs. 80.5A and B). The patient's inspiratory effort causes the ventilator to increase the flow to the patient to maintain the same pressure during inspiration. During expiration, the flow out of the exhalation valve maintains the expiratory pressure fairly uniform. No mechanical positive pressure breaths are given.

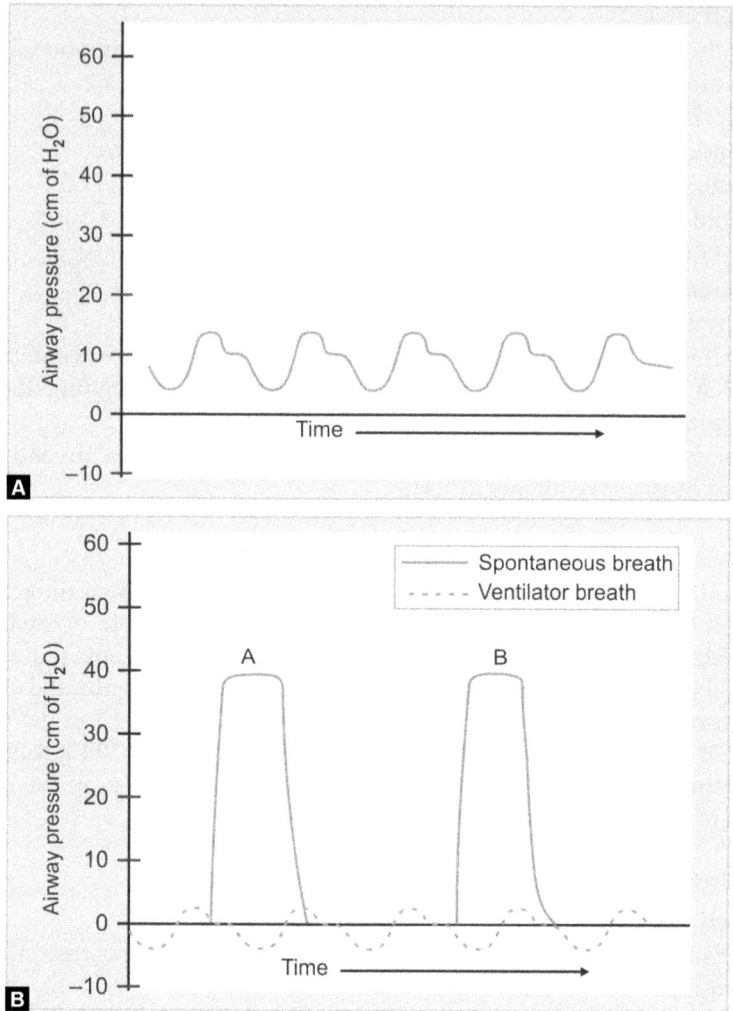

Figs. 80.5A and B: Graphical presentation of continuous positive airway pressure (CPAP) of 14 cm of H_2O.

Indications

This approach is frequently used to assess the patient's ability to breathe without ventilatory support. The advantages of CPAP over T-piece breathing are:
- Improved oxygenation.
- Detection of low minute ventilation and apnea (as ventilator alarms remain in place).
- The patient's spontaneous VTs and rate can be easily read.
- The work of breathing is reduced, if auto-PEEP is present.

Bileveled Positive Airway Pressure

Conceptually, bileveled positive airway pressure (BiPAP) is a mode which combines PEEP with PS and is used more in context of noninvasive ventilation (NIV) using a nasal or oronasal mask. In this mode, both expiratory positive airway pressure (EPAP) as well as inspiratory positive airway pressure (IPAP) are adjustable. IPAP helps in improving alveolar ventilation, normalization of $PaCO_2$ and reduction in work of breathing, whereas EPAP improves oxygenation by reducing intrapulmonary shunting. Inspiration is triggered at the inspiratory flow of greater than 40 mL/sec for more than 30 ms. Expiratory flow is detected when the inspiratory flow decreases below a manufacturer determined threshold level (flow cycled) or when IPAP is longer than 3 s (time cycled).

Indications

Bileveled positive airway pressure is useful in preventing endotracheal intubation in cases of respiratory failure due to several conditions, such as COPD, pulmonary edema, pneumonia, acute lung injury, and ARDS. It is also helpful in weaning and avoiding intubation in patients with respiratory failure during post-extubation period.

NEWER MODES OF MECHANICAL VENTILATION

Inverse Ratio Ventilation

Inverse ratio ventilation (IRV) is not a different mode but a maneuver to improve oxygenation in cases with severe hypoxic respiratory failure.

High-frequency Ventilation

High-frequency ventilation (HFV) used more commonly in neonates and infants with neonatal respiratory failure, provides very high respiratory frequency with smaller VT which is less than the volume of anatomic dead space. It includes high frequency oscillatory ventilation (HFOV) and high frequency jet ventilation (HFJV).

Airway Pressure Release Ventilation

Airway pressure release ventilation (APRV) is similar to CPAP, in which a patient is allowed to breathe spontaneously. During APRV, the clinician sets a "pressure high", "pressure low" and a time at each level (time high and time low). Ventilation occurs during the release from pressure high to pressure low.

Proportional Assist Ventilation

This is a form of partial ventilatory support which avoids many adverse effects of CMV, such as excessive ventilation, use of sedative/paralytic agents and muscle disuse atrophy. During partial support, the pressure applied to the respiratory system (P_{rs}) is contributed by the pressure produced by the respiratory muscles (P_{mus}) and the ventilator (P_{aw}), the latter of which represents the amount of assistance delivered.

Advantages

Proportional Assist Ventilation (PAV) is shown to be effective to unload the respiratory muscles, without imposing a fixed breathing pattern, in enhancing patient comfort, and patient-ventilator interaction.

Complications

Proportional assist ventilation has limited use for ventilatory treatment in the clinical setting. Most importantly, it is important to have knowledge of the mechanical characteristics of the respiratory system for proper adjustments of PAV settings. This information is not usually available in patients receiving partial support.

Proportional Assist Ventilation Plus and Proportional Pressure Support

Proportional assist ventilation plus (PAV+) and proportional pressure support (PPS) are forms of synchronized ventilatory assistance. In these modes, the ventilator generates pressure in proportion to the patient's effort, i.e. the greater the effort, the more the pressure the ventilator generates.

Neurally Adjusted Ventilatory Assist

The electrical activity of the inspiratory muscles is used as an index of the inspiratory neural drive. The neural drive is measured as crural diaphragm electrical activity (EAdi) to express global diaphragm activation with the help of esophageal bipolar electrodes.

Biologically Variable Ventilation

Biologically variable ventilation (BVV) was designed to improve the management of ARDS. It mimics spontaneous breath-to-breath variability and incorporates natural variable noise into volume-targeted CMV. The ventilator has a program to modulate respiratory rate and VT, while maintaining a fixed minute ventilation based on a previously generated data file.

Hybrid or Mixed Modes

Some ventilators allow combinations of modes though there is little reason to use such a hybrid mode. The hybrid mode of SIMV plus PSV is commonly used as a means to add sighs to PSV, an option not generally available. SIMV plus PSV has the advantage of guaranteeing some backup minute ventilation (which PSV does not). It is sometimes used for difficult to wean patients.

INITIATING MECHANICAL VENTILATION

Initial Ventilator Settings

The initial ventilator settings for each critically ill patient depend on the goals of ventilation set for the patient: full respiratory muscle rest (versus partial exercise), the patient's respiratory system mechanics and the required minute ventilation. Some common clinical scenarios are described below:

Patients with Normal Lung Mechanics and Gas Exchange

These patients may require mechanical ventilation because of:
- Loss of central drive to breathe (drug overdose or structural injury to the brainstem)
- Due to neuromuscular weakness (high cervical myelopathy, myasthenia gravis)
- Treatment of shock (as adjuvant therapy)
- To achieve hyperventilation (treatment of raised intracranial pressure).

Following are the acceptable initial settings after intubation:
- FiO_2 of 0.5–1.0
- VT 8–12 mL/kg, of 8–12/min
- Inspiratory flow rate of 40–60 L/min.

In patients with preserved respiratory drive and without profound weakness, PSV can be used. The PS is adjusted (usually 10–20 cm H_2O above PEEP), to bring the respiratory rate down in the low 20s, usually corresponding to VTs of about 500 cc. It should be noted that PSV is entirely spontaneous, with no machine backup. Therefore, hypoventilation may occur despite the use of PSV, if there is further deterioration of muscle strength or blunting of respiratory drive. Once stabilized, effort should be made to bring down FiO_2 less than 0.6. For hyperventilation, the initial respiratory rate should be increased to the range of 16–20 breaths/min.

Patients with Severe Airflow Obstruction

Bronchial asthma: Patients with acute severe asthma who require mechanical ventilation are extremely anxious and distressed. Deep sedation should be routinely given to reduce respiratory workload. Some patients may also require therapeutic paralysis. Reduced respiratory work helps to reduce oxygen consumption (and hence carbon dioxide production). Sedation also helps lower airway pressures and reduce the risk of self-extubation. Use of paralytic drugs may occasionally cause long lasting weakness.

The targets should be, to minimize alveolar overdistention (P_{plat} less than 30) and dynamic hyperinflation (auto-PEEP below 10 cm H_2O or end-inspiratory lung volume less than 20 mL/kg), a strategy that largely prevents barotrauma. A low minute ventilation generally causes a rise in PCO_2 to above 40 mm Hg, (permissive hypercapnia), often to 70 mm Hg or higher. Sedation will be required to tolerate permissive hypercapnia. Careful attention should be paid to the inspiratory flow and flow profile. The flow changes, which have little effect in normal individual without airflow obstruction, can have a dramatic impact in obstructed patients. Specifically, reduction in the inspiratory flow or switching to a decelerating flow profile, reduces the airway pressures and the amount of ventilator alarming. But the same actually worsens auto-PEEP, by prolonging inspiration. Therefore, a close watch should be kept on auto-PEEP and expiratory flow profile.

Chronic obstructive pulmonary disease: The expiratory flow limitation in COPD patients arises largely from loss of elastic recoil of lungs. Though the peak airway pressures on the ventilator tend not to be extraordinarily high, the auto-PEEP and its consequences are common.

The initial ventilator settings in this situation to achieve the goal of rest and relative hypoventilation may consist of: VT of 5–7 mL/kg; respiratory rate of 24–28 breaths/min with either an SIMV or an A/C mode, set on minimal sensitivity. Usually, good oxygenation can be achieved with a FiO_2 of 0.4. Inspiratory flow rates may be adjusted for patient comfort, but usually in the range of 60 L/min. PEEP should be used, when the patient is triggering the ventilator, but is not required in sedated patient. Biochemical and functional changes associated with muscle fatigue are restored usually after 2–3 days of rest, but 24 hours is probably not sufficient.

Patients with Adult Respiratory Distress Syndrome

Ventilation in these patients is aimed to reduce shunt and avoid toxic concentrations of inspired oxygen. Ventilator settings should be chosen which do not amplify the preexisting lung damage. The initial FiO_2 is kept at 1.0 because of the typically extreme hypoxemia. PEEP beginning with 15 cm H_2O, should be immediately instituted. It is rapidly adjusted thereafter either to produce an arterial saturation of 90% on an FiO_2 of less than 0.6 (least PEEP approach), or a value 2 cm H_2O higher than the lower inflection point of the inflation pressure-volume curve (open-lung approach).

The VT should be 5–7 mL/kg on A/C or SIMV, since higher VTs usually overdistend the lung at end inspiration, as judged by the upper inflection point of the respiratory pressure-volume curve, which may even contribute to systemic inflammation. Alternatively, PCV can be used with a P_{insp} (PEEP plus the pressure increment) of 30–35 cm H_2O. This will generally drive VT of 350–550 mL/kg. In both modes the respiratory rate of 24–28 breaths/min is acceptable, as long as there is no auto-PEEP. The combination of high levels of PEEP (especially when the open-lung approach is used) and low end-inspiratory pressures, leaving only a small range for tidal ventilation is called as lung protective ventilatory (LPV) strategy. A common consequence of LPV is hypercapnia (permissive hypercapnia).

COMPLICATIONS OF MECHANICAL VENTILATION

Mechanical ventilation is associated with multiple complications some of which may be related temporally and not caused by ventilatory support per se (Table 80.1).

TABLE 80.1: Common complications associated with mechanical ventilation.

Endotracheal intubation	Complications
• During intubation	Trauma to teeth and soft tissue Esophageal intubation Vomiting and aspiration Hypoxia Arrhythmia Bradycardia
• While intubated	Obstruction Pneumonia and atelectasis Aspiration Kinking of endotracheal tube (ET) tube Mucosal injury Improper position Accidental extubation
• Post-extubation	Aspiration Laryngospasm Hoarseness Laryngeal or subglottic edema Laryngeal stenosis Tracheal stenosis
Positive pressure ventilation	
• Pulmonary	Barotrauma Ventilator associated pneumonia Deconditioning of respiratory muscles Oxygen toxicity
• Extrapulmonary	Raised intracranial tension Hypotension Stress ulcer and cholestasis Renal dysfunction

A successful outcome of mechanical ventilation depends upon the avoidance and presentation of complications. Comprehensive intensive care of patient can therefore be considered as essential component of mechanical ventilation.

CHAPTER 81

Noninvasive Ventilation

GC Khilnani, Vijay Hadda

INTRODUCTION

Noninvasive ventilation (NIV) refers to technique of augmenting alveolar ventilation without an endotracheal airway. Technically, NIV involves inspiratory pressure support plus positive end-expiratory pressure (PEEP) via a nasal or face mask. Continuous positive airway pressure (CPAP) is also considered as a form of NIV, when used as a therapy for respiratory failure although it is neither a ventilatory support mode nor does it actively assist inspiration.

TECHNICAL ASPECT OF NONINVASIVE VENTILATION

Types of Noninvasive Ventilation

Noninvasive mechanical ventilation support can be either negative pressure ventilation or positive pressure ventilation.

Negative Pressure Ventilation

Negative pressure ventilation consists of the application of external subatmospheric pressure to the chest wall, causing its expansion during inspiration, expiration occurs passively when the pressure around the chest wall returns to normal atmospheric level. Tidal volume is related to peak inspiratory negative pressure, more the negative pressure, more the tidal volume. In this form of ventilation, the pressure waveform, a square wave produces a greater tidal volume than a half sine wave generated by the ventilator pump. Negative pressure ventilation is used in patients with respiratory failure due to chest wall deformity, neuromuscular diseases or central hypoventilation. The negative pressure ventilators were widely used during polio epidemics in Europe in 1950s.

Noninvasive Positive Pressure Ventilation

Noninvasive positive pressure ventilation (NIPPV) requires a mechanical ventilator to deliver the continuous or intermittent positive airway pressure through the upper airway to actively assist ventilation. The ventilator is connected by tubing to an interface (nasal, orofacial and other types of mask) applied to the patient.

Equipment of Noninvasive Positive Pressure Ventilation

Ventilator Device

The primary requirement for NIPPV is the equipment to deliver positive pressure ventilation (ventilator). This can be achieved with either large bedside critical care volume ventilators or the specially designed ventilators meant for NIV. The critical care ventilators have options of different modes of ventilation. Moreover, there is better oxygen blending. The specialty ventilators have fewer options, but are more leak tolerant. With corrections of ventilatory options, range of support and leak tolerance, the modern-day ventilators are not much different.

Interfaces

The interface consists of a tight-fitting mask of silicone. Various kinds of interfaces include the nasal and orofacial masks, full face masks, mouthpieces, nasal pillows, and helmets. Orofacial masks are the most commonly used interfaces. Use of these masks compared with nasal masks lead to faster correction of blood gases. Orofacial masks are preferred in patients who are less cooperative, have a higher severity of illness, are mouth breathers or pursed lips breathers, edentulous and those requiring more effective ventilation. Nasal masks are used in patients with a lesser severity of illness. These do not produce claustrophobic, allow speaking, drinking, coughing and secretion clearance. There is lesser risk of aspiration and emesis. But there are more chances of air leaks especially in edentulous patients and mouth-breathers. They are less effective in patients with nasal deformities or blockade. Nasal masks are best suited for more cooperative patients.

It is important that the mask is properly sized and tightly fits to prevent air leak. An appropriate mask and its proper application are of paramount importance for effective ventilation. Leak is the most important problem of all of interfaces. On the other hand, excess pressure is discomforting as well as increases the risk of pressure necrosis. Some amount of air leak is always likely but most of the machines have facility for leak compensation. It is important to be careful to minimize excess pressure on the face or nose. Straps should allow passage of one or two fingers between the face and the straps.

Various Modes of Ventilation

Noninvasive positive pressure ventilation usually provides a form of assisted ventilation, where every breath is supported by the ventilator. Two types of breaths can be used, either volume targeted or pressure targeted:
1. Volume-targeted NIPPV
2. Pressure-targeted NIPPV.

Volume-targeted Noninvasive Positive Pressure Ventilation

A predetermined tidal volume is delivered over a fixed inspiratory time. It is generally recommended to set higher than usual tidal volume to compensate for possible leaks (12–14 mL/kg). The usually set peak-flow rate of 45–60 L/min is required to decrease the patient's inspiratory effort. Excessive peak-flow rates can increase the sense of dyspnea (the patient receives "too much air"). Modern ventilators are designed to provide volume-targeted NIPPV; the delivered volume is reduced in the case of leaks without any adaptation by the ventilator.

Pressure-targeted Noninvasive Positive Pressure Ventilation

The ventilator maintains a constant preset pressure after the breath is triggered by the patient. It stops when the flow is supposed by the end of the patient's effort or after a fixed, preset inspiratory time (assist pressure control). The advantages of a pressure-targeted NIPPV are: (1) The preset pressure is maintained in case of leaks, so an appropriate volume is delivered; (2) The likelihood of leaks and the problems thereof are reduced because the pressure in the mask is limited; (3) There is good synchrony between the patient and the ventilator; (4) The combination of PSV and PEEP is very efficient to reduce the work of breathing.

Pressure-targeted ventilation with CPAP is the most basic level of support. CPAP is most frequently used for management of cardiogenic pulmonary edema and obstructive sleep apnea. Most patients on NIPPV require pressure support mode of ventilation with PEEP (popularly called bilateral positive airway pressure BiPAP) when the patient receives ventilatory support during both phases of respiration, i.e. preset inspiratory positive airway pressure (IPAP) and expiratory positive airway pressure (EPAP). The difference between IPAP and EPAP is a reflection of the amount of pressure support ventilation provided to the patient. EPAP is actually synonymous with PEEP. Some noninvasive ventilators have facilities of proportional-assist ventilation (PAV), which provides flow and volume assistance with each breath.

The pressure-targeted modes are generally preferred because they provide better patient comfort and synchrony. They are also more tolerant of the leaks due to ventilatory interfaces.

Mechanism of Action of Noninvasive Positive Pressure Ventilation

Intermittent positive pressure is transmitted to the alveoli, increasing transpulmonary pressure, causing lung inflation and assisting alveolar ventilation. NIPPV improves daytime ventilatory muscle function by reducing chronic respiratory muscle fatigue, improving respiratory system compliance through reversal of microatelectasis of lung and preventing nocturnal hypoventilation by resetting the respiratory center's sensitivity to carbon dioxide.

STEPS TO SUCCESSFUL PROVISION OF NONINVASIVE POSITIVE PRESSURE VENTILATION

It is important to have proper selection of patient, ventilator settings [intensive care unit (ICU)/ward/home], and the type of interface and patient's cooperation for success of NIPPV. Of course, the underlying disease is an important parameter of success.

Choosing the Patients

It is important to ensure that patient is able to understand the instructions. Although altered level of consciousness is a relative contraindication, patients with chronic obstructive pulmonary disease (COPD) with impaired consciousness may be given a trial of NIPPV for 30–60 minutes; quite often, there is improvement in the level of consciousness. Other contraindications to its use include hemodynamic instability, presence of copious respiratory secretions, impaired swallowing reflex, active upper gastrointestinal bleeding, and orofacial trauma.

Hemodynamic parameters are important considerations; presence of hemodynamic instability or associated organ failure in a patient with respiratory failure carries a risk of failure of NIPPV. History of recent facial surgery, trauma or deformity are obvious contraindications. Patients should be carefully assessed for contraindications before the decision to initiate NIPPV is taken (Box 81.1).

Location of Noninvasive Positive Pressure Ventilation Application

Initially, it was recommended that NIPPV should be initiated only in the ICU since some proportion of patients would require endotracheal intubation. It has now been recognized that this modality can be used in general wards. The location of NIPPV therapy is largely determined by the severity of the illness.

BOX 81.1: Contraindications to use of noninvasive positive pressure ventilation (NIPPV).

- Uncooperative/obtunded patient
- Agitated patient
- Hemodynamic instability or presence of organ failure
- Severe comorbidity
- Recent facial/upper airway trauma
- Recent upper gastrointestinal tract surgery
- Intestinal obstruction
- Excessive secretions in the airways
- Undrained pneumothorax

Explanation and Evaluation

Physician should explain to the patient about the breathing support being provided to him and its benefits. Patients should also be provided a feel of the interface. It is useful to inform the patient that some discomfort might occur in the beginning due to tight-fitting mask and the repeated gush of air with each inspiration.

Initial Ventilator Settings and Adjustments

The primary goals of NIPPV are: adequate ventilation and oxygenation, correction of respiratory failure, adequate patient tolerance and comfort. Adequate tidal volume usually in the range of 5–7 mL/kg is essential in the initial settings. Additional support may be needed to reduce the respiratory rate to less than 25 breaths/min. Inspired oxygen is adjusted to achieve hemoglobin oxygen saturation of more than 90% for adequate oxygenation.

All patients should be initiated on a pressure support that is lower than the target level. To start with, an IPAP of 6 cm of water with EPAP of 2 cm of water is a reasonable setting. A pressure difference of 4 cm of water between IPAP and EPAP is desirable. Pressure may be augmented every few minutes by 2 cm of water, to reach a target level to achieve the therapeutic end points. The maximum recommended level of IPAP is 24 cm of water, whereas that of EPAP is 16 cm of water. If any patient requires higher IPAP/EPAP support, one should strongly consider endotracheal intubation. Oxygen should be supplemented through a port provided in the mask or in the NIPPV machine at a flow rate, so as to maintain oxygen saturation above 90%.

Monitoring of Patients on Noninvasive Positive Pressure Ventilation

Patient should be monitored for patient–ventilator asynchrony, deterioration of sensorium, gastric distention and development of air leaks as patient changes posture or speaks. Pulse rate, blood pressure, respiratory rate, signs of respiratory distress and oxygen saturation should be monitored during the first hour. Arterial-blood gases (ABGs) must be repeated within the first hour and monitored as and when necessary. A rising $PaCO_2$ with a fall in pH should be taken as a sign of NIPPV failure when invasive ventilation should be considered.

Predictors of Response to Noninvasive Positive Pressure Ventilation

Trials of NIPPV are usually given for a period of 1–2 hour duration. Extended trials without significant improvement only delay optical treatment with intubation and mechanical ventilation. NIPPV trial should not exceed 2 hours if patients fail to improve but may be as short as of a few minutes in a patient where there is an immediate failure.

Objective criteria for discontinuation are important to limit trials in patients in whom NIV ultimately fails. The patients who are fulfilling these criteria are best managed by invasive mechanical ventilation, hence also referred as intubation criteria.

CLINICAL USES OF NONINVASIVE POSITIVE PRESSURE VENTILATION: EVIDENCE AND RECOMMENDATIONS

Hypercapnic Respiratory Failure

Chronic Obstructive Pulmonary Disease

NIPPV in acute exacerbation of COPD: Use of NIPPV for management of acute respiratory failure (ARF) secondary to acute exacerbation of COPD is now the standard of care. NIPPV acts primarily by reducing the patient's effort and work of breathing in patients with COPD presenting with acute exacerbation. NIPPV also leads to reduced rate of nosocomial pneumonia and other complications related to endotracheal intubation. Patients with type II respiratory failure secondary to COPD with altered level of consciousness improve within 30-60 minutes with NIPPV. Therefore, such patients should get the therapy under close monitoring.

NIPPV in chronic stable COPD: The possibility that NIPPV might aid patients with severe chronic COPD has intrigued clinicians for decades. Earlier investigators thought that the intermittent use of NIPPV might give rest to the mechanically disadvantaged respiratory muscles, relieving chronic fatigue and enhance ventilatory and overall functions. NIPPV led to improvement in ABGs and unloading of respiratory muscles when pressures were set according to the patients comfort and improvement in ABGs. Use of nocturnal NIPPV in chronic stable COPD patients with CO_2 retention leads to significant improvement in daytime blood gases and sleep quality, compared with those receiving oxygen therapy alone.

Noninvasive positive pressure ventilation significantly reduces ICU admissions, improves alveolar ventilation, exercise capacity, quality of life. Nocturnal NIPPV provides significant physiological and clinical benefits to stable patients with severe COPD with significant hypercapnia. NIPPV may be more effective in selected patients with hypercapnia and hypoxemia. Recently, the use of NIPPV among patients with stable COPD and hypercapnia was shown to have significantly lower death rate as compared with standard treatment.

Facilitating Extubation in Chronic Obstructive Pulmonary Disease

Based on success of NIPPV in managing patients with ARF, there have been efforts to try the same in patients on conventional mechanical ventilation, in order to facilitate weaning and prevent reintubation in patients with COPD. In these patients, NIPPV can be used in three ways: (1) after early extubation, in order to reduce duration of invasive mechanical ventilation; (2) as a prophylactic measure to avoid respiratory failure and reintubation; and (3) in patients who develop respiratory distress after extubation.

Noninvasive positive pressure ventilation weaning is shown to be significantly associated with reduced mortality, fewer episodes of ventilator-associated pneumonia, lesser length of ICU stay and hospitalization, total days of ventilation, duration of invasive ventilation and need for tracheostomy. Trial of extubation to NIPPV should always be considered in patients intubated for hypercapnic respiratory failure due to COPD who fail spontaneous breathing trials. This approach should be used for patients who are good candidates for NIPPV and are able to tolerate levels of pressure support via mask (i.e. 15 cm H_2O). Difficult intubation is a contraindication for this approach.

Bronchial Asthma

As in COPD exacerbations, there is increased airway obstruction, dynamic hyperinflation and impaired ventilatory effort leading to respiratory muscle fatigue in asthma exacerbations. But there are few randomized controlled trials on the use of NIPPV in asthma. Initial positive results are reported with both CPAP and BiPAP in a limited number of reports or uncontrolled studies.

A trial of NIPPV for acute asthma and respiratory failure should be considered before intubation and mechanical ventilation in selected patients who can tolerate and cooperate with this therapy. In view of lack of strong data, NIPPV should only be used under close observation of the experienced respiratory therapists, nurses, and physicians and in an area with facility of immediate intubation, if needed.

Hypoxemic Respiratory Failure

Cardiogenic Pulmonary Edema

Noninvasive positive pressure ventilation has been used in patients with cardiogenic pulmonary edema; both CPAP and BiPAP have been used. The favorable effects on lung mechanics include improvements in alveolar recruitment and functional residual capacity and reduction in anatomic shunting. It also reduces the work of breathing by decreasing the preload and afterload. There is a suggestion that patients with cardiogenic pulmonary edema secondary to acute myocardial infarction get maximum benefits from this therapy. There is always a concern of recurrence of myocardial infarction in these patients, though there is enough evidence that the use of NIPPV does not add to the risk of myocardial infarction and should not be considered as a contraindication to this therapy. It may be avoided in patients who require emergency lifesaving procedure, such as percutaneous coronary intervention. NIPPV use has been shown to be associated with reductions in intubation and mortality rates.

Pneumonia

Variable results of NIPPV use are reported in patients with pneumonia and ARF. NIPPV is shown to reduce intubation rates, ICU length of stay and mortality rate. Patients with underlying COPD are reported to respond better than others. But the evidence to support the routine use of NIPPV in ARF due to pneumonia is not strong.

Acute Lung Injury/Acute Respiratory Distress Syndrome

Patients with acute respiratory distress syndrome (ARDS) require conventional mechanical ventilation. NIPPV has been tried in these patients in an effort to avoid endotracheal intubation. But the benefits of this modality are not well documented in these trials. Therefore, NIPPV should be used in these patients with caution; endotracheal intubation should not be delayed.

Respiratory Failure in Immunocompromised Patients

Immunocompromised patients who require endotracheal intubation have higher rate of ventilator-associated pneumonia. The use of NIPPV in such patients leads to reduced rate of nosocomial infection which results in reduced mortality and ICU stay. The current recommendations strongly favor (level A) the use of NIPPV in immune-compromised patients with ARF.

Postoperative Respiratory Failure

Noninvasive positive pressure ventilation is widely used during postoperative period in patients with abdominal and thoracic surgery. It is believed that it provides better patient comfort and oxygenation after extubation. The current evidence shows only some usefulness of this modality, it does not strongly support the routine use of CPAP or NIPPV in postoperative patients, either prophylactically in high-risk patients or as an early therapy of respiratory insufficiency.

Weaning or Postextubation Respiratory Failure

Noninvasive positive pressure ventilation during weaning or postextubation period has been used in three ways: (1) A *facilitation technique* for early extubation in patients who fail to meet standard extubation criteria; (2) A *rescue or curative technique* for avoiding reintubation in patients who fail extubation; and (3) A *preventive or prophylactic technique* for preventing extubation failure. NIPPV helps to avoid reintubation and improve outcomes in patients with failed weaning. The benefit of facilitating ventilator weaning and early extubation is greatest for COPD patients. But early indiscriminate use in all patients with different risk factors is not recommended. Patients who fail extubation and are treated with NIPPV should be closely monitored for delays in intubation.

Palliative Care and 'Do Not Intubate' Status

Noninvasive ventilation may be particularly useful in patients who have given 'Do Not Intubate' (DNI) consent. NIPPV use is reserved primarily for COPD and congestive heart failure patients if the patient and/or family desires to prolong survival. But it can be used for other diagnoses as well if the goal is to palliate, relieve dyspnea or to delay the death.

Other Intensive Care Unit Applications of Noninvasive Positive Pressure Ventilation

Preoxygenation before Intubation

Preoxygenation by face mask is standard of care for improving the oxygen status for the patients requiring endotracheal intubation. NIPPV might be a useful preoxygenation technique in the hypoxemic critically ill patient. The current evidence is insufficient to suggest the routine use of NIPPV for this purpose and further studies are required before reaching any conclusion.

Before Fiberoptic Bronchoscopy

Fiberoptic bronchoscopy (FOB) is an important tool for determining the etiological diagnosis of pneumonia. Arterial oxygen tension routinely decreases by 10–20 mm Hg in patients after they undergo uncomplicated FOB, may complicate hypoxemia in patients with already compromised oxygen status which categorizes them as high risk for developing respiratory failure or serious cardiac arrhythmias. NIPPV seems a logical approach in such situations. There are some data to suggest that its use is associated with improved oxygenation and reduces post-procedure respiratory failure in patients with severe hypoxemia undergoing bronchoscopy.

Chronic Ventilation Failure

Chronic ventilation failure is the observed in many conditions, including the chest wall diseases, neuromuscular disease, and sleep apneas. Mechanical ventilatory support in form of NIPPV, especially at night, may be helpful in improving ventilation in these conditions. The benefits of this modality include a reduction in need of hospitalization for respiratory illness, improvement in daytime ABGs, respiratory muscle strength and improvement in activities of daily living. Data also suggest a good long-term survival benefit of home ventilation with NIPPV. For sleep apnea syndrome, NIPPV is the standard modality of therapy.

In conclusion, there is the strong evidence to support the use of NIPPV for the initial management of ARF due to COPD exacerbations and acute cardiogenic pulmonary edema. It is also useful in the immunocompromised patients and to facilitate extubation in patients with COPD with failed spontaneous breathing trials. A limited trial of NIPPV is also justified in carefully selected patients with asthma exacerbations, postoperative respiratory failure, extubation failure or a 'do not resuscitate' status. The early response to NIPPV after the first hour or two is the best predictor of eventual outcome. The clinician should consider intubation in case the patient does not show a favorable initial response.

CHAPTER 82

Blood Gas Monitoring

Inderpaul Singh Sehgal, Ritesh Agarwal

INTRODUCTION

Monitoring of arterial blood gases (ABGs) provides information regarding oxygenation, acid-base and ventilatory status that is essential for patient care. It is important to recognize blood gas abnormalities before the appearance of clinical symptoms or signs. A patient may appear well oxygenated; however he/she may be hypoxic and demonstrate low PaO_2 values on blood gas measurements. Therapeutic interventions are required after careful monitoring of blood gases. Venous sample though easy and safer to obtain, is not helpful for blood gas monitoring. Blood sample from any artery represents the sample from the left ventricle. On the other hand, venous sample is affected by the metabolism, blood flow and many other factors of different tissues. However, central venous samples have been shown to correlate well with arterial samples with respect to pH, PCO_s and base excess in mechanically ventilated trauma patients to reach clinically reliable conclusions. But central venous sample cannot substitute arterial samples for resuscitation and management.

ARTERIAL SAMPLING

Arterial blood is needed for ABG analysis. Although many arteries including femoral, brachial, or *dorsalis pedis* can be used for sampling, radial artery is the most commonly used site for obtaining an arterial sample due to the ease of access, positioning and patient comfort. Moreover, there is a good collateral vascular network minimizing the risk of vascular interruption in case of complications, such as vascular spasm, intraluminal clotting or periarterial hematoma formation, which can compromise the blood supply. Radial artery can also be fixed against the radius bone for obtaining sample, and compressed in case of continued ooze.

It is important to ensure adequate collateral circulation before performing arterial puncture. In case of the upper extremity, this can be done with the help of a simple and reliable test, the Allen's maneuver. In this, the hand is clenched to form a fist; pressure is applied to obstruct the radial and ulnar arteries at the wrist. The hand is relaxed (but not fully extended) when the palm and finger are seen to blanch. Thereafter, the pressure from ulnar artery is removed. The thumb and index finger get flushed within 6 seconds, followed by flushing of the entire hand. This is a positive Allen test indicating adequacy of collateral circulation, i.e. ulnar artery alone is capable of supplying the hand. If the test is negative, it implies the inability of ulnar artery to supply the entire hand. In this situation, the radial artery should not be used for arterial puncture. In an uncooperative or unconscious patient who cannot clench the fist, the test is done in a similar fashion by obstructing both the arteries, raising the patient's hand above the level of the heart until blanching occurs. The hand is then lowered below the level of the heart and pressure removed from the ulnar artery.

ARTERIAL CANNULATION

Indwelling arterial catheters are used to sample arterial blood for ABG and for invasive hemodynamic monitoring. The preanalytical errors related to improper sampling, handling and storage are minimal with samples obtained from arterial cannulae. Arterial cannulation is however, associated with risks like thrombosis of the cannulated artery, thrombus embolism leading to digital gangrene, air embolism, local infection, and systemic sepsis.

Arterial cannulation should be done under sterile conditions. The artery is located by palpating the arterial pulse and cannulated after ensuring collateral circulation. In patients in whom artery cannot be located by palpation, ultrasound can be used to located and guide the arterial cannulation. For arterial cannulation, internal-guidewire, separate-guidewire or a direct puncture technique can be used.

Oxygen Analysis

There are several techniques to analyze oxygen in the dissolved form. The methods include manometric and volumetric measurements, chemiluminescence method, gas chromatography, physical methods using paramagnetic properties of oxygen and electrochemical techniques. It is the membrane-covered oxygen electrode employing the principle of polarography, which is most useful and employed in clinical laboratories.

The electrode system is covered by a polypropylene membrane that allows a slow diffusion of oxygen from the blood into the electrode. The membrane is a slow diffusion membrane to prevent oxygen depletion during the measurement. The ease with which oxygen molecules can pass through the membrane depends upon its permeability coefficient expressed in terms of the number of moles of the gas passing through a specific area and thickness at a given temperature and pressure difference across the membrane.

A galvanic electrode has also been used for oxygen analysis. It is based on a principle similar to the Clark electrode. The voltage for cathode reduction is produced internally by the galvanic cell. The cathode is usually composed of gold, the anode of lead, and the electrolyte solution is potassium hydroxide.

Some of the technical difficulties in using the polarographic method of gas analysis include the alteration in the electrolyte layer thickness, changes in electrolyte concentration causing dryness, deposition of silver on the platinum cathode, artifacts due to the presence of gas bubbles in solution and changes in the sensitivity of the membrane. The response time, i.e. the time required in sensitivity of the membrane or the time required for the output to change following a change in the partial pressure of oxygen (PO_2) of the electrode depends upon the membrane thickness and the permeability coefficient.

Calibration of the electrode is done with an oxygen concentration of 0% and either of 12% or 20%. The calibration of gases for PO_2 and partial pressure of carbon dioxide (PCO_2) are generally combined for purposes of conveniences and economy.

PCO_2 Electrode

Partial pressure of carbon dioxide (PCO_2) is measured with the help of Severinghaus electrode. It utilizes the principle of Henry's law, i.e. the amount of gas (CO_2) diffusing across a semipermeable membrane is directly proportional to the pressure gradient (i.e. PCO_2) in contact with the membrane. The PCO_2 electrode consists of a silicon elastic membrane containing a measuring half-cell (silver-silver chloride) and a similar reference half-cell. It is calibrated each time with a gas mixture containing 5% and 10% CO_2 concentrations. As stated earlier, gas mixture of 5% CO_2 plus 12% or 20% O_2 (remainder nitrogen) and 10% CO_2 plus 90% N_2 can be used to calibrate both O_2 and CO_2 electrodes.

pH Electrode

The modern pH electrode is an ultramicro Sanz electrode consisting of a pH sensitive glass rolled into a fine capillary tube that draws in a very small quantity of blood to be tested. It maintains anaerobic and thermostatic conditions essential for pH measurement. It is important to know the pH of the buffer solution in the measuring half-cell for purposes of calibration. When the measuring half-cell contains the buffer solution with pH of 7.384 the difference between the two half-cells is 0.554 pH units and a 33.5 mv potential difference is predicted. Thus, the voltmeter measures 33.5 mv and a slope potentiometer sets the display at 7.384. Two point calibrations are generally sufficient.

NONINVASIVE BLOOD GAS MONITORING

Blood gas analysis requires repeated arterial punctures or cannulation. Several noninvasive methods have emerged in the last quarter of a century as fairly reliable alternatives to arterial sampling.

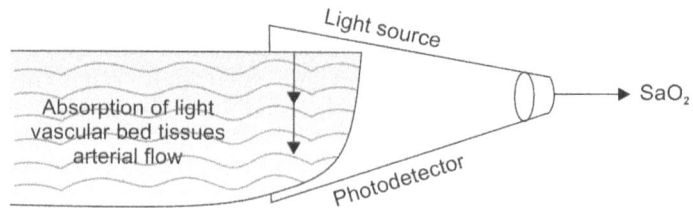

Fig. 82.1: Light of known wavelength is passed through the fingertip and measured by photodetector.

Oximetry

Oximetry involves assessment of arterial oxygen saturation. It allows assessment of hemoglobin saturation without the need of repeated arterial punctures and is an important monitoring tool for critically ill patients. The concept of pulse oximetry is based on three principles (Fig. 82.1): (i) spectrophotometry, (ii) Lambert–Beer law, and (iii) Optical plethysmography.

Pulse oximeters use only two wavelengths; therefore, cannot distinguish between the relative concentrations of each type of hemoglobin derivative present in the blood. A pulse oximeter thus measures the *functional saturation,* i.e. the relative concentration of oxyhemoglobin expressed as a fraction of the total amount of hemoglobin able to bind oxygen, namely, the ratio of the concentration of oxyhemoglobin and the concentrations of oxyhemoglobin and deoxyhemoglobin. The ratio of absorbencies at these two wavelengths is calibrated empirically against direct measurements of arterial blood oxygen saturation (SaO_2) in volunteers, and the resulting calibration algorithm is stored in a digital microprocessor within the pulse oximeter to give the estimated patients' oxygen saturation (SpO_2).

Limitations

Pulse oximeters have several limitations which need to be considered while interpreting SpO_2:
- SaO_2 bears a physiological relationship to arterial oxygen tension expressed with the sigmoid-shaped oxygen-hemoglobin dissociation curve. Therefore, even large changes in PaO_2 in the upper and lower horizontal portions of curve cause only minimal changes in SaO_2. On the other hand, errors of only a few percentage in SaO_2 measurements could easily represent a large and significant error in the oxygen tension values. Because the oxygen-hemoglobin dissociation curve is flattened at saturation values more than 90–95%. Factors that affect the oxygen-hemoglobin dissociation curve, such as pH, temperature, $PaCO_2$ affect the relationship between oxygen saturation and PaO_2.
- Pulse oximeters also give us no information about the acid-base or the ventilatory status of the patient and hence should not be used as an alternative to blood gas monitoring.

- Low perfusion states, such as hypotension, vasoconstriction, hypothermia or cardiopulmonary bypass and cardiac arrest, produce a signal that is too small to be processed, and make it difficult for the sensor to distinguish a true signal from background noise. Increased venous pulsations as seen in right heart failure can lead to artificially lower SpO_2 readings.
- The presence of abnormal hemoglobins can lead to erroneous pulse oximetry measurements. Oximetry overestimates the SpO_2 in the presence of elevated carboxyhemoglobin levels. Methemoglobin which contributes to light absorption at both 660 nm and 940 nm increases red and infrared light absorptions, which correlates with a saturation of 85%. The difference in the optical absorbance of adult and fetal hemoglobins is too small (<3%) to affect the clinical accuracy of oximetry measurements.
- Nail polishes, (specifically blue, green or black colors) have light absorbance near 660 nm and may cause falsely low readings of SpO_2. A number of dyes and pigments can also interfere with the accuracy of pulse oximetry. Hyperbilirubinemia as well as polycythemia have not been shown to affect SpO_2.
- High frequency radio interference from electrocautery units and high-intensity light sources (such as infrared, xenon, and fluorescent lamps) may also affect SpO_2. Motion artifact is a significant source of error and false alarms.

Clinical Applications

Pulse oximetry is a noninvasive, simple, and cheap method to measure monitor oxygen saturation. It is widely used during anesthesia, surgery, critical care, hypoxemia screening, exercise, and transport from the operating room to the recovery and the emergency room. SpO_2 monitoring for preterm neonates, pediatric and ambulatory patients is also quite feasible with the small, lightweight optical sensors. Pulse oximeter has made it simple to monitor patients during various procedures (bronchoscopy, endoscopy, cardiac catheterization, exercise testing, and sleep studies). Oximetry is also routinely used during labor and delivery for both the mother and infant.

In critically ill patients, noninvasive monitoring can decrease the distress caused by repeated arterial punctures, and assist in titrating the FiO_2 and ventilatory settings. Continuous monitoring also provides information on trends in patient's condition, to assist the clinician in assessing the response to therapeutic procedures. Hypoxemia is detected more frequently and early during anesthesia and in the recovery rooms with the use of pulse oximetry. With SpO_2 monitoring, one can detect the occurrence of complications like bronchospasm, atelectasis, and bradycardia early and more frequently. It is also a valuable tool to determine the need to prescribe or to withhold oxygen therapy in patients with end-stage diseases.

The accuracy of most noninvasive pulse oximeters is generally acceptable for a wide range of clinical applications. Pulse oximetry has largely replaced transcutaneous oxygen tension monitoring earlier popular in neonatal intensive care. Intrapartum fetal oximetry is also shown to compare well with fetal scalp blood gas assessment in neonatal management.

Transcutaneous Oxygen Measurement

Partial pressure of oxygen in blood perfusing the skin transcutaneous oxygen ($PtcO_2$) has been used as an estimate of arterial PO_2. This can be measured with a modified Clarke electrode, which uses a platinum cathode and a silver anode in a potassium chloride solution. Response of $PtcO_2$ electrode to a rapidly changing PaO_2 is slow. These problems are minimized in neonates and infants in view of the thin skin with lower metabolism. Local heating may lead to thermal injury to the skin and the site of the electrodes may need to be changed frequently. Accuracy is affected by low perfusion states, hemoglobin concentration, capillary density, and hydration of the epidermis. It has a potential role in monitoring in neonates and infants in critical care, but in adults the use of $PtcO_2$ measurement is limited.

Transcutaneous PCO_2 Measurement

Transcutaneous CO_2 ($PtcO_2$) measurement reflects $PaCO_2$ in the arterial blood in a similar fashion as the $PtcO_2$, which reflects PaO_2. The electrode senses the PCO_2 by monitoring changes in either the pH of bicarbonate containing electrolyte solution or the infrared absorption from a sample chamber. In view of a much higher solubility of CO_2 in the tissues, $PtCO_2$ estimation is less dependent upon cutaneous perfusion than $PtcO_2$. Therefore heating the skin to 40°C suffices. The electrode can be left in place for up to 48 hours without the risk of thermal injury. Heating causes a temperature dependent rise in the PCO_2 and an overestimation of $PaCO_2$.

Transcutaneous PCO_2 measurement can be also used to diagnose apnea, for example in brain dead patients. A $PtcCO_2$ of 60 mm Hg accurately predicts a $PaCO_2$ of 60 mm Hg which helps to reduce the duration of apnea test. Combined O_2-CO_2 electrodes are also available. But there is a problem of change in the pH of the electrolyte solution for PCO_2 sensing because the OH^- ions produced by O_2 reduction accumulate in these electrodes. Some of the electrodes are designed to consume the accumulated OH^- ions preventing the pH shift.

SUMMARY

In summary, the assessment of ABG pressures is the gold standard to diagnose oxygenation status and respiratory failure. However, there are increasing applications of noninvasive assessments with pulse oximeters for both diagnosis and monitoring. Transcutaneous measurements of both O_2 and CO_2 are also fairly simple and reliable.

CHAPTER
83

Cutaneous Capnography

Preyas Vaidya, Arvind H Kate, Prashant Chhajed

INTRODUCTION

Arterial blood gas analysis is the gold standard for assessment of arterial partial pressure of carbon dioxide ($PaCO_2$) but repeated sampling is difficult for routine clinical use. There is also a chance of preanalytical errors due to venous sampling and presence of air bubbles. End-tidal carbon dioxide tension ($PetCO_2$) is shown to correlate with $PaCO_2$ in patients with endotracheal intubation. $PetCO_2$ estimate of $PaCO_2$ may be inaccurate in case of ventilation or perfusion mismatch in patients with obstructive lung disease and acute respiratory distress syndrome.

On the other hand, measurement of cutaneous carbon dioxide tension ($PcCO_2$) is used as a noninvasive surrogate measure of $PaCO_2$. The measurement is done with electrodes based on Severinghaus principle. $PcCO_2$ is performed by placing a heated surface electrode on the skin to increase blood flow into the arteriovenous anastomoses and the venous plexus, i.e. arterialization of capillary blood.

Transcutaneous PCO_2 is a safe and reliable tool especially for trend-monitoring, provided there is no major vasoconstriction. Although $PcCO_2$ monitoring has been there for several years, it did not find common usage in clinical practice. There is increased usage now with availability of newer devices that have features like automatic calibration, shorter response, and equilibration times.

SITE FOR MEASUREMENT

The earlobe sensor detects the $PcCO_2$ change 9–48 seconds faster than a cutaneous sensor fixed at the upper arm. The heated sensor increases the blood flow at the measurement site. The arterialization time of the earlobe (i.e. the time until the cutaneous value reflects the arterial value) is significantly shorter at the earlobe (2.5 ± 1 min) than at the inner arm (7 ± 2 min). Warming the earlobe with the sensor not only increases the blood flow which is required for $PcCO_2$ measurement but also improves the quality of the peripheral oxygen saturation (SpO_2) signal, which has been questioned at the earlobe. Digital ear pulse oximetry (part of combined SpO_2 and $PcCO_2$ sensor) is reported to have a shorter SpO_2 response times than conventional, analogue ear pulse oximetry. Due to these factors the delay to the detection of hypoxemia may be shortened. Other measurement sites, such as the forehead, anterior abdominal wall, chest, and infraclavicular site have been successfully used to accurately measure $PcCo_2$. This becomes particularly important when measurements are sought in infants and neonates, as they do not have earlobe to place the sensor.

FACTORS INFLUENCING $PcCO_2$ MONITORING

The success of $PcCO_2$ monitoring depends on technical and patient factors. The technical factors which may affect the accuracy of the measurement include improper application of the sensor membrane, trapped air bubbles in the electrolyte solution under the membrane, damaged sensor membranes, delayed changing of sensor membrane, calibration gas leaks leading to an improper calibration and excessive force on the ear lobule in case of ear clips. The patient factors which may influence $PcCO_2$ values include hypoperfusion at the site of measurement, shock, edema, skin thickness, thickness of the ear lobule for ear clips, and drugs causing vasoconstriction.

MEDICAL APPLICATIONS OF $PcCO_2$ MONITORING

End-tidal Carbon Dioxide Monitoring

Measurement of $PetCO_2$ is a noninvasive method of estimating $PaCO_2$. For the estimation of pulmonary dead space, there is an excellent correlation between $PaCO_2$-$PetCO_2$ gradient and the ratio between dead space and tidal volume (VDS/VT). Its use to confirm correct placement of endotracheal tube in the airway has a sensitivity and specificity of up to 100%. This method cannot be used to detect bronchial or some hypopharyngeal misplacements. With the established relationship between $PaCO_2$-$PetCO_2$ and VDS/VT, the research for the detection of pulmonary embolism is promising but incomplete.

Advantages

Inadvertent esophageal intubation is an important complication with catastrophic consequences. While direct visualization of the endotracheal tube, endotracheal tube condensation, observation of chest wall movement, and auscultation of breathe sounds are helpful to confirm endotracheal placement, these are not foolproof. Addition of CO_2 detection with the use of the disposable partial pressure or maximal concentration of carbon dioxide detector is a useful clinical adjunct for determination of endotracheal tube position. The detector also helps to assess the return of spontaneous circulation as well as prognosticate short-term survival in adults and children.

Limitation

- It is not possible to diagnose hypocarbia or hypercarbia, right mainstem bronchus intubation, or oropharyngeal intubations with colorimetric $EtCO_2$ detectors in spontaneously breathing patients.
- The results are unreliable if the colorimetric detector is contaminated with acidic gastric contents or drugs.
- Humidity decreases the clinical lifespan of detector.
- During cardiopulmonary resuscitation, a positive test confirms correct placement of the tube within the airway, but a negative test may point to either esophageal placement or airway intubation with poor or absent pulmonary blood flow. An alternative means to assess endotracheal tube placement is needed in this situation.

CLINICAL SETTINGS FOR THE USE OF CUTANEOUS CAPNOGRAPHY

Both $PcCO_2$ and $PetCO_2$ monitoring have independent indications, which may in fact be complimentary to each other.

Use in Emergency Room

There is concordance between the $PcCO_2$ measurement and the arterial blood gas values ($PaCO_2$) in patients presenting with acute respiratory failure in the emergency department.

Operation Room

The $PcCO_2$ monitoring provides better estimates of $PaCO_2$ during various surgical procedures. End-tidal PCO_2 ($PetCO_2$) may not be accurate to monitor carbon dioxide concentrations during general anesthesia, because of ventilation or perfusion mismatch. $PcCO_2$ is a good value addition to capnography in such patients with an increased $PetCO_2$ or $PaCO_2$ difference and in situations requiring continuous, noninvasive and precise control of carbon dioxide level (e.g. one lung ventilation).

Pulse oximetry, widely used to monitor patients postoperatively, provides no information on ventilator status. On high concentrations of supplemental oxygen, oxygenation can be maintained with inadequate alveolar ventilation because of the diffusion of oxygen molecules from the airways into the alveoli. In this setting, severe hypercapnia and respiratory acidosis may result.

Intensive Care Unit

The potential applications of $PcCO_2$ measurement in the ICU include monitoring patients receiving mechanical ventilation, noninvasive ventilation, and postextubation. The aim in these situations is mainly to monitor the trends of change in PaCO$_2$ by monitoring PcCO$_2$. PetCO$_2$ is commonly used in patients receiving mechanical ventilation. PetCO$_2$ cannot be applied to patients receiving noninvasive ventilation because of airflow through the mask. The response time of PcCO$_2$ values to a change in noninvasive ventilation has been shown to be compatible with the aim of clinical monitoring.

Neonatal Intensive Care Unit

Noninvasive monitoring of arterial oxygen saturation (SaO$_2$) and PaCO$_2$ is necessary for continuous estimation of the respiratory status and avoid repeated blood gas analyses. Transcutaneous measurement of PCO$_2$ represents a simple and noninvasive method to monitor ventilation in a continuous manner.

Carbon dioxide monitoring is also important in children receiving noninvasive respiratory support especially at home since nocturnal hypercapnia may often occur in children. Monitoring of nocturnal pulse oximetry and daytime arterial blood gas estimation alone are not sufficient to diagnose nocturnal hypercapnia.

Transcutaneous CO$_2$ monitoring, initially introduced in the neonatal intensive care units, can now be used in infants, children, and also adults. It is shown to be as accurate as end-tidal CO$_2$ in patients with normal respiratory function and even more so in patients with shunt or ventilation-perfusion inequalities.

Transcutaneous CO$_2$ monitoring is of particular help in situations in which end-tidal CO$_2$ monitoring is not helpful such as high frequency ventilation, apnea testing, and noninvasive ventilation. It has also been used in spontaneously breathing children with airway and respiratory problems (such as croup and severe acute asthma), as well as to monitor metabolic status during treatment of acidosis. It may not replace arterial blood sampling but can help in monitoring a trend in PCO$_2$ where clinically significant. Also, it serves as an important tool in gauging the microcirculation in patients with septic shock and may signify outcome of such patients. It should be viewed as a complementary technology and may be used in combination with end-tidal CO$_2$ monitoring in an ICU.

Endoscopy Room

The British Thoracic Society guidelines suggest that PcCO$_2$ monitoring may be useful in patients with chronic obstructive pulmonary disease (COPD) having hypercapnic respiratory failure. The combined SPO$_2$/PcCO$_2$ monitoring at the earlobe is a novel approach to detect hypoventilation accompanied with significant elevation of PcCO$_2$ that occurs during bronchoscopy. PcCO$_2$ may provide an early indication of respiratory depression during flexible bronchoscopy and therefore might improve patient safety during sedation.

It may also be used to titrate the administration of sedative drugs to prevent unintentional deep sedation or anesthesia.

Flexible Bronchoscopy

Combined oximetry and cutaneous capnography effectively monitor ventilation during flexible bronchoscopy in patients with COPD. Possibly, COPD patients with elevated baseline $PaCO_2$ or a low baseline SpO_2 will benefit more from better monitoring of ventilation with cutaneous capnography.

Assessment of long-term Oxygen Therapy

Assessment of carbon dioxide (measured invasively or noninvasively) is also essential in hypercapnic patients on both short-term and long-term oxygen supplementation. Hypercapnia frequently gets precipitated or aggravated on uncontrolled oxygen therapy. Recognition of hypercapnia is important to regulate oxygen therapy in such patients. $PcCO_2$ is used both to estimate $PaCO_2$ and to determine trend changes. Combined cutaneous capnography and oximetry (SpO_2) are now possible with a single earlobe sensor.

Sleep Laboratory

Nocturnal capnometry helps capture features of sleep apnea (such as the balance of apnea and postapnea duration), which are not picked up by the apnea–hypopnea index. The application of continuous $PcCO_2$ monitoring to overnight studies is limited due to the change of the skin site of the probe after 4 hours and recalibration to prevent thermal injuries to the skin. This is a time-consuming procedure; the acquisition of the $PcCO_2$ values is further delayed by the equilibration time of up to 20 minutes. As discussed earlier, continuous $PcCO_2$ monitoring between 5–8 hours has been shown to be reliable in adults at a probe temperature of 43°C. The possibility of performing continuous an 8-hour $PcCO_2$ monitoring (with validation studies) will allow to study the ventilation patterns during polysomnography and also be a tool for optimal titration of nocturnal noninvasive ventilation pressures in patients with chronic respiratory failure.

Lung Function Laboratory

A suspected diagnosis of hyperventilation can be confirmed or excluded by the use of $PcCO_2$ monitoring. $PcCO_2$ monitoring might be helpful for oxygen titration especially in patient with severe chronic obstructive pulmonary disease. Therefore, multiple arterial blood gas sampling can be avoided.

Cardiopulmonary Exercise Testing

Cutaneous estimations of PCO_2 and SPO_2 can be used in cardiopulmonary exercise testing, circumventing the need for arterial cannulation.

Other Uses

Transcutaneous carbon dioxide monitoring is also finding its way in home care and palliative therapy. It has a role in detecting early hypercapnia in neuromuscular disorders and help initiate therapy. As home management of chronic respiratory failure is increasing with the use of noninvasive ventilations, its efficacy and monitoring may improve its optimal use in these patients. Transcutaneous carbon dioxide tension monitoring will help to know the trend of carbon dioxide in these patients noninvasively and continuously. It has also helped in proving efficacy of opioids in palliation of respiratory symptoms without worsening of gaseous parameters.

In summary, $PcCO_2$ monitoring is now less cumbersome than before. Combined $PcCo_2$ and SpO_2 measurement has great potential to improve patient safety by better monitoring of ventilation during conscious sedation and general anesthesia, including postoperative surveillance.

CHAPTER 84

Nutritional Management and General Care in the Intensive Care Unit

Inderpaul Singh Sehgal, Navneet Singh

INTRODUCTION

Malnutrition arises from an imbalance between nutrient intake and nutrient requirements. Diseases especially critical illnesses are unique in that they cannot only affect nutritional intake and requirements but also increase the nutrient losses (urinary, gastrointestinal or from other sites). In fact, in majority of the malnourished critically ill patients, multiple mechanisms are believed to operate simultaneously. Further, presence of malnutrition can hinder recovery and increase morbidity and mortality.

MALNUTRITION IN CRITICAL ILLNESS

Prevalence and Epidemiology

The prevalence of malnutrition among hospitalized patients, including those in the intensive care units (ICUs), has increased steadily over the years because of several reasons including an increasing age of the general population, development of newer and often aggressive medical and surgical treatment modalities for different chronic debilitating diseases, and finally progress achieved in intensive care management. The prevalence of malnutrition among hospitalized patients is estimated to be as high as 30–50%. There are four discrete phases of any critical illness: acute critical illness (ACI), prolonged acute critical illness (PACI), chronic critical illness (CCI), and recovery from critical illness (RCI).

A patient can be malnourished either on admission itself or develop it subsequently during his illness due to multiple factors. During ACI, myriad of endogenous substances comprising hormones (adrenocorticotropic hormone, catecholamines, glucagon, growth hormones, vasopressin, and others), cytokines, and chemokines that cause a shift from an anabolic state to catabolic state. These metabolic abnormalities further lead to physiologic changes, reduced tissue function, and finally loss of body mass. ACI is followed by a persistent proinflammatory state (PACI) representing contrasting physiology characterized by blunted hypothalamic-pituitary responses. Some patients develop a chronic constant state of CCI, manifested by a paradigm of disease entities like kwashiorkor, marasmus, hypoproteinemia, hyperglycemia, immune suppression, and neurocognitive dysfunction like delirium, depression or psychosis. RCI is marked by deliverance from mechanical ventilation and a return of anabolic physiology.

Malnutrition can affect the pulmonary system directly by causing a reduction in diaphragmatic muscle mass, respiratory muscle strength, maximum voluntary ventilation, and functional residual capacity which make the process of weaning difficult. Optimal nutritional supplementation provides an opportunity to slow down or even halt the catabolic process and thus prevent malnutrition which, in turn, can favorably alter the hospital course of such patients.

Differentiation of Catabolism in Critical Illness from Starvation

One of the fundamental differences between the two is that in the former the basal metabolic rate (BMR) is elevated while, in contrast, it is depressed in the later. Ketogenesis is a prominent feature of starvation but not critical illness (Table 84.1).

Effect of Malnutrition on Clinical Outcomes in Critically Ill Patients

There is significantly a higher incidence of complications, length of hospital stay, and in-hospital mortality rates in critically ill patients who are malnourished than those who are well-nourished. Furthermore, presence of malnutrition has been shown to be associated with worse outcomes even with a lesser severity of critical illness.

TABLE 84.1: Differentiation of catabolism in critical illness from starvation.

Feature	Critical illness	Starvation
BMR/REE	↑	↓
Respiratory quotient	(0.8–0.9)	(0.6–0.7)
Cytokine levels	↑	↓
Primary fuels	Mixed	Fat
Proteolysis	+++	+
Ureagenesis	+++	+
Urinary nitrogen losses	+++	+
Gluconeogenesis	+++	+
Ketone production	+	+++

(BMR, basal metabolic rate; REE, resting energy expenditure)

REFEEDING SYNDROME

Refeeding syndrome represents maladaptive response to abrupt feeding after starvation and is characterized by dyselectrolytemia, respiratory failure, heart failure, and death. Refeeding may be associated with one or more of the following symptoms or signs: unintentional weight loss of more than 15% within previous 3-6 months, body mass index of less than $16\,kg/m^2$, inadequate nutrition intake of more than 10 days, and low potassium, phosphate, and magnesium before feeding. It is important to recognize refeeding syndrome as it has been associated with higher risk of cardiac arrhythmias, heart failure, respiratory failure, and difficult weaning.

ASSESSMENT OF NUTRITIONAL STATUS IN CRITICALLY ILL PATIENTS

Assessment of nutritional status includes evaluation of clinical, anthropometric, chemical, and immunologic parameters. Apart from details of disease states (chronic debilitating diseases, history of inadequate food intake over prolonged periods of time, drug abuse, alcoholism, and chronic psychiatric disorders), nutritional history comprises three key components that include actual weight and height (BMI), recent (3-6 months) weight loss, and recent decrease in nutrient intake. Although history constitutes most important role, it may not be possible to obtain a reliable history from critically ill patients. Physical examination should specifically focus on nutrition parameters, anthropometry, and body composition/circumference measurements.

There is no single test that alone is sensitive and specific to detect malnutrition in critically ill patients. Various measurements (body weight, anthropometry, hepatic secretory proteins such as albumin, prealbumin, transferrin, retinol-binding protein and other proteins secreted by liver, total lymphocyte count and delayed cutaneous hypersensitivity, blood or serum levels of electrolytes like potassium, phosphorus, calcium, etc.) have their own limitations. Multiparameter nutritional indices include subjective global assessment, prognostic nutritional index, and prognostic inflammatory and nutritional index. However, even though these multiparameter indices are objectively designed, they again rely on the values of different clinical and laboratory parameters and hence are limited by the same concerns as the individual parameters themselves.

GOALS AND PRINCIPLES OF NUTRITIONAL SUPPORT

General goals of providing nutritional support to critically ill patients include:
- Nutritional support to the patient should be provided depending upon several considerations, such as the following:
  - Underlying medical condition
  - Current nutritional status
  - Current metabolic requirements
  - Route available for administration of nutrients.

- Treatment and prevention of nutrient deficiencies (both macro and micro)
- Avoidance of complications likely to occur with nutritional support
- Improvement in patient outcomes related to disease morbidity.

TIMING OF INITIATION OF NUTRITIONAL SUPPORT

Many patients, especially those who are previously well nourished, can tolerate short periods of starvation (usually less than 1 week) during a critical illness. However, even in well-nourished patients, nutritional supplementation is necessary if they are unable to resume oral nutrition or if their oral intake is insufficient for more than 3-4 days. Early institution (within 24 hours of admission) of enteric feed has been shown to have beneficial effects on the intestinal epithelium. Enteral nutrition increases the intestinal oxygen demand, hence causing concerns regarding its use in hemodynamically unstable patients. The current evidence suggests that early institution of enteral feed in unstable patients also increases intestinal blood flow and improves intestinal function, and may protect against bowel-related complications. A delay in provision of nutrition in the presence of a hypercatabolic state even for a short period of time is likely to be associated with increased morbidity and mortality. Enteral nutritional support can thus be started as early as 12-48 hours of admission to the ICU. In most critically ill patients oral feeding may not be feasible and hence enteral nutritional support should be attempted after placement of a nasogastric (or in some cases nasojejunal) tube.

ROUTE OF ADMINISTRATION OF NUTRITIONAL SUPPORT

Both enteral and parenteral route can be used depending upon the feasibility. Enteral route is preferred in the presence of a functional gut. Enteral nutrition also helps in modulation of the host's immune response besides providing energy and protein to maintain gut integrity. Enteral nutrition favors maintenance of structure and functioning of intestinal villi (both by reducing the incidence of mucosal atrophy and decreasing the abnormal increase in intestinal permeability) and thus promotes gut motility that eventually helps in initiating oral feeding.

Enteral nutrition causes stimulation of gut epithelial cell metabolism by direct contact with nutrients, increase in mucosal blood flow, and secretion of immunoglobulin A and enterotrophic hormones like gastrin and enteroglucagon. Lack of enteral nutrition leads to atrophy of intestinal villi, bacterial overgrowth, and increases permeability of the gut mucosa causing bacterial translocation. Provision of parenteral nutrition leads to a rapid atrophy of gut mucosa; it also impairs both humoral and cellular immunity. Parenteral nutrition also leads to increased free radical formation, thus causing further damage. In addition to being more physiological, enteral nutrition is also less expensive. It leads to improved utilization of nutrients, and possibly helps to avoid some of the infectious complications associated with parenteral nutrition, one of the mechanisms being reduction in translocation of bacteria from the gut.

There is no denying the fact that parenteral nutrition remains "a valuable yet challenging weapon in our therapeutic armory in the presence of gastrointestinal feed intolerance or failure. It should be used wisely and not indiscriminately because most intensive care patients with a fully functional gastrointestinal tract can be fed safely with enteral nutrition".

Addition of Parenteral Nutrition to Enteral Nutrition

There is a school of thought among intensivists that adding parenteral nutrition to enteral nutrition leads to improvement in calorie delivery and therefore may positively influence patient outcomes. Published literature seems to suggest otherwise.

Contraindications to Enteral Nutrition

Enteral feeding remains the preferred route of administration of nutritional support in patients in whom there is no obvious contraindication. It is not uncommon to encounter absolute and relative contraindications for administration of enteral nutritional support. Enteral nutrition is absolutely contraindicated in patients with a nonfunctional gut due to intestinal obstruction, anatomic disruption, generalized peritonitis or severe intestinal ischemia. Normally, splanchnic blood flow increases in response to nutrient load taken orally or administered enterally. This response is lacking in patients who have reduced gut perfusion due to severe or prolonged shock. Even if it occurs, it may not be sustained and this ultimately leads to hampered digestion and absorption. In fact, early feeding during hemodynamic compromise or shock can further contribute to mesenteric ischemia, infarction, and even perforation.

Enteral nutrition should start only after hemodynamic stability. Presence of abdominal distension with enteral feeds, localized peritonitis, intra-abdominal abscess or severe pancreatitis form relative contraindication to enteral feeding. Similarly, enteral nutrition should wait in patients at high risk of aspiration due to a terminal disease, coma, and those with short bowel (<30 cm).

QUANTITY AND VOLUME OF NUTRITION SUPPORT

Recommendations and practice guidelines have been given and revised from time to time in relation to the quantity of nutritional support to be administered to critically ill patients.

Energy (Calorie) Requirements

For most patients, provision of calories in the range of 20–30 kcal/kg/day is appropriate. Factors that should be taken into consideration while deciding the optimal amount for a given patient include gender, age, presence or absence of preexisting malnutrition, type and severity of critical illness as well as the phase of critical illness (acute vs. recovering). It is desirable to achieve the goal of providing the entire energy requirements by the enteral route alone within the first 7–10 days of hospitalization.

Protein Requirements

Protein requirement consists of 1.2–1.5 g/kg body weight/day (maximum 2.0 g/kg body weight/day). Patients with significant protein losses (e.g. extensive burns, digestive or urinary losses) can be given higher amounts.

Volume Requirements

In general, approximately 1 mL of water is needed per kcal while administering enteral feeds. However, fluid requirements and restrictions vary from patient to patient and therefore the total volume to be administered may need to be individualized. The total amount of calories can be administered in a volume that is appropriate for the patient by changing the relative concentrations of the different constituents namely carbohydrates, proteins, and fats. It needs to be mentioned that the recommended proportion of carbohydrates, fats, and proteins is 30–70%, 15–30%, and 15–20%, respectively of total calories. For nonprotein calories, carbohydrates and fat should be in a ratio ranging from 1.5:1 to 2.5:1.

Issues Related to Body Weight

Determination of body weight is an important issue for critically ill patients. If direct weighing is not feasible, ideal body weight can be estimated from height and anthropometric tables. The body weight used for calculating energy and protein requirements often needs to be modified according to the baseline nutritional status. Malnourished and obese patients generally require calorie delivery based upon determination of an "optimal" body weight.

Issues Related to Estimation of Energy Requirements

By using the Harris–Benedict equation, the resting energy expenditure (REE) can be calculated and subsequently the total energy expenditure (TEE) by multiplying REE with a stress/activity factor (normally 1.2–1.4 in critically ill patients). Indirect calorimetry is another method used for this purpose and is probably more accurate method than either the equations or simple formulae.

DELIVERY OF ENTERAL NUTRITION AND ITS DETERMINANTS

The quantity of enteral feeds administered has been shown to be significantly lower than what is prescribed in as high as 40% of all hospitalized patients. Use of formulations with a higher energy and protein density has been suggested to enhance the total nutritional intake.

Feeding interruptions because of diagnostic or therapeutic procedures remain an important reason for reduced intake. Other common reasons for decreasing or discontinuing feeds after initiation included high gastric residual volumes and mechanical feeding tube problems. Potential factors implicated for intolerance to feeds include the admission diagnosis, preexisting illnesses, electrolyte and metabolic abnormalities, advanced age, and use of drugs (such as narcotics or catecholamines) and shock. Elevated plasma cholecystokinin concentrations have also been shown to correlate with feed intolerance.

Position of Feeding

Adoption of a semirecumbent position while feeding patients is likely to have the best effect in terms of both tolerance to enteral feeds and patient outcomes. The frequency of clinically suspected and microbiologically confirmed pneumonia has been shown to be lower among patients fed in the semirecumbent position as compared to those in the supine position.

Nasogastric versus Nasojejunal Feeding

Enteral nutrition is most commonly given with nasogastric feeding. After placement of a nasogastric tube, check abdominal X-rays should be done to detect any malpositioning of the feeding tube (looping inside the oral cavity or in the lower esophagus, or introduction into the trachea). Nasojejunal feedings has been shown to be associated with improved tolerance of enteral nutrition, and therefore with a reduction in the requirement for parenteral nutrition.

Although nasojejunal feeding leads to lesser gastrointestinal complications mainly because of a lesser incidence of high gastric residual volumes, it is also associated with increased frequency of tube-related complications (occlusion, accidental withdrawal, and dislodgement) and these can often negate its advantage (s) over nasogastric feeding.

Residual Volumes

Gastric residual volumes should be measured ideally prior to administration of each feed or earlier, if indicated. It is advisable to have minimal residual volumes (ideally <150 mL) in order to reduce the risk of aspiration of feed contents into the tracheobronchial tree.

In the presence of high gastric residues, a reduction in the frequency and volume of enteral feeds may be necessary along with more frequent monitoring of gastric residual volumes. Prokinetic agents (metoclopramide, cisapride or erythromycin) can be used to improve gastric emptying although the relative efficacy of one drug over the other or use of a combination versus a single drug is debatable. In most cases, it is gastric motility that is hampered (gastroparesis or gastric atony) and true ileus (dilated and nonfunctional small intestine) is rare.

Role of Bowel Sounds

Bowel sounds should not be used as a criterion to determine initiation or interruption or discontinuation of enteral feeding. The reasons proposed are:
- They do not correlate well with gut motility in critically ill patients.

- Bowel sounds are produced due to movement of air through the small intestine and require the presence of both gastric air and gastric emptying. Critically ill patients who have nasogastric tubes in situ may not have either or both of these and hence there may be minimal or no movement of air from the stomach into the small intestine and hence decreased or absent bowel sounds even in the presence of a normally functioning small intestine.
- Most clinicians do not listen for bowel sounds for more than few seconds while one needs to listen for them for 2–4 minutes in each of the abdominal quadrants. Passage of flatus or stool is also not required for initiation of enteral feeding.

Diarrhea and Enteral Nutrition

Patients on enteral nutritional support who develop diarrhea that persists for more than 3 days may need evaluation for *Clostridium difficile* infection after other common causes have been excluded since these patients are usually receiving broad-spectrum antibiotics. Frequency and volume of enteral feeds may need to decrease in these cases. Parenteral nutrition may be needed for some time to ensure adequate nutritional support. Antidiarrheal agents or probiotics (like *Saccharomyces boulardii*) can also be considered.

In conclusion, the evidence available so far supports that the enteral route should be used for administration of nutritional supplementation. Conventional strategies for enteral feeding are preferred to parenteral nutrition or modified enteral feeding strategies since there is no clear cut evidence that any of the latter two are associated with improvement in patient outcomes.

GENERAL CARE IN ICU

For most critically ill patients, supportive measures including the "ABCs" (airway, breathing, circulation) are required (Box 84.1). Ensuring patency of the airway is a must for all patients admitted to the ICU. Endotracheal intubation is not always necessary when there is adequate presence of cough and gag reflexes as well as of spontaneous ventilation. However, if there are

---

BOX 84.1: Key components of general care of the critically ill patients.

- Hemodynamic and respiratory monitoring
- Judicious use of sedatives, analgesics, and neuromuscular paralyzing agents
- Periodic assessments for weaning and tracheostomy
- Prophylaxis against stress-related mucosal disease
- Prophylaxis against deep venous thrombosis
- Glycemic control—avoid intensive insulin therapy
- Prevention of pressure ulcers
- Implementation of infection prevention strategies
- Avoid unnecessary transfusions

any concerns regarding airway protection and/or clinical deterioration, it is advisable to have the airway secured preemptively since endotracheal intubation reduces the risk of aspiration. Intubation is also indicated in cases of acute (or sometimes in acute-on-chronic) respiratory failure for providing assisted mechanical ventilation. Two important issues related to management of critically ill patients need mention here—prophylaxis against deep venous thrombosis (DVT) and stress-related mucosal disease (SMRD).

Deep Venous Thrombosis Prophylaxis

In the absence of any specific contraindications, some form of DVT prophylaxis is advocated for most ICU patients. Studies have shown DVT and pulmonary embolism to be an underdiagnosed entity among patients admitted to ICUs.

Stress-related Mucosal Disease Prophylaxis

Stress-related mucosal disease (SRMD) or stress-related mucosal ulceration is an important and frequently occurring gastrointestinal complication among ICU patients. This can be responsible for increased length of stay in the hospital as well as adversely influence other clinical outcomes. Suppression of gastric acid production to prevent stress-related mucosal ulceration and gastrointestinal bleeding is achieved with drugs which include sucralfate, histamine 2-receptor antagonists (H2 blockers), and proton pump inhibitors (PPIs).

Both enteral and intravenous PPIs consistently maintain gastric pH more than or equal to 4.0 and are therefore as safe and as efficacious as H2 blockers or sucralfate for prevention of bleeding. Sucralfate can protect the gastric mucosa without raising gastric pH. However, the benefit of SRMD prophylaxis as a routine in all ICU patients has not been convincingly proven. An increased risk of nosocomial pneumonia with use of H2 blockers and PPIs as well as of reduced absorption of concomitantly administered oral medications with sucralfate has led to several authors recommending against routine prophylaxis against SMRD in the ICU. There is a need to carry out a risk–benefit assessment for each critically ill medical patient prior to initiation of SRMD prophylaxis.

Bedsore Prevention

Another common problem in intensive care settings is the occurrence of pressure ulcers (previously called "bedsores"). There is a wide variation in the reported prevalence (4%–49%). Age, duration of mechanical ventilation, bowel incontinence, presence of diabetes mellitus, spinal cord injury, and renal failure are proven risk factors for its occurrence. Specialized mattresses (alternating pressure air, low air loss and foam) should be used for prevention of pressure ulcers. Significantly lower incidence of new pressure ulcers in patients with acute lung injury is reported with enteral diet enriched in eicosapentaenoic acid, gamma linolenic acid, and vitamins A, C and E.

Appropriate pressure ulcer care results in a significant and sustained decrease in the development of grade II-IV pressure ulcers in these ICU patients. Timely transfer to a specific pressure-reducing mattress prior to the occurrence of a pressure ulcer is the most important factor. A multidisciplinary team approach is required for prevention as well as treatment.

Essentially speaking, ICU care involves a coordinated, multidisciplinary approach with active involvement of nursing staff, pharmacists, and other staff members. Recovery and rehabilitation measures should start as soon as the patient is admitted in the ICU ward.

CHAPTER 85

Management of Complex Airways Diseases

Rubal Patel, Atul C Mehta

INTRODUCTION

In the acutely decompensating patient, securing the airway in a timely manner with the best practice approach is crucial to ensure an optimal outcome. The initial evaluation should include historical, clinical, and anatomic components in order to consider important factors, such as the neurological status, level of consciousness, hemodynamic status, and respiratory reserve.

The difficult airway is defined as "the clinical situation in which a conventionally trained anesthesiologist experiences difficulty with facemask ventilation of the upper airway, difficulty with tracheal intubation, or both". There is greater likelihood of adverse events (such as airway injury, hypoxic brain injury and even death) in cases of failure to recognize risk factors and inadequate management of the difficult airway.

DIFFICULT AIRWAY SITUATIONS

The difficult airway may be described using the following scenarios:
- *Difficult facemask or supraglottic airway (SGA) ventilation*: Inadequate ventilation results from inadequate mask or SGA seal, excessive gas leak, or excessive resistance to the ingress or egress of gas. Examples of signs of inadequate ventilation include absent or inadequate chest movement, absent or inadequate breath sounds, auscultatory signs of severe obstruction, cyanosis, gastric air entry or dilatation, decreasing or inadequate oxygen saturation, absent or inadequate exhaled carbon dioxide, hemodynamic changes associated with hypoxemia or hypercarbia (e.g. hypertension, tachycardia, and arrhythmia).

- *Difficult SGA placement*: SGA placement requires multiple attempts, irrespective of tracheal pathology.
- *Difficult laryngoscopy*: Inability to visualize the vocal cords after multiple attempts at conventional laryngoscopy.
- *Difficult tracheal intubation*: Multiple attempts at tracheal intubation irrespective of tracheal pathology.
- *Failed intubation*: Failure to place endotracheal tube (ETT) on multiple attempts.

Complication rates are higher in the intensive care unit (ICU) environment than in the operating room. ICU patients have limited physiologic reserve and multiple comorbidities. Moreover, a thorough anatomical evaluation may not be always possible in the ICU patients. Difficult intubations can arise from inadequate visualization of the larynx or anatomic abnormality (distortion or narrowing of the larynx or trachea).

INDICATIONS FOR ARTIFICIAL AIRWAY

The first step in the airway management algorithm consists of establishing the indication for intubation. Restoration of sufficient oxygenation and ventilation is of greatest importance regardless of the underlying cause.
Indications for endotracheal intubation are:
- Hypoxic or hypercapnic respiratory failure
- Inability to protect the airway (e.g. neurologic insults, such as stroke or drug overdose)
- Airway obstruction from any cause
- Inability to clear secretions, blood, or foreign material.

There are three principal methods of mechanical ventilation in a critically ill patient: noninvasive positive pressure ventilation (NIPPV) via facemask, extraglottic airway, and the endotracheal route. NIPPV is useful in patients with acute exacerbations of obstructive airway disease or cardiogenic pulmonary edema. Endotracheal intubation is the mainstay of mechanical ventilatory support for most patients in the intensive care unit.

Training Strategies

Proficiency in airway management is achieved through various educational tools.

The knowledge of the airway anatomy and its variants is essential to assess for the type of intubation approach and to predict the level of difficulty that may be encountered during the procedure. Airway models and virtual simulators are essential tools to teach trainees basic information regarding airway intubation and equipment without direct patient contact. Communication with the entire team is paramount when dealing with complex airway issues.

Anatomy

A key component to competency in complex airway management is familiarity and understanding of airway anatomy. The airway is divided into the upper (nares to glottis) and lower (trachea and conducting bronchi) airway.

Upper Airway

Evaluation of the patient for endotracheal intubation begins with examination of the oral cavity and the pharynx. The oral cavity (teeth, tongue, hard palate, and soft palate) is assessed for clues that may impede a smooth intubation process.

Lower Airway

The lower airway is comprised the trachea and conducting bronchi. The trachea is a fibrous, muscular tube that extends approximately 10–12 cm in length and 2 centimeters in width in the adult, from the cricoid cartilage to the carina.

Tracheal Blood Supply

Branches of the inferior thyroid artery provide blood supply to the upper trachea and bronchial arteries supply the lower trachea. Vascular perfusion to the trachea may adversely affect critically ill patients with hypotension. Pressure trauma from the endotracheal cuff may result in ischemic necrosis in these situations.

Preintubation Assessment

It is imperative for the experienced practitioner to consider comorbidities in predicting problems that may be encountered during endotracheal intubation. The best predictor of difficult intubation is the history of a previous difficult intubation.

There is likelihood of six basic problems that may occur alone or in combination:
1. Difficulty with patient cooperation or consent
2. Difficult mask ventilation
3. Difficult SGA placement
4. Difficult laryngoscopy
5. Difficult intubation
6. Difficult surgical airway access.

Environment

Operating room with well-stocked intubation tools offers the most controlled environment. The environment should be altered to make it as conducive as possible to administer care to the patient. Personnel should be limited to essential providers and spectators should be asked to leave.

Conditions for intubation in the ICU should be close to ideal. Availability of the following essentials should be assured prior to attempting intubation: supply of 100% oxygen, a well-fitting mask with attached bag-valve device, suction equipment, and oral and nasal airways of appropriate sizes. The bed positioning should allow the patient's head at the level of the physician's mid-chest.

Patient History

A focused airway history is a paramount in anticipating the possibility of a difficult airway. A variety of congenital diseases, such as Dwarfism or trisomy 21, Pierre Robin syndrome, Treacher Collins syndrome, and Goldenhar syndrome have been reported to have difficulty with laryngoscopy or intubation. Multiple acquired conditions have also been associated with a difficult airway. A dry cough, hoarseness, stridor or wheezing may be suggestive of a tumor causing intrinsic or extrinsic compression of the trachea or tracheal deviation. Disease states, such as arthritis, cervical disk abnormalities, diabetes mellitus, and scleroderma impact on neck and mandibular mobility making it difficult to properly position the patient for intubation. In addition, previous surgery, burns or radiation to the neck may cause scarring and contractures which may limit tissue mobility. The presence of a tracheostomy stoma or a scar from a previous tracheostomy may be suggestive of subglottic stenosis or an indication of a previous airway complication. Morbidly obese individuals may have a history of snoring and obstructive sleep apnea due to a short, thick neck and excessive soft tissue of the neck and upper airway, which will consequently complicate endotracheal intubation.

Insertion of the laryngoscope may also be more difficult in obese individuals. Pregnancy may also increase the risk of aspiration and bleeding from swollen oral mucosa. Infections in the mouth, salivary glands, tonsils or pharynx may cause pain, swelling or muscle spasms and limit one's ability to easily intubate. Persons with acromegaly may have enlargement of the tongue, epiglottis, and vocal cords causing a narrowed glottic opening. A history of recent trauma may trigger suspicion of an intracranial injury, a basilar skull fracture or injury to the airway or cervical spine.

Physical Examination

A thorough inspection of the patient's posture, habitus, face, mouth, neck, and jaw is essential prior to undergoing endotracheal intubation if possible.

Inspection

Mallampati classification system of the oropharynx is commonly used to predict endotracheal intubation difficulty. The open mouth is examined with the head in neutral position and the tongue protruded. The distance between the base of the tongue to the uvula and soft palate and pharyngeal pillars is rated:
- *Class I:* Uvula, soft palate, and pharyngeal pillars are easily visible
- *Class II:* Soft palate and pharyngeal pillars are visible

- *Class III:* Soft palate alone is visible
- *Class IV:* Only hard palate is visible.

The opening of the mouth and thyromental distance (distance from the mandibular mentum to the superior thyroid notch during neck extension) should be assessed. Difficult airway is suggested by the mouth opening of less than two finger widths and a thyromental distance less than three finger width. An alert patient should be able to bend his head forwards to touch the chin to chest, hyperextend, and turn the head from side to side without pain or paresthesia. Cervico-occipital extension of less than 160° angle at the hyoid bone limits proper positioning of the mouth and pharynx to visualize the glottis for endotracheal tube placement. A careful evaluation of the mouth should also include examination for any prominent or protruding teeth blocking the view of the glottis. The presence of loose teeth, dental caps and bridges add to the risk of aspiration from dislodgement or damage to the teeth.

Palpation

The hyoid bone, superior thyroid notch, and cricothyroid ligament should be palpated prior to attempting intubation. The neck should also be palpated for evidence of thyroid enlargement or masses, which could potentially obstruct the airway or impede visualization of the glottis.

Auscultation

Auscultation of the neck and chest for stridor or adventitious breath sounds is also an important component of the preintubation assessment. The use of bronchodilators or steroids may be indicated if airway obstruction is suspected.

TECHNIQUES

Airway management may be achieved by definitive or nondefinitive methods. The nondefinite techniques include utilization of assist devices, such as an oral or nasal airway or SGA. The definite methods enable control of ventilation, administration of high levels of oxygen, and protection against aspiration. There are three major methods of obtaining a definitive airway: orotracheal, nasotracheal, and the surgical airway.

Laryngoscopy

Direct laryngoscopy remains the most commonly used method for endotracheal intubation. With this, one can directly visualize the vocal cords and glottis to confirm the ETT placement. The choice of blade shape (the curved Macintosh or the straight Miller blade) depends on personal preference. Video laryngoscopy can also provide an indirect view of the vocal cords and glottic inlet. A fiberoptic or digital laryngoscope is inserted transorally and the images displayed on a monitor. The magnified images allow for detailed examination of the larynx. Video-assisted laryngoscopy is reported to result in higher intubation success rates in the ICU setting. It provides improved grade of laryngoscopic view and reduces the esophageal intubation rate in comparison to direct laryngoscopy.

Endotracheal Tube

Commonly, one selects an ETT of about 7.0–7.5 mm in diameter for an average adult female and 7.5–8.0 mm for an average adult male. Traumatic complications, such as perforation or laceration of the pharynx, larynx, trachea or the esophagus can sometimes occur during endotracheal intubation. Occasionally, there can be vocal cord injury and dislocation of the arytenoid cartilages. Malpositioning of the ETT includes mainstem bronchus intubation causing contralateral lung atelectasis and should be readily identified on physical examination and chest radiograph. Examples of other complications occurring during the peri-intubation period include aspiration pneumonitis, hypotension, arrhythmias, hypoxia, hypercarbia, laryngeal spasm, bronchospasm, and adverse events from anesthesia.

Orotracheal Intubation

Orotracheal intubation is the most commonly performed procedure to secure an airway. Removal of obstruction is the most important step. Relief from obstruction by the tongue is attempted by head tilt, chin lift or jaw thrust maneuvers. Facemask or nasal cannula is then used to give supplemental oxygen.

Nasotracheal Intubation

Nasotracheal intubation provides an alternate route to secure the airways, particularly in case of oral trauma. The tube is inserted in the nose, against the nasal septum with the curvature of the tube directed along the larynx until it is visualized in the oropharynx. The tube is advanced through the glottic opening with the aid of a laryngoscope and Magill forceps. The nasal tube can also be inserted over an intubating bronchoscope. Nasal intubation is contraindicated in patients with basilar skull fractures and in apneic patients. Complications, such as epistasis, laryngospasm, damage to the turbinates, and nasal perforation can occur with nasal intubation. Sinusitis is another serious complication.

Confirmation of Tube Placement

It is vitally important to confirm proper tube positioning after endotracheal intubation. Correct ETT placement may be confirmed by several methods. The most confirmatory test is direct visualization of the ETT passing through the vocal cords. Fogging of the ETT is another sign of tracheal intubation; however, it has been reported to occur with esophageal intubations as well. Capnography and colorimetric detection of carbon dioxide are other commonly used methods for confirmation of endotracheal intubation.

ALTERNATIVE AIRWAY TECHNIQUES

It may be difficult to obtain an artificial airway in certain clinical scenarios by conventional techniques. Examples include cervical and oropharyngeal trauma and difficult anatomy, such as excessive supraglottic redundant soft tissue. In order to prepare for such situations, it behooves the intensivist to become skilled in performing alternative techniques. Various tools and equipment that facilitate alternative techniques include fiberoptic, video, optical and mechanical methods for better viewing of the larynx to expedite the passage of an ETT into the trachea. These devices, such as stylet, lighted stylet introducer—gum elastic bougie designed to facilitate management of difficult and failed airways are useful for the management of the difficult or failed airway as well as for routine intubations.

Supraglottic Airway Device

Extraglottic airway devices for supralaryngeal ventilation include cuffed, orally inserted hypopharyngeal airways and cuffed, orally inserted esophageal airways (Combitube™).

Flexible Bronchoscopy

The use of a bronchoscope can be instrumental in the placement of an ETT through the mouth or the nose. The ETT is placed over the bronchoscope; the scope is passed through the glottis for direct visualization of the vocal cords and advanced beyond the vocal cords into the trachea. Flexible bronchoscopy is a successful tool for difficult airway intubations. It is particularly useful when upper airway anatomy is distorted due to tumors, trauma or congenital anomalies as well as in patients with cervical injuries. It also allows awake intubation with topical anesthesia. Bronchoscopy is also helpful in identifying causes of acute hypoxia and to remove secretions or blood from the airway.

Transtracheal Jet Ventilation

Transtracheal jet ventilation is performed by a large bore catheter (14-gauge) through the cricothyroid membrane into the trachea (needle cricothyroidotomy), which is confirmed by aspiration of air before connecting to the ventilation system. Complications, such as aspiration, bleeding, barotraumas, and inadequate ventilation can sometimes occur.

Retrograde Intubation

Retrograde intubation is done by placing a guide wire into the pharynx in a retrograde fashion through a puncture in the cricothyroid membrane. An 18-gauge (or larger) needle attached to a 20 mL syringe partially filled with saline is advanced midline through the cricothyroid membrane to aid placement of an ETT. When the trachea is entered, a large volume of air will be seen in the syringe. The needle is then aimed superiorly and the syringe is removed. A guidewire is threaded through the needle into the oropharynx, the wire tip retrieved with Magill forceps and the ETT advanced down the trachea over the guidewire. Retrograde intubation is contraindicated in the presence of complete upper airway obstruction and laryngeal trauma. It is a time-consuming procedure and therefore not done in cases of urgent intubation.

Surgical Airway

A surgical airway is required when other means of establishing an airway are not successful, such as in case of laryngeal and facial injuries. This may also be needed for long-term need for ventilatory support.

Cricothyroidotomy: Cricothyroidotomy establishes an airway through cricothyroid membrane. This is the preferred method of a surgical airway in situations with supraglottic obstruction and can be lifesaving.

A cricothyroidotomy is absolutely contraindicated when the patient can be safely orally or nasally intubated. Complications to this technique include bleeding, infection, vocal cord damage, posterior tracheal or esophageal rupture, and tracheal stenosis.

Tracheostomy (percutaneous vs. surgical): Tracheostomy is a commonly performed procedure for prolonged mechanical ventilation. The timing of tracheostomy should be individualized and based on the likelihood of benefit and predicted need for prolonged ventilation. Early tracheostomy has been advocated in the literature to improve survival and decrease ventilator days. Tracheostomy may be performed by an open surgical approach or by percutaneous dilatation technique.

Percutaneous tracheostomy is a common procedure performed at the bedside or in the operating room. Successful performance of the bedside percutaneous procedure is related to the expertise of the operator and ancillary personnel. Percutaneous tracheostomy requires less time to perform and is less expensive than a surgical approach.

Disadvantages of percutaneous tracheostomy compared to surgical tracheostomy include an increased risk of anterior tracheal injury and posterior tracheal wall perforation. It is contraindicated in the presence of an uncorrectable bleeding diathesis, gross distortion of the neck from masses, scarring from previous neck surgery, infection in the soft tissues of the neck, and inability to extend the neck. Complications such as infections, bleeding, accidental extubation, pneumothorax, tracheal ring fracture, and tracheal stenosis can occur following tracheostomy.

Surgical tracheostomy is usually done 2 cm above the suprasternal notch. A vertical tracheostomy is done between the second and fourth tracheal ring after midline incision. A tracheostomy tube is placed through the dilated stoma.

CONCLUSION

In summary, acquiring expert knowledge in securing the airway is a critical step when caring for patients in the ICU. A multidisciplinary team approach further improves outcomes, given the heterogeneous patient populations that exist in the intensive care setting.

CHAPTER 86

Analgesia and Sedation in the ICU

Karan Madan, Ritesh Agarwal

INTRODUCTION

Critically ill patients experience a wide variety of stress in the intensive care unit (ICU) environment. Patient discomfort may be attributed to trauma and invasive procedures or related to prolonged immobility, nursing care, and various forms of monitoring and therapy. Pain, presence of catheters or tubes, and disruption of sleep are important sources of distress to the patients in the unfamiliar ICU enclosure. Also, a number of patients in the ICU develop delirium which may be associated with increased long-term morbidity and poor psychological outcomes, like post-traumatic stress disorder. Delirium is found to be common in patients on longer duration of ventilation and hospitalization.

TEAMWORK (MULTIDISCIPLINARY MANAGEMENT) AND PATIENT-FOCUSED CARE

The choice of medication and the target level of sedation and analgesia need to be individualized. The core principle of patient-focused care is based on the varying needs of sedative and analgesic medications in different patients at different times. Higher levels of sedation and even neuromuscular blockade are required when using nonconventional techniques, such as high frequency oscillatory ventilation or positioning the acute respiratory distress syndrome patient prone. Nursing staff play an extremely important role as they interact with the patients most frequently.

INITIAL EVALUATION AND MEDICATION RECONCILIATION

Initial interventions should be targeted at appropriate management of the predisposing conditions along with sedative, analgesic, and antipsychotic medications as deemed appropriate according to the clinical situation. The concept of medication reconciliation is extremely important when patients move into and out of the ICU. As many as 50% of all medication errors occur at the time of ICU admission or discharge. In approximately 60% of the patients, regular medications are discontinued at the time of admission to the ICU. In the context of sedation and analgesia, omission of medications like antidepressants, anxiolytics, analgesics or antipsychotics can lead to many undesirable consequences. There are also risks of precipitation of withdrawal symptoms.

CONSEQUENCES OF OFF-TARGET SEDATION AND ANALGESIA

Improper assessment and inadequate treatment of pain and agitation in the ICU is associated with a number of adverse consequences (Box 86.1).

Need for Frequent Patient Assessment

A large proportion of ICU patients are oversedated as observed in epidemiological surveys. An important finding was the demonstration that during nighttime, an extremely low proportion of nursing staff perceived their patients to be oversedated.

ASSESSMENT OF PAIN, SEDATION, AND AGITATION IN THE ICU

Assessment of pain, level of consciousness, agitation, and cognition are central to patient management. Decisions regarding change in medication can be done accordingly.

BOX 86.1: Consequences of off-target sedation and analgesia.

- *Consequences of inadequate pain relief and agitation:*
  - Self-extubation and removal of other tubes and catheter devices
  - Violent behavior
  - Patient ventilator dyssynchrony
  - Excessive pain leading to increased agitation and anxiety
  - Precipitation of myocardial ischemia in susceptible patients
  - Pain-related immunosuppression
- *Consequences of oversedation:*
  - Pressure nerve palsies due to neural compression
  - New-onset delirium
  - Prolonged duration of mechanical ventilation
  - Prolongation of intensive care unit and hospital length of stay
  - Pressure sores and infections
  - Increased incidence of ventilator-associated pneumonia

Use of Validated Scales and Tools

The use of validated assessment methods like sedation scales, pain assessment tool, and delirium assessment tool provides homogeneity of assessment between different caregivers; enhances communication, and provides objective measurement, therefore cardinal to patient-focused care. In addition, the use of scales permits medication titration to the desired levels thereby minimizing the risk of oversedation and provision of adequate analgesia.

Assessment of Pain

Experiencing pain is extremely distressing for any individual. Relatively simple procedures that occur frequently in the ICU, such as suctioning and repositioning, are usually reported as the greatest source of discomfort to the ICU patients.

Pain Assessment Methods

- *Communicative patients:* Patient's self-report is the gold standard for assessment of pain.
  - Numeric rating scale or numeric pain scale (NPS): It utilizes rating of pain on a 0–10 scale with 0 indicating no pain and 10 being the worst pain experienced. A body outline diagram along with the NPS can help to localize the site of pain
- *Noncommunicative patients*: A number of other scales rely on the patient's behavioral and physiologic parameters to signify the presence of pain in the noncommunicative adults.

The COMFORT scale and the FLACC (face, legs, activity, cry, consolability observational tool) scale were meant for use in the pediatric population. The PAIN (pain assessment, intervention, and notation) algorithm incorporates observation of pain-related variables but is too cumbersome in its original form for routine ICU use. The behavioral pain scale (BPS) and the critical care pain observation tool (CPOT) are objective pain assessment scales which can be used in ICU patients during mechanical ventilation. Both have been tested for validity and reliability.

Other Methods for Assessment of Pain

Pain risk profile: It is based on the identification of various individual and environmental factors which may contribute to pain in ICU patients. Early identification of susceptible individuals may allow early initiation of appropriate analgesic therapy.

Surrogate reporting: This method relies on the information provided by the surrogates, usually family members.

Analgesic response: This is based on the principle of therapeutic challenge with analgesics. It can be tried when the patient is unable to self-report and there is likelihood of presence of pain.

> **BOX 86.2:** Various sedation scales.
>
> - Ramsay sedation scale (RSS)
> - Richmond Agitation–Sedation Scale (RASS)
> - Sedation agitation scale (SAS)
> - Motor activity assessment scale (MAAS)
> - Adaptation to the intensive care environment (ATICE) instrument
> - Minnesota Sedation Assessment Tool (MSAT)
> - Vancouver Interaction and Calmness Scale (VICS)

Assessment of Sedation and Agitation in the ICU

Use of a sedation scale is associated with improved quality of sedation and a statistically significant reduction in the hours of oversedation. A number of scales have been developed (Box 86.2).

Assessment of several other variables as below should also be done.

Cognition

- Cognition refers to the ability to follow commands.
- Ramsay sedation scale (RASS) and adaptation to the intensive care environment (ATICE) include the simultaneous assessment of cognition.
- The RASS additionally permits the assessment of sustainability.

Agitation

Agitation is assessed by many scales. It is measured as a separate subscale in ATICE and Vancouver Interaction and Calmness Scale (VICS). Agitation assessment is incorporated into a single scale in sedation agitation scale (SAS), motor activity assessment scale (MAAS), and RASS.

OBJECTIVE MEASUREMENT OF THE CEREBRAL ACTIVITY IN THE ICU

Objective measurement of the brain activity can be done using the cerebral function monitors. These monitors record the electroencephalography (EEG) signals from the cerebral cortex, process them through various algorithms, in order to yield a dimensionless numeric value, which ranges from 0 (complete EEG suppression) to 100 (awake). The various available systems are the bispectral index (BIS), patient state index (PSI), narcotrend index, and the cerebral state index (CSI). BIS values in the ICU are often erroneous because of the electromyography interference or electrical current-related artifact.

Brain function in the ICU can be monitored objectively with response entropy, state entropy, and auditory-evoked potentials. BIS may also be useful for assessment of consciousness in patients under deep sedation and those paralyzed with neuromuscular blocking agents.

MANAGEMENT OF ANALGESIA AND SEDATION IN THE ICU

Most patients in the ICU require the administration of sedative-analgesic medications for optimizing comfort. The most important group comprises

> **BOX 86.3:** Dosing of the selected sedative analgesic medications.
>
> Drug loading dose or maintenance dose:
> - Morphine 2–4 mg intravenous (IV) bolus or 0.07–0.5 mg/kg/hr
> - Fentanyl 25–50 µg IV bolus or 0.7–10 µg/kg/hr
> - Hydromorphone 0.2–0.6 mg IV bolus or 7–15 µg/kg/hr
> - Midazolam 2–5 mg IV bolus or 0.04–0.2 mg/kg/hr
> - Lorazepam 2–4 mg IV bolus or 0.01–0.1 mg/kg/hr
> - Diazepam 0.03–0.1 mg/kg
> - Propofol 5–80 µg/kg/min
> - Dexmedetomidine 0.5–1 µg/kg over 10 minutes or 0.2–0.7 µg/kg/hr
> - Remifentanil 1 µg/kg over 1 minute or 0.6–15 µg/kg/hr

the mechanically ventilated patients, many of whom face the extremes of physiologic stress. In them, sedatives and analgesics are required to improve patient ventilator synchrony and oxygenation.

Intravenous (IV) route is the preferred route of administration, as it allows better dose titration, has a faster onset of action, and higher bioavailability than other routes (Box 86.3). Intermittent therapy should be used wherever possible and continuous infusions should be avoided since continuous IV sedation is associated with prolonged duration of mechanical ventilation and increased length of stay (LOS) in the ICU.

Analgesic Medications

Pharmacotherapy with opioid analgesic agents is the mainstay of provision of analgesia to patients in the ICU. Acetaminophen and the nonsteroidal anti-inflammatory agents possess weak analgesic activity and may lead to adverse effects in patients who are critically ill. Acetaminophen has a limited role in critically ill patients in provision of relief from mild to moderate pain or discomfort and use as an antipyretic agent.

Opioid Analgesics

Mechanism of action of opioids: Opioids stimulate the opioid receptors (μ, κ, and δ) which are widely distributed throughout the peripheral tissues and the central nervous system. The main μ receptor is subdivided into the μ_1 and the μ_2 subtypes. μ_1 receptors are responsible for the mediation of analgesia, whereas μ_2 receptor binding leads to constipation, nausea, and respiratory depression. κ receptor binding mediates spinal analgesia, pupillary constriction, and the sedative effects of opioids.

It is important to note that although opioid administration may lead to mild to moderate anxiolytic effect, they do not produce amnesia. Opioids have an excellent cough suppressant action. In addition, they provide a marked relief in the subjective sense of dyspnea. By a combination of these two effects, they may be particularly helpful in mechanically ventilated patients. Morphine, fentanyl, and hydromorphone are the most commonly used opioid analgesic agents in the ICU.

Morphine: Morphine is a μ receptor agonist, possesses weak κ and δ receptor agonistic activity. The excretion of both morphine and the active metabolites occurs through the kidney. Morphine should be avoided in renal insufficiency, to prevent drug accumulation.

Fentanyl: Fentanyl, a μ receptor agonist, has high lipid solubility and a rapid onset of action (<1 minute). Fentanyl is the preferred agent for rapid-onset analgesia in acutely distress.

Hydromorphone: Hydromorphone, a μ receptor agonist, is similar to morphine in duration of action and half-life. However, its hepatic metabolism (by glucuronidation) leads to inactive metabolites (hydromorphone-3-glucuronide) making hydromorphone the opioid of choice in patients with end-stage renal disease.

Remifentanil: Remifentanil, an ultrashort-acting selective μ receptor agonist, is emerging as a promising opioid analgesic for use in the critically ill patients. Because of the short duration of action, remifentanil may be preferable for analgesia in patients requiring frequent neurological assessments. Although the ultrashort action is beneficial in avoidance of prolonged drug effects, pain may rapidly emerge after drug discontinuation and longer acting agents may need to be administered to patients with ongoing pain.

Other agents: Meperidine with an onset of action and half-life similar to morphine should not be routinely used for analgesia in the ICU. It has an active metabolite, normeperidine, a central nervous system (CNS) stimulant which can cause neuroexcitation, manifested as tremors and seizures.

Side effects of opioids:
- Respiratory depression*:* Opioids lead to dose-dependent, centrally mediated respiratory depression with respiratory rate decreased initially with preserved tidal volumes. As the dosage increases, tidal volume also is reduced and ventilatory response to hypoxia is obtunded.
- Hypotension: Opioid-induced hypotension is of particular concern in hypovolemic and hemodynamically unstable patients and can occur in euvolemic patients also. By blunting the sympathetic tone, vagally mediated bradycardia, histamine release, and increase in systemic venous capacitance, opioids can cause a precipitous fall in blood pressure.
- Gastric retention and ileus*:* Routine use of stool softeners and stimulant laxatives may minimize opioid-induced constipation but is often ineffective, small bowel intubation for feeding may be required in view of gastric hypomotility.

Other side effects: Muscle rigidity, urinary retention, nausea, and pruritus.

Sedative Drugs

Benzodiazepines

Benzodiazepines, the most commonly used sedative agents in intensive care, have anxiolytic and anticonvulsant properties. They are potent inducers of anterograde amnesia but do not cause retrograde amnesia. The pharmacologic effect depends on the degree of GABA receptor (gamma-aminobutyric acid) binding. Approximately, 20% binding is associated with anxiolysis, 30–50% with sedation, and 60% with hypnosis.

Benzodiazepines are associated with a dose-dependent respiratory depression which is particularly marked when coadministration is done with opioids.

They can lead to hypotension particularly in hypovolemic patients. They can modulate the anticipatory pain response thereby can lead to reduction in the dose of opioids administered (an opioid-sparing effect).

Midazolam

Midazolam is a rapidly acting, water-soluble benzodiazepine (onset of action within 5 minutes) which has a short duration of action. The primary metabolite is 1-hydroxymidazolam glucuronide, a CNS depressant which can cause prolonged sedation especially if kidney failure is present, as it is renally excreted. Obese patients and patients with hypoalbuminemia can also have prolonged sedation after midazolam administration. CYP 3A4 inhibiting drugs like ketoconazole, itraconazole, and erythromycin can lead to prolongation of sedative effects of midazolam.

Midazolam infusions are recommended for short-term use only because of the unpredictable awakening and time to extubation if continued for longer than 48–72 hours. Midazolam is a preferred agent for rapid sedation of acutely agitated patients.

Lorazepam

Lorazepam effect starts within 5–20 minutes and lasts for up to 6–8 hours. Unlike midazolam, lorazepam hepatic metabolism produces inactive metabolites excreted by the kidney. An important concern with lorazepam administration is propylene glycol toxicity. Propylene glycol is used as a solubility enhancer of the drug for IV preparations. The toxicity may manifest as hyperosmolar states, worsening metabolic acidosis, and acute tubular necrosis. Monitoring of serum osmolal gap should be done in patients receiving 50 mg/day and greater or more than 1 mg/kg of lorazepam per day. An osmolal gap greater than 10–15 indicates significant accumulation of propylene glycol. Treatment involves discontinuation of lorazepam infusion. In severe cases, hemodialysis provides effective removal of propylene glycol.

Lorazepam use in the ICU was found to be an independent risk factor for transition to delirium, even after adjusting for covariates. Fentanyl, propofol, and morphine were also associated with higher odds ratio but not reaching statistical significance, in the same study.

Although lorazepam is recommended for the sedation of most patients via intermittent IV administration or continuous infusion, in view of the possible concerns regarding prolonged emergence times, risk of propylene glycol toxicity and possible increased risk of delirium, prolonged infusions of lorazepam should be used cautiously. Midazolam is a better option in patients with normal renal and liver function parameters.

Propofol

Propofol (2,6 di-isopropylphenol) is a widely used ICU sedative. Like the benzodiazepines, it possesses sedative and hypnotic properties and provides amnesia. However, its site of binding on the GABA receptor is different from that of the benzodiazepines. It lacks analgesic properties therefore patients may require a greater dose of opioids for pain relief if receiving propofol rather than benzodiazepines.

It is profoundly lipophilic, therefore, crosses the blood–brain barrier, and rapid redistribution after infusion discontinuation leads to quick emergence times. Propofol is preferred agent for rapid awakening for example for neurological assessment. It reduces cerebral blood flow causing decrease of the intracranial pressure. It is metabolized in the liver but its clearance is not significantly altered by hepatic or renal disease. Clearance of the drug is slow in the elderly patients. Propofol causes profound respiratory depression, can also cause hypotension, especially in hypovolemic patients. Airway should be secured or intubation should be at standby whenever administering propofol.

Propofol is a caloric source and provides 1.1 kcal/mL from fat. Prolonged infusions may be associated with hypertriglyceridemia and also pancreatitis; therefore serum triglyceride levels should be monitored. Triglyceride concentrations should be monitored after 2 days of propofol infusion. Moreover, nutrition support prescription should include total caloric intake from lipids.

Propofol infusion syndrome: It is a rare complication of infusion of propofol, characterized by acute refractory bradycardia leading to asystole in the presence of one or more of the following: metabolic acidosis (base deficit >10 mmol.L^{-1}), rhabdomyolysis, hyperlipidemia, and enlarged or fatty liver. This potentially fatal condition may occur at doses higher than 4 mg/kg.h^{-1} for greater than 48 hours duration. Treatment involves immediate discontinuation of propofol and supportive treatment with hemodialysis or hemoperfusion, as the clinical setting dictates.

Dexmedetomidine

The drug possesses anxiolytic, sedative, and analgesic properties. There is no significant respiratory depression with its use. There is also mounting evidence to suggest that dexmedetomidine may have some protective effects against ischemic and hypoxic injury.

The onset of action occurs after approximately 15 minutes of IV injection, the drug distribution occurs rapidly from the brain, leading to a short terminal half-life. Hepatic metabolism by glucuronidation leads to production of inactive metabolites. Dose reductions are required in the presence of both renal and liver disease. The drug is apparently remarkably safe when administered as the sole agent, with oversedation which spontaneously recovers on drug discontinuation being the only reported adverse event on accidental infusion of large doses. However, on coadministration with sympatholytic or cholinergic agents in the settings of vagal stimulation, there is a risk for excessive bradycardia and even sinus arrest.

Dexmedetomidine can provide excellent sedation without respiratory depression during fiberoptic intubation or other difficult airway procedures. In these settings, it has added benefits of decreasing saliva production and airway secretions. In high infusion doses, it has been used as a sole agent to anesthetize patients with tracheal stenosis, as it preserves spontaneous ventilation. The most important treatment-related adverse effect of dexmedetomidine is bradycardia.

Volatile Anesthetic Sedation

Volatile anesthetic agents offer the advantage of quick onset and offset of action and ease of titration of effect. The route of delivery and elimination are primarily the lungs, therefore, hepatic or renal dysfunction has little impact on the duration of effect and emergence times. Excellent control of the drug effect can be done by monitoring the end-tidal concentration or fraction. Adverse effects can be immediately reversed by decreasing the inspired concentration of the agent. Isoflurane, desflurane, and sevoflurane have been used for ICU sedation. The major obstacles to the use of volatile anesthetics for ICU sedation are cost, concerns for environmental pollution, and the need of anesthetic expertise. The requirement of a cumbersome circuit for delivery hinders their use.

The use of volatile anesthetic sedation has demonstrated shorter emergence times (isoflurane vs. midazolam or propofol), shorter times to extubation and hospital LOS postcardiac surgery (sevoflurane vs. propofol), better cognitive functions after emergence (desflurane vs. propofol), and a trend towards lesser propensity to develop delirium (isoflurane vs. midazolam). Volatile anesthetic sedation may become an attractive alternative to routine use of IV sedative agents in the ICU in future.

Peripherally Acting µ-opioid Receptor Antagonists

Opioids can cause a number of gastrointestinal side effects such as constipation, ileus, and delayed gastric emptying. Peripherally acting µ-opioid receptor antagonists (PAM-ORAs) can be used to antagonize the peripheral side effects of opioids, importantly constipation and ileus. They do not cross the blood–brain barrier to antagonize the central effects of opioids, hence preserving the analgesic effects.

Use of Patient-targeted Sedation: Analgesia Protocols and Daily Interruption of Sedation

Use of Sedation Protocols or Algorithms

Use of protocols for ICU sedation and analgesia involves assessment of pain and levels of sedation, using validated assessment tools and integration of the same into an algorithm according to which changes in the medication dosage are done. Patient management regarding ICU sedation and analgesia is multidisciplinary; therefore, this area is particularly well suited to a protocolized and structured approach.

The primary aim of these approaches is to avoid accumulation of medications and their active metabolites which can be associated with a slower rate of recovery from critical illness. Critically ill patients are susceptible to prolonged effects of sedative analgesic medications, owing to a number of factors like alterations in volume and protein-binding status and presence of renal or hepatic dysfunction and other factors. Use of protocols has also been associated with reduction in diagnostic studies for unexplained changes in mental status, a reduction in the side effect of medications, and reduction in hospitalization costs. Less patient ventilator dyssynchrony and decreased incidence of VAP have also been found to be associated with the use of a sedation algorithm or protocol.

Analgesia-based Sedation Protocols or Cosedation

Recently, there has been interest in strategies that focus primarily on provision of analgesia, with addition of a sedative or hypnotic agent as and when required—termed as "analgesia based" or "cosedation" strategies. Two approaches have been used in trials. In one, initially titration of analgesic infusion is done prior to the addition of a sedative drug. In the other approach, coinfusion of both sedative and analgesic drugs has been done.

Analgesia-based strategies have been demonstrated to reduce the duration of mechanical ventilation, lead to better sedation with more "on-target" sedation, less patient ventilator asynchrony, and faster awakening for neurological assessment in neurotrauma patients.

Daily interruption of sedation (DIS): The underlying principle of this strategy is to provide a daily drug-free period to minimize the chances of drug accumulation and allow the patient to awaken. A reassessment can be done to the actual level of pain, level of agitation, and the readiness of the patient to tolerate spontaneous breathing. The strategy incorporating DIS (midazolam or propofol) and analgesic (morphine) medications until the patient was agitated or able to follow simple tasks, led to significant reductions in the duration of mechanical ventilation, use of less number of diagnostic tests for unexplained altered level of consciousness, and a shorter ICU LOS.

Daily interruption of sedation has also been associated with a reduction in the risk of several well-known complications of critical illness like ventilator-associated pneumonia, upper gastrointestinal bleed, bacteremia, cholestasis, barotraumas, venous thromboembolism, and sinusitis requiring surgical intervention. A careful clinical observation is required while practicing the DIS strategy. If the patient develops signs of increasing distress and agitation, a bolus administration of the drugs can be done and infusions restarted at half the previous rates. Patients who, after the daily interruption of medications, do not develop signs of increased agitation and are awake, should have their drugs restarted only when needed, not routinely.

RECENT DEVELOPMENTS AND NOVEL APPROACHES

"No Sedation" Protocols

This strategy appears promising but findings will need to be confirmed in large, multicenter trials, before it can be widely adopted. Nonetheless, this approach may provide a shift in paradigm for the future research trials to using as less sedation in the ICU as possible.

Patient-controlled Sedation for Mechanical Ventilation

Based on the demonstration that patients who self-administer analgesics, i.e. patient-controlled analgesia, eventually have lesser drug requirements and achieve better symptom control; it was hypothesized that patient-controlled sedation in mechanically ventilated patients, an untested approach till now, might lead to reduced sedative requirements, and eventually may be associated with better clinical outcomes.

Sedation and Analgesia Withdrawal

Symptoms of acute withdrawal syndrome can occur following prolonged administration of these agents in the ICU. Also, frank withdrawal symptoms may not be obvious all the time; patient may manifest clinical signs only. Withdrawal symptoms and even physical dependency have been documented, particularly in critically ill pediatric population with almost any agent. Development of withdrawal syndrome may have potential deleterious consequences and has also been linked to the development of ICU delirium. One should carefully monitor for nonspecific indicators of withdrawal such as hypertension, tachycardia, fever, nausea, insomnia, delirium, agitation, and diaphoresis. Gradual reduction of sedative and analgesic medications is important in patients at high risk, particularly the children.

Delirium in the ICU

Delirium, seen in about 35–80% of the ICU patients, is diagnosed by the presence of an acute change mental status, inattention, disorganized thinking, and fluctuation in the level of consciousness. Agitation may also be present. Delirium is independently associated with a longer hospital stay, increased mortality and higher economic costs. Delirium is classified as hypoactive, hyperactive, or mixed. Hypoactive delirium characterized by psychomotor retardation is associated with the worst prognosis. Unlike hyperactive delirium which is easily recognized, hypoactive delirium is difficult to detect.

Assessment of Delirium in the ICU

Assessment of delirium should be routinely done in critically ill patients even in calm and apparently nonagitated patients. Clinical history and examination forms the gold standard for the diagnosis of delirium. This method of assessment is usually not possible in critically ill and ventilated subjects because of the inability to speak and write and, therefore, other tools for assessment of ICU delirium have been developed. These tools can be used for delirium assessment by trained ICU staff and not necessarily by psychiatrists.

Prevention and Treatment of Delirium

Delirium prevention in the ICU: The strategies for prevention of delirium may be divided into nonpharmacologic, pharmacologic, and combined approaches. Use of certain nonpharmacologic approaches has demonstrated favorable outcomes in non-ICU patients. These strategies based on the underlying principles of reorientation, communication, mobilization, and minimization of drug exposure may be used in ICU subjects too. Pharmacologic approaches to reduce delirium in the ICU have not been evaluated extensively. No studies have been done to assess the role of prophylactic haloperidol in the ICU patients. Dexmedetomidine appears to be a promising drug which may assume an important role in ICU delirium management. A combined approach using both pharmacologic and nonpharmacologic methods has been tried, with a reduction in subsyndromal delirium. These strategies are difficult to implement, may not be appropriate for use in all patients.

Treatment of delirium: Pharmacologic therapy remains the mainstay of management of delirium in the ICU. Attention should first be paid to the recognition of an underlying correctable cause. Antipsychotic agents are the most commonly used and recommended drugs for the management of delirium. Both conventional and atypical antipsychotic agents are apparently effective.

Haloperidol, olanzapine, and quetiapine have been used in the management.

Haloperidol is the drug of choice for the treatment of delirium. It is usually administered by intermittent IV injections with a starting dose of 2 mg IV followed by repeated doubling doses every 15–20 minutes. The loading dose is meant for the control of acute agitation. Afterwards, intermittent doses (25% of the loading dose) may be given every 6 hours followed by gradual tapering.

Monitoring should be done for electrocardiographic changes (QT interval prolongation and arrhythmias) when receiving haloperidol. Development of extrapyramidal syndrome (EPS) is another known complication of administration of neuroleptic agents. If EPS develops, haloperidol should be stopped and a trial of diphenhydramine or benztropine should be given.

Prior to hospital discharge, cognitive function assessment is preferable in all the patients with proper neuropsychiatric advice and rehabilitation during follow-up, if required.

In conclusion, teamwork and patient-focused care play a key role in the management. Adequate pain relief should always take priority oversedative administration and adequacy of analgesia should be determined using patient self-report, if possible. Protocol-based sedation and DIS are strategies which are backed up with good quality evidence to be associated with better patient outcomes. Delirium assessment using validated delirium assessment tools should be included as a part of the patient assessment and delirium should be appropriately managed.

CHAPTER
87

Weaning from Mechanical Ventilation

Ajmal Khan, Ritesh Agarwal

INTRODUCTION

Weaning is the process of withdrawal of ventilatory support. It includes discontinuation of mechanical ventilation (MV) as well as removal of artificial airway, if any. Weaning can be either abrupt or gradual depending upon the clinical condition of the patient. The weaning process may represent almost 40–50% of the total duration of MV; the time involved in weaning is likely to be higher in patients with slowly resolving underlying diseases.

The process of weaning begins when the patient has started recovering from acute respiratory failure, maintaining balance aggressiveness with safety while making a clinical decision. The assessment for weaning generally begins from the first day of ventilation. Not only delayed weaning is associated with increased costs of intensive care unit (ICU) care but the risks of nosocomial pneumonia, iatrogenic lung injury, and death are also increased. On the other hand, a premature weaning attempt carries the risk of compromised gas exchange and airway protection, muscle fatigue, difficulty in re-establishing the airway, and 6–12-fold increased risk of mortality.

Weaning can further be classified as:
- *Simple weaning*: Initiation of weaning to successful extubation on the first attempt without any significant problem.
- *Difficult weaning*: Failure to tolerate initial spontaneous breathing trial (SBT); successful weaning after up to three SBTs or up to 7 days from first SBT.
- *Prolonged weaning*: Failure of at least three SBT or weaning after more than 7 days of the first SBT.

Both difficult and prolonged weaning increase the duration of hospitalization and carry a higher ICU mortality of approximately 25%.

PATHOPHYSIOLOGY OF WEANING

In a patient being mechanically ventilated, a complex interaction of control of breathing, lung and chest wall mechanics, respiratory muscles, gas exchange properties of the lung, and the cardiovascular hemodynamics determines the process and timing of weaning. Disturbance at any level can potentially lead to weaning failure.

Altered Control of Breathing

Central drive is depressed due to metabolic alkalosis and the use of sedative or hypnotic drugs. This can occur secondarily to either a structural lesion, such as brainstem strokes, central apneas or metabolic factors (such as electrolyte disturbances or sedation or narcotic usage).

Additionally, structural or metabolic abnormalities, including drugs affecting the peripheral nerves will also result in altered afferent or efferent output and ventilator dependence.

Altered Respiratory Mechanics

Physiological variables most commonly altered during weaning process are the resistance, elastance, and air trapping. Four factors account for the increase in resistance; these are increased inspiratory flow, decrease in lung volume, accumulation of secretions, and bronchoconstriction. Auto-positive end-expiratory pressure (auto-PEEP) increases the pressure gradient required to inspire irrespective of whether patient is triggering the ventilator or breathing spontaneously. The increase in inspiratory threshold raises the work of breathing and weaning failure.

Respiratory Muscle Dysfunction

Respiratory muscle weakness occurs commonly in the critically ill patients as a consequence of:
- Atrophy and remodeling from inactivity
- Critical illness neuropathy and myopathy
- Drugs (neuromuscular blockers, aminoglycosides, and corticosteroids)
- Metabolic factors like nutrition, electrolytes, and hormones
- Imbalance between respiratory muscle capacity and the load.

Inadequate nutrition causes increased protein catabolism leading to a loss of muscle performance. Similarly, in semistarvation conditions, normal hypoxic ventilatory response and hypercapnic ventilatory response deteriorate. In contrast, overfeeding leads to excess CO_2 production that may impair the ventilator withdrawal by further increasing the ventilation loads on ventilatory muscles.

Electrolyte imbalance such as deficiency of phosphate and magnesium impedes ventilatory muscle function. Severe hypothyroidism and myxedema also depress the diaphragmatic function as well as blunt the ventilatory responses to hypercapnia and hypoxia. Beside thyroid hormone, insulin/glucagon and adrenal corticosteroids are also important for optimal muscle function, deficiency of any of them may cause respiratory muscle dysfunction.

Cardiovascular Performance

All the ventilatory work during respiration is performed by respiratory muscle without getting fatigued. Thus they depend on an efficient transport of oxygen by the cardiovascular system. Cardiovascular dysfunction during the transition from MV to spontaneous breathing occurs due to increased metabolic and circulatory demands, increased venous return due to displacement of blood from the abdomen to thorax by contracting diaphragm and increased left ventricular after load imposed by negative pleural pressure swings.

OUTCOME OF WEANING

Weaning failure is defined as any of the following: (1) Failure of the weaning process; (2) Intolerance indicated by objective indices (such as tachypnea, tachycardia, hypertension, hypotension, hypoxemia or acidosis, arrhythmia) and subjective indices (such as agitation or distress, depressed mental status, diaphoresis, and evidence of increasing effort); (3) The need for reintubation within 48 hours following extubation.

ASSESSMENT FOR WEANING

The evaluation of patients' readiness for weaning begins with the resolution of respiratory failure and/or the disease entity that prompted the initiation of MV as well as the presence of a basic level of physiological readiness like intact airway reflexes, afebrile state, and cardiovascular stability. The patient's capacity to breathe spontaneously is often underestimated by the subjective criteria and clinical judgment. To facilitate the process of assessment, various objective criteria have been established. Nevertheless, the objective criteria only need to assist physician's clinical judgment, and many patients may be weaned even if they do not fulfill these criteria.

Indices to Predict Weaning Success Prior to SBT

Even prior to the implementation of an SBT, there are certain simple indices that are used to predict the outcome of the weaning trial.

Simplified Weaning Index (SWI)

$SWI = F_V \times (IP - PEEP)/MIP \times 40 \times PaCO_2$

A SWI less than 9 per minute is 93% predictive of successful weaning in the patient whereas a SWI greater than 11 per minute is 95% predictive of weaning failure.

CROP Index (Compliance, Rate, Oxygenation, Pressure)

The CROP index incorporates several measures: dynamic respiratory system compliance (Crs), spontaneous breathing frequency (f), arterial to alveolar oxygenation [partial pressure of arterial oxygen (PaO_2)/partial pressure of alveolar oxygen (PAO_2)], and PI_{max}:

$$CROP\ index = C_{dyn} \times MIP/f \times (PaCO_2/PACO_2)$$

The CROP index measures the relationship between the demands placed on the respiratory system and the ability of the respiratory muscles to handle them. A CROP index of more than 13 mL/breaths/min predicts successful weaning.

Rapid Shallow Breathing Index

Rapid shallow breathing index, i.e. the ratio of frequency to tidal volume obtained during the first minute of a T-piece trial at a threshold value of less than or equal to 105 breaths/min/L, predicts weaning outcomes significantly better than other "classic" and commonly used parameters. But RSBI has certain pitfalls: (i) excessive false positive predictions and (ii) a less predictive power in chronic obstructive pulmonary disease (COPD) and elderly patients as well as those who need ventilatory support for more than 8 days. In such patients who have RSBI of less than or equal to 105 breaths/min/L, one may use SBT of 30–120 minutes to further assess patient readiness for weaning.

Rapid shallow breathing index is also influenced by the ventilatory settings, has a limited value when measured during trials of pressure support ventilation (PSV). It should only be used when patients is disconnected from the ventilator and spontaneously breathe for 1 minute. It can easily be applied at the bedside to readily identify patients who are candidates for SBT.

Muscle Load Indices

These require more sophisticated measurements, such as pleural pressure (estimated from esophageal pressure) to calculate the pressure time product and pressure time index (PTI). PTI can be a useful predictor of fatigue when it is more than 0.1.

TECHNIQUES OF WEANING

Once the patient has passed the predictor test, patient can be immediately extubated. Because of the high rates of postextubation distress and reintubation rates of approximately 40%, this approach is not recommended and there is need for a formal weaning trial before extubation. Weaning trials also improve the patient's likelihood of tolerating extubation because of the improved reconditioning of the respiratory muscles. The major techniques used for weaning from MV is simply to initiate a trial of unassisted spontaneous breathing in the form of either a T-piece trial, low level continuous positive airway pressure (CPAP) trial, synchronized intermittent mandatory ventilation (SIMV) trial, PSV trial or a combination of these trials. As long as the principle of "Do Not Exhaust" is followed, the decision on which trial to use, remain largely a matter of physician preference and the local protocols. SBTs are used to test

readiness for weaning as well as to implement a weaning protocol that involves increasing periods of unsupported spontaneous breathing interspersed with periods of full ventilatory support.
Available methods of weaning are:
- Conventional methods:
  - Spontaneous breathing trials
  - Pressure support ventilation
  - Synchronized intermittent mandatory ventilation
  - SIMV with PSV.
- Newer modes:
  - Automatic tube compensation
  - Adaptive support ventilation
  - Automode ventilation
  - Airway pressure release ventilation
  - Volume-assured pressure support
  - Proportional assist ventilation
  - Noninvasive positive pressure ventilation.

Spontaneous Breathing Trials

These consist of disconnection from the ventilator and putting the patient on T-piece with supplemental oxygen. It is mainly used to assess the readiness for extubation but it can also be used for weaning. The length of each SBT is gradually increased and ventilatory support is decreased. SBT can be given without disconnecting the patient from the ventilator so that ventilatory support may be immediately reinstituted in case of SBT failure. SBT can be performed at low level of CPAP (5 cm H_2O) or pressure support (PS) (7 cm H_2O).

Prolongation of a failing SBT may precipitate muscle fatigue, hemodynamic instability, discomfort or worsened gas exchange. The initial few minutes of an SBT should be closely monitored because the adverse effects usually occur early. To assure safety, SBT may be continued for about 30 minutes but not more than 120 minutes. Failure of SBT is defined by the appearance of tachypnea, tachycardia, arrhythmia, hypertension, hypotension, hypoxemia or other evidence of agitation or distress, depressed mental status, and diaphoresis.

Prompt search should be made for other causes or complicating factors in a case of a failed spontaneous breathing and appropriate medical management is optimized. SBTs during the next day are not helpful because the failures are often due to persistent mechanical abnormalities of the respiratory system (especially the muscle fatigue) which are not likely to reverse rapidly. The process of weaning can be expedited with the help of computer driven assessments and clinician feedback tools to perform SBTs and sedation optimization strategy.

Pressure Support Ventilation

In this method of weaning, PS is gradually reduced and the patient's inspiratory effort is recognized. It ensures appropriate delivery at the time of inspiration and cycles to the expiratory phase with passive patient exhalation. Breath is flow cycled to the expiratory phase when the flow decelerates to 5 L/min or 25% of the peak inspiratory flow. Flow deceleration is determined by resistance and compliance of the respiratory system which decelerates slowly in patients with airflow obstruction. Active exhalation is stimulated if the flow needed to cycle is not reached. During weaning, PSV is started at around 10–20 cm of H_2O and reduced by 2–4 cm H_2O at least twice daily till very low values can be tolerated. PSV is useful to counteract the extra work imposed by breathing through an endotracheal tube.

Synchronized Intermittent Mandatory Ventilation

Weaning by SIMV is achieved by gradually decreasing the mandatory breathing rate by 2–4 breaths per minute and allowing the patient for spontaneous breathing effort to maintain the minute ventilation. As traditionally believed, respiratory muscle rest does not occur during mandatory breath of SIMV. In fact, respiratory center output and respiratory muscle activity are as great during the mandatory breaths as the spontaneous breaths.

Continuous Positive Airway Pressure

Continuous positive airway pressure by itself is not a mode as it does not provide any inspiratory support. CPAP when applied during spontaneous breathing in patients with acute respiratory insufficiency, reduces mean intrathoracic pressure, has beneficial effects on right and left ventricular performance, improves oxygenation, and reduces the work of breathing. Although combinations of CPAP and PSV are commonly applied during the weaning period, there is also a lack of prospective randomized controlled trials to suggest that CPAP is superior to other techniques, such as PSV alone or T-tube in the process of weaning from invasive MV.

Role of Noninvasive Ventilation in Weaning

Mechanical ventilation once instituted, can be withdrawn abruptly in majority of patients. Approximately one-third of the patients require gradual weaning. Among them, 13–19% need reintubation because of postextubation respiratory failure. The need for reintubation is an independent predictor of mortality even though it does not imply an increased severity of illness. Therefore, strategies that prevent the development of respiratory failure after extubation and subsequent reintubation are needed. One such strategy is the application of noninvasive ventilation (NIV) that has been applied in patients with difficult weaning as well as used for the prevention and treatment of postextubation respiratory failure.

Noninvasive ventilation is shown to decrease duration of MV, ICU, and hospital stays in patients with chronic respiratory failure due to COPD. It is also associated with lesser incidence of nosocomial pneumonia, decreased need for tracheotomy, facilitate weaning, as well as an improvement in survival. A longer time from extubation to reintubation is associated with worse outcome. Therefore, the delay in reintubation correlates with worse survival rates in patients who had received NIV for established postextubation respiratory failure.

Early use of NIV to avert respiratory failure after extubation in patients at risk is shown to decrease the reintubation rate and ICU mortality compared to standard therapy, even though it does not improve the hospital mortality. It can be concluded that NIV is useful to facilitate weaning in hypercapnic respiratory failure as well as to prevent postextubation respiratory failure in high-risk patients, such as the elderly, those with multiple comorbidities, weaning failures, chronic heart failure, and with APACHE II (Acute Physiology And Chronic Health Evaluation II) score more than 12 on the day of extubation.

Automated Weaning

There are a number of feedback systems that automatically reduce the level of applied pressure (in pressure-support breaths) for patients recovering from respiratory failure. These algorithms may incorporate different targets such as the simple tidal volume, tidal volume with rate and inspiratory/expiratory time considerations, and tidal volume with rate and end-tidal CO_2 considerations.

Role of Tracheostomy

Tracheostomy is useful for long-term airway access in patients requiring prolonged MV. Tracheostomy has several advantages: (i) improved patient comfort and better articulated speech, (ii) effective airway suctioning, (iii) decreased airway resistance due to short length of tracheostomy tubes, (iv) better patient mobility, and (v) greater airways security and ability to eat orally. As a result, there occur fewer ventilator-related complications and accelerated weaning from MV. Tracheostomy reduces the work of breathing and may also decrease the need for sedation.

SUMMARY

In summary, both disease factors and management factors may lead to difficult weaning that requires a good assessment for the readiness of weaning. It is important to choose appropriate mode(s) of ventilatory support which maintain a favorable balance between respiratory system capacity and load, attempt to avoid diaphragm muscle atrophy, and aid in the weaning process. The SBT is the "gold standard" for ventilator withdrawal. It is advisable to wait for 24 hours before attempting a new trial of spontaneous breathing. A failed trial can precipitate respiratory muscle fatigue. Decision to extubate in successful SBT requires further assessment of patient's ability to protect the airway. Pressure support or assist-control ventilation modes are preferred in patients failing initial trial or trials. We generally use gradual reduction of PS in these patients with PS reduced by 2 cm H_2O every 6 hours. NIV trial to facilitate weaning is warranted in selected patients especially those with hypercapnic respiratory failure.

CHAPTER 88

Hyperbaric Oxygen Therapy

PS Tampi, SK Jindal

INTRODUCTION

Hyperbaric oxygen (HBO_2) therapy is defined as the administration of oxygen at a greater than one atmospheric pressure at sea level. Hyperbaric medicine owes its origin to the problems encountered by deep-sea divers, exposed to high-pressure diving sports, commercial or military expeditions at depths of 10 m or more. In clinical medicine, this is simulated by exposing a patient to hyperbaric atmosphere in a closed monoplace or multiplace chamber. In both situations, the partial pressure of arterial oxygen (PaO_2) approaches 1,500 mm Hg at a pressure equivalent to 33 fsw (feet of seawater).

RATIONALE OF HYPERBARIC OXYGEN

An increased atmospheric pressure increases the partial pressure of O_2 in the alveolar air and arterial blood, provided the fractional concentrations of oxygen remain the same. Since the oxygen dissolved in the plasma depends upon PaO_2, the dissolved O_2 content of blood is also increased. This is independent of hemoglobin levels of the blood. Therefore, under hyperbaric conditions the total oxygen-carrying capacity of the blood is significantly more. At 1 atmosphere (sea level), with a person breathing 100% O_2, the PaO_2 is about 670 mm Hg and the total oxygen content of 18.7 mL/dL. Increasing the pressure to 3 atmospheres, the PaO_2 increases to about 1,700 to 1,800 mm Hg and the total O_2 content to 22 mL/dL. Of this, about 25% (i.e. 5.5 mL/dL) is dissolved in plasma. This, in fact, is equivalent to the total oxygen content of blood under normal conditions, at much lower hemoglobin level of 4 g%. Therefore, under hyperbaric conditions, it is possible to maintain adequate oxygen content of blood as well as delivery to the tissues with a very low or no hemoglobin at all. However, it should be remembered that the whole of the tissue oxygen requirements can be met by dissolved oxygen, only if PaO_2 is around 2,025 mm Hg.

OTHER PHYSIOLOGICAL EFFECTS OF HYPERBARIC OXYGENATION

- *Effect on $PaCO_2$*: An increased hemoglobin saturation of venous blood reduces its ability to carry CO_2, and results in carbon dioxide accumulation (Haldane effect).
- *Vasoconstriction*: Occurs due to increase in PaO_2, and has a therapeutic value.
- *Angiogenesis*: The mechanism by which this occurs is not known but occurs only when oxygen is administered at more than 1 atmosphere absolute (ATA) pressure. and does not occur with 100% oxygen at 1 ATA.

BENEFICIAL EFFECTS OF HBO_2

Hyperbaric oxygen administration achieves two principal objectives:
1. It increases PaO_2 and tissue PO_2 to levels higher than those obtained at 1 atmosphere. This has several potential therapeutic benefits. The oxygen delivery to the tissues is increased, which may promote healing; the phagocytosis and antibiotic action on the microorganisms are augmented. Hyperoxia induces vasoconstriction, which reduces tissue edema. Finally, the oxygen dissolved in the plasma is available to the tissues, without any increase required in the hemoglobin level. This is not associated with any increase by blood transfusions. Problems of increased blood viscosity are therefore avoided.
2. There is an increase in the ambient pressure which increases interstitial tissue pressures as well. This is used to treat decompression sickness (DCS), which may occur in divers. Similarly, presence of air or gas in the blood either injected accidentally during some procedure or due to embolization can be absorbed with HBO_2 therapy.

MECHANISM OF ACTION OF HBO_2

- Hyperbaric oxygen increases dissolved oxygen in the plasma, which readily diffuses into the hypoxic tissues.
- Increased oxygenation results in vasoconstriction at the site, resulting in induced transudation, reduction in capillary pressure, and thereby reducing the tissue edema.
- The reduction in tissue edema reduces compression of the cells, thereby enhancing the reabsorption of fluid.
- With edema being less, barriers of diffusion are reduced and oxygen diffusion to the tissues improves, resulting of improvement in tissue functions.

- Improved vascularization due to neovascularization results in speedy recovery of tissues and gives way to tissue regeneration.
- Oxide, hydroperoxide, and superoxide radicals of oxygen are toxic, and interfere with cell metabolism of bacteria, and thereby destroy the bacteria.
- Hyperbaric oxygen modulates the immune system and helps in the faster elimination of viruses.
- Bacterial killing effect of leukocytes is impaired in the hypoxic state. Increased oxygenation will enhance the killing power of leukocytes.

INDICATIONS

Indications for HBO_2 are highly variable. DCS, air embolism, gas gangrene, and carbon monoxide (CO) poisoning are the only clearly defined indications.

Decompression Sickness

Decompression sickness occurs when the ambient air pressure is allowed to lower rapidly after a prolonged exposure to a higher pressure. This is commonly seen in the deep sea or scuba divers, after emerging from a diving juggernaut, and occasionally in the aviators or astronauts on reaching the outer atmosphere or space. Due to a sudden lowering of pressure, the inert gases dissolved in body fluids bubble out in both intravascular and extravascular compartments resulting in multiple symptoms.

The common clinical manifestations can be classified into three types: Type I includes musculoskeletal pains, skin and lymphatic tissue, often fatigue. Type II includes neurological symptoms (either central or peripheral such as paresthesias and sensorimotor deficits), cardiorespiratory (such as substernal pain, cough, and dyspnea), audiovestibular (such as nausea, vomiting, nystagmus, tinnitus, and hoarseness of voice), and shock. Type III syndrome is characterized with severe symptoms of DCS and arterial gas emboli (AGE). Sometimes, it is refractory to recompression and proves fatal. The bubbles in DCS injure the vascular endothelium, cause platelet aggregation, denatured lipoproteins, and activation of leukocytes. These changes are followed by capillary leaks and other proinflammatory events.

Hyperbaric oxygen decreases the size of the bubbles by increasing the pressure as well as by creating an oxygen gradient. In DCS type I, the mainstay of therapy consists of hyperbaric oxygen and recompression to about 60 fsw for two 20-minute periods, with a slow decompression to 30 fsw for another 20 minutes. For DCS type II and III, patients are placed at 60 fsw (2.8 ATA) for at least three 20-minute intervals and are then slowly decompressed to 30 fsw. The duration to keep a patient at 60 or 30 fsw depends on the patient's response to therapy. Both steps help in the reduction and resolution of the bubbles and maintenance of tissue oxygenation. Increased occurrence of oxygen toxicity under higher pressure conditions limits the duration of use of hyperbaric oxygen. Relapse may occur after discontinuation of the therapy. Short-term observation, especially in patients with neurological symptoms for at least

6 hours, is generally recommended. Some people advocate the provision of observation units for about 24 hours after hyperbaric therapy.

Air Embolism

Air bubbles may form in the venous circulation, due to sudden decompression (e.g. DCS) or more commonly get introduced during central venous instrumentation, invasive medical and surgical procedures, hemodialysis, chest trauma or positive pressure ventilation, and employing high levels of positive end-expiratory pressures. These air bubbles finally end up in the lungs, causing obstruction of pulmonary circulation, and presenting a picture of pulmonary air embolism. It may occasionally be fatal if a large pulmonary vessel gets blocked. Bubbles may also form in the arterial circulation, but are rare because of the higher hydrostatic pressure in the larger vessels. AGE due to pulmonary barotrauma causes symptoms within seconds to minutes of the event and can include loss of consciousness, confusion, neurological deficits, cardiac arrhythmias or cardiac arrest. Cerebral air embolism is uncommon but more serious in nature.

Treatment of air embolism employs resuscitative and restorative measures for pulmonary circulation through removal and/or absorption of air from the pulmonary vessels. Attempts to remove the air bubbles include direct needle aspiration, Trendelenburg position or removal through a central venous catheter. Administration of 100% oxygen helps reabsorption of air. Hyperbaric oxygen administration rapidly reduces the bubble size. Generally 50% O_2 at a pressure of 165 feet is administered initially for a few minutes followed by intermittent periods of 100% oxygen at a lower pressure of 65 feet.

Gas Gangrene and Other Necrotizing Infections

There is an increased evidence to suggest a major role of HBO_2 on inflammatory cytokines and mediators. It is shown to cause cytokine downregulation and growth factor upregulation. HBO_2, therefore, is likely to promote wound healing by suppressing inflammation and facilitating repair. It also augments the antibacterial action of leukocytes, which gets otherwise inhibited under hypoxic conditions and thereby improves the efficacy of antibiotics. These effects have been shown in a few clinical trials and clinical experience, when used as an adjunct treatment for gas gangrene, nonhealing wounds (e.g. diabetic foot), osteomyelitis, and necrotizing fasciitis. It is also shown to shorten the treatment with antibiotics for soft tissue infections. Angiogenesis occurs in response to high oxygen concentration through fibroblast proliferation and collagen synthesis. HBO_2 also likely stimulates growth factors and has direct and indirect antimicrobial activity thereby increasing intracellular leukocyte killing.

Carbon Monoxide Poisoning

Carbon monoxide, a byproduct of incomplete combustion of coal, is a colorless and odorless poisonous gas. It is a common cause of death in miners and other personnel working with coal furnaces in foundries and factories. CO poisoning, in India, occurs in people burning indoor coal for heating and cooking during winter months in ill-ventilated houses. Deaths in this scenario are commonly reported in individuals sleeping in closed rooms. Malfunctioning air conditioning systems in cabins have been occasionally blamed for CO poisoning.

Carbon monoxide poisoning is generally insidious. Neurological complications are most frequent. Some of the common symptoms include headache, confusion, dizziness, nausea, and vomiting. In more serious forms, syncope, seizures, and coma may precede the death. Cardiac arrhythmias and pulmonary edema may also occur.

Carbon monoxide affinity for hemoglobin is almost 300 times that of oxygen. Immediately on exposure to CO, therefore, there is displacement of oxygen and formation of carboxyhemoglobin (HbCO). CO also shifts the oxygen dissociation curve to the left (the Haldane effect), thereby restricting oxygen delivery to tissues. CO is also known to bind cytochrome oxidase aa3/C and myoglobin promoting reperfusion injury due to release of free radicals and lipid peroxidation.

Treatment of CO poisoning needs to be prompt and aggressive. A great degree of evidence supports that hypoxia occurs late in CO poisoning. But the treatment of both, the actually poisoned persons and the environmental exposures, is based on a hypoxic theory of toxicity. Oxygen therapy is the mainstay of therapy besides other supportive care.

Adjunct to Treatment of Cancers

Hyperbaric oxygen may improve the treatment of malignant tumors by increasing the tumor sensitization to radiotherapy. A significant improvement is reported with HBO_2 followed by radiotherapy for local tumor control, mortality for cancers of the head and neck, and local tumor recurrences in cancers of head, neck, and uterine cavity. It also improves the response to photodynamic and chemotherapy, possibly by raising intratumoral oxygen tension. It was also shown to improve survival in locally advanced breast cancer undergoing neoadjuvant chemotherapy. HBO_2 may also promote neovascularization and stimulate healing of radiation-induced tissue injury especially in areas with reduced oxygen tension.

Miscellaneous Conditions

- *Acute insults*:
  - Asphyxiation: Drowning, near-hanging, and smoke inhalation
  - Orthopedics trauma conditions such as crush injury, compartment syndrome, and soft tissue sports injuries
  - Hemodynamic shock, myocardial ischemia, and as an aid to cardiac surgery
  - Acute neurological conditions: Stroke, cerebral edema, spinal cord injury and vascular diseases of the spinal cord, brain abscess, and radiation myelitis

- Obstetrics: Complicated pregnancy, diabetes, eclampsia, heart disease, placental hypoxia, fetal hypoxia, and congenital heart disease of the neonate
- Hematology: Sickle cell crises and severe blood loss anemia
- Acute occlusion of central artery of retina
- Gastrointestinal: Gastric ulcer, necrotizing enterocolitis, and paralytic ileus, pneumatoides, cystoides intestinalis, and hepatitis
- Lung diseases: Lung abscess and pulmonary embolism (adjunct to surgery)
- Otorhinolaryngology: Sudden deafness, acute acoustic trauma, and labyrinthitis
- *Subacute and chronic conditions*:
  - Nonhealing wounds and venous leg ulcers: HBO_2 improves survival of skin flaps with poor circulation
  - Management of burns (reimplantation surgery), as an adjunct
  - Nonhealing fractures and bone grafts
  - Osteoradionecrosis
  - Subacute or chronic neurological conditions: Multiple sclerosis, migraine, multi-infarct dementia, and peripheral neuropathy
  - Deep coma—vegetative state
  - Chronic pain from fibromyalgia syndrome and myofascial pain syndrome
  - Migraine and cluster headache
  - Meniere's disease and malignant otitis externa (chronic infection)
  - Endocrines: Diabetes
  - Aid to rehabilitation: Spastic hemiplegia of stroke, paraplegia, chronic myocardial insufficiency, and peripheral vascular disease.

HBO_2 IN PEDIATRIC AGE GROUP

Since the proportion of surface area to body mass is much greater in children than in adults, and as the temperature within the chamber can fluctuate, the child needs to be kept warm without causing hyperthermia. Tympanostomy tube placements may be considered to prevent middle ear trauma.

POTENTIAL NEW INDICATIONS

Bisphosphonates-associated Osteonecrosis

Bisphosphonates are used in the treatment of bone metastases, osteoporosis, Paget's disease, and acute hypercalcemia. However, their use may lead to osteonecrosis in these patients. The pathophysiology leading to osteonecrosis is unknown. No reliable treatment for this condition is available at present.

CONTRAINDICATIONS

Contraindications for HBO_2 therapy can be divided into the absolute contraindications, which include untreated tension pneumothorax; and, relative contraindications, which include upper respiratory infections, bronchial asthma, emphysema with CO_2 retention, symptomatic pulmonary lesions seen on chest X-ray, history of thoracic or ear surgery, Eustachian tube disorders, congenital spherocytosis, pacemakers, epidural pain pump, uncontrolled high fever, pregnancy, claustrophobia, seizure disorders, and malignant diseases.

COMPLICATIONS

Hyperbaric oxygen toxicity is primarily related to pressure changes and the toxic effects of oxygen. Important complications include barotrauma to the ear, sinuses, and lungs. Trauma to ears or sinuses may be avoided with slow compression, the use of decongestants, and patient education. Very rarely, myringotomy may be done in severe and refractory cases. Pulmonary barotrauma is very rare, perhaps occurring 1 in 50,000 treatments. It can be prevented by careful pretreatment screening for pulmonary blebs, air trapping caused by bronchospasm or secretions, preexisting pneumothorax, central lines, and ventilatory support.

Oxygen toxicity with occurrence of grand mal seizures is noticed beyond a depth of 3 ATA (66 feet or 20 m of sea level). Damage of lung tissue, manifested by decrement in vital capacity and irritation to large airways, may occur due to oxygen toxicity following HBO_2. Increased pressure causes increased gas density and airway resistance. This produces an altered voice called the "Donald Duck voice", and an increased awareness of breathing. Hypoventilation may result especially in a patient with the underlying obstructive lung disease. Increased partial pressure of nitrogen causes symptoms of mild euphoria at pressure of 2.5 ATA, progressing to frank intoxication, and decreased performance at over 4 ATA.

Accumulation of O_2 may occur in the event of an exposure for several days. Hyperpnea and occasionally respiratory acidosis may result. Other toxic substances or pollutants, that may continue to accumulate in a closed chamber and reach toxic pressures, include alcohol (from disinfectant solution), sulfur dioxide, hydrocarbons, CO, volatile substances, and mercury vapors. A regular monitoring is required for their concentrations. The nursing and medical personnel looking after the patient in a hyperbaric chamber may suffer from DCS due to tissue bubble formation. The risk is rather low because the chamber is kept warm; exposure is short, and decompression rate is slow. Risk of an accidental fire is greater in hyperbaric conditions.

All inflammable material should, therefore, be kept away. Refractive changes and cataract in the lens of the eye may occur as a complication of prolonged HBO_2 therapy.

Claustrophobia may be a problem in up to 10% of patients, especially in the monoplace chamber.

In conclusion, the indications for HBOT have expanded significantly in the recent years. This is especially so for serious and non-responsive problems. But there are a number of complications which should be kept in mind whenever it is tried for doubtful and unproven indications.

CHAPTER
89

Pleura: Anatomy and Physiology

Srinivas Rajagopala

The pleural cavity is akin to a sealed, wet, and stretchable elastic bag inserted between the lung and thoracic wall which helps to decrease the friction generated between the lung and thoracic wall during respiratory movements. It comprises the serous, elastic pleural membranes with a smooth and lubricating surface which line the inner surface of the thoracic cage and the outer surface of the lungs and mediastinum.

ANATOMY OF THE PLEURA

The pleura is divided into the visceral pleura which covers the lung parenchyma, including the interlobar fissures and the parietal pleura which lines the inside of the thoracic cavities. The parietal pleura can be arbitrarily classified into the costal, mediastinal, and diaphragmatic pleura according to the structure it invests. The visceral and the parietal pleurae meet and fuse at the lung root. The surface area of the visceral pleura of one lung (approximately 1,000 cm) is similar to that of the parietal pleura of one hemithorax.

The balance of elastic recoil pressures of the chest wall and the lung, generate the pleural pressure which in humans is approximately -5 cm H_2O at mid-chest at Functional Residual Capacity (FRC) and -30 cm H_2O at Total Lung Capacity (TLC). The pleural pressure is also influenced by the pressure of pleural fluid, the regional pleural surface deformation, and weight of lung in dependent areas. The pleural space in health contains about 0.5–2 mL fluid on each side, allowing for close apposition of the visceral and parietal layers.

DEVELOPMENT OF THE PLEURAL MEMBRANES

The coelomic cavity in the fetus becomes partitioned into the pericardium and the pleural canals (cephalad portion) and into the peritoneal canals by the septum transversum (caudally) at three weeks of gestation. At 9-week development, the pleuropericardial and the pleuroperitoneal membranes divide the pericardial and pleural cavities and unite with the septum transversum. This leads to completion of the partition between each pleural cavity and the peritoneal cavity. This newly formed pleural cavity is fully lined by a mesothelial membrane that develops into the parietal pleura. The primordial lung buds bulging into the pleural cavities carry with them a covering of the lining mesothelium, which later develops into the visceral pleura.

HISTOLOGY OF THE PLEURA

The histology of the parietal pleura is fairly constant across species whereas that of the visceral pleura varies significantly. The parietal pleura has five layers and has a mean thickness of 20–25 µm. The layers include the innermost mesothelium, a submesothelial loose connective tissue layer, a superficial elastic layer, a subpleural highly vascularized loose connective tissue layer, and an outer fibroelastic layer. Mesothelial cells may have a variety of functions important to pleural biology. Mesothelial cells can secrete extracellular matrix components and also organize them. They also secrete neutrophil and monocyte chemotactic factors. Mesothelial cells also produce several cytokines like transforming growth factor-β, epidermal growth factor, and platelet-derived growth factor that are important in pleural inflammation and fibrosis. Microvilli are present on the surface of mesothelial cells and serve to increase surface area for metabolic activity. Lymphatic plexus of the costal pleura drains along the intercostal nodes; those in the mediastinal pleura drain to the trachea-bronchial and mediastinal nodes. The diaphragmatic pleura drains into the parasternal, middle phrenic, and posterior mediastinal nodes.

The visceral pleura may be thick (humans, sheep, cows, pigs, and horses) which is supplied by the bronchial circulation (systemic) or thin (dogs, cats, and monkeys) which depends on the lung parenchyma for nutrition. Sensory nerve fibers, supplied by the intercostal and phrenic nerves, are present in only the parietal pleura. Therefore, any pain from pleural inflammation indicates the involvement of the parietal pleura.

PLEURAL FLUID: NORMAL VOLUME AND CELLULAR CONTENTS

There is always a small amount of pleural fluid that is physiologically present in the pleural cavity. The fluid is maintained according to the Starling's forces and lymphatic drainage. Fluid exchange across the pleural membranes can be defined by the following relationship:

$$\text{Fluid movement} = L \times S [(P_{cap} - P_{pl}) - \sigma (\Pi_{cap} - \Pi_{pl})]$$

where P and C are the hydrostatic and osmotic pressures respectively, within the capillaries (cap) and pleural space (pl), L is the hydraulic conductivity of the membrane, S is the surface area, and Π is the osmotic coefficient for proteins.

Normal pleural fluid consists of a microvascular filtrate which is formed from the parietal pleura capillaries. It is drained predominantly via the parietal pleura lymphatic stoma; the absorptive gradient in the visceral pleural capillaries and the active transport across mesothelial cells play only a small role. The pleural fluid formed has characteristics of interstitial fluid (protein 1-2 g/100 mL and total leukocyte cell counts of 1,000-2,500/µL). Most of the protein is composed of albumin (50%), globulins (35%), and fibrinogen. The pleural fluid lines along the pleural surface with an average thickness of 20 µm (thicker in dependent portions). The pleural fluid protein ratio is low (i.e. 0.15-0.2) indicating exudation of protein from the pleural microvasculature.

There are two possible mechanisms to explain the regional differences in pleural pressure and fluid accumulation: (1) The *hydrostatic equilibrium model*, i.e. the vertical pressure gradient due to the viscous flow generates a continuous column of fluid throughout the pleural space and therefore creates a vertical gradient of 1 cm H_2O/cm height; (2) The *viscous flow model*, i.e. the pleural fluid pressure is always equal to pleural surface pressure. The thin layer of fluid formed due to hydrostatic forces separates the pleural surfaces; the pleural space is thus a "real" and not a potential space; as the pleural fluid accumulates, the viscous resistance to flow falls rapidly and the gradient approaches the hydrostatic pressure gradient of 1 cm H_2O/cm height. The pleural space is 20 µm across and pressures (Ppl) cannot be accessed without creating deforming forces in health. As effusions accumulate, however, Ppl can be measured. While measuring Ppl, the zero reference level is the top of the effusion. Placement of the needle at the most dependent level will prevent damage to lungs and helps to remove the largest amount of pleural fluid.

PHYSIOLOGY AND PATHOPHYSIOLOGY OF PLEURAL FLUID TURNOVER

Pleural fluid is formed at the parietal pleura capillaries. The constant pleural liquid production across species with differing visceral pleural thickness, the closer distance of parietal pleural microvessels (10-15 µm vs. 20-25 µm in visceral pleura) and the higher venous pressure in the parietal pleural side all favor a systemic (parietal pleural) origin of pleural fluid. Also the pleural fluid protein decreases as systemic blood pressure increases and also decreases with age (blood pressure increases and pulmonary resistance decreases with age), favoring the systemic circulation as the site of its formation. Fluid thus filtered enters the pleural space because of the leaky nature of the mesothelial surface and the strongly negative pleural pressures. In health, the pleural fluid production from parietal fluid capillaries in humans is about 0.01 mL/kg/hr.

Pleural fluid is absorbed by bulk flow at the lymphatic stoma (2-6 µm) in the parietal pleura. Diffusion, active transport, and transcytosis also contribute minimally to physiological turnover of pleural fluid. The importance of "bulk flow" as a mode of absorption is that pleural fluid protein remains constant with absorption (and does not increase as in diffusion). This permits the use of concentration of protein in the pleural fluid to differentiate between exudates and transudates. Transudative effusion results as a result of an imbalance between fluid formation at the parietal pleura capillaries and via visceral pleura in conditions of interstitial fluid excess and removal via parietal lymphatics. Exudative effusions result from an abnormality in the pleural surfaces and an exudation of protein-rich fluid in the pleura. Most of the parietal pleural stomas are distributed dorsocaudally and the visceral pleura is devoid of stoma. Parietal pleura lymphatics can absorb 0.28 mL/kg/hr, yielding a safety factor that is 28-fold before accumulation can occur.

PHYSIOLOGICAL CHANGES WITH A PLEURAL EFFUSION

When the pleural space is occupied by fluid, the pleural pressure becomes positive. The increase in volume of pleural fluid will be accompanied by an increase in the size of thoracic cavity (distending pressure = $P_{atm} - P_{pleura}$) and/or a decrease in size of the heart or lungs (distending pressure = $P_{alv} - P_{pleura}$).

In experimental settings, the lung volume decreases by 30% at functional residual capacity and 20% at TLC with addition of saline in the pleural cavity. Therapeutic drainage of every 1,000 mL fluid is shown to increase FEV_1 (forced expiratory volume in 1 second) and FVC (forced vital capacity) by 200 mL. After thoracocentesis, there is a greater increase in maximal inspiratory pressures than the improvement in lung volume. This is possibly due to relief from the downward displacement of the diaphragm. Pleural effusion leads to an ipsilateral intrapulmonary shunt and this does not change significantly post-thoracocentesis. Consequently, partial pressure of arterial oxygen does not increase post-thoracocentesis and may actually paradoxically decrease. Exercise limitation in pleural effusions results from decline in lung volumes and cardiac function, as reflected by a reduced oxygen pulse. Therapeutic thoracocentesis, however, does not lead to any immediate improvement in exercise capacity.

PHYSIOLOGICAL CHANGES WITH PNEUMOTHORAX

When a pneumothorax occurs, the pleural pressures become uniformly positive unlike a pleural effusion in which a gradient from bottom to top exists. Therefore, the upper lobe is affected more than the lower lobe with a pneumothorax, whereas the lower lobes are more affected with pleural effusion. In pneumothorax, the increase in the volume of a hemithorax is fourfold less than the decrease in the volume of the lung. Hypoxemia occurs because of an intrapulmonary shunt and due to reduced cardiac output in tension pneumothoraces.

PLEURAL MANOMETRY

Clinical application of pleural physiology begins with measurement of intrapleural pressures. Pleural manometry can be performed with a vertical-column water manometer or a hemodynamic transducer connected to a standard physiologic system. Pleural manometry can also be performed in the absence of complex equipment using central venous pressure manometers connected to a thoracentesis catheter inserted in the most dependent portion of the pleural effusion.

There are three possible pleural elastance curves which reflect the relationship between change in pressure for volume removed. These are: a large volume removed with minimal change in pressure (normal), a normal initial elastance with a rapid drop in pressure (lung entrapment), and an initial negative pressure with a rapid drop in pressure (trapped lung). In general, pressures of less than −5 cm H_2O or pleural elastance (pressure change divided by the amount of fluid removed) more than 25 cm H_2O/L suggest trapped lung. An initial normal pressure with subsequent drop suggests pleural entrapment by malignancy or inflammation, extensive parenchymal disease or endobronchial obstruction. Pleural elastance can also guide therapeutic thoracocentesis because reperfusion pulmonary edema does not occur till pleural pressures are less than −20 cm H_2O. Also, an elastance more than 19 cm H_2O/L can predict the failure of pleurodesis as pleural opposition is unlikely if lung entrapment exists.

PLEURAL ULTRASOUND

The presence of pleural fluid provides an excellent acoustic window. Ultrasound therefore allows examination of the parietal and visceral pleura, as well as the effusion. Pleural fluid is usually hypoechoic (darker) and the air-filled lungs are hyperechoic (brighter). Ultrasound has a very good sensitivity for diagnosing effusions and guiding thoracentesis when used in real time.

CHAPTER 90

Tubercular Pleural Effusion

Pranab Baruwa, Kripesh Ranjan Sarmah

Pleural involvement in tuberculosis (TB), the second most common form of extrapulmonary TB, is reported in approximately 5% of all TB patients. TB pleural effusion is a common presentation in acquired immunodeficiency syndrome or human immunodeficiency virus (AIDS or HIV) in about 15–90% patients. Without treatment, TB pleuritis may resolve spontaneously but most of them develop active TB at a later date.

PATHOLOGY AND PATHOGENESIS

Pleural TB can be a manifestation of primary or postprimary disease. In primary disease, rupture of subpleural foci occurs as the initial event. Postprimary form is frequently associated with parenchymal disease like consolidation or cavity formation. TB pleural effusion in the absence of radiologically evidence of TB is more commonly due to primary infection. TB bacilli are only rarely seen in the pleural effusion, since it occurs mostly due to delayed hypersensitivity. Tubercular protein after entering the pleural space following tubercular infection initiates hypersensitive reaction and interacts predominantly with $CD4^+$ T cells. The resultant inflammation results in fluid formation due to increased capillary permeability. Moreover, the pleural stomata get occluded causing impediment of lymphatic clearance. For the first 24 hours, the pleural fluid predominantly contains neutrophils which appear to secrete a monocyte chemotaxin. Further, there is recruitment of monocytes to the pleural space, contributing to the formation of granulomas. From this period onwards, the lymphocytes become the predominant cells. The late phase is denoted by marked $CD4^+/CD8^+$ cell response with release of interferon-γ and granuloma formation.

CLINICAL FEATURES

Most cases of pleural TB effusion manifest with acute features of less than 1 week duration in one-third of patients and for less than 1 month in the other two-thirds. Asymptomatic effusion can rarely occur. Pleural TB is generally a disease of young age even though there are increasingly reported cases among middle-aged people; about 19% cases are due to reactivation. In general, patients with TB pleuritis are younger than patients with parenchymal disease. Patients with pleural effusion secondary to reactivation TB are generally older than those with primary tubercular effusion.

The common symptoms in pleural TB consist of cough (71–94%), fever (71–100%), chest pain (78–82%), and dyspnea. Commonly, the pleuritic pain precedes the cough. Patients are generally febrile with temperature of mild to moderate degree while some may have normal temperature. TB effusion is typically unilateral and small to moderate in amount which usually occupies less than two-thirds of hemithorax. HIV-positive patients with tubercular effusion are usually older and more likely to have *Mycobacterium tuberculosis* (*Mtb*) positive smear and culture from the fluid. HIV-positive patients also tend to show positive pleural biopsy. These patients have higher incidence of disseminated disease than the non-HIV cases with more frequent symptoms of fever, dyspnea, night sweat, fatigue, diarrhea, and tachypnea. Hepatosplenomegaly and lymphadenopathy are also more common in HIV-positive patients.

Physical examination of chest in a case of TB effusion is similar to that in any other type of pleural effusion. The percussion note over an effusion is usually dull. Auscultation characteristically reveals decreased or absent breath sounds. Near the superior border of the fluid, however, breath sounds may be bronchial in character and accentuated in intensity. This phenomenon has been attributed to the increased conductance of breath sounds through the partially collapsed lung, compressed by the fluid. In case of a loculated effusion, the typical findings of pleural effusion may not be present.

DIAGNOSIS

Pleural Fluid Analysis

Tuberculosis pleural fluid is usually clear and straw colored, it can be turbid or serosanguineous, but rarely bloody. Effusion is usually exudative (Box 90.1).

Pleural fluid lactate dehydrogenase (LDH) is usually high, in most cases more than 200 U/dL, the pH ranges from 7.3 to 7.4 (rarely over 7.4), although it can be less than 7.3 in approximately 20% cases. The glucose concentration is more than 60 mg/dL in 80–85% cases and less than 30 mg/dL in the rest of cases.

The cell counts range from 100 per dL to 5,000 per dL with more than 90% lymphocytes in two-thirds of cases. There may be neutrophil predominance in the initial stages of illness (up to 1–2 weeks) which is replaced with lymphocyte predominance after repeated thoracenteses. Chronic pleural inflammation prevents exfoliation of mesothelial cells into the pleural cavity making the

> **BOX 90.1:** Criteria for diagnosis of exudative effusion.
> - Pleural fluid protein of >3 g/dL, or
> - Light's criteria; at least one of the following:
>   - Pleural fluid to serum fluid protein ratio >0.5
>   - Pleural fluid to serum fluid lactate dehydrogenase (LDH) ratio >0.6
>   - Pleural fluid LDH more than two-thirds of upper limit of normal serum LDH, or
>   - Pleural fluid to serum fluid albumin gradient ($\leq$1.2 g)

> **BOX 90.2:** Elevated adenosine deaminase levels in lymphocyte-rich pleural fluid diseases in various.
> - Tuberculosis
> - Rheumatoid arthritis
> - Bronchoalveolar carcinoma
> - Mesothelioma
> - *Mycoplasma pneumoniae* and *Chlamydia pneumoniae*
> - Psittacosis
> - Paragonimiasis
> - Infectious mononucleosis
> - Brucellosis
> - Mediterranean fever
> - Histoplasmosis and coccidioidomycosis
> - Most patient with empyema

presence of more than 5% mesothelial cells as almost incompatible seen with TB pleural effusion. HIV-infected patients may have numerous mesothelial cells. Pleural fluid eosinophilia of more than 10% is also less likely seen in TB, except when the patient has concomitant pneumothorax or a previous traumatic thoracentesis that caused hemorrhage within pleural space.

Adenosine Deaminase Enzyme Activity

Adenosine deaminase (ADA) present in abundance in activated T lymphocytes rises in patients with TB pleural effusion. ADA of more than 70 IU/L is highly suggestive of TB while less than 40 IU/L virtually excludes the diagnosis. Specificity of ADA increases when the ADA concentration of more than 50 IU/L is present in conjunction with the pleural fluid lymphocyte to neutrophil ratio of more than 0.75. Sensitivity and specificity of ADA are reported to be high in countries with high TB burden. Raised ADA in lymphocyte-rich pleural fluid is also seen in some other diseases (Box 90.2).

Radiological Investigations

Radiological findings are usually similar in pleural effusion of different etiologies. They can be suggestive but not specific to TB. Chest X-rays reveal usually unilateral small-to-moderate effusion. The classical X-ray picture in posteroanterior projection is the obliteration of the lateral costophrenic (CP) angle with high density laterally with a gentle, medial, downward curve and a smooth, meniscus-shaped upper border which terminates at the mediastinum (Fig. 90.1). In addition, there is loss of hemidiaphragm silhouette, apical capping, elevation of hemidiaphragm, decreased visibility of lower lobe vasculature, and accentuation of minor fissure. An amount of 175–525 mL of fluid produces noticeable increase in density over lower lung zone on supine radiograph. Sometimes, pleural effusion may present as subpulmonic or loculated effusion. Rarely, pleural TB may present as pleural nodules and thickening.

On computed tomography (CT) scan, the typical finding of free flowing pleural fluid is seen as a sickle-shaped opacity in the most dependent part of the thorax, posteriorly. CT scan is also helpful to demonstrate pleural loculation as well as to see the associated parenchymal and pleural pathology. Associated parenchymal lesions are seen in 20–50%, or even in 67% patients. CT scan can help to detect other findings such as pleural thickening, calcification, loculated effusion, empyema, empyema necessitans, and bronchopleural fistula (BPF).

Ultrasonography (USG) is a useful modality in the evaluation of pleural diseases. It helps to differentiate pleural fluid from pleural thickening, helps in guided thoracentesis, identification of loculations, and differentiate pyopneumothorax from lung abscess. USG is also useful to demonstrate fibrin bands of varying lengths, mobile delicate septations, encysted pleural effusions, pleural thickenings, and pleural nodules. Positron emission tomography CT in pleural effusion sensitivity of 100% and specificity of 96% is helpful for identifying malignant pleurisy. This may be helpful in identifying TB from malignant effusion.

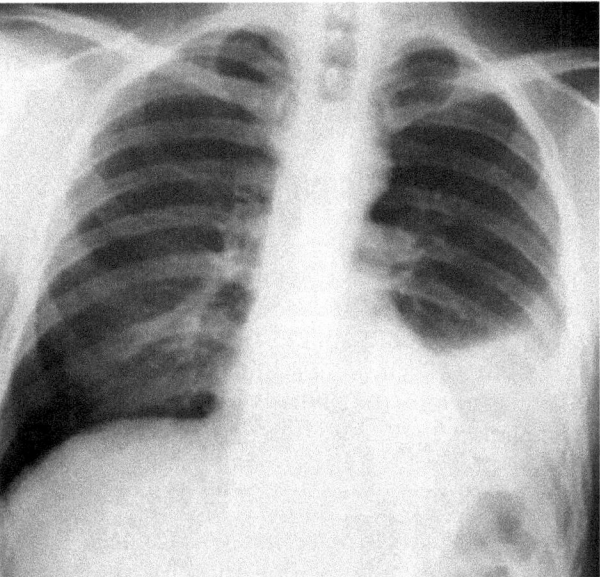

Fig. 90.1: Posteroanterior view showing left-sided moderate pleural effusion.

Sputum Examination

Smears of sputum are rarely positive in primary cases, cultures are positive in only 25–33% of patients, especially if there is an associated underlying lung disease.

Tuberculin Test

Positive tuberculin test constitutes a supportive evidence for TB. Negative tuberculin test may be negative in the presence of immunosuppression, malnourishment, and recent infection.

Pleural Fluid Culture and Smear

Pleural effusion is a paucibacillary disease. Fluid examination may detect acid-fast bacilli (AFB) in less than 10% of cases. The yield for *Mtb* is over 20% in patient with HIV coinfection. Liquid culture methods give higher yield than solid media. Bedsides, inoculation of fluid in the liquid media can be used to increase the culture sensitivity.

Pleural Biopsy

Granulomas are seen on pleural biopsy in 50–97% of patients. The diagnostic yield is high (from 60–95%) when both biopsy and culture methods are used together. Differential diagnosis of granulomatous pleuritis includes sarcoidosis, rheumatoid arthritis, fungal disease, and nocardial infection.

Thoracoscopy

Thoracoscopy is used for direct visualization and pleural biopsy. TB pleuritis may be seen as the presence of yellow white tubercles, reddening, and adhesions. Thoracoscopy is the most accurate tool to establish the diagnosis with a diagnostic accuracy of 100% on histology and 76% positive on culture.

Miscellaneous Indirect Investigations

Interferon-γ Release Assay

Interferon-γ release assay (IGRA) tests (QuantiFERON-TB gold, T-spot TB) are being used for diagnosis of latent TB and recommendations are similar to that of tuberculin test. The sensitivity of T-spot TB in pleural effusion is higher than IGRA in peripheral blood or ADA in pleural effusion. This may be due to higher level of Culture Filtrate Protein-10 (CFP-10) and Early Secretory Antigenic Target-6 (ESAT-6) in pleural fluid.

Polymerase Chain Reaction

Polymerase chain reaction (PCR) can detect as few as 10 bacilli. For diagnosis of pleural TB, the test shows a sensitivity ranging from 20% to 90% and specificity 78% to 100%.

Xpert MTB or rifampicin assay: It is an automated system which uses real-time PCR and molecular beacon probes to determine the presence of MTB complex DNA and *rpoB* gene mutation. Xpert MTB or rifampicin assay in tubercular pleural effusion has shown sensitivity and specificity of 25% and 100%, respectively.

Immunodiagnosis

Several immunological markers of TB such as immunoglobulin A (IgA) against MPT-64 and MT-10.3, anti-IgM and IgG antibodies against anti-A60, and others have been evaluated for diagnosis. Serum antibody levels against TB antigens have poor sensitivity and specificity, the performance of serological tests for diagnosis of TB pleuritis has been disappointing, regardless of HIV coinfection.

HIV Infection and Pleural TB

Patients of TB effusion with HIV or AIDS tend to have a longer duration of illness and lower incidence of chest pain. Systemic signs and symptoms as well as the concomitant parenchymal lesions are significantly more common. The pleural fluid is more likely to be smear and culture positive for AFB. If CD4 count is less than 100, about 50% will have positive smear for AFB in their pleural fluid; these patients have significantly lower lymphocyte count.

Multidrug-resistant Tuberculosis and Pleural Effusion

Drug resistance in pleural TB follows similar pattern to that of parenchymal TB. Therefore, drug susceptibility testing is sought in areas where there is high incidence of resistance. Multidrug-resistance occurs in only 1% of patients with pleural TB and any first-line drug resistance occurs in less than 10%.

MANAGEMENT

The major objectives of treatment lie in the resolution of effusion, healing of active lesion, and prevention of subsequent reactivation of TB. The other objectives of management are to prevent development of pleural fibrosis and to treat complications that may develop due to pleural effusion. A large majority of patients require only the medical treatment.

Medical Management

Tubercular pleural effusion is a type of extrapulmonary paucibacillary disease. With adequate antitubercular treatment, most cases resolve completely with fewer chances of recurrence. New patients should receive an intensive phase of all the four primary drugs (rifampicin, isoniazid, pyrazinamide, and ethambutol) followed by the maintenance phase of 4 months with three drugs (rifampicin, isoniazid, and ethambutol). The drugs are administered either daily or intermittently, i.e. thrice a week. Under the Revised National Tuberculosis Control Programme, intermittent regimens are used and each dose should be directly observed.

The penetration of isoniazid in the pleural fluid is excellent, as of pyrazinamide is very poor, whereas the penetration of rifampicin is intermittent. An average patient with TB pleural effusion becomes afebrile within 2 weeks of starting chemotherapy, but temperature elevations may persist for as long as 2 months. Patients do not require any bedrest and need isolation only when there is associated parenchyma disease with positive sputum. The incidence of pleural thickening at 6–12 months after beginning of therapy is approximately 50%. Residual pleural thickening is not related to the initial pleural fluid findings; patients with low glucose, high LDH, and high cytokine level are only slightly more likely to have residual thickening. However, in patients with loculated pleural effusion, there can be delayed resorption, even after completion of 6 months of treatment.

Role of Corticosteroid

Prednisolone (0.5–1 mg/kg/day) has been used for a period ranging from 4 weeks to 12 weeks, for an early resolution of clinical symptoms and signs (fever, chest pain, and dyspnea). There is a trend towards less residual fluid at the end of treatment with use of steroid. No difference is, however, seen in the development of residual pleural thickening or adhesion. The use of steroids in HIV or AIDS-associated TB pleural effusion is not currently recommended because of the lack of survival benefit and an increased risk of Kaposi sarcoma.

Role of Surgery

Surgical intervention is required in a few cases of failure of medical therapy, complication of scarring, and to establish a proper diagnosis. Pleural effusion remains undiagnosed in 25% cases after routine investigations; this can be reduced to 4% by thoracoscopic biopsies. Diagnostic as well as therapeutic thoracentesis is the most common surgical procedure. Decortication is required when pleural thickening persists and causes significant clinical symptoms. Surgical interventions are also required for complications of empyema, BPF, and others.

COMPLICATION OF TB PLEURAL EFFUSION

Pleural Thickening and Fibrothorax

Tubercular pleural effusion can lead to residual changes ranging from minimal pleural thickening to fibrothorax. Commonly, it causes symptoms of dull ache, heaviness, and chest pain. Extensive fibrothorax may cause volume loss of the underlying lung, breathlessness, and ventilatory impairment.

Empyema (Chronic Persistent Pleural Effusion)

Chronic TB empyema represents chronic active infection of pleural space. Such complication can occur due to progress of primary TB effusion that is usually moderate to large in size. Empyema can also form due to direct extension of infection from thoracic lymph nodes or subdiaphragmatic foci, through hematogenous spread and following pneumonectomy. Chronic TB empyema may present as an abnormality on routine chest X-ray with BPF or as empyema necessitans. Besides anti-TB chemotherapy, intercostal tube drainage is necessary. Decortication, extrapleural pneumonectomy or thoracoplasty may also be required.

Empyema Necessitans

Empyema necessitans is formed by the break of empyema through the parietal pleura for spontaneous discharge of its content. It is usually formed in the subcutaneous tissues of the chest wall, but may sometimes occur at other sites, such as the esophagus, breast, retroperitoneum, flanks, groins, pericardium, and vertebra. Surgical drainage is required, along with routine antitubercular treatment. Certain rare complications of TB include pseudochylothorax and chylothorax formation.

Bronchopleural Fistula

It is the direct communication between the pleural cavity and the bronchial tree or the lung parenchyma. Due to the effective modern antitubercular chemotherapy, BPF is an uncommon complication in current era. Fistulas are seen with old healed TB and after therapeutic pneumothorax, not followed by proper treatment. Patients present with variable amounts of sputum production and fluctuating air fluid levels on serial X-rays. Confirmation of diagnosis can be made by injecting the methylene blue dye in the pleural space and demonstrating its presence in sputum or in the trachea-bronchial tree. Treatment requires adequate anti-tuberculosis drug therapy, followed by surgical management.

CHAPTER 91

Parapneumonic Effusion and Empyema

Devasahayam J Christopher

INTRODUCTION

Pleural effusion frequently accompanies bacterial pneumonia in up to 40% of hospitalized patients. Hospitalized patients with pleural effusion, accompanying bacterial pneumonias, are 2.7 times more likely to have treatment failures than those without accompanying effusion. Although parapneumonic effusion (PPE) normally responds to antibiotic therapy, nonresponsive effusions may progress to become purulent.

DEFINITIONS

Empyema

Empyema is described as the presence of pus in the pleural cavity. This results from bacterial invasion of the pleural cavity though the lung parenchyma, systemic circulation or from the chest wall. It is however not necessary for each infected pleural effusion to progress to empyema.

Parapneumonic Effusion

Any pleural effusion associated with bacterial pneumonia, lung abscess or bronchiectasis.

Complicated Parapneumonic Effusion

Effusions that do not resolve without therapeutic thoracentesis or tube thoracostomy are called complicated PPEs. Some of these are purulent (empyemas), while others have nonpurulent pleural fluid.

PATHOGENESIS

Infection of the pleural space is the result of a complicated interaction of the host defense mechanisms and the organisms. There are three distinct pathophysiological stages in the development of PPE. The distinctions between the stages are not sharply demarcated. There are different characteristics of pleural fluid seen during different stages of PPE.

Exudative Stage

Exudative stage is characterized by formation of fluid within the pleural space formed in response to inflammation induced by bacterial infection in the lung parenchyma and the pleural membranes. The fluid at this stage is sterile but contains a host of locally released proinflammatory cytokines, such as interleukin-8 and tumor necrosis factor-alpha. These cytokines cause increased tissue and capillary permeability through their action on the mesothelial cells and the capillaries within the visceral and the parietal pleura. At this stage, the pleural fluid is not infected and consists of a combination of interstitial tissue fluid and the microvascular exudates. It is characterized with low lactate dehydrogenase (LDH) and normal glucose levels. The effusion at this stage is likely to resolve without the need for intercostal drainage if appropriate antibiotic therapy is instituted.

Fibrinopurulent Stage

The fibrinopurulent stage follows the exudative phase usually as a consequence of inadequate or inappropriate therapy. In the initial stages, the fluid contains polymorphs, bacteria, and cellular debris. Fibrin clots and septae develop later due to the presence of clotting factors. This loculation of pleural fluid becomes difficult to drain with the intercostal tube. With further progression of infection, the pleural fluid pH and glucose levels go down and LDH level goes up with formation of pus due to the lysis of bacteria and inflammatory cells.

Organizational Stage

The last stage is characterized by fibroblast proliferation and formation of an inelastic "pleural peel" due to deposition of fibrous tissue on both the visceral and the parietal membranes—in the pleural peel causes restriction of lung expansion and impairment of gas exchange in severe cases. Occasionally, the untreated chronic infection may result in the penetration of the purulent fluid into the lung with formation of a bronchopleural fistula and/or into the chest wall empyema necessitans. Following pleural organization, some individuals may undergo spontaneous healing with resolution of pleural thickening, while others are left with pleural thickening or peel.

EPIDEMIOLOGY

Pleural infection most commonly occurs as a complication of bacterial pneumonia. Some of the important and independent risk factors include diabetes mellitus, gastroesophageal reflux, alcohol, and intravenous drug abuse. Children and the elderly are more prone to develop empyema. Poor dental hygiene and aspiration may predispose to lung infection in particular with anaerobic organisms. It should also be appreciated that empyema can occur without an underlying bacterial pneumonia. These may occur as a complication of surgery and pleural procedures, such as thoracentesis or tube thoracostomy, presumably from unsterile technique.

BACTERIOLOGY

Published reports of PPEs have shown substantial variations in the bacteriology of isolated aerobes. It is likely that the introduction of antibiotics may have at least partially contributed to this variation. Over the years, the most commonly isolated organisms have varied between *Streptococcus pneumoniae, S. haemolyticus,* and *Staphylococcus aureus.* In children, bacteriology is slightly different than in adults, *Haemophilus influenzae* being the most commonly isolated aerobe, the anaerobes being much less frequent. Anaerobes require stringent transport process to preserve viability; the investigators with interest in culturing anaerobes have had greater success.

CLINICAL FEATURES AND DIAGNOSIS

Patients with empyema usually present with an acute febrile illness and features of pneumonia, such as cough, purulent sputum, and dyspnea. Pleuritic chest pain is present in around 60% of patients but its absence does not exclude the diagnosis of pleural infection. Presence of an anaerobic infection may be frequently indolent with weight loss, anorexia, and malaise.

There are few clinical parameters that can distinguish between pneumonia with or without PPE. Therefore, PPE should be considered while evaluating all patients with pneumonia, particularly those who are unresponsive to antimicrobial therapy. Further, not all patients with PPE have an acute illness.

Radiological Investigations

Chest radiograph can detect significant effusion and is often the only required imaging for its detection. Effusion may be free or loculated, may show evidence of air-fluid level. Empyema may give the appearance of pleural mass or tumor within the lung, when the collection occurs within a fissure. Computed tomography (CT) scan of the chest is used to detect and quantitate minimal effusion. In resource limited settings, blunting of the costophrenic angle on a lateral chest radiograph or obscuration of the dome of the diaphragm is considered sufficient to detect the presence of pleural fluid. Decubitus views may complement the information obtained from the erect chest radiographs.

In the lateral decubitus film, the amount of fluid can be roughly quantitated by measuring the distance between the chest wall and the lower part of the adjacent lung. If the length is less than 10 mm, the effusion is deemed to be too small to be clinically significant. Such effusions resolve with antibiotics alone. CT evidence of pleural thickening is present in 80–100% of the empyemas; so, its presence would favor this diagnosis, when PPE is being evaluated. "Split pleura sign" on contrast CT enhancement of visceral and parietal pleura differentiates empyema from a peripherally situated lung abscess.

Ultrasonography is an excellent method to assess pleural effusion. It can also help quantify the amount of effusion by assessing the depth of fluid. It can also be used at the bedside, for example, in the intensive care units. Empyema results in dense echogenicity and loculations which are detectable on ultrasonogram. It is also helpful in ensuring successful pleural fluid aspiration in as high as 97% of the cases (Fig. 91.1).

Thoracocentesis

Clinical features and routine blood tests are poor predictors of the need for drainage; the delay in instituting adequate drainage increases the morbidity. It is thus recommended that diagnostic pleural aspiration should be performed in all patients with PPE. The exception to this rule is a small pleural effusion (<10 mm on a lateral decubitus chest radiograph), which may resolve with antibiotics alone. When the effusion is small and does not completely cover the dome of the diaphragm in a chest radiograph (posteroanterior view), it is safer to perform an ultrasound-guided aspiration which is more accurate.

The drainage of frank pus on thoracentesis is diagnostic of empyema. The pleural fluid should be examined for microbiological and biochemical studies. In case of frank pus from empyema, microbiological cultures should be done for the choice of antibiotics. Tuberculous etiology should always be kept in mind while evaluating empyema in high TB prevalence settings.

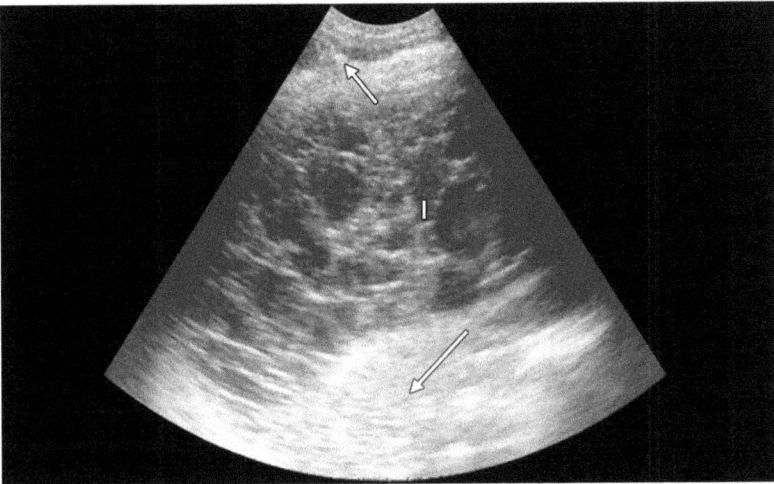

Fig. 91.1: Ultrasonogram of chest showing multiple loculations. Short arrow indicates needle performing biopsy of the parietal pleura. Long arrow indicates collapsed lung.

Pleural Fluid Analysis

In parapneumonic effusion, the fluid may vary between clear or straw colored and odorless to thick, purulent, and foul smelling. Only around 11% of effusions exhibit foul smell. Foul odor could indicate an anaerobic or mixed (aerobic and anaerobic) etiology. Absence of foul smell however does not rule out an anaerobic infection. After gross examination, the pleural fluid is tested for proteins, LDH, glucose, and pH. Another sample is sent for microbiological studies—Gram stain, aerobic cultures, mycobacterial and fungal cultures, as deemed necessary. If the resources permit, anaerobic cultures too should be done on all exudative effusions of undetermined etiology. Acid-fast bacilli smears and mycobacterial cultures are also important. Predominance of lymphocytes in the fluid may suggest the possibility of malignancy or tuberculosis. Purulent fluid should always be drained.

It is well understood that PPE with an acidic pH (<7.20) is more likely to run a complicated course with loculated fluid collections and empyema, when compared to an effusion with pH greater than 7.20. Intercostal drainage is instituted to avert this complication, antibiotic treatment alone may not suffice. Furthermore, there is more likelihood of the need for surgical intervention in those with an acidic pH (<7.20).

Measurement of pH should not be performed on obviously purulent pleural fluid; it may damage the blood gas analyzer. Moreover, tube drainage should be instituted regardless of the pH value in case of purulent effusion. The PPE caused by *Proteus* is known to present paradoxically with alkalotic pleural fluid pH, because the *Proteus* split urea to produce ammonia.

TREATMENT

Prompt recognition is essential for optimal management of pleural infection. Antibiotic therapy and drainage of fluid collection constitute the cornerstone of management.

Antibiotic Treatment

All patients suspected of having pleural infection need treatment with antibiotics. While it is ideal to prescribe antibiotics based on the results of pleural and/or blood cultures, this causes a delay in the commencement of treatment. Therefore, appropriate "empiric" antibiotic treatment should commence for all patients. Selection of antibiotics should be based on Gram stain results, presence of hospital-acquired versus community-acquired infection, and on the clinical severity of the illness. Antibiotic penetration into the pleural space is variable in the descending order from metronidazole, penicillin, clindamycin, vancomycin, ceftriaxone to gentamycin, and other aminoglycosides.

Cultures do not always grow pathogens, but may remain negative in up to 42% of the cases. *S. milleri, S. pneumoniae,* staphylococci, and *H. influenzae* are more commonly seen in case of community-acquired infection. Most of these organisms except *S. milleri* group are resistant to β-lactams. Pleural infection is rarely caused by atypical bacteria, while 10% of cases may occur anaerobic infection. When cultures are negative, antibiotics should cover community-acquired or hospital-acquired pathogens as the case may be; anaerobes should be covered too. Antibiotic choice should be directed by local policy guided by standard international and national recommendations.

Empirical antibiotic regimen should be appropriately changed after the culture results have become available. Continuation of antianaerobic therapy is usually necessary since the anaerobic organisms are difficult to culture. There is no definitive data to show how long to treat empyema. Generally, antibiotic treatment should continue for at least 3 weeks, with at least 1 week of intravenous antibiotics.

Closed Intercostal Drainage

There is consensus of opinion regarding the need of pleural space drainage under the following circumstances:
- Frank pus or turbid/cloudy fluid within the pleural space
- Presence of organisms identified by Gram stain or culture from (nonpurulent) effusion
- Effusion fluid with a pH less than 7.2
- Large uncomplicated effusions for relief of dyspnea.

Repeated thoracentesis is an alternative, albeit a less popular strategy compared to intercostal drain insertion. It facilitates increased mobility and lower complication, in particular infection rates. This management strategy has support from experimental and clinical trials.

In loculated effusions, the tube can be placed under guidance into the biggest locula. The role of suctioning and flushing the drainage tube with around 30 mL of sterile saline four times daily can be helpful, particularly when a small bore chest tube is used. The optimal timing of drain removal is unknown, although clinical response is clearly the most important parameter. It is our practice to remove the drainage tube, when the drainage is less than 50 mL; provided the fluid is clear and nonturbid. If on the other hand the fluid is turbid, we remove it only after the drainage reduces to less than 10 mL. If there is inadequate drainage or failure of resolution with a single chest drain, there may be a need to reposition the tube after radiological assessment or placement of additional tubes. Failure of chest tube drainage heralds increased morbidity and mortality.

Intrapleural Fibrinolytics

The apparent benefit of fibrinolytics was supported by five randomized studies in adults which showed success rates between 60% and 95%. Although fibrinolytics conferred benefits, such as decreased hospital stay, improved radiographic appearance, and decreased rate of surgery; the benefits were variable and inconsistent.

While there was only limited success with intrapleural fibrinolytic agents, the observation that DNA is the main cause of viscosity of empyema fluid has led to the hypothesis that intrapleural administration of the enzyme deoxyribonuclease (DNase) might reduce empyema fluid viscosity and thus improve the drainage of pleural fluid.

Surgical Treatment

Medical therapy alone is not successful in up to 30% of patients with empyema. Surgical management is required in these patients even though there is no good quality data on the indications and optimum timing of surgery. Surgical interventions may help patients who do not improve clinically and radiologically after 7 days of standard treatment. Video-assisted thoracic surgery (VATS) is the recommended method of choice for patients with failed tube drainage. VATS will help to divide the adhesions and septae to aid drainage. Thoracotomy and decortication is required in cases with multiple loculi and adhesions with success rates of up to 95%. Decortication is likely the only treatment modality in chronic empyema and pleural thickening with persistent sepsis.

Rib resection and open surgical drainage under local anesthesia are done in patients who are unfit for general anesthesia.

Nutrition

Maintenance of good nutrition is an important component of treatment because of the highly catabolic state. Patients with low serum albumin have poor outcome. An aggressive nutritional support is required for these patients.

SUMMARY

PPE and empyema indicate the presence of pleural infection more commonly seen in patients with one or more risk-factors. Early recognition of infection and the causative organisms is important to make therapeutic decisions. Adequate drainage and appropriate antibiotic therapy are important for early resolution. Chronic and/or complicated empyemas may need additional surgical management.

CHAPTER
92

Malignant Pleural Effusions and Pleurodesis

Srinivas Rajagopala

INTRODUCTION

Malignant pleural effusion (MPE) is the second most common cause of exudative pleural effusions in countries with high prevalence of tuberculosis; while in most of the Western countries, MPE is the topmost cause. Metastatic etiology is several times more common than the primary pleural malignancy.

ETIOLOGY OF MALIGNANT EFFUSIONS

About 50–65% of MPEs are associated with lung and breast cancer. Another 25% are associated with lymphoma, gastrointestinal, and genitourinary cancers. Sarcomas (including melanomas), germ cell tumors, and prostatic carcinoma together account for another 10% of all MPEs. The primary cancer is unknown in 7–15% cases; the diagnosis of pleural malignancy is the first indication of cancer in about 10% of effusions. Primary pleural malignancy is an uncommon cause of MPE; metastatic MPEs are 25-fold common than mesothelioma even in areas where the latter is relatively common. Pleural effusion in lung cancer is a sign of metastatic stage IVA disease with poor prognosis.

About 30–43% of all MPEs occur secondarily to lung cancer—the most common cause; breast cancer being the second most common cause. Adenocarcinomas are the most common lung cancers associated with MPEs, but effusions may also occur with other histopathological types. The risk of pleural effusion in patients with lung cancer is more in patients with anti-p53 positivity. It takes about 2 years but can be up to 20 years for MPE to develop in breast cancer from the time of initial diagnosis. MPE generally occurs on the same side as the underlying lung or breast cancer (70%). It can, however, occur on the contralateral side (20%) or may be occasionally bilateral (10%). About 3% of effusions related to Hodgkin disease and 20% of effusions related to non-Hodgkin lymphoma are chylothoraces. Not all patients with MPEs are symptomatic; patients may have asymptomatic stable effusions that do not require management throughout their disease course.

PATHOGENESIS OF METASTASIS AND EFFUSIONS

There are several mechanisms to explain the development of pleural metastases: (1) invasion of pulmonary vascular system with tumor emboli which cause seedling of the visceral pleural surface and thereafter of the parietal pleura; (2) direct tumor invasion; (3) hematogenous spread to the parietal pleura from the extrapulmonary primary malignancy; and (4) lymphatic involvement. In lung cancer, the first mechanism is the more likely cause in most cases. Pleural metastases are sometimes seen without the presence of effusion. Increased pleural permeability secondary to production of vascular endothelial growth factor (VEGF) is largely responsible for the development of MPE. Lymphatic blockade in the parietal pleura stoma and at the lymph nodes also contribute to generation of MPE and pleural involvement and intrathoracic lymphadenopathy correlate with pleural effusions related to malignancy in autopsy studies. In general, direct involvement of pleura by the malignancy makes it inoperable and the treatment approaches are predominantly palliative. However, "paramalignant" causes of effusion, especially pneumonia, pulmonary embolism, and atelectasis may be operative in about 17% of cases and this should be ruled out before palliation alone is considered.

CLINICAL PRESENTATION

Breathlessness is the most common symptom with which the patients present. Dyspnea due to a large pleural effusion occurs due to decreased chest wall compliance and diminished lung expansion, contralateral mediastinal shift causing compression of the normal lung, and decreased ipsilateral lung volume. Breathlessness is partly due to reflex stimulation of the receptors from the chest wall and lung parenchyma. Nonproductive cough is another important symptom of pleural effusion. Both dyspnea and cough are relieved promptly by thoracentesis; failure of improvement suggests atelectasis, pneumonia, lymphangitis carcinomatosa, pulmonary embolism or another associated medical condition (congestive cardiac failure) as the etiology.

Patients with lung entrapment by the pleural malignancy will have an improvement in dyspnea without complete lung expansion; the inhibition of stretch receptors by the fluid removal is believed to mediate this. Patients may also have systemic manifestations such as malaise, anorexia, and weight loss that are related to the advanced stage of malignancy. A constant dull, aching chest pain may be seen in MPE; however, this is more common in patients with mesothelioma. Chest pain is caused by malignant infiltration of the parietal pleura, ribs, and intercostal structures. The presence of hemoptysis suggests an endobronchial growth as the primary symptom responsible for the MPE. A history of smoking and occupational exposure to asbestos may suggest the diagnosis of MPE. Symptoms for more than a month, absence of fever, massive effusion, and serosanguineous fluid on thoracentesis also favor the possibility of malignancy.

RADIOLOGICAL FINDINGS

Typically, symptomatic MPE at presentation occupies half to two-thirds of the hemithorax. While about 10% of patients have small effusions, it is massive in additional 10% of patients. A massive effusion is likely to cause mediastinal shift to the contralateral side. But the contralateral mediastinal shift with an apparent large pleural effusion may be absent in case of bronchogenic carcinoma of the mainstem bronchus causing ipsilateral lung collapse, malignant mesothelioma, mediastinum fixation (e.g. due to malignant lymph nodes) or lung entrapment by extensive pleural malignancy. Multiloculation at presentation is unusual in malignant effusions (as opposed to parapneumonic effusions) because of the high fibrinolytic activity of the metastatic tumor lesions. Chest radiographs of patients primary lung cancer and an effusion often demonstrate associated abnormalities; these might sometimes be apparent after a therapeutic thoracentesis.

Computed tomography (CT) of the chest is helpful in the evaluation of patients with an MPE. CT of chest will delineate pleural abnormalities, mediastinal lymphadenopathy, and parenchymal disease. CT is also useful to look for chest wall and airway involvement that cannot be detected on standard chest radiograph. CT of the chest should include the upper abdominal cuts should be obtained to visualize possible adrenal and hepatic deposits. The diagnosis is favored by the presence of parietal pleural thickening of greater than 1 cm malignant pleural thickening. Malignancy is also suggested by circumferential and nodular pleural thickening as well as by mediastinal pleural thickening (specificity 94–100%). CT appearances of mesothelioma are quite similar to metastatic pleural effusion. Mesothelioma is suspected by the presence of concomitant pleural plaques (20%), asbestosis, and extensive chest wall invasion. Mesothelioma should also be considered if there is circumferential nodular lung encasement, pleural thickening with irregular pleura-pulmonary margins or nodules, and interfissure thickening. Magnetic resonance imaging is generally not done in patients with MPE; it may help in the evaluation of chest wall involvement in mesothelioma. Positron emission tomography provides information on the extent of involvement in malignant mesothelioma but does not offer any etiological help.

DIAGNOSIS

Pleural Fluid Analysis

Malignant pleural effusion is generally hemorrhagic while about 50% of MPEs are nonhemorrhagic with raised red blood cell counts of less than

10,000 cells/μL. The fluid is almost always an exudate with elevated lactate dehydrogenase. Fluid cytology is composed mainly of lymphocytes (50–70% of all cells), macrophages, and mesothelial cells with low nucleated cell count, generally less than 3,000/μL. The presence of pleural eosinophilia does not exclude the possibility of pleural malignancy—prevalence of malignancy is almost similar in eosinophilic and noneosinophilic effusions.

The pleural glucose level is less than 60 mg/dL in about 20% of MPE. Impaired glucose transfer to pleural fluid and glucose utilization by tumor burden contribute to the observed low-glucose levels. Lactic acid generated by anaerobic glycolysis in the pleural space and impaired carbon dioxide movement from the pleural space are responsible for low pH generation. Low pleural fluid pH (<7.30) and low pleural fluid glucose (<60 mg/dL) carry a higher sensitivity of diagnosis by initial cytology examination. These findings generally indicate the presence of an advanced disease and decreased survival and lesser chances of successful pleurodesis. Increased amylase concentration is seen in 10–14% of patients with MPE, especially adenocarcinoma of the lung and ovary, usually due to increased salivary isoenzyme concentration. The routine assay of amylase is unhelpful in the diagnosis of exudates of undetermined etiology and should be measured only if there is a pretest suspicion of acute pancreatitis, chronic pancreatic disease or esophageal rupture.

Pleural Cytology

The diagnosis of MPE is established by demonstrating malignant cells in the pleural fluid or in the pleura tissue. Pleural fluid cytology is diagnostic in up to 55–60% of patients with MPE depending on the tumor load and the histopathological type of the primary malignancy. Pleural cytology is rarely positive in squamous cell carcinoma (SCC) because bronchial obstruction and lymphatic involvement are frequent causes of pleural effusion in this setting. At least two samples are submitted for cytology and these need not exceed 50 mL in quantity. Use of a cellblock analysis increases the yield of positive tests and enables immunohistochemistry. A positive cytology establishes malignancy, but provides no information about the site of primary. This is evaluated by subsequent imaging, endoscopy or markers (prostate-specific antigen, cancer antigen-125, etc.).

Pleural Biopsy

The sensitivity of percutaneous blind pleural biopsy using Abrams' biopsy needle varies from 40% to 75% depending on the extent of parietal pleural involvement, number and adequacy of biopsies, and operator experience. If blind biopsy is performed without cytology, one-third of patients who would otherwise be diagnosed will be missed. CT-guided percutaneous pleural biopsy has a yield similar to thoracoscopic biopsy and may be performed when confirmation of the diagnosis (without the need for pleurodesis) is the dominant clinical problem or where thoracoscopy is unavailable.

Medical thoracoscopy has a yield exceeding 95% for malignancy; further, this can be combined with complete drainage of the effusions, adhesiolysis, and talc poudrage with a greater percentage of successful pleurodesis. Medical thoracoscopy can be performed under local anesthesia with conscious sedation in an endoscopy suite. Use of nondisposable rigid or semirigid instruments in these settings helps to make the procedure as less invasive and cheaper than video-assisted thoracoscopic surgery. Thoracoscopy is safer with more than 95% diagnostic yield and accuracy. Major complications with thoracoscopy are seen in less than 2–3% of cases, procedure-related death is exceedingly rare (0.4%). Pleuroscopy may be performed with a rigid or semirigid pleuroscope. The use of rigid pleuroscope is associated with a greater need for sedation, analgesia, and scar size but is associated with higher yield, bigger biopsy size, ease of biopsy, and quality of imaging. Either of these could be combined with therapeutic poudrage during the diagnostic procedure.

Pleural fluid levels of tumor markers like carcinoembryonic antigen (CEA), carbohydrate antigens (CA) 15-3, 19-9, 549 and 72-4, neuron-specific enolase, SCC antigen, cytokeratin 19 fragments (CYFRA21-1), and sialyl state-specific mouse embryonic antigen (SSEA-1) have been evaluated for separating benign and malignant effusions. In general, these markers are not specific enough and have no role in daily practice. Clonality of lymphocytes demonstrated by flow cytometry on fluid samples establishes the diagnosis of lymphoma.

Immunohistochemistry is routinely used to differentiate adenocarcinomas from mesothelioma. Metastatic adenocarcinomas stain positive with CEA, MOC-3.1, B72.3, Ber-EP4, and BG-8, whereas mesotheliomas (and benign mesothelial cells) stain positive with calretinin and cytokeratin. A panel of four markers is usually employed in clinical practice. Staining for thyroid transcription factor-1 in fluid and tissue can help to establish pulmonary origin of adenocarcinomas.

MANAGEMENT

The initial step is to establish malignancy and the site of the primary. This guides subsequent chemotherapy and/or hormonal therapy and radiotherapy. The major indication for palliative treatment in patients with an MPE is relief of dyspnea. The main considerations affecting management decisions include the patient's degree of breathlessness, functional status, duration of expected survival, type of primary tumor (and expected response to chemotherapy), and lung expansion following thoracentesis. The below modalities are used in isolation or combined as the clinical situation dictates.

Observation

Observation is appropriate when patients are asymptomatic and neither therapeutic thoracocentesis nor pleurodesis is indicated in patients diagnosed with asymptomatic mild to moderate MPEs.

Chemotherapy and Radiation

Malignant pleural effusions from small-cell lung cancer, breast carcinoma, and lymphoma may respond favorably to chemotherapy alone. If the effusion is mild-to-moderate, a trial of chemotherapy may be performed as a modality to control the effusion. In chylothorax from lymphoma, mediastinal radiation is effective. Chemotherapy is not useful in isolation to control the effusion, however, in most patients with MPEs secondary to carcinoma lung. Anti-VEGF antibody bevacizumab is used as a triplet-combination therapy in nonsquamous lung cancer. Pleurodesis should precede this treatment since VEGF is essential for successful pleurodesis. In patients undergoing systemic chemotherapy, pleural effusions should be aspirated before chemotherapy is given because the antineoplastic drugs may accumulate in the pleural space and lead to increased systemic toxicity. Pleurodesis always precedes chemotherapy because the intercostal drain may become a potential nidus of infection.

Therapeutic Thoracentesis

Therapeutic thoracentesis is performed in all dyspneic patients with MPE for relief of breathlessness. The initial therapeutic thoracentesis is always combined with pleural manometry and pleural elastance measurement. Caution should be exercised when draining more than 1.5 L in a single session because of the potential of Reperfusion Pulmonary Oedema (REPO) and using pleural manometry to limit the procedure when pressure falls to −20 cm H_2O can guide safe thoracentesis in this setting. The amount of fluid evacuated by pleural aspiration should also be guided by the presence of cough or chest discomfort.

Mechanisms proposed for REPO include reperfusion injury of the underlying hypoxic lung, increased capillary permeability, and local production of neutrophil chemotactic factors such as interleukin-8. Caution must be exercised especially when the underlying lung has been collapsed for more than a week and large (>1.5 L) effusions are being drained without manometry; reperfusion edema complicates 2–7% such procedures. REPO can also complicate thoracoscopic drainage of effusions. Therapeutic thoracocentesis alone has a high rate of symptom recurrence at 1 month and alternate options must be explored in all symptomatic patients. Repeated thoracentesis in a patient who should undergo pleurodesis should be discouraged as this leads to formation of adhesions and hinders complete pleural evacuation (and subsequent pleurodesis).

Pleurodesis

Pleurodesis is devised to cause symphysis of the pleural surfaces by chemical or mechanical means for symptom relief. Primarily it aims to prevent reaccumulation of the effusion. Following intrapleural administration of the pleurodesic agent, there occurs injury to the pleural surfaces, followed by diffuse inflammation and local activation of coagulation with fibrin deposition and subsequent development of fibrosis with obliteration of the pleural space. Efficacy of pleurodesis is diminished because of high intrapleural fibrinolytic activity, high tumor burden, and concomitant use of steroids or possibly NSAIDs. However, the mechanism of pleurodesis is highly complex, involves the intrapleural procoagulant-fibrinolytic milieu and angiogenesis pathways and differs from agent to agent.

Patient Selection, Initial Preparation and Procedure

The *sine qua non* for successful pleurodesis is apposition of the pleural surfaces. While the exact amount of apposition required for a successful pleurodesis is unknown, it is usual to attempt pleurodesis after at least 50–70% apposition is visible on frontal radiographs. Suction may be applied if apposition does not occur; however, this is usually unnecessary and excessive use of suction may increase the risk of REPO. Lack of apposition may be due to a thick visceral peel (lung entrapment), pleural loculation, proximal large airway obstruction or a persistent air leak. If thick visceral peel is evident on initial imaging, consideration is given to tunneled catheters as the definitive initial procedure. If pleural loculations are evident, thoracoscopic drainage, adhesiolysis, and pleurodesis are the procedure of choice. If this is unavailable, surgical pleurectomy or intercostal tube drainage, fibrinolysis, and subsequent slurry instillation after pleural apposition can be attempted.

Presence of proximal airway obstruction is a relative contraindication for initial intercostal tube drainage; the endobronchial obstruction is first alleviated by airway interventions. Pleural suction can be attempted for incomplete lung expansion due to persistent air leak. It is recommended to use high-volume and low-pressure systems with a gradual increment in pressure to about −20 cm H_2O. Mild sedation with midazolam should be given prior to pleurodesis. Lignocaine 3 mg/kg (21 mL of 1% solution for a 70 kg male, maximum of 250 mg) is instilled intrapleurally just prior to the sclerosant. This achieves good analgesia with safe peak serum levels of lignocaine. The chemical sclerosant is then instilled in the pleural space either through an intercostal tube as a solution or during thoracoscopy with an atomizer, following complete drainage of the effusion. The intercostal drain is clamped for an hour after the procedure. Position changes during this time may be advised but is unnecessary as pleurodesis is virtually instantaneous.

Choice of Sclerosant

An ideal sclerosant should have high molecular weight and chemical polarity, low regional and rapid systemic clearance. It should also show a steep dose-response curve with good tolerance and minimal or no side effects. The choice of a sclerosant is determined by the efficacy, safety, ease of administration, number of administrations for a desirable outcome and cost. There are a number of agents available for use but there is no ideal sclerosant. Graded talc as slurry or poudrage is the most widely used and the most effective agent for pleurodesis currently. Problems with use of *medical* talc in India include its unavailability, cost, and need for appropriate sterilization prior to use. Sterilized commercial talc (face talc, Johnson & Johnson) which has been batch analyzed for impurities (asbestos) and particle size has been used for pleurodesis effectively during thoracoscopy or as slurry. This is another acceptable option for pleurodesis provided that batch analysis and sterilization can be ensured.

Iodopovidone is an iodine-based topical antiseptic agent. It is rapidly absorbed from mucosal surfaces with a 100-fold increase in serum iodine concentration following topical administration. Iodopovidone is excreted unchanged without undergoing any significant metabolism. Tetracycline was widely used in the past; however, the production of parenteral tetracycline has ceased in most countries and this agent is no longer available. Bleomycin is an antineoplastic agent used in pleurodesis. Its mechanism of action is predominantly as a chemical sclerosant similar to talc. The recommended dose is 60,000 units intrapleurally. Bleomycin is expensive and relatively ineffective compared to talc for achieving pleurodesis. Nitrogen mustard and mitoxantrone are other antineoplastic agents which have been used for successful pleurodesis and are cheaper alternatives to bleomycin.

Silver nitrate causes caustic injury to the mesothelium and results in pleural adhesions and pleurodesis. Quinacrine is an antimalarial agent that has been used for pleurodesis.

The search for more effective and safe agents for pleurodesis is ongoing. Transforming growth factor-β is a unique cytokine with potent profibrotic as well as anti-inflammatory activity. It upregulates collagen production and does not cause any inflammatory pleural response in animal models. It appears to be a more effective pleurodesis agent than talc in animals and human trials are awaited.

Thoracoscopic Poudrage versus Intercostal Tube Drainage and Pleurodesis

Thoracoscopic talc poudrage may be more effective when compared to talc slurry. However, the evidence base of the superiority of talc poudrage is weak; several trials suggest that talc slurry is as efficacious as poudrage.

Other Issues in Pleurodesis

Drainage with small bore drain (10–14 Fr) catheter is normally the initial choice for pleurodesis because of the ease of performance and less discomfort to the patient. Moreover, it is as effective as larger drains (24–32 Fr). Pleurodesis is performed once the amount of drain drops to less than 150 mL/day and the lung is fully expanded. The chest drain is removed once the output is less than 150 mL/day postpleurodesis. This leads to longer hospital stays and greater costs. Rapid pleurodesis involves placing a 9–14-Fr catheter under guidance, achieving complete drainage, and then attempting pleurodesis immediately. If loculations or fluid reaccumulation is detected, sonographically guided thoracentesis and pleurodesis through the thoracentesis needle is performed.

This has been shown to be effective and can be performed with small drains in less than 24 hours.

The amount and duration of fluid draining after sclerosant instillation does not indicate pleurodesis success, and the length of stay is significantly reduced when the chest drain is removed at 24 hours (4 vs. 8 days). In the absence of excessive fluid drainage (>250 mL/day), the intercostal tube is removed within 24–48 hours of pleurodesis. The use of rotation and position change to disperse sclerosant after instillation through the chest drain is not supported by evidence. Unlike mesothelioma, malignant seeding of biopsy sites and drain site is extremely uncommon in metastatic pleural effusions and routine radiation to these sites is not recommended.

Long-term Ambulatory Pleural Drainage

Incomplete lung re-expansion due to a thick visceral pleural peel (lung entrapment) prevents pleural apposition and prevents successful pleurodesis. Unlike patients with "trapped lung", these effusions are exudative, associated with ongoing pleural malignancy or inflammation and may increase in size. The best management option for this situation is the insertion of a tunneled pleural catheter. This is 15.5 F silicone rubber catheter, 66 cm in length, with fenestrations along the proximal 24 cm and is inserted into the pleural space using the Seldinger technique under local anesthesia. A one-way valve prevents air from entering and permits drainage into a vacuum bottle at regular intervals.

PROGNOSIS

Survival is primarily determined by the performance status of the patient, the site of the primary cancer, and the stage of malignancy. Mortality is significantly associated with the performance status; the median survival is 1.1 months in patients with Karnofsky score less than 30 and 13.2 months with a score more than 70. In general, lung carcinoma with MPE has the shortest survival while ovarian carcinoma has the longest survival.

CHAPTER 93

Pneumothorax

Uma Devraj, GA D'Souza

INTRODUCTION

Pneumothorax or the air in the pleural space is classified as "spontaneous", which occurs without an obvious cause, or "traumatic", which occurs from direct or indirect trauma. Traumatic pneumothorax is further subcategorized as "Iatrogenic pneumothorax", that is a type of traumatic pneumothorax following a diagnostic or therapeutic pleural puncture. Spontaneous pneumothorax is classified as primary spontaneous pneumothorax (PSP) which occurs in otherwise healthy individuals and secondary spontaneous pneumothorax (SSP) which occurs as a complication of an underlying lung disease. Many PSP patients may also have occult lung disease as evidenced by demonstration of subpleural blebs on computed tomography (CT) scans.

DEFINITIONS

Recurrent pneumothorax: A recurrent pneumothorax is one that occurs on the same side within 7 days of initial resolution. A pneumothorax is considered "persistent" if the air leak lasts for more than 5 days.

Closed pneumothorax: A closed pneumothorax is one in which the alveolar pleural communication is sealed.

Tension pneumothorax: When the intrapleural pressure is above atmospheric pressure, it is called tension pneumothorax.

Open pneumothorax: An open pneumothorax communicates with the atmosphere and results in pendulum breathing (shunting of the physiological dead space between the two lungs) in addition to lung collapse.

PATHOPHYSIOLOGY

The pressure in the pleural space is negative with reference to the atmospheric pressure during the entire respiratory cycle attributable to. Air reaches the pleural space either due to (A) rupture of subpleural bulla or bleb; (B) rupture of overdistended alveoli into the adjacent bronchovascular sheath medially to produce pneumomediastinum (Macklin effect), which may be accompanied by subcutaneous emphysema or pneumothorax, or (C) rupture of overdistended alveoli that can dissect air from alveoli to the peripheral portion of the lung.

The pleural pressure is always less than the alveolar pressure and the atmospheric pressure owing to the elastic recoil of the lung. Air will flow into the pleural space if a communication develops between the pleural space and an alveolus or between the pleural space and the atmosphere.

With pneumothorax, the thoracic cavity enlarges and the lung proportionately collapses. This results in a decrease in vital capacity and arterial partial pressure of oxygen (PO_2). The reduction in arterial PO_2 is caused by areas with low ventilation-perfusion ratios, anatomic shunts, and, occasionally, alveolar hypoventilation. The decreased vital capacity is usually well tolerated in patients with PSP whereas it can precipitate respiratory failure in patients with SSP. The total lung capacity, functional residual capacity, and diffusing capacity are also reduced, although less than the vital capacity.

When perfusion to the collapsed lung is preserved, there is an increase in the pulmonary shunt and substantial hypoxemia. If perfusion to the collapsed lung is reduced by hypoxic vasoconstriction, hypoxemia may be minimal. In general, pneumothoraces occupying less than 25% of the hemithorax are not usually associated with significant shunts. Redistribution of pulmonary blood flow results in improvement of hypoxemia within 24 hours, despite the size of the pneumothorax.

RESOLUTION OF PNEUMOTHORAX

When there is air, it is reabsorbed from the pleural space by simple diffusion into the venous blood. The rate of gas resorption depends on: (1) the pressure gradient for the gases between the pleural space and venous blood; (2) the diffusion properties of the gases present in the pleural space; (3) the area of contact between the pleural gas and pleura; and (4) the permeability of the pleural surface.

The net gradient for gas absorption, from pleural space into capillary blood, is only 54 mm Hg (760–706) on assuming that the pleural pressure is approximately zero when there is pneumothorax. To hasten the absorption of a pneumothorax, the patient can be made to breathe 100% oxygen.

ETIOLOGY

Pneumothorax can occur as a complication of an underlying lung disease when it is labelled as scondary pneumothorax (Table 93.1). On the other hand, primary spontaneous pneumothorax by definition occurs in people without

TABLE 93.1: Etiology of secondary spontaneous pneumothorax.

Infection:
- Tuberculosis (most common cause in India)
- *Pneumocystis jirovecii* pneumonia
- Acute bacterial pneumonia

Obstructive lung disease:
- Chronic obstructive lung disease
- Asthma

Interstitial lung disease:
- Idiopathic pulmonary fibrosis (usual interstitial pneumonitis)
- Nonspecific interstitial pneumonitis
- Eosinophilic granuloma
- Lymphangioleiomyomatosis
- Sarcoidosis
- Langerhans cell granulomatosis
- Radiation pneumonitis or fibrosis
- Histiocytosis X

Malignancy:
- Primary lung carcinoma
- Pulmonary metastasis (especially sarcomas)
- Complications of chemotherapy

Connective tissue disease:
- Rheumatoid arthritis
- Ankylosing spondylitis
- Marfan syndrome
- Ehler–Danlos syndrome
- Polymyositis or dermatomyositis
- Scleroderma

Other:
- Catamenial pneumothorax
- Pulmonary infarction
- Pulmonary hemorrhage
- Pulmonary alveolar proteinosis
- Tuberous sclerosis
- von Recklinghausen's disease
- Wegener's granulomatosis

an underlying lung disease. But, subpleural blebs or bullae can be found in almost 75% of these patients undergoing thoracoscopy. It is unclear whether these are actually the site of air leakage. Only a small number of blebs are found ruptured at the time of thoracoscopy or surgery. In the remaining, air leaks into the pleural space through "pleural porosity" of visceral pleura, i.e. the areas of disrupted mesothelial cells replaced by a porous inflammatory elastofibrotic layer.

The development of blebs, bullae, and areas of pleural porosity may be attributed to distal airway inflammation, hereditary predisposition, and anatomical abnormalities. Some of the other risk factors include the low-body mass index, caloric restriction, abnormal connective tissue, and ectomorphic physiognomy where the intrapleural pressures are more negative and therefore the relative apical ischemia. Smoking is also an important risk factor. Patients with PSP are usually tall and thin. Catamenial pneumothorax during menstrual periods is seen in about 3% of PSP in women. There are few reports of pneumothorax during pregnancy. Lymphangioleiomyomatosis is an important cause of recurrent pneumothorax seen exclusively in women.

Genetic Factors

Genetic abnormalities play an important part in the development of PSP. Autosomal dominant gene with incomplete penetrance has been shown in some cases. Association to an X-linked recessive gene has also been shown. Other associated genetic conditions are lymphangioleiomyomatosis, alpha$_1$-antitrypsin deficiency, and cystic fibrosis (CF). It is more frequent in Marfan syndrome, Ehlers–Danlos syndrome, and homocystinuria.

Clinical Manifestations

Primary spontaneous pneumothorax is commonly seen between 20 years and 40 years. It may occur both at rest and exertion. The main symptoms are acute-onset chest pain, cough, and dyspnea. Occasionally, there may be hemoptysis, orthopnea, and Horner's syndrome.

Small pneumothoraces (occupying <20%) may not be possible to detect on physical examination. The vital signs are usually normal in small and moderate pneumothorax. Presence of tension pneumothorax is considered if the pulse rate is more than 140 beats/min or if there is associated hypotension, cyanosis, or electromechanical dissociation.

On physical examination, the hemithorax on the side of pneumothorax is larger with diminished respiratory movements, hyperresonant percussion note, and absent or reduced breath sounds. The liver may be pushed inferiorly in case of a right-sided pneumothorax. With a large pneumothorax, the trachea may be shifted toward the contralateral side. Hamman's sign, i.e. a crunching or clicking noise heard synchronous with the heartbeat, may be auscultated with a pneumothorax (particularly on the left side) or pneumomediastinum and is influenced by respiration and body position.

LABORATORY INVESTIGATIONS AND DIAGNOSIS

An upright posteroanterior chest radiograph confirms the diagnosis in most of the cases, demonstrating a pleural line. Chest radiograph findings include the presence of hyperlucency and absence of pulmonary vascular markings, in the area of pneumothorax between the outer margin of lung and the chest wall. The lateral decubitus radiograph is superior to erect or supine chest radiograph and is as sensitive as CT scanning in detecting a pneumothorax.

Currently, thoracic ultrasound is being increasingly used in diagnosis of pneumothorax, especially in critical care and to check postprocedure for pneumothorax. "Lung sliding" (movement of visceral pleura against parietal pleura), or "seashore sign" (sand-like grainy image in M mode) on ultrasound indicates that the lung touches the chest wall. Absence of lung sliding in

B-mode and "stratosphere" or "bar code sign" in M mode suggests presence of pneumothorax. Identification of a "lung point" confirms presence of pneumothorax with 100% certainty. In expert hands, lung ultrasound is more sensitive than chest X-ray, to detect pneumothorax.

Thin-walled cysts or avascular bullae can be mistaken for pneumothorax. Skin fold, clothing, tubing, or chest wall artifact scan mimic pneumothorax on the chest radiograph. CT scan in patients with severe bullous lung disease will help to differentiate emphysematous bullae from pneumothoraces.

Pleural effusions may accompany pneumothorax in 20–25% of cases. A hemopneumothorax occurs in 2–3% of spontaneous pneumothoraces. This is due to bleeding from rupture or tearing of vascular adhesions between the visceral and parietal pleura as the lung collapses.

Electrocardiographic changes may be seen due to mechanical effects of a pneumothorax. A left-sided pneumothorax may mimic anterolateral myocardial infarction showing rightward shift of the frontal QRS axis, diminution of precordial R voltage, decrease in QRS amplitude, and precordial T-wave inversion. Absence of significant Q wave and ST-segment elevation helps differentiate ECG changes due to pneumothorax from that due to myocardial infarction. With a right-sided pneumothorax changes mimicking a posterior myocardial infarction may be seen: diminution of precordial QRS voltage, right-axis deviation, and a prominent R wave in lead V_2 with associated loss of S-wave voltage.

Arterial PO_2 is usually less than 80 mm of Hg in 75% of patients.

RECURRENCE RATES

Recurrence of pneumothorax may occur soon after the initial episode either on the same side or on the contralateral side. The rate of recurrence increases with each successive pneumothorax; 33% after the first episode, 62% after the second episode, and 83% after the third episode.

TREATMENT

Primary Spontaneous Pneumothorax

Treatment is aimed to clear the air from the pleural space as well as to prevent recurrence. A number of therapeutic options are there for the treatment of PSP (Box 93.1).

BOX 93.1: Treatment options for primary spontaneous pneumothorax.

- Observation
- Oxygen treatment
- Simple manual aspiration
- Small catheter drainage
- Chest tube drainage
- Medical thoracoscopic talc poudrage or pleural abrasion
- Video-assisted thoracoscopic surgery (VATS) with bleb or bullectomy
- VATS with pleural abrasion or partial pleurectomy
- Axillary thoracotomy

Supplemental Oxygen

Supplemental oxygen administration hastens the rate of air absorption. This is especially used in hospitalized patients who are not subjected to aspiration or tube thoracostomy.

Simple Aspiration

Manual aspiration is usually the first-line of treatment in PSP patients with a good success rate which varies between 50% and 80%. There are no significant complications. Recurrence rates are similar to those with standard chest tube drainage. Patient at professional risk of developing recurrence (aviation personnel, divers) and those with a prolonged air leak (>14 days) should also have recurrence prevention treatment. An anxious patient is a relative indication.

Tube Thoracostomy

Tube thoracostomy is done if simple aspiration is ineffective and thoracoscopy is not readily available; it rapidly causes re-expansion of the underlying lung. A water seal is used along with intercostal tube drainage.

Persistent Air Leak

In PSP, air leak ceases in two-thirds at the time of presentation and in 88% within the next week. Instillation of 1% taurolidine solution through the chest tube causes cessation of air leak within 24 hours. This is successful in 66% with postoperative air leak lasting 4 days or more. Intervention with video-assisted thoracoscopy (VATS) or open thoracotomy should be considered when the air leak persists beyond 5 days in PSP.

Pleurodesis

The goal of pleurodesis is to prevent recurrence in both PSP and SSP. It consists of tube thoracostomy with instillation of a sclerosing agent. Pleurodesis is a procedure that causes symphysis of the two pleural membranes. Medical intervention consists of chemical pleurodesis using agents, such as quinacrine, silver nitrate, talc or tetracycline derivatives. Chemical pleurodesis creates an intense inflammatory reaction which obliterates the pleural space. Parenteral preparation of tetracycline (35 mg/kg) or doxycycline (10 mg/kg), or 20 mL 10% iodopovidone in 80 mL normal saline solution is effective in producing pleurodesis. Since severe chest pain is a common side effect with tetracycline pleurodesis, adequate analgesia is indicated prior to the procedure.

Talc slurry (100 mg/kg) also results in effective pleurodesis but may be associated with acute respiratory distress syndrome (ARDS), hypoxia, and hypotension in a minority. ARDS is probably more common if smaller talc particles (<10 μm) are used.

Recurrence rates can be reduced from approximately 40%–25% by pleurodesis and to 5% by stapling of pleural bleb and pleural abrasion through a thoracoscope. Hence, the latter is preferred when available. But in most centers, it would not be available and chemical pleurodesis is an acceptable alternative.

Thoracoscopy

Video-assisted thoracoscopic surgery is being increasingly used in patients with PSP or SSP to prevent recurrence. The advantages are the entire lung can be inspected and a search for the cause of air leak carried out. There is 2–14% recurrence with VATS after resection of large bullous lesions. Endostapling or suturing followed by pleurodesis by pleural abrasion may be done in case there are pleural blebs responsible for pneumothorax.

Open Thoracotomy

Open thoracotomy, suturing of the blebs, and pleural abrasion are done if VATS is not available. Operative management is indicated in case of recurrence, high-risk professions or lifestyles, (such as pilots or scuba divers), and bilateral or tension pneumothorax. It is also indicated for persistent air leak after 72 hours, incomplete re-expansion of the lung following conservative treatments, and in patients from remote areas with poor access to medical care.

Secondary Spontaneous Pneumothorax

Secondary spontaneous pneumothorax requires hospitalization and air evacuation followed by recurrence prevention after the very first episode. Air evacuation is better achieved with chest tube drainage. Rapid improvement in symptoms results after evacuation of pneumothorax even if small.

Small-bore chest tube or a pigtail catheter is usually sufficient; large-bore chest tubes are required when large air leaks are suspected or when positive pressure ventilation is required. Persistent air leak is more common in SSP, particularly in the elderly. Recurrence prevention should preferably by VATS; in case a visible air leak is present (e.g. a ruptured emphysematous bulla), it should be closed by electrocautery or stapling. In all cases, pleurodesis should be done using talc poudrage, pleural abrasion or partial pleurectomy.

Pneumothorax Secondary to Tuberculosis

Tuberculosis was the most common cause in India; 41% and 50% of SSP in studies from north and south India, respectively. SSP associated with tuberculosis should be treated with tube thoracostomy and often requires prolonged periods of chest tube drainage. Surgery should be delayed if possible till he or she has received antituberculous therapy for at least 6 weeks.

Pneumothorax in Patients with Acquired Immunodeficiency Syndrome

Pneumothorax in patients with acquired immunodeficiency syndrome (AIDS) is associated with multiple etiologies. *Pneumocystis jirovecii*, pyogenic infections, Kaposi's sarcoma, cytomegalovirus, pulmonary Cryptococcus, coccidioidomycosis, and mycobacterial disease have all been associated with spontaneous pneumothoraces. Most patients have a CD4+ count less than 100 cells/mm^3. Approximately 5% of patients with AIDS who receive prophylactic pentamidine develop a spontaneous pneumothorax. This population also has higher risk of contralateral pneumothorax and iatrogenic pneumothorax, because of frequent pulmonary procedures or need for ventilation. SSP associated with *P. jirovecii* is notoriously difficult to treat due to the necrotizing nature of the pneumonia. All patients with SSP due to associated AIDS should undergo tube thoracostomy. Heimlich valve or VATS is indicated if air leak persists for more than a few days.

Chronic Obstructive Pulmonary Disease and Asthma

Pneumothorax potentially is a lethal complication of emphysema. In adults with acute asthma, it is reported in less than 2% of cases. Besides other forms of treatments, use of endobronchial valves is an effective and minimally invasive intervention in patients with persistent air leaks, who are poor surgical candidates.

Cystic Fibrosis

Pneumothorax in patients with CF is associated with significant mortality. The risk of pneumothorax increases with age and poor pulmonary function (forced expiratory volume in 1 second). The risk of pneumothorax increases with presence of microorganisms, such as *Pseudomonas aeruginosa*, *Burkholderia cepacia*, and *Aspergillus* in the airways attributable to increased inflammation, airway secretions, and air trapping. Preventive measures should be adopted with the first episode itself due to the high recurrence rates.

Catamenial Pneumothorax

Pneumothorax that occurs during menstruation is described as catamenial pneumothorax. Respiratory symptoms in such cases develop within 24-48 hours of onset of menstrual flow. Episodes of catamenial pneumothorax are possibly due to transperitoneal migration of endometrial tissue from the pelvis to the pleural cavities through small defects in the diaphragm. More commonly seen on the right side, the defects may sometimes be left-sided or even bilateral pneumothoraces. Catamenial pneumothorax tends to be recurrent.

The treatment of catamenial pneumothorax is aimed at treating endometriosis, by suppressing the ectopic endometrium. This can be attempted by suppression of ovulation with oral contraceptives or by suppression of gonadotropins with danazol or gonadotropin-releasing hormone to produce a medical oophorectomy. Alternatively, the blebs can be stapled, and the diaphragmatic defects can be closed followed by parietal abrasion or pleurectomy, or chemical pleurodesis using VATS.

Iatrogenic Pneumothorax

Iatrogenic pneumothoraces are common, most often due to transthoracic needle aspiration especially in the presence of underlying chronic obstructive pulmonary disease or if the lesion is deep within the lung. This is also more likely when the angle of the needle route is wide. Other causes include transbronchial biopsy, thoracentesis, pleural biopsy, and central vein catheterization. Pneumothorax may sometimes develop during mechanical ventilation with high levels of positive end-expiratory pressure or following other invasive procedures, such as tracheostomy, intercostal nerve block, mediastinoscopy, liver biopsy, and cardiopulmonary resuscitation.

Diagnosis of iatrogenic pneumothorax gets frequently delayed following a procedure. This can be avoided by doing bedside lung ultrasound immediately after the procedure. Small asymptomatic pneumothoraces usually resolve spontaneously without any treatment. Evacuation of air is required for large or symptomatic pneumothoraces, with simple manual aspiration or placement of a small catheter or chest tube attached to a Heimlich valve. Larger tube drainage may be necessary in patients with emphysema or when mechanical ventilation is indicated.

Traumatic (Noniatrogenic) Pneumothorax

A traumatic pneumothorax is commonly caused by either penetrating or nonpenetrating chest trauma. A pneumothorax results whenever there is rupture of either the visceral or the mediastinal pleura.

Tube thoracostomy is required for most traumatic pneumothoraces at least in the beginning. Tube thoracostomy may however be unnecessary if there is an occult pneumothorax or if the distance between the lung and chest wall is less than 1.5 cm, unless the patient is on mechanical ventilation. Immediate thoracotomy is indicated whenever there is fracture of the trachea, a major bronchus or traumatic rupture of the esophagus. Rupture of the esophagus may also be accompanied by hydropneumothorax. Pleural fluid amylase concentration is raised in such case and mortality approaches 100% in the absence of urgent surgical treatment.

Tension Pneumothorax

Tension pneumothorax is said to be present if the intrapleural pressure is greater than the atmospheric pressure throughout expiration and frequently during inspiration. Tension pneumothorax usually develops in patients receiving positive pressure to their airways and occasionally in spontaneously breathing patients with a one-way valve mechanism permitting air to enter the pleural space during inspiration but not exit during expiration.

Onset of tension pneumothorax is abrupt with sudden deterioration in the cardiopulmonary status of the patient. Cardiac output falls due to an impaired venous return and profound hypoxia occurs due to ventilation–perfusion mismatch. The severe cardiopulmonary impairment in patients with tension pneumothorax is responsible for the clinical features of distress, cyanosis, diaphoresis, tachycardia, hypotension, and labored breathing. Immediate treatment is warranted in such cases especially in the mechanically ventilated patients.

Treatment should include high concentrations of supplemental oxygen to alleviate hypoxia and drainage of air. Air evacuation is generally achieved with a large-bore (14- to 16-gauge) catheter inserted into the pleural space through the second anterior intercostal space. An audible gush of air from the pressurized pleural space immediately following insertion of the needle confirms the diagnosis. Alternatively, air is aspirated with the use of a needle fitted with a partially sterile water-filled syringe. The needle is generally inserted through the second anterior space, though the lateral fifth intercostal space may be safer. Intercostal tube drainage should be placed immediately thereafter.

Malignant Pleural Mesothelioma

Arun S Shet, Girish Raju, GA D'Souza

INTRODUCTION

Mesothelioma is the primary neoplasm of the pleural and peritoneal cavities and rarely the tunica vaginalis, or the pericardium. Around 70% of cases of pleural mesothelioma are associated with documented asbestos exposure.

EPIDEMIOLOGY

The annual incidence of malignant pleural mesothelioma in India is not known. Considering the consumption of asbestos in India which has greatly increased to approximately 300,000 tons per year in 2007, the incidence is likely to be significant. There is an increase in the risk of malignant mesothelioma proportionate to the cumulative exposure. Asbestos is extensively used in India. It is predicted that mesothelioma incidence will rise in India similar to what happened in the United States in the past 50 years.

Radiation Therapy

Ionizing radiation to supradiaphragmatic fields may be a risk factor for the subsequent development of mesothelioma, with a long latent period between the initial treatment and the diagnosis of the second malignancy.

Viral Oncogenes

Several lines of evidence have implicated the simian virus 40 (SV40) as a cofactor in oncogenesis related to mesothelioma. SV40 is an oncogenic virus in human and mammalian cell systems. Sequences of DNA of the virus have been found in lymphomas, brain and bone tumors, and mesothelioma.

Nanomaterials

There is an increase in the use of nanomaterials in several industries. Data from animal models implicated carbon nanotubes in the development of peritoneal mesothelioma.

PATHOGENESIS

Mesothelial cells form the lining of the parietal and visceral pleura where they normally facilitate the free movement of the lung during the process of respiration. Any form of injury to these cells can result in proliferation that occurs in response to the release of local growth factors. Asbestos can induce changes in these cells by several processes that can ultimately lead to malignant proliferation. One of these mechanisms is by irritation as a result of physical properties. This irritative process can span from pleural plaques to a frank mesothelioma-like process. Similarly, asbestos fibers can pierce individual cells and cause rupture of the mitotic spindle apparatus disrupting mitosis and resulting in chromosomal damage to the cells. Another form of injury induced by asbestos is the production of reactive oxygen species, which cause oxidant stress and damage to DNA, proteins, and lipids. Finally, asbestos can also induce phosphorylation of kinases such as mitogen-activated protein (MAP), extracellular signal-regulated kinase (ERK) that can increase the expression of early response proto-oncogenes (*fos* and *jun*) and activate certain transcription factors [activator protein 1, (AP1)] promoting cellular activation and proliferation.

Thus, the development of mesothelioma appears to be a culmination of several events that act in concert to produce the eventual clinical phenotype exhibited by patients with mesothelioma.

PATHOLOGY

Early stage mesothelioma due to its slow growth can present as multiple small nodules that occur characteristically on the parietal pleura but can also involve the visceral pleura. These nodules coalesce and form a thickened rind of tumor engulfs the parietal and visceral pleurae. At the advanced later stage, the tumor encases the entire lung as well as extends along the interlobar fissures with minimal invasion of the underlying lung parenchyma. The tumor can be either firm or gelatinous to feel. Invasion of the adjacent structures, chest wall, pericardium, and diaphragm can occur and a large number of patients are shown to have mediastinal lymph node involvement at autopsy.

Mesotheliomas are classified into three broad subtypes: epithelioid, sarcomatoid, and biphasic (mixed). The epithelioid variant is the most common with tubulopapillary, acinar (glandular), adenomatoid, and solid epithelioid patterns. The differential diagnosis includes reactive mesothelial hyperplasia, metastatic carcinomas, and other epithelioid tumors. Biphasic or mixed mesotheliomas have epithelioid and sarcomatoid features.

There is no single marker with high sensitivity and specificity for malignant mesothelioma, which makes it essential to use a panel of markers (both positive and negative). Pancytokeratin stains are very useful in diagnosis and will stain the vast majority of mesothelioma. If the tumor is pancytokeratin negative, then the screening panel should be broadened to include stains to exclude lymphoma, melanoma, angiosarcoma or epithelioid hemangioendothelioma.

CLINICAL PRESENTATION

Mesothelioma is most commonly diagnosed in the fifth to seventh decades of life. History of exposure to asbestos may have actually happened in childhood. Dyspnea and nonpleuritic chest pain are the most common presenting symptoms. It can be rarely asymptomatic seen as unilateral pleural effusion detected incidentally on routine chest radiograph.

The clinical picture may also be accompanied by a variety of paraneoplastic syndromes such as: (A) disseminated intravascular coagulation; (B) migratory thrombophlebitis; (C) thrombocytosis; (D) Coombs-positive hemolytic anemia; (E) hypoglycemia, and (F) hypercalcemia associated with secretion of a parathyroid hormone-like peptide.

DIAGNOSTIC APPROACH

Malignant mesothelioma is commonly misdiagnosed initially. Thoracentesis or closed pleural biopsy is needed to establish the diagnosis of pleural malignancy, but it may not be adequate to distinguish mesothelioma from lung adenocarcinoma. Closed pleural biopsy is also not sufficiently reliable to define the histological subtype of mesothelioma, a potentially important factor in choosing therapy. In addition, negative results do not exclude a diagnosis of mesothelioma. Although rarely indicated, surgical intervention (via video thoracoscopic biopsy or open thoracotomy) has a higher diagnostic yield.

Cytological and Histopathological Diagnosis

Once a sample of pleural fluid or tissue is obtained, a panel of multiple immunohistochemical markers is important to diagnose malignant mesothelioma.

TREATMENT

Surgery may be needed for diagnostic, palliative, or rarely, curative purposes. Aggressive surgical intervention is not feasible in majority of patients who have locally advanced disease, advanced age, or other comorbid medical illnesses. Surgery is helpful for palliative treatment while a survival benefit is seen in selected patients.

Pleurectomy and extrapleural pneumonectomy have been used to try to definitively treat the primary tumor, although neither of these approaches has been shown to increase the survival. These procedures can be considered in patients to obtain symptom control, especially for lung entrapment syndrome. Surgery is best performed in conjunction with other forms of treatment.

However, the greatest challenge in surgical management appears to be in selecting the most appropriate procedure bearing in mind the clinical stage of the disease and the functional assessment of the patient along with a judicious consideration of neoadjuvant therapy.

Pleurodesis

Persistent dyspnea from large, unilateral pleural effusions is the most common and bothersome symptom in mesothelioma. Complete drainage of fluid followed by pleurodesis is the most helpful palliative procedure. This can be achieved with tube thoracostomy or video thoracoscopy and introduction of a pleurodesic agent into the pleural space.

Instilling of agents (tetracycline, doxycycline, bleomycin, and talc), pleurectomy, pleuroperitoneal shunting, and radiation are other treatments that have been described for malignant pleural effusions. The general recommendations for pleurodesis in mesothelioma are to use sterile talc and perform this procedure early in the disease. There is an increasing use of indwelling pleural catheter (IPC) drainage to improve symptoms without doing pleural symphysis.

Thoracoscopic application (poudrage) is more successful than other methods of pleurodesis (e.g. tube thoracostomy). Trials have not made comparisons between different methods of attaining pleural symphysis or different chemical agents to achieve this goal.

Chemotherapy

Although previously results of chemotherapy were disappointing and survival rates less than 10 months, the appearance of several new antineoplastic agents has resulted in improvements in objective response rates and overall survival. Currently, two chemotherapeutic strategies appear to have shown favorable results including adjuvant chemotherapy and induction chemotherapy.

Single-agent Adjuvant Chemotherapy

Cisplatin, gemcitabine, pemetrexed, anthracycline, and vinca alkaloids have shown substantial benefits in phase II studies. Cisplatin is the most effective single agent which constitutes the backbone for combination chemotherapy regimes.

Combination Adjuvant Chemotherapy

Platinum-based dual agent chemotherapy significantly prolongs survival compared with single agent chemotherapy.

Any combination of doublet-based chemotherapy is currently considered the standard therapy for first-line treatment of mesothelioma.

Overall, a very careful evaluation of the socioeconomic status, overall performance status, and patient willingness for chemotherapy may help further delineate patients that would benefit most from chemotherapy.

Induction Chemotherapy

Induction chemotherapy has acceptable response rates of 30–40%. After induction chemotherapy, there are good resectability rates for extrapleural pneumonectomy.

Second-line Chemotherapy

Several-second line agents have been shown to have a response in the setting of mesothelioma that is unresponsive to primary combination chemotherapy. Exceptionally, well-preserved patients in whom financial status does not impact treatment decisions may elect to undergo salvage therapy in which case our most preferred agent is pemetrexed or vinorelbine. Ideally, such patients should be enrolled in a clinical trial.

Radiotherapy

Malignant mesothelioma is traditionally resistant to radiotherapy. Furthermore, the diffuse nature of the tumor prevents localized radiation therapy. However, local radiotherapy can be delivered to surgical sites with questionable margins or to prevent seeding of tumor and can also be used to palliate symptoms. Fractionated radiotherapy using intensity modulation is the technique that has shown some success and is generally used after surgical resection of malignant melanoma. Other radiotherapeutic approaches have also been tried but the results have been disappointing.

Novel Approaches

Molecularly targeted therapies (thalidomide, bevacizumab, gefitinib, imatinib, and erlotinib), immunotherapy (interferon and interleukins), and gene therapy have been investigated with varying but limited degrees of success. Most of these therapies have not yielded dramatic results; although with the small numbers that have been studied, assessment of results tends to be somewhat conflicted. In general, such treatments should be attempted only in the setting of a clinical trial.

Palliative Therapy

Recurrent pleural effusions are best managed by drainage of all fluid, followed by chemical or surgical pleurodesis.

There are several types of pain in malignant mesothelioma associated with local involvement of the chest wall, intercostal nerve or vertebral invasion or organ invasion. Opiates, or nonsteroidal anti-inflammatory drug in addition to an opiate, are often required. Neuropathic pain requires additional drugs such as carbamazepine, gabapentin or sodium valproate. Intrathecal analgesia or nerve block is required in some patients. Palliative radiotherapy for pain relief may also be considered in cases of painful chest wall infiltration or nodules.

Dyspnea due to encasement of the lung by tumor is difficult to treat; a combination of palliative therapies including blood transfusions (for anemia), diuretics (for fluid overload), centesis (for effusion), and oxygen may be tried.

Psychosocial factors are important in the palliation of malignant mesothelioma. In the setting of limited resources, it is especially important to pay attention to palliative care provided in the form of a team of doctors and nonmedical staff including, surgeons, chest physicians, oncologists, pain and palliative care specialists, psychologists, and physiotherapists to ensure that this occurs in a timely and meaningful manner.

CHAPTER

95

Pulmonary Involvement in Connective Tissue Diseases

Om P Sharma, Aditya Jindal

INTRODUCTION

Connective tissue diseases (CTDs) also called as collagen vascular diseases (CVDs) can involve any part of the thorax, including the lung parenchyma, pleura, airways, blood vessels, lymph nodes, lymph channels, chest wall musculature, and the diaphragm. In these multisystem disorders, the lung involvement can be a part of the multisystem illness, or it may be the only manifestation of the systemic illness. Occasionally, the lung involvement may herald the onset of the systemic illness. Respiratory system is commonly involved in rheumatoid arthritis (RA), systemic sclerosis (SSc), systemic lupus erythematosus (SLE), polymyositis, dermatomyositis, Sjögren's syndrome (SS), and mixed connective tissue disorder.

RHEUMATOID ARTHRITIS

Rheumatoid arthritis primarily affects the joints, but can also involve the lungs and pleura, eyes, skin, heart, and peripheral nerves. Pleuropulmonary disease is more commonly seen in patients with severe chronic articular disease, high titers of rheumatoid factor, presence of subcutaneous nodules, cutaneous vasculitis, myopericarditis, ocular inflammation, and Felty's syndrome. Pleuropulmonary abnormalities associated with the rheumatoid process are many and the differential diagnosis is wide (Box 95.1).

Pleural Involvement

Pleural involvement can cause pleural effusion, empyema, chylothorax, pleural thickening, fibrothorax, and lung entrapment. Pleural effusion can be caused

> **BOX 95.1:** Pulmonary complications of rheumatoid arthritis: Tissue-involved manifestation.
>
> - Pleura effusion
> - Empyema
> - Pleural thickening
> - Calcification
> - Pneumothorax
> - Parenchyma necrobiotic nodules
> - Caplan's syndrome
> - Pneumonitis
> - Interstitial fibrosis
> - Bronchiolitis obliterans organizing
> - Pneumonitis (BOOP)
> - Apical bullous disease
> - Airway obstruction
> - Bronchiolitis
> - Bronchiectasis
> - Blood vessels, vasculitis
> - Pulmonary hypertension
> - Thoracic muscle cage dyspnea, muscle weakness

by inflammation or by necrosis, cavitation, and rupture of a nodule into the pleural space. Pleural disease has a remarkable predilection for men, although RA is more common in women in a ratio of 2:1 to 3:1. Pleural involvement mostly remains subclinical or asymptomatic. When symptoms occur, dyspnea, fever, and chest pain are most common. Physical examination may reveal a pleural friction sound and diminished breath sounds over the affected lung field.

Pleural fluid analysis usually reveals a white cell count less than 5,000/mm^3, pleural fluid glucose of less than 0.3 g/L, pleural fluid glucose to serum glucose ratio less than 0.5, pH less than 7.3, and high pleural fluid lactate dehydrogenase (LDH) level (i.e. >700 IU/L). Low glucose levels are nonspecific, may occur in tuberculosis and malignant mesothelioma. Less commonly, patients with RA and a long-standing pleural effusion may develop cholesterol effusion, known as a pseudochylous or chyliform effusion. Cholesterol effusion has the appearance of an empyema, but is sterile. The milky appearance is due to an elevated cholesterol level (always >65 mg/dL and sometimes over 1,000 mg/dL); cholesterol crystals, identifiable with polarized light, may also be present. Cytological examination of rheumatoid pleural fluid often reveals slender or elongated or round multinucleate macrophages and giant multinucleated cells and phagocytes or "RA cells".

Rheumatoid pleuritis and pleural effusions commonly resolve spontaneously. The reported useful treatment options include nonsteroidal anti-inflammatory drugs (NSAIDs), glucocorticoids (oral or intrapleural), pleurodesis, and decortication. When treatment is required due to the presence of pleuritic chest pain or the size of effusion, the initial choice is an NSAID, such as indomethacin. In refractory cases of pleural effusion, a moderate dose of oral glucocorticoids, e.g. 10–20 mg of prednisone daily, may be beneficial. If the patient is intolerant of the side effects due to systemic glucocorticoids, intrapleural glucocorticoids, e.g. 120–160 mg of depo-methylprednisolone acetate, can be tried. Use of chemical pleurodesis and decortication is reserved for refractory effusions and fibrothorax.

Interstitial Lung Disease

Diffuse pulmonary fibrosis of RA has features similar to those seen in idiopathic pulmonary fibrosis (IPF) patients. However, rheumatoid pulmonary fibrosis is a separate entity, because the lungs of these patients, in addition to the usual changes of IPF, show specific features of hyaline collagen nodules, often with necrosis, along with a surrounding palisade of fibroblasts. The symptoms of rheumatoid interstitial lung disease (ILD) are nonspecific, namely dyspnea, dry cough, and basal lung crepitations. Finger clubbing may also be present.

In established cases, chest X-ray films show small lungs with diffuse bilateral reticulonodular infiltrates with lower lobe predominance. Progression of disease results in cystic spaces, honeycombing, and fibrosis. High-resolution computed tomography (HRCT) of the chest shows similar lesions, but with higher sensitivity. There is a good correlation of HRCT findings of ground glass appearances with activity of RA. HRCT patterns of usual interstitial pneumonia (UIP) are common.

Erythrocyte sedimentation rate is usually raised and serum rheumatoid factor is positive. Rheumatoid ILD has a better prognosis and slower rate of deterioration than IPF. Spontaneous remission can occur. No optimal therapeutic approach has been established for RA-related ILD. Often corticosteroids are used as the first-line treatment. Initial dose of prednisone is 1 mg/kg per day for 6–8 weeks with subsequent tapering based on clinical and lung function monitoring. Response to corticosteroids is variable. Drugs, like methotrexate, azathioprine, cyclophosphamide, have been used alone and in combination with prednisone. Cyclosporine has been proved beneficial in selected cases. Several new biological agents have been used for treatment. Some of the drugs, such as methotrexate, tacrolimus, and biological (e.g. abatacept) are themselves known to cause drug-induced ILD.

Rheumatoid Nodules

Rheumatoid nodules are the specific pulmonary manifestation of RA. There are two types of rheumatoid lung nodules: (i) intrapulmonary necrobiotic nodules and (ii) Caplan's syndrome.

Necrobiotic Nodules

These may occur in any part of the lung, but are generally frequent in subpleural areas and in association with interlobular septa. The histology of a rheumatoid pulmonary nodule is similar to that of rheumatoid nodules at other sites, with central necrosis, palisading epithelioid cells, a mononuclear cell infiltrate, and vasculitis. These nodules may shrink, disappear, cavitate or become fibrotic. The prognosis is good.

Caplan's Syndrome (Rheumatoid Pneumoconiosis)

In 1953, Caplan first reported the occurrence of lung nodules in coal miners who also had RA. Caplan's syndrome can also occur in patients with RA exposed to both asbestos and silica. Histologically, the findings are similar to necrobiotic nodules, but are surrounded by pigmented cells. There is no effective treatment for Caplan's syndrome. The prognosis is good.

Organizing Pneumonia

Organizing pneumonia complicating RA, presents with cough, dyspnea, malaise, weight loss, and fever. Crackles are heard on auscultation. Transbronchial lung biopsy or thoracoscopic lung biopsy is required for diagnosis. Patchy intraluminal polypoid plugs of immature fibroblast tissue may be seen in the respiratory bronchioles.

The prognosis of OP is generally good, but spontaneous improvement is rare. Most patients with OP respond rapidly to oral glucocorticoid therapy. Treatment is started with prednisone (1-1.5 mg/kg/day using ideal body weight) to a maximum of 100 mg/day given as a single oral dose in the morning for 4-8 weeks. Prednisone is thereafter reduced to 0.5-1.0 mg/kg/day for another 4-6 weeks and gradually tapered to zero if the patient remains stable or is improved after 3-6 months. Chest radiography and pulmonary function testing is done every 6-8 weeks during the first year. Treatment should be reinstituted aggressively in case of any recurrence. An alternate choice consists of using cyclophosphamide (1-2 mg/kg/day given as a single daily dose) not exceeding 150 mg/day, for a period of 3-6 months.

Airway Obstruction

Upper Airway Obstruction

Upper airway disease, such as cricoarytenoid abnormalities are more commonly seen patients with long-standing disease. Upper airway obstruction occurs due to rheumatoid nodules on the vocal cord or vasculitis involving the recurrent laryngeal or vagus nerves. Early symptoms of upper airway disease may include a hoarse voice, odynophagia, tenderness of throat, and pain on coughing or speaking. Diagnosis of upper airway obstruction is made by laryngoscopy and flow volume loops.

Obliterative Bronchiolitis

Obliterative bronchiolitis (OB) is a rare and usually fatal condition characterized by progressive concentric narrowing of membranous bronchioles. An OB is more common in women patients with positive rheumatoid factor test and SS. It can also occur in patients with RA who receive D-penicillamine, gold and sulfasalazine treatment. Patients typically present with the rapid onset of dyspnea and dry cough.

Constitutional symptoms, such as fever and malaise are not usually seen. Inspiratory crackles and a mid-inspiratory squeak are heard over the lungs on auscultation. Evidence of airflow obstruction, normal diffusing capacity for carbon monoxide (DLCO), and hypoxemia are generally there on lung function tests. Trial therapy is indicated with high-dose corticosteroids (prednisone, 1–1.5 mg/kg/day).

Bronchiectasis

Although an association between bronchiectasis and RA has been noted, it does not appear to be clinically significant in most patients.

Apical Bullous Disease

Apical fibrotic and cavitary lesions similar to those in ankylosing spondylitis (AS) have been reported in patients with RA.

Thoracic Cage Involvement

Abnormalities of thoracic cage mobility, similar to those seen with AS, can occur.

Pulmonary Hypertension

Pulmonary arterial hypertension (PAH) is rare in patients with RA. Its clinical manifestations and prognosis are similar to those with idiopathic PAH in the absence of RA. Secondary pulmonary hypertension usually associated with severe ILD has also been reported in patients with RA.

Lung Cancer

The risk of lung cancer is slightly greater in patients with RA than in the general population.

SYSTEMIC SCLEROSIS

More than 80% of patients with SSc have lung involvement. ILD and pulmonary hypertension are the two major pulmonary complications. Other less common pulmonary complications include pleural effusions, aspiration pneumonia, spontaneous pneumothorax, bronchiectasis, hemoptysis, drug-induced pneumonitis, and lung cancer (Box 95.2).

Interstitial Lung Disease

Interstitial lung disease in SSc is the most frequent cause of mortality. Commonly, there are symptoms, such as fatigue, breathlessness, dry cough, and chest pain; hemoptysis is rare. Presence of bilateral fine inspiratory crackles or rales at the lung bases is the most characteristic physical sign.

> **BOX 95.2:** Pulmonary complications of systemic sclerosis.
>
> *Common:*
> - Nonspecific interstitial pneumonitis
> - Usual interstitial pneumonitis or fibrosis
> - Pulmonary hypertension
> - Alveolar cell carcinoma
> - Pleural thickening
>
> *Uncommon:*
> - Pleural effusion
> - Pneumothorax
> - Bronchiectasis
> - Lung cancer
> - Vascular aneurysm

The symptoms, physical findings, and radiographic characteristics of SSc-associated ILD are similar to other types of ILD. The classic radiographic features of established ILD comprise of symmetric, reticular opacities. These are usually most pronounced at the lung bases. Thin section (3 mm or less) HRCT scanning of the lung can demonstrate the character and distribution of fine structural abnormalities not seen on chest radiographs.

The extent of ILD seen on HRCT, inversely related to forced vital capacity (FVC), is a predictor of survival. The FVC is reduced and there is a proportional reduction of the forced expiratory volume in 1 second (FEV_1). The FEV_1/FVC ratio remains normal. The total lung capacity (TLC), functional residual capacity (FRC), and residual volume (RV) are decreased in ILD. The patients with SSc who have a near-normal FVC at initial presentation have low-risk for progression to severe lung disease. Diffusion capacity is reduced in over 70% of the patients and its decrease correlates with the severity of ILD seen on HRCT. A reduction in DLCO accompanied by relatively normal spirometry and lung volumes suggests pulmonary vascular disease. The value of the 6-minutes walk test (6MWT) is more limited in SSc, as it does not discriminate well between patients with lung involvement and those without.

The common pathological patterns of SSc-associated ILD are Nonspecific Interstitial Pneumonia (NSIP) and UIP. Fibrotic NSIP is the most frequent finding on lung biopsy. Intimal thickening of pulmonary arteries and resulting luminal narrowing may be there. Lung biopsy is generally not required for the SSc-associated lung disease. Broncho-Alveolar Lavage (BAL) fluid shows increase in counts of neutrophils, eosinophils, lymphocytes, and mast cells. The clinical significance of these findings is controversial.

Pulmonary Arterial Hypertension

The prevalence of PAH in SSc varies 7–50%. It may occur as an isolated pulmonary complication of SSc, or can coexist with ILD. SSc is frequently associated with the CREST syndrome (calcinosis, Raynaud phenomenon, esophageal dysmotility, sclerodactyly, and telangiectasia). Early PAH is asymptomatic, but exertional dyspnea is a common initial symptom. There may be chest pain (due to right ventricular angina) and near-syncope or syncope on exertion due to reduced cardiac reserve in patients with advanced PAH. On physical examination, one may find prominent a-waves in the jugular venous pulse, loud pulmonic second heart sound, right ventricular gallop, murmur of tricuspid regurgitation, and palpable right ventricular heave.

On a chest radiograph, PAH produces an enlarged pulmonary artery and attenuation of the smaller pulmonary vessels. The presence of PAH may be suspected if pulmonary function tests show a significant decrease in DLCO (<65% of the predicted value) in the presence of normal spirometry.

Doppler echocardiography permits estimation of pulmonary artery pressures when tricuspid regurgitation is present. The test cannot be relied upon to exclude PAH in high-risk patients due to its limited sensitivity and technical limitations. Right heart catheterization is the gold standard for identification and evaluation of PAH.

A new screening test for PAH in SSc is measurement of serum levels of brain natriuretic peptide (BNP) and/or N-terminal probrain natriuretic peptide (NT-proBNP). Elevated NT-proBNP levels have a sensitivity and specificity of 90%, respectively for the presence of PAH.

Aspiration Pneumonitis

Gastroesophageal reflux, present in most patients, may cause recurrent aspiration of gastric contents and lung injury.

Pleural Disease

Pleural effusion and spontaneous pneumothorax are rare complications.

Bronchiectasis

Cylindrical bronchiectasis is a common finding on HRCT scanning of the lungs of patients with SSc. In one study comprising 22 patients, bronchiectasis was present in 59% of cases.

Lung Cancer

There is increased risk of lung cancer in SSc patients with diffuse skin involvement. Corticosteroids offer no benefit in the course of established ILD. Colchicine also does not affect the scleroderma lung disease. Cyclophosphamide may significantly improve dyspnea and lung functions.

SJÖGREN'S SYNDROME

Sjögren's syndrome is associated with lymphocytic infiltration of lacrimal and salivary glands. Typically, there are symptoms of dryness of the eyes (keratoconjunctivitis sicca) and dryness of the mouth (xerostomia). The disease can exist as a primary disorder or as a secondary condition along with other autoimmune diseases, such as RA, SLE, and scleroderma.

> **BOX 95.3:** Pulmonary complications of Sjögren's syndrome.
>
> - Nonspecific interstitial pneumonitis
> - Usual interstitial pneumonitis
> - Lymphocytic interstitial pneumonitis
> - Pulmonary lymphoma
> - Diffuse pulmonary amyloidosis

Primary Sjögren's syndrome (pSS) primarily affects women between 50 years and 70 years of age. The prevalence of pulmonary disease in SS has not been established, and the reported incidences vary greatly. In one study, the prevalence of respiratory disease in patients with pSS was found to be as high as 75%.

An ILD, the most common lung abnormality in SS, occurs in about 25% of all patients. It is particularly seen in patients who have both glandular and extraglandular features of SS. The most common type of ILD in pSS is NSIP (Box 95.3).

Dyspnea and dry cough are two principal symptoms; the presence of bibasilar crackles is the most frequent sign. Asymptomatic patients can have detectable abnormalities on pulmonary function testing or HRCT. The chest radiograph may be normal, or may show a fine reticular or nodular pattern with basilar prominence on chest radiograph in 10–20% of cases. The HRCT is more sensitive than chest radiograph for interstitial disease.

In patients with interstitial opacities on chest radiograph, pulmonary function tests commonly reveal a restrictive pattern with a low diffusing capacity. The combination of a restrictive defect and a low DLCO appears to be more common in pSS than in secondary SS. Anti-Ro antibody-positive patients have significantly lower diffusing capacity than anti-Ro antibody-negative patients.

In patients without clinical or radiographical evidence of pulmonary disease, BAL may show evidence of inflammation. A pure lymphocytic alveolitis is common; neutrophil predominance is also observed in some cases. A wide-spectrum of histological changes, including a mild inflammatory response, NSIP, end-stage fibrosis, honeycombing, and OP, is seen. A feature common in SS is lymphocytic infiltration causing follicular bronchiolitis, lymphocytic interstitial pneumonia, nodular lymphoid hyperplasia, and lymphoma. Occasionally, in SS, lung biopsy specimens may reveal noncaseating granulomas, a finding suggestive of sarcoidosis.

In symptomatic patients with SS and ILD and functional deterioration, the standard treatment is oral prednisone in the dosage of 1 mg/kg/day with subsequent tapering, continued for at least 6 months. The patients who do not improve with systemic glucocorticoids should receive azathioprine, cyclophosphamide, and cyclosporine.

SYSTEMIC LUPUS ERYTHEMATOSUS

During the course of their illness, most patients with SLE show signs of pulmonary involvement (Box 95.4). Pulmonary manifestations include the

> **BOX 95.4:** Pulmonary manifestations of systemic lupus erythematosus.
> - Acute lupus pneumonitis
> - Chronic lupus pneumonitis
> - Vanishing lung syndrome
> - Alveolar hemorrhage
> - Cryptogenic organizing pneumonia
> - Pleural effusion
> - Linear atelectasis
> - Acute reversible hypoxemia
> - Veno-occlusive disease
> - Adult respiratory distress syndrome
> - Pulmonary hypertension

presence of pleuritis and pleural effusion, interstitial lung disease, Vanishing Lung Syndrome (VLS), pulmonary hemorrhage, and thromboembolic pneumonia. Chest pain, cough, and dyspnea are often the first symptoms. Pleural inflammation may cause chest pain in the absence of a friction rub or radiographic evidence of a pleural effusion. The pain is often aggravated by deep breaths and change of position. Chest pain may also arise from the inflamed muscles and the connective tissue.

Pleural Disease

The effusions, when present, are small, recurrent, and often bilateral. The pleural fluid is an exudate with elevation of pleural fluid LDH. The total white cell count is low and pleural fluid glucose concentration is only slightly lower than serum blood levels. The complement levels and protein concentration are characteristically low in lupus effusions. Pleural disease and pain in SLE generally responds well to local heat, NSAIDs, and topical analgesics. Steroids in moderate to high dose may be used if there is no response within a few days. Immunosuppressive drugs are rarely required. Fibrothorax and lung entrapment are uncommon.

Acute Lupus Pneumonitis

Acute lupus pneumonitis may be seen in 1–12% of the patients. Commonly, the patient complains of fever, chest pain, cough, and dyspnea. Rarely, hemoptysis may be present. Pleural effusion is another common clinical feature present in about 50% of the patients. Pathologically, lupus pneumonitis is characterized by acute alveolar wall injury, alveolar hemorrhage, alveolar edema, hyaline membrane formation, and immunoglobulin and complement deposition. Diagnosis of alveolitis is usually made by the presence of late inspiratory crackles, and CT scan abnormalities. Acute lupus pneumonitis is difficult to distinguish from alveolar hemorrhage on clinical grounds along. Video-assisted thoracoscopic or open lung biopsy may be required. The patients with lymphocytosis on BAL have the best prognosis, whereas, the predominance of eosinophils or neutrophils in lavage fluid portends high mortality rate. Lupus pneumonitis developing in the postpartum period has a poor prognosis.

Acute lupus pneumonitis needs prompt and aggressive treatment with prednisone around 1–1.5 mg/kg/day in divided doses. If no response is seen within 72 hours, the administration of intravenous pulse glucocorticoids (1 g of methylprednisolone per day for 3 days) and addition of slower acting immunosuppressive drugs, such as cyclophosphamide, should be considered.

Chronic Lupus Pneumonitis

Chronic (fibrotic) lupus pneumonitis occurs in less than 10% of patients with long-standing SLE, and those with anti-Ro antibodies are more likely to develop chronic pneumonitis. These patients frequently suffer from chronic nonproductive cough, dyspnea, and recurrent pleuritic chest pain. Pulmonary function studies show a restrictive pattern with reductions in lung volumes, DLCO, and arterial blood oxygen tension. Chest radiographs reveal changes of chronic pneumonitis. The HRCT, BAL, and 67-gallium scintigraphy are the important tools to diagnose lupus pneumonitis. In undiagnosed cases, lung biopsy may become necessary.

Treatment of chronic lupus pneumonitis is begun with oral prednisone in a dose of 1 mg/kg/day. Patients treated with glucocorticoids tend to improve slowly and stabilize with time. Symptomatic improvement may not always be reflected in DLCO improvement. Immunosuppressive agents are considered if no response is seen within a few months of beginning steroid therapy. The optimal choice of immunosuppressant is uncertain, but cyclophosphamide, azathioprine or mycophenolate have all been utilized.

Pulmonary Hypertension

Mild-to-moderate pulmonary hypertension occurs in more than 50% of patients. Dyspnea, chest pain, and chronic nonproductive cough are the frequent symptoms. Fatigue, weakness, palpitations, and edema may also occur. Physical findings are similar to pulmonary hypertension from any other cause. Laboratory abnormalities include hypoxemia, enlarged pulmonary arteries with clear lung fields on chest radiography, reduced lung volumes and a reduced carbon monoxide diffusing capacity, and electrocardiographic evidence of right ventricular hypertrophy. The typical histopathological features of lupus-induced pulmonary hypertension include plexiform angiomas, thickening of the muscular wall of the pulmonary arteries, and immunoglobulin and complement deposition in the arterial walls.

Management of patients with secondary pulmonary hypertension and SLE is similar to that in idiopathic PAH. The echocardiography-based definitions of PH are useful in predicting 6-year mortality.

Vanishing Lung Syndrome

This syndrome is characterized by dyspnea, pleuritic chest pain, and a progressive decrease in lung volume without any significant lung or pleural disease on chest CT. The most likely cause of VLS is a myositis or myopathy that affects the diaphragms. However, some patients with VLS may have normal diaphragmatic muscle strength. The syndrome should always be considered in patients with SLE who have dyspnea, clear chest X-rays, and elevated diaphragms. Corticosteroids, theophylline, and/or immunosuppressive therapy may improve symptoms and pulmonary function.

Pulmonary Hemorrhage

Alveolar hemorrhage is an uncommon complication in SLE. Rarely, it may be the presenting manifestation of SLE, but most commonly it occurs during the course of an already diagnosed lupus.

The patient complains of dyspnea, hemoptysis, and cough. Chest X-ray films may reveal bilateral alveolar infiltrates. Hemorrhage may sometimes be suggested on findings seen on pulmonary magnetic resonance imaging due to the paramagnetic effects of iron in hemorrhagic blood which result in preferential T2 shortening. The BAL fluid is bloody with hemosiderin-laden macrophages. Pulmonary diffusing capacity for carbon monoxide is significantly elevated; the diagnosis can be established definitively by lung biopsy.

High-dose corticosteroids, cyclophosphamide, plasmapheresis, antibiotics, and mechanical ventilation have improved survival rate.

Cryptogenic Organizing Pneumonia

The cryptogenic organizing pneumonia (COP) is characterized by the presence of fibrous tissue plugs in bronchioles and alveolar spaces. Clinically, the patient may present with dry cough and multiple infiltrates on chest X-ray. The diagnosis is confirmed by lung biopsy. Treatment with oral prednisone (1 mg/kg/day) is usually effective.

Acute Reversible Hypoxemia

Acute hypoxemia as a manifestation of SLE is characterized by hypoxemia, a normal chest radiograph, and no evidence for pulmonary emboli. Plasma C3a levels are markedly elevated. In addition, upregulation of adhesion molecules, such as E-selectin, vascular cell adhesion molecule-1 and intercellular adhesion molecule-1, occurs suggesting that there is excessive complement activation and leukocyte-endothelial cell adhesion and leuko-occlusive vasculopathy. Glucocorticoids alone or with aspirin are effective.

Pulmonary Veno-occlusive Disease

Pulmonary veno-occlusive disease, a rare cause for pulmonary hypertension seen in SLE, is characterized by intimal fibrosis, occlusion of the pulmonary veins, and edema in the interlobular septa. HRCT shows thickened interlobular septa, lymph node enlargement, and ground glass opacities.

Adult Respiratory Distress Syndrome

When adult respiratory distress syndrome (ARDS) develops, it is commonly due to bacteremia or sepsis with gram-negative bacilli and more likely occurs in those who had been treated with glucocorticoids. It has a poor prognosis.

DERMATOMYOSITIS AND POLYMYOSITIS

Four principal types of lung disease have been described in dermatomyositis-polymyositis (DM-PM) (Box 95.5).

Interstitial Lung Disease

When sought systematically in all patients, using techniques, such as HRCT of the chest, the prevalence of ILD is about 40% in DM-PM. Several histological patterns of ILD occur in DM-PS.

Patients with ILD typically present with dyspnea and a nonproductive cough, fever, and arthralgias. Chest auscultation usually reveals dry bibasilar crackles. ILD can precede the diagnosis of myositis by months or years, or be the predominant feature at the time of presentation. The course of ILD varies amongst different patients. In patients with symptomatic ILD, the pulmonary disease determines prognosis; it is worse than in the patients who do not have ILD. The prognosis and response to treatment are worse in patients with DM.

The diagnosis of ILD in DM and PM can be established by the clinical presentation, chest X-ray, high resolution CT scan, and pulmonary function tests. The major radiographical finding is diffuse reticulonodular interstitial changes found predominantly in the lung bases. Thin-section or high resolution chest CT is an excellent technique for characterizing nonspecific interstitial changes on chest X-ray. Typical patterns include ground glass opacification, basilar consolidation, septal thickening, honeycombing, and irregular linear opacities. The Jo-1 antigen, precipitating antibody to an acidic nuclear protein antigen, is an important marker of the PM-DM-associated ILD.

Treatment of ILD in patients with myositis almost always requires glucocorticoids, regardless of whether pulmonary or muscle disease is the predominant feature of the patient's illness. Since ILD is a fatal disease, a second agent is added from the beginning of therapy in patients with DM or PM complicated by ILD. Options for this second agent in patients with mild ILD include azathioprine and methotrexate; azathioprine is preferred because of its favorable side effect profile. In patients with moderate-to-severe ILD, cyclophosphamide is given. In patients with inexorable disease, rituximab and intravenous immune globulin are the most commonly used treatment options.

BOX 95.5: Four types of lung disease in dermatomyositis or polymyositis syndrome.

- Interstitial lung disease
- Respiratory muscle weakness
- Infection
- Drug-induced pneumonitis

Respiratory Muscle Weakness

Respiratory muscle weakness occurs in 4–8% of patients with DM or PM. Typical inflammatory myopathic changes have been seen in the diaphragm, intercostal muscles, and accessory muscles. Respiratory muscle weakness can cause mild dyspnea, linear or plate-like changes on chest X-ray, respiratory failure, and hypercapnic coma. The patients with expiratory muscle strength less than 30% of normal and FVC less than 55% of predicted normal are prone for developing hypercapnia.

Lung infection is common in DM and PM. Prophylaxis with trimethoprim-sulfamethoxazole against *Pneumocystis jirovecii* is given to the patients with DM or PM-ILD who are treated with high-dose glucocorticoids and immunosuppressive agents.

ANKYLOSING SPONDYLITIS

Ankylosing spondylitis primarily affects the sacroiliac joints and the axial skeleton. It is a chronic progressive inflammatory disease that is 2–3 times more common in men than in women. The disease is strongly associated with human leukocyte antigen-B27, a histocompatibility antigen I. There is a wide range of pulmonary manifestations seen in AS (Box 95.6).

Upper Lobe Fibrosis

Upper lobe fibrosis is the most common extra-articular manifestation of AS. Occurring predominantly in men, the infiltrate may be unilateral, bilateral, acute or chronic, solid, or cavitary. The cavities may become colonized with fungi or mycobacterial agents. The HRCT imaging, however, reveals higher prevalence of apical fibrosis. The clinical significance of the HRCT abnormalities that are common in asymptomatic AS patients is uncertain (Box 95.7).

BOX 95.6: Pulmonary manifestations of ankylosing spondylitis.

- Upper lobe fibrosis
- Upper lobe cavities with fungus balls
- Interstitial lung disease
- Pleural effusion or thickening
- Sleep apnea syndrome
- Pneumothorax

BOX 95.7: High-resolution computed tomography abnormalities in ankylosing spondylitis-related lung disease.

- Apical fibrosis
- Thin-walled cavities
- Fungus ball
- Nonspecific parenchymal abnormalities
- Hilar or mediastinal adenopathy
- Emphysema
- Pleural changes

The pathogenesis of the apical fibrosis and other lung abnormalities seen in AS lesion is not known. Histological features include hyaline and elastic degeneration with interstitial fibrosis. Granulomas and vasculitis are absent.

Sleep Apnea Syndrome

The prevalence of sleep apnea syndrome is higher in AS patients than in general population. It has been suggested that AS predisposes to sleep apnea via different mechanisms that include restriction of the oropharyngeal airway due to cervical spine or temporomandibular arthritis, compression of medullary centers or by restrictive lung disease. Fatigue, a common symptom of AS, may be related to sleep apnea syndrome.

Pneumothorax

A rare manifestation of pulmonary involvement in AS is due to rupture of fibrocystic foci. Due to the tendency of recurrence, prophylactic measures should be undertaken.

Respiratory Muscle Weakness

Maximum inspiratory pressure, maximum expiratory pressure, and maximum voluntary ventilation are reduced. There is diminished chest expansion due to the reduced respiratory muscle strength.

MIXED CONNECTIVE TISSUE DISEASE

Mixed connective tissue disease (MCTD) refers to a systemic autoimmune disease characterized by overlapping features of two or more CTDs. The pathogenesis and pathophysiology of MCTD are not well known. The clinical, radiological, and physiological features of lung involvement in MCTD are similar to those observed in progressive SSc in particular and other CTDs in general. PAH and ILD occur in long-term follow up and affect the disease progression.

Interstitial Lung Disease

Histopathological features of ILD in MCTD include alveolar septal infiltration by lymphocytes, plasma cells, and type III collagen fibers. These are similar to those seen in IPF. Treatment in the acute inflammatory state consists of corticosteroids and cytotoxic agents, such as chlorambucil and cyclophosphamide.

Pleural Effusion

Pleuritis occurs in about one-third of all the patients with MCTD. Occasionally, bilateral pleural inflammation is the initial event of MCTD; the fluid is usually exudative. Pleural thickening is uncommon.

> **BOX 95.8:** Common drugs employed for treatment of connective tissue-related lung diseases.
> - Corticosteroids, cyclophosphamide, methotrexate and azathioprine, and biological agents are the main drugs
> - Rheumatoid arthritis-related interstitial lung disease responds to corticosteroids and methotrexate
> - Corticosteroids are not useful in scleroderma-related lung disease; cyclophosphamide is the drug of choice
> - Acute lupus pneumonitis responds to corticosteroids
> - Collagen vascular disease-related organizing pneumonia or cryptogenic pneumonia has good prognosis and responds to corticosteroids
> - Polymyositis-dermatomyositis-related lung disease is fatal; corticosteroids and cyclophosphamide should be used

Pulmonary Hypertension

Progressive pulmonary hypertension is the most serious pulmonary complication of MCTD. It is often accompanied by severe systemic vasculitic lesions. In one study, out of all the patients studied, 67% had pulmonary hypertension. In these patients, elevated pulmonary vascular resistance was associated with impairment of diffusion capacity. Lung biopsy specimens reveal muscular hypertrophy of the small pulmonary arteries. Plexogenic angiopathy and intimal thickening of medium-sized arteries has been observed. Fatal pulmonary hypertension has been reported in MCTD patients.

Treatment

Most CTDs require anti-inflammatory and immunosuppressant drugs. The commonly employed drugs for CTD-related pulmonary disease are listed in Box 95.8.

CONCLUSION

Pulmonary involvement is common in CVDs. It is necessary to differentiate the primary lung disease related to the disease process from the superimposed secondary infections and drug-induced changes. The treatment options are limited and include corticosteroids, immunosuppressive drugs, and newer biological agents.

CHAPTER 96

Pulmonary Manifestations of Other System Diseases

Ajmal Khan, SK Jindal

INTRODUCTION

The lungs with their dual blood circulation and an open airway system exposed to the environment are liable to get involved in diseases of other organ systems. The spectrum of these pulmonary manifestations is wide—a major source of morbidity and mortality.

PART I

CARDIOVASCULAR DISEASES

The heart and the lungs in the thoracic cavity complement the action of each other due to their embryological and anatomical relationships. Any deviation of pressure and volume in the heart or the gas exchange in the lungs will have deleterious consequences on the other. Increase in pressure or volume in the pulmonary vasculature as a consequence of left heart dysfunction induces secondary abnormalities in gaseous exchange. Similarly, decreased pressure downstream curtails the force and endurance of the respiratory muscles disposing them to mechanical disadvantage and ventilatory defects. On the other hand, an intrinsic defect in the parenchyma, airways or the vascular bed of the lungs produces right heart dysfunction that ultimately leads to altered geometry of the interventricular septum and compromised left heart function.

Heart Failure

There is linear increase in blood flow from apex to base of the lung under physiological conditions. Increase in left atrial pressure secondary to left heart failure causes shift of linear flow of blood to more uniformly distributed flow through distension and recruitment of capillaries. Additional safety mechanisms that prevent edema formation are low permeability and active transport of alveolar epithelial cells, resorption into blood vessels, as well as lymphatics, mediastinal, and pleural drainage. Higher pulmonary venous and capillary filling pressures promote vascular distension and perivascular, peribronchiolar, interstitial, and alveolar edema leading to symptom complex of dyspnea, wheezing, and exercise intolerance (Box 96.1).

The diagnosis of heart failure is largely based on history and physical examination supported by ancillary tests such as chest radiograph, electrocardiogram, and echocardiography. Raised jugular venous pressure indicates a state of volume overload. A chest radiograph is helpful to distinguish heart failure from primary pulmonary disease. Plasma concentrations of brain natriuretic peptide are raised in cases of dyspnea of cardiac causes. Described below are the pulmonary abnormalities commonly seen in heart failure.

Ventilatory Abnormalities

Left-sided heart failure of any cause leads to fluid accumulation in the lungs responsible for changes in their mechanical and gas-exchanging properties. In general, total lung capacity (TLC) and functional residual capacity (FRC) are reduced whereas the residual volume may be normal or slightly increased. Variable degrees of obstructive defects alone are more prevalent during periods of decompensation that improve with diuresis predominantly due to reduction in extravascular lung water and pulmonary and bronchial blood flow. In stable patients, obstructive defects are related to adequacy of treatment, normal aging, and smoking habits.

Ventilatory abnormalities improve following correction of cardiac abnormalities. The exact cause of restrictive defects in chronic heart failure remains elusive. Reduced lung compliance owing to cardiac size augmented by increased interstitial fluid accumulation, general muscle weakness, and wasting likely accounts for restrictive changes seen in heart failure. Additionally, parenchymal changes induced by increased levels of circulating cytokines like tumor necrosis factor-α or pulmonary vascular remodeling due to chronic high left atrial pressures lead to altered lung compliance and consequently restrictive changes in lung mechanics.

Diffusion Abnormalities

A fall in lung perfusion and reduction in the conductance of the alveolar-capillary membrane in case of heart failure causes alterations of respiratory

BOX 96.1: Mechanisms of dyspnea and exercise limitation in heart failure.
- Decreased lung compliance
- Bronchial hyperresponsiveness
- Ventilation perfusion mismatch
- Stimulation of lung stretch receptors
- Respiratory muscle weakness

mechanics and gas exchange capacity. The lung diffusion abnormalities in heart failure are attributable to the presence of interstitial edema, hydrostatic injury of alveolar-capillary membrane, and altered alveolar fluid clearance. These mechanisms are responsible for remodeling and a persistent reduction in alveolar-capillary membrane conductance and lung diffusion capacity.

Sleep Abnormalities

There is significantly high prevalence of breathing abnormalities during sleep heart failure. Depending on the severity of heart failure, about 37–75% of patients have central sleep apnea (CSA), and an additional 10–25% have obstructive sleep apnea (OSA). The presence of CSA may promote progression of cardiac disease and an increased risk of mortality which is independent of underlying cardiac dysfunction.

Apneas result in recurrent hypoxia, arousal, and large swings in intrapleural pressure leading to sympathetic surge, oxidative stress, vascular endothelial dysfunction, and mechanical effects on the heart and vessels leading to development of cardiovascular disease. Cheyne–Stokes respiration or periodic breathing characterized by alternating periods of central apneas or hypopneas with hyperpnea is the predominant form of CSA observed in the setting of heart failure.

In heart failure, abnormalities in any of these parameters result in repetitive arterial oxyhemoglobin desaturations and arousals from sleep leading to increase in sympathetic neural drive causing further worsening of an already compromised heart. Ventilatory instability due to increased circulation time and increased loop gain in the metabolic control of ventilation is largely responsible for CSA while predominantly upper airway collapse during sleep leads to OSA in heart failure.

Symptoms of heart failure and sleep apnea may overlap. The clinical clues for sleep apnea in patients with heart failure include the following: presence of hypocapnia, atrial fibrillation, ventricular tachycardia, a low left ventricular ejection fraction, a high New York Heart Class (III and IV), and excess premature ventricular beats and couplets. Polysomnography needs to be done to confirm the diagnosis.

NEUROMUSCULAR DISEASES

The function of respiratory system is accomplished by the ventilatory apparatus (lung and the chest wall) controlled by the neurochemical network. Neuromuscular diseases produce respiratory manifestations due to altered function of central nervous system, spinal cord, peripheral nerves, neuromuscular junction, and muscles. There is respiratory muscle weakening, particularly the diaphragm causing hypoventilation. Involvement of muscles of expiration results in the impairment of cough and bulbar functions disrupting cough, swallowing, and speech. Common final abnormality in these disorders is primarily ventilatory failure, pulmonary hypertension, and cor pulmonale. The pattern, prognosis, and treatment of neuromuscular disorders causing respiratory dysfunction depend on the level of neuromuscular impairment, natural course of the primary disorder, and availability of curative therapy.

Assessment of Respiratory Muscle Function

Clinical presentation of patients with respiratory neuromuscular disorders can vary from totally asymptomatic to overt respiratory failure.

Gas Exchange

The initial manifestation of mild to moderate respiratory muscle weakness is that of alveolar hypoventilation with a normal or elevated pH. Arterial carbon dioxide (pCO_2) tension may decrease due to increased ventilator drive. In patients with mild to moderate muscle dysfunction, one cannot rely on pulse oximetry or blood gas estimation. Carbon dioxide retention rises progressively with the disease progression because of the decrease in the respiratory muscle strength to less than 50% of the predicted values. Chronic hypercapnia is also aggravated by other factors such as altered control of breathing compounded by blunted hypercapnic and hypoxic ventilatory drive, atelectasis, and abnormal chest wall compliance. Arterial tension of oxygen (pO_2) and the alveolar-arterial oxygen tension gradient [pO_2 (A–a)] are usually normal unless there is concomitant parenchymal or alveolar abnormality.

Pulmonary Function Tests

Integrated function of respiratory muscle, nerves, airways, and lung parenchyma can be assessed noninvasively by measuring TLC, vital capacity (VC), and maximum voluntary ventilation (MVV). Alterations in the function of respiratory muscles and nerves limit the ability to lower intrathoracic pressure and reduce the ability to generate a full inspiration, leading to restrictive defects. Furthermore, rapid and shallow breathing pattern due to neuromuscular weakness leads to increased dead space to tidal volume ratio that compromises their ventilatory function.

Reduction in lung volumes is appreciated only in cases with severe impairment of respiratory muscle strength (>50%). This is possibly explained on the basis of the sigmoid shape of the pressure–volume relationship of the respiratory system. In patients with bilateral diaphragmatic palsy, there is significant positional variation in VC which may be reduced by more than 30% in the supine position. This is a more sensitive indicator of respiratory muscle weakness than the upright measurement of TLC and VC alone. This is not true in individuals without diaphragmatic palsy in which situation there is potential for false positive results.

In neuromuscular disorders, reduction in forced vital capacity is proportional to the increase in forced expiratory volume in 1 second so that the ratio is preserved unless concomitant obstructive processes are also present. This preserved ratio is largely because of above normal lung recoil and patent airways. In the presence of normal expiratory flow rates, MVV is an index of respiratory muscle endurance which correlates better than VC to predict respiratory muscle strength.

Respiratory Muscle Strength Assessment

Neuromuscular diseases are diagnosed on the basis of respiratory muscle weakness. Respiratory muscle strength is assessed by maximal static inspiratory and expiratory pressures (PI_{max} and PE_{max}). Measurements of both pressures are done at the airway opening during a voluntary contraction against an occluded airway. PI_{max} is measured during a maximal, static inspiratory effort (Muller maneuver) initiated at either FRC or RV while PE_{max} is measured during a maximal, static expiratory effort (Valsalva maneuver) at TLC. Both PI_{max} and PE_{max} are reduced in generalized neuromuscular weakness.

Diaphragmatic Paralysis

Diaphragm is the most important muscle of ventilation which consists of noncontractile central tendon and contracting muscle fibers attached to the inner surface of the thoracic cage. The diaphragm alone is responsible for most of the inspiratory effort during supine breathing. Diaphragm is supplied by the phrenic nerve (C_3–C_5) which may be involved in different neuromuscular diseases. Diaphragmatic paralysis may involve one leaflet (unilateral paralysis) or the whole diaphragm (bilateral paralysis) due to several diseases (Table 96.1).

Clinical Features

The degree of symptoms of diaphragmatic paralysis is variable depending upon the underlying lesion (a unilateral or bilateral paralysis), rapidity of onset, concurrent lung or heart disorders, and the degree of obesity (Table 96.2). In unilateral disease, only shortness of breath upon undertaking of strenuous physical exertion or total absence of symptoms may be present. Occasionally, Hoover's sign (i.e. an uninhibited movement of costal margin away from the midline on the side of the injury) or unilateral abdominal paradox at the affected side is observed.

TABLE 96.1: Etiologies of diaphragmatic paralysis.

Neurological disorders	Myopathic disorders	Miscellaneous
Multiple sclerosis	Limb-girdle muscular dystrophy	Phrenic nerve injury: • Blunt trauma • Cardiac surgery
Amyotrophic lateral sclerosis	Acid maltase deficiency	Infection: • Pleurisy • Herpes zoster
Spinal cord transection	Hypothyroidism or hyperthyroidism	Inflammatory: • Vasculitis • Chronic inflammatory demyelinating polyneuropathy
Guillain–Barré syndrome	Systemic lupus erythematosus	Diabetic neuropathy
Poliomyelitis	Mixed connective-tissue disease	

TABLE 96.2: Differences between unilateral and bilateral diaphragm paralysis.

	Unilateral paralysis	Bilateral paralysis
Dyspnea	Absent or only on exertion	Always present
Orthopnea	Occasional	Unable to lie supine
Hypoxemia	Rare	Common
Hypercarbia	Rare	Common
Forced vital capacity	Normal	Drop of >30% from upright to supine
Chest X-ray	Eventration of diaphragm	Bilateral small lungs due to atelectasis
Fluoroscopy	Sniff test positive	Absence of caudal displacement
USG	Findings of paralysis restricted to the side of involvement	Findings of paralysis on both sides

Bilateral paralysis occurs as part of severe generalized muscle weakness, but it may present in isolation as the first manifestation of a more generalized neuromuscular syndrome with later involvement of other muscles. These patients often present with dyspnea on mild activity especially that requires expiratory muscle recruitment like bending or lifting and sensing suffocation in the supine position. A unique symptom is dyspnea with immersion in water due to decrease in VC of more than 30% as compared to less than 10% in normal individuals. With disease progression, dyspnea worsens and progressive hypercapnia and hypoxemia develop that are worse during sleep.

Diagnosis

Clinical examination: Under normal condition, expansion of abdomen and rib cage occurs synchronously during inspiration while in supine position; there is greater expansion of anterior abdominal wall during inspiration due to enhanced abdominal compliance. Diaphragmatic paralysis leads to inward movement of abdomen as the rib cage expands during inspiration, a phenomenon known as paradoxical respiration. These paradoxical motions can be detected noninvasively using magnetometry or respiratory inductance plethysmography.

Pulmonary function tests: For screening significant diaphragmatic impairment, simpler test like VC in upright and supine position may be used. In bilateral diaphragmatic paralysis, characteristically the decreases in VC from erect to supine position are 30–55%. Isolated diaphragmatic dysfunction may be suspected if the predominant abnormality is a low PI_{max} (<60 cm H_2O) with relatively preserved PE_{max}, however, a normal PI_{max} due to the preserved strength of accessory muscles may also be seen in these individuals.

Maximal transdiaphragmatic pressure: Contraction of diaphragm lowers the intrathoracic pressure while it increases the intra-abdominal pressure. Pressure developed specifically by the diaphragm can be measured as the difference between abdominal and pleural pressures. Abdominal and pleural pressures are measured with balloon-tipped gastric (P_{ga}) and esophageal catheters (P_{es}). Transdiaphragmatic pressure (P_{di}) is calculated as $P_{di} = P_{ga} - P_{es}$. During tidal respiration, P_{es} becomes more negative as pleural pressure drops, whereas P_{ga} rises as abdominal contents are compressed with the descend of the diaphragm. Thus the pressure tracings move in opposite directions. The P_{es} and P_{ga} move in the same directions and transdiaphragmatic pressure is zero in the presence of complete diaphragm paralysis. Although P_{di} specifically assesses diaphragmatic function, the requirement to place esophageal and gastric pressure transducers in patients with swallowing impairment and a complex procedure to generated maximum P_{di} obviates it as a useful maneuver.

Phrenic nerve stimulation: The phrenic nerve is accessible transcutaneously for direct stimulation either by electric or magnetic impulses as it traverses the neck. In contrast to the electric impulse which selectively stimulates phrenic nerve, magnetic impulses tend to stimulate cervical nerve roots as well that may activate rib cage muscles and give false-positive results. Once stimulated, both conduction time to assess the integrity of phrenic nerve and P_{di} to assess the mechanical output of diaphragm can be measured.

Diaphragm imaging: Chest radiography allows visualization of the elevated hemidiaphragms but additional testing is required to exclude other pathologies. In addition, it also detects other pulmonary pathologies as cause of respiratory symptoms. Fluoroscopy provides a real-time examination of diaphragm dome motion; best seen when both hemidiaphragms are visualized simultaneously in a lateral projection. A cephalad motion of diaphragm during inspiration is characteristic.

Fluoroscopic sniff test is not sensitive for bilateral diaphragm paralysis. In case of unilateral paralysis, the Kienbock's sign is positive on fluoroscopy, i.e. the affected diaphragm moves paradoxically upward with a vigorous sniff. At least 2 cm of upward motion is considered abnormal.

Ultrasound examination helps to visualize and diagnose the diaphragmatic palsy. This is done with a 7–10 MHz transducer placed over the lower rib cage between the seventh and ninth intercostal spaces in the midaxillary line. The diaphragm muscle in the zone of apposition is represented as a nonechogenic central structure bordered by two echogenic lines: the peritoneal and diaphragmatic pleurae. One can also measure the diaphragm thickness (t_{di}) at end-expiration along with the change in t_{di} during inspiration.

Treatment

In most patients with unilateral diaphragm paralysis, there is a compensatory increase in motor output to the intercostal muscles and increased output to the normal hemidiaphragm. These compensatory mechanisms maintain adequate ventilation and gas exchange.

In unilateral disease, main aim of treatment is exclusion of serious underlying intrathoracic pathology. Prognosis is good in patients with mild symptoms; routinely they do not need treatment. In patients with disproportionate symptoms, surgical plication of the affected hemidiaphragm may provide excellent results. Surgical plication causes improved lower lobe expansion and prevention of paradoxical motion leading to improved efficiency of remaining innervated respiratory muscles.

The treatment of bilateral diaphragmatic paralysis depends on the cause of paralysis. In bilateral disease, in the absence of myopathy and preserved phrenic nerve, phrenic nerve pacing with radiofrequency signaling can be used. Even in patients with nonfunctional phrenic nerve, if the intercostal nerve is functional and can be anastomosed, pacing can be done. Once pacer is implanted, retraining of deconditioned diaphragm requires expert and careful monitoring. Diaphragmatic pacing is limited by potential to fail abruptly, induction of diaphragm fatigue, upper airway obstruction, and high cost.

In patients with nocturnal hypercapnia, some form of mechanical ventilatory support is required. Mechanical support can be provided by rocking bed, cuirass respirator, nasal continuous positive airway pressure (CPAP) or intermittent positive pressure ventilation by nasal mask and/or appliances. Noninvasive ventilation rather than mechanical ventilation is preferred for respiratory support in case of respiratory failure due to isolated diaphragm paralysis and no other neuromuscular impairment.

Sleep Abnormalities in Neuromuscular Diseases

Sleep-associated breathing problems are fairly common, seen in up to 42% of individuals in patients with neuromuscular diseases. Nocturnal breathing abnormalities often precede respiratory failure during wakefulness by months or even years.

In normal subjects, there is a fall in minute ventilation and oxyhemoglobin saturation (SaO_2), whereas arterial carbon dioxide tension rises with the onset of sleep. These changes can be attributed to the withdrawal of wakefulness drive to breathe and reduction of protective reflex systems. Physiologically, ventilation decreases by ±10% during sleep due to:

- Reduced wakefulness ventilatory drive stimulation at the respiratory centers
- Reduced ventilatory response to chemical stimuli (hypercapnia and hypoxia)
- Rapid eye movement (REM) sleep-related muscle paralysis
- Increased upper airway resistance due to reduced neural input to airway dilator muscles.

Distribution of respiratory muscle involvement dictates the nature of sleep-associated breathing disorders. An obstructive defect is likely to predominate in patients with intact diaphragm but weak upper airway or intercostal muscles. In contrast, hypoventilation and gaseous exchange abnormalities will predominate in severe diaphragm dysfunction due to suppression of intercostal and accessory muscles in REM sleep.

Central hypopneas are the most frequently reported discrete sleep-related breathing events in patients with respiratory muscle weakness. These events are more frequent and prolonged in REM sleep. In neuromuscular diseases, there are abnormalities of ventilatory control that may also reduce respiratory drive and ventilation via mechanisms unrelated to respiratory muscle weakness. Screening sleep studies are therefore commended in these patients. Polysomnography is the gold standard to identify abnormal breathing and other events during sleep.

PART II

ENDOCRINE DISORDERS

Endocrine diseases can present with different respiratory symptoms. Respiratory problems may occur indirectly because of an increased risk of infection (as in diabetes) or due to upper airway obstruction secondary to goiter. Alterations in pulmonary function associated with disorders of the endocrine system can also occur because of the direct involvement of the respiratory system or its components.

Diabetes Mellitus

Diabetes is a systemic disease that produces structural and functional changes in many tissues, particularly in the connective tissues, leading to end organ damage in eyes, kidneys, and nervous system. The alveolar capillary network in the lung constitutes the largest microvascular organ in the body; it is highly susceptible to systemic microangiopathy. Owing to a large physiological reserve of gas exchange, clinical manifestation and disability develop later in the lung than in the smaller microvasculature, such as the kidney and retina.

Diabetes can cause several clinical and functional respiratory complications concerning lung volume, pulmonary diffusing capacity, control of ventilation, and bronchomotor tone (Box 96.2). Although the clinical implications of these changes are mild, the presence of simultaneous diabetic complications

BOX 96.2: Pulmonary complications of diabetes mellitus.

- Functional abnormalities:
  - ↓Vital capacity
  - ↓Total lung capacity
  - ↓Diffusion capacity for carbon monoxide
  - ↓Inspiratory muscle strength
  - ↓Cough reflex
- Increased risk of infection:
  - Tuberculosis
  - Fungal infections
  - *Legionella* pneumonia
- Aspiration pneumonia
- Neuromuscular abnormalities:
  - Sleep-disordered breathing
  - ↓Bronchomotor tone
  - ↓Ventilatory response to hypoxia and hypercapnia

involving the heart and kidneys could determine severe respiratory derangements. Diabetic lung involvement is best characterized as a loss of physiological reserves because of the long-term progression of subclinical dysfunction. Its interaction with normal aging and cumulative microvascular injury independently compromise alveolar gas exchange and lung function.

Diabetes and Lung Function

Both type 1 and type 2 diabetes are associated with modestly impaired restrictive pulmonary function. This functional impairment has been shown primarily through cross-sectional associations between diabetes status and pulmonary function measures, including the forced vital capacity, forced expiratory volume in 1 second, and their ratio.

Considering large vascular network rich in collagen and elastin, the lungs are prone to microvascular damage and nonenzymatic glycation in diabetes leading to reduction in alveolar gas transport, as manifested by reduced diffusing capacity of lung for carbon monoxide (DLCO). Although a few studies have reported a normal lung DLCO, majority reported a reduced diffusing capacity among diabetic patients which is correlated with microangiopathy in other organs, duration of diabetes, and microalbuminuria. Because the DLCO reflects the interplay of vascular and parenchymal factors, the measurement of postural changes (sitting and supine) in DLCO could be more reliable method of assessing these early abnormalities than the simple DLCO measurement in sitting position in diabetes.

Subclinical autonomic dysfunction can occur within a year of diagnosis in type 2 and within 2 years in type 1 diabetes. Reduced or absent cough reflex, diminished perception of inspiratory loading, sleep-disordered breathing, and aspiration are all associated with autonomic dysfunction in diabetics. Similarly, central disorder of the respiratory control leading to sleep apnea and blunted hypoxic and hypercapnic drive has been consistently shown in diabetes with autonomic dysfunction. The presence of subtle abnormalities in the lungs of diabetes and the limitation to detect these changes early are necessary to identify and control the risk factors like smoking, poor glycemic control, and cardiovascular disease to preserve the condition of near normal lung function.

Diabetes and Tuberculosis

Diabetes is associated with an increased risk of active tuberculosis (TB) both in case–control and in cohort studies. There is little evidence to suggest that diabetes increases susceptibility to TB infection, with an overall relative risk (RR) of 3.11 for TB, regardless of different study designs, background TB incidence, or geographic region of the study. In elderly patients, the increased risk is limited to those with uncontrolled diabetes with hemoglobin A1c (HbA1c) more than or equal to 7%.

Diabetes patients with TB have high mycobacillary burdens at diagnosis, which they clear more slowly with current treatments leading to higher rates of relapse; and higher rates of multidrug-resistant TB. Similarly, radiological predilection for lower lung fields, tendency to cavitate, and multilobar involvement are more frequently found in diabetics. At clinical level, it is difficult to make early diagnosis of the combination as the symptoms of the complicating disease are quite often masked by the primary illness. Thus, the delayed and missed diagnosis of each disease is likely to complicate and worsen the natural history and outcome for the other disease.

Thyroid Dysfunction

Thyroid hormones play a crucial role in lung development, surfactant synthesis, and lung defenses. Consequently, both hyper- and hypothyroidism may alter the functions of respiratory systems resulting into several complications (Box 96.3). Both the excess and the deficiency of thyroid hormones can contribute to dyspnea and exercise limitation through common mechanism of congestive heart failure or myopathy leading to respiratory muscle weakness and respiratory failure. Pleural effusion due to hypothyroidism per se or secondary to pericardial involvement may cause respiratory symptoms which resolve with treatment of hypothyroidism.

Obstructive manifestations such as dyspnea, stridor, wheezing, hoarseness or cough produced by goiter can occur by direct compression of extrathoracic or intrathoracic trachea. Compression or irritation of recurrent laryngeal nerves may also result in airway obstruction due to vocal cord paralysis. One of the most consistent findings in hypothyroidism is its influence on central ventilatory control. Both hypoxic ventilatory drive and hypercapnic ventilatory response are depressed in hypothyroidism. The blunting is more marked in myxedema which can be effectively improved with thyroid hormone replacement. Blunted ventilatory response is an important cause of increasing failure; approximately 3% of the mechanically ventilated patients who have weaning failure are subsequently detected to have hypothyroidism.

In hypothyroidism, respiratory disturbances due to sleep apnea are observed in up to 50–100% patients besides the fact that the prevalence of hypothyroidism in sleep apnea is very low. Both central apnea due to blunted ventilatory response to hypoxia and obstructive apnea secondary to deposition

BOX 96.3: Pulmonary complications of thyroid dysfunction.

- Functional abnormalities:
  - Dampening of flow volume loop in goiter
  - ↓Inspiratory muscle strength due to myopathy
  - Blunted ventilatory response to hypoxia
  - Blunted hypercapnic ventilatory response
- Sleep apnea:
  - Central
  - Obstructive
- Pleural effusion:
  - Hypothyroid pleural effusion
  - Hypothyroid-associated effusion due to pericardial involvement
- Aspiration pneumonia

of mucopolysaccharides in the oropharynx and tongue leading to narrowing of upper airway during sleep can occur in hypothyroidism. Although hormone replacement leads to normalization of sleep apnea, a few patients may require continuous positive airway pressure support on long-term basis.

Acromegaly

Acromegaly is characterized by excessive bony growth, soft tissue hypertrophy, and facial coarsening consequent to excessive release of growth hormone, most commonly from a pituitary adenoma. Macroglossia, nasal polyps, oropharyngeal airway narrowing, and vocal cord dysfunction are common features which predispose to respiratory disturbances and sleep apnea. Inspiratory pharyngeal collapse during sleep due to hypertrophy of parapharyngeal and retropharyngeal soft tissue and an enlarged tongue are some of the important causes of obstructive sleep apnea. Neck circumference of greater than 41 cm and the circumference of the index finger of above 8.5 cm were found as good predictors of development of sleep apnea. Other respiratory problems which are commonly seen in acromegaly are extrathoracic airway obstruction, difficult intubation, and vocal cord dysfunction.

GASTROINTESTINAL DISEASES

Because of close anatomical proximity and continuity of abdominal viscera to the thorax, any intra-abdominal pathology can secondarily involve the lungs. Because of similar embryological development, diseases of the gut and lungs are quite often complicated by each other. Involvement of diaphragm by an intra-abdominal inflammation can compromise ventilation without affecting the lung. More commonly, few diseases have simultaneous and pronounced pulmonary manifestations.

Gastroesophageal Reflux Disease

Gastroesophageal reflux disease (GERD) may trigger, exacerbate or possibly cause many pulmonary diseases (Box 96.4). Despite extensive studies addressing the pathophysiological link between respiratory symptoms and reflux disease, the true relationship remains uncertain. Mechanisms by which GERD leads to respiratory symptoms are:
- Microaspiration from the proximal esophagus
- Reflux of acid from the lower esophagus

BOX 96.4: Pulmonary disorders associated with gastroesophageal reflux disease.
- Chronic cough
- Bronchial asthma
- Aspiration pneumonia, lung abscess, and bronchiectasis
- Vocal cord dysfunction
- Chronic bronchitis
- Idiopathic pulmonary fibrosis

- Presence of an anatomical or physiological abnormality in the lower esophageal sphincter.

Patients with chronic cough and asthma have a high prevalence of GERD. There is clear documentation of higher prevalence of GERD in asthma and chronic cough than in the general population with around 75–80% of asthmatics showing reflux symptoms. In addition, GERD has been postulated as a potential trigger for asthma.

Furthermore, physiological alterations associated with asthma or its treatment may themselves promote gastroesophageal reflux. Transient lower esophageal sphincter relaxation and negative pressure generated during episode of coughing or bronchoconstriction and flattening of diaphragm secondary to hyperinflation are commonly seen in asthmatics and are associated with change in pressure gradient between the thorax and the abdomen. Similarly, beta agonists and theophylline dilate the smooth muscle throughout the body including at the lower esophagus disrupting the gastroesophageal physiological barrier. Both of these factors may lead to GERD in asthma.

Only a specific subgroup of patients with respiratory symptoms respond to therapy for GERD, which includes a combination of antireflux measures such as the weight reduction, avoidance of meals before bedtime, eating low-fat diet, and acid-suppressive therapy.

Acute Pancreatitis

Pulmonary complications are the most frequent and potentially the most serious systemic complications of acute pancreatitis. The spectrum of pulmonary sequelae of acute pancreatitis ranges from subclinical arterial hypoxemia to frank acute respiratory distress syndrome (ARDS) (Box 96.5). When present, these sequelae are associated with significant mortality. Respiratory dysfunction precedes the occurrence of heart, liver, and renal failure, responsible for early deaths in severe acute pancreatitis.

Arterial Hypoxemia and Respiratory Failure

Hypoxemia in acute pancreatitis is predominantly caused by ventilation-perfusion mismatch resulting in right to left intrapulmonary shunting. Changes in pulmonary vascular permeability and reduction in oxygen affinity of hemoglobin related to increase in circulating fatty acids are the other mechanisms responsible for hypoxemia in acute pancreatitis.

BOX 96.5: Pulmonary complications of acute pancreatitis.
- Pleural effusion
- Atelectasis
- Mediastinal abscess
- Pneumonitis
- Pulmonary infarction
- Acute respiratory distress syndrome

Subclinical arterial hypoxemia is frequently seen during early stages of acute pancreatitis. Arterial hypoxemia [partial pressure of arterial oxygen (PaO_2 <80 mm Hg)] can be seen in up to 55–65% of patients during the first 48 hours without any obvious clinical or radiological abnormality and is associated with significantly higher mortality. The mortality rises to 14% at PaO_2 less than 60 mm Hg, from a mortality of 6% at PaO_2 less than 70 mm Hg. Mortality of 60% was observed in as high as 22% patients of acute pancreatitis with severe respiratory insufficiency.

Acute Respiratory Distress Syndrome

The most serious pulmonary complication of acute pancreatitis is ARDS seen in approximately 15–20% patients with an associated mortality of 50–75%. Usually, persistent and refractory hypoxemia evolves to overt ARDS in 2–7 days, but it may have rapid onset and course. Rapid appearance and progression to multilobar infiltrates is classically noted on chest radiography. Although the exact mechanism of lung injury is poorly understood, pancreatic enzymes and inflammatory mediators appear to play a key role in its pathophysiology. Pancreatic enzyme phospholipase A_2 binds to pulmonary capillaries and has the potential to induce enzymatic degradation of phospholipid component of surfactant leading to increased vascular permeability and alveolar collapse. Free fatty acids released from triglycerides by pulmonary lipases lead to capillary and alveolar wall damage and alveolar edema.

Pleural Effusion

Pleural effusion is a frequent complication of both acute and chronic pancreatitis with an associated mortality of 20–30%. When present, the effusions are usually small, left-sided, occasionally bloody, and indicative of severe disease. Effusion is usually exudative, serosanguineous in appearance with high amylase, protein, and lactate dehydrogenase. The main mechanisms proposed for effusion in acute pancreatitis are:
- Increased permeability of lymphatics
- Impaired lymphatic drainage
- Increased permeability of diaphragmatic capillaries
- Pancreaticopleural fistulae.

Pancreatitis-related effusions are usually self-limited and resolve spontaneously without any therapeutic intervention when the pancreatic inflammation subsides. Persistence of effusion indicates the occurrence of complications like pancreatic abscess or pseudocyst formation. Symptomatic effusions may be drained with thoracentesis or tube thoracotomy, while chronic effusions often require drainage of the pseudocyst and abscess or excision of the fistulous tract.

Inflammatory Bowel Disease

Inflammatory bowel disease (IBD) can involve the airway at various levels; parenchyma or pleura can develop at any time in the history of the IBD.

Surgical intervention like colectomy or proctocolectomy is a risk factor of IBD-related airway inflammation. Sudden onset and rapid progression of respiratory symptoms within a few days, weeks or months are also defined following proctocolectomy.

Pulmonary function testing in these patients reveals obstructive defects and decrease in gas transfer factor. Small airway obstruction can be found in patients with normal lung function suggesting subclinical abnormalities in the airway. Variable degrees of inflammation and mucosal changes on bronchoscopic examination can be found in nearly all patients with major airway involvement.

Steroids, given by inhalation or by mouth, are the treatment of choice which rapidly controls the symptoms.

HEPATIC DISORDERS

Respiratory dysfunction manifested by dyspnea is commonly seen in patients with chronic liver disease. Pulmonary disorders associated with liver disease include complications of cirrhosis and portal hypertension, such as fluid retention (ascites and hepatic hydrothorax) and muscular wasting, cardiopulmonary disorders associated with specific liver diseases, and pulmonary vascular disorders including hepatopulmonary syndrome (HPS) and portopulmonary hypertension (PoPH).

Hepatic Hydrothorax

In the absence of a coexisting cardiopulmonary disease, development of transudative pleural effusion (>500 mL) in cirrhotic patient with portal hypertension is termed as hepatic hydrothorax. It can complicate approximately 4–6% of cirrhotic liver disease irrespective of the underlying etiology. Movement of fluid from the abdomen cavity to the pleural space via small defects in the diaphragm due to pressure gradient between the abdominal and the pleural cavities is the predominant mechanism of hydrothorax. The negative intrathoracic pressure favors the transfer of fluid across these defects, and patients usually have minimal or mild ascites. Additionally, intravascular volume expansion secondary to sodium retention and hypoalbuminemia, collateral anastomoses between portal and azygous systems, and passage of fluid via transdiaphragmatic lymphatics contribute to the development of hydrothorax.

Diagnosis of hepatic hydrothorax can be made on the basis of unilateral effusion in patients with advanced cirrhosis; diagnostic thoracentesis is mandatory to rule out alternative diagnosis. In an appropriate background, the similarity in the composition of pleural fluid and the ascetic fluid establishes the diagnosis. Sometimes, ultrasonography or nuclear scan is required to establish the presence of ascites. Spontaneous infection within the pleural fluid is known as spontaneous bacterial empyema which should be considered in patients with hydrothorax who develop new-onset fever, pleuritic pain, encephalopathy or unexplained deterioration in clinical status.

Liver transplantation is the definitive treatment of choice. Sodium restriction, diuretics, thoracentesis, transjugular intrahepatic portosystemic shunt, pleurodesis, and video-assisted thoracic surgery are alternative options to alleviate symptoms and prevent complications. Chemical pleurodesis by itself in hydrothorax is a promising approach but limited by low success rate, rapid reaccumulation of fluid, and scant inflammatory responses. The use of continuous positive airway pressure which decreases the negative pleural pressure and thus prevents shifting of fluid from peritoneal cavity is an effective approach in selected patients with refractory hepatic hydrothorax.

Hepatopulmonary Syndrome

The triad of liver disease with impaired arterial oxygenation induced by intrapulmonary vasodilation is known as hepatopulmonary syndrome. HPS is not dependent on the severity of liver disease, can occur without cirrhosis or in acute liver failure. It is usually diagnosed in fifth or sixth decades of life with no gender predilection. Prevalence of HPS in liver transplant centers ranges from 5% to 32% due to different cutoffs use for gas exchange abnormalities.

Clinical Features

Most patients have features of advanced liver disease such as jaundice, ascites, palmar erythema, enlarged liver, and spleen. Extensive cutaneous spider nevi which are seen more commonly in patients with HPS are considered as a cutaneous marker of both systemic and intrapulmonary vasodilatation. Specific pulmonary features consist of dyspnea, platypnea, orthodeoxia, cyanosis, and digital clubbing. Increased dyspnea in the upright position, i.e. platypnea and orthodeoxia (decrease in PaO_2 from the supine to the upright position) are the characteristics, but not pathognomonic features of HPS.

Diagnosis

In patient with chronic liver disease, presence of platypnea, orthodeoxia, and clubbing strongly suggest a diagnosis of HPS (Box 96.6). Hyperkinetic circulation, systemic hypotension, and low or normal pulmonary artery

BOX 96.6: Diagnostic criteria for hepatopulmonary syndrome.

Essential features:
- Chronic liver disease
- Normal or near normal chest radiograph
- Gas exchange abnormalities - ↑(A – a) partial pressure of oxygen of ≥ 15 mm Hg with or without concomitant arterial hypoxemia (partial pressure of arterial oxygen <80 mm Hg)
- Positive contrast-enhanced echocardiogram or abnormal intravenous radiolabeled perfusion lung scan or both

Additional features:
- ↓Diffusing capacity of lung for carbon monoxide
- Dyspnea with or without platypnea and orthodeoxia
- Hyperkinetic circulatory state with normal or low pulmonary artery pressure

pressure with normal or low pulmonary vascular resistance are its characteristic hemodynamic features.

Treatment

Orthotopic liver transplantation has been shown as an effective measure for complete resolution of HPS in approximately 80% of patients. Alternatively, medical management with agents like bismesylate almitrine and propranolol has been tried to reduce the shunt but the results are disappointing. Supplemental oxygen therapy when PaO_2 is less than 60 mm Hg should be administered to all patients as this is the only proven effective therapy.

Portopulmonary Hypertension

Portopulmonary hypertension is defined as an elevated mean pulmonary arterial pressure (mPAP) more than 25 mm Hg, an increased pulmonary vascular resistance >240 dynes/sec/cm^5, and a normal pulmonary artery occlusion pressure (<15 mm Hg) in a patient who has portal hypertension with or without cirrhosis. PoPH generally presents during the fifth decade of life after 4–7 years of diagnosis of portal hypertension. The condition is both pathophysiologically and clinically different from HPS (Table 96.3).

Clinical picture in PoPH is indistinguishable from that of primary pulmonary hypertension, appears late in the evolution of disease. Predominantly, patients have exertional dyspnea. As the severity increases, peripheral edema, fatigue, abdominal bloating, palpitation, and syncope may appear.

Treatment aimed at lowering pulmonary artery pressure and resistance is indicated in all symptomatic patients. Diuretic administration is required

TABLE 96.3: Differentiation between hepatopulmonary syndrome and portopulmonary hypertension.

	Hepatopulmonary syndrome	Portopulmonary hypertension
Causes	Liver disease with or without cirrhosis	Liver disease with portal hypertension
Pathophysiology	Pulmonary vasodilation	Pulmonary vasoconstriction
Symptoms	Platypnea, orthodeoxia	Dyspnea, edema
Partial pressure of arterial oxygen	Hypoxemia, orthodeoxia	Hypoxemia at late stages
Chest X-ray	Usually normal	Signs of pulmonary hypertension
Contrast ECHO	Late (>3–6 cardiac cycles) appearance of microbubbles in left atrium	Usually negative
Cardiac output	Increased	Normal or decreased
Pulmonary vascular resistance	Decreased	Increased
Shunt	>10%	Nil

for associated cor pulmonale and volume overload. Anticoagulation is often contraindicated because of the associated hemorrhagic diathesis related to liver disease and its complications. Supplemental oxygen to maintain saturation above 90% is beneficial for all patients.

Drugs with vasodilating and vasomodulating effects can be given but there are no randomized controlled trials specific to this population. Use of these drugs should be individualized, depending upon the severity of disease and prospects for liver transplantation.

Orthotropic liver transplantation can be beneficial in a highly selected subset of patients but the resolution of pulmonary hypertension after transplantation is not universal. Both intraoperative and immediate postoperative complications of liver transplantation are also high because of the associated comorbidities and deranged hemodynamics.

RENAL DISEASES

Renal Failure

Chronic renal failure usually affects the lung indirectly by affecting other organ systems of the body such as through raised pulmonary venous pressure and anemia. A transient respiratory gas exchange abnormality following hemodialysis is also a frequent occurrence.

The common renal complications are discussed here (Box 96.7).

Pulmonary Edema

Subclinical or overt pulmonary edema is common in renal failure due to a number of different mechanisms:
- Fluid overload
- Hypoproteinemia with reduced plasma colloid pressure
- Depressed myocardial function
- Increased microvascular permeability.

The characteristic distribution of edema in the more central part of the lungs is explained by diversion of flow through the shortest arterial pathway. Hypertension, diabetes mellitus, anemia, and ischemic heart disease, commonly seen in end-stage renal disease, may also adversely affect the lungs.

BOX 96.7: Pulmonary complications of renal failure.

- Pulmonary edema
- Pleural diseases:
  - Pleural rub
  - Pleural effusion
  - Fibrosing uremic pleuritis or fibrothorax
- Pulmonary calcifications
- Sleep apneas
- Hemodialysis-induced gas exchanges abnormalities

Pleural Effusion

Pleural effusion is seen in approximately 3% of patients of renal failure. The exact mechanism of pleural disease is not understood; it is probably similar to that of pericarditis seen in uremia. Almost half of patients with pleural effusion are symptomatic with fever, chest pain, cough or dyspnea; the degree and severity of uremia has no correlation with the occurrence of effusion. Both transudative and exudative effusions can occur, most commonly it is an exudate which is frequently serosanguineous or frankly hemorrhagic. Lymphocytes are the predominant cells; pleural biopsy characteristically reveals chronic fibrinous pleuritis. Transudative effusions are seen in the fluid overload states or congestive heart failure. Confident diagnosis of uremic pleuritis requires exclusion of other common causes of effusion like pleural infection, malignancy, and pulmonary embolism.

Effusion routinely disappears with dialysis in 4-6 weeks in most cases. In 25% of patients it may persist, progress or recur. In a small number of patients, progressive pleural thickening may lead to ventilatory defects requiring surgical decortication.

Hemodialysis-induced Pulmonary Gas Exchange Abnormalities

Arterial hypoxemia during dialysis is commonly seen. A fall in arterial PaO_2 of 10-15 mm Hg is observed within a few minutes of dialysis, reaches a plateau after 45-60 minutes and persists for the duration of dialysis. Hypoxemia may occur due to:
- Shift in oxyhemoglobin dissociation curve due to procedure-related rise in pH
- Alkalosis-induced depression of central ventilatory drive
- Impairment of oxygen diffusion
- Ventilation-perfusion mismatching due to pulmonary leukostasis
- Loss of carbon dioxide via dialysate-induced hypoventilation.

Hypoxemia during hemodialysis is considered a predictable effect of loss of carbon dioxide (CO_2). Removal of CO_2 during hemodialysis leads to decrease in minute ventilation. The diffusion of CO_2 into the dialysis fluid is substantially more with acetate buffer than with bicarbonate buffer.

Due to the large cardiopulmonary reserve, the reduction in arterial PaO_2 has no significant effect in patients with normal cardiopulmonary function. In patients with compromised function, supplemental oxygen during hemodialysis should be given. Composition of dialysis membrane and the dialysate buffer should also be appropriately changed.

CHAPTER
97

Pulmonary Involvement in Tropical Diseases

Sanjay Jain, SK Jindal

INTRODUCTION

Tropical diseases encompass all those conditions that occur solely, or principally, in the tropics. In practice, the term refers to infectious diseases that thrive in hot, humid climatic conditions. Many of these diseases involve the lungs directly or indirectly through various mechanisms. Theoretically, almost any tropical infection can involve the respiratory system (Box 97.1), but a few which are more common and important are included in this chapter.

MALARIA

Malaria is a very important cause of mortality in the developing countries. Pulmonary involvement occurs in 3–10% cases, most commonly in malaria due to *Plasmodium falciparum*. Different clinical forms of pulmonary complications have been described in malaria (Box 97.2).

BOX 97.1: Tropical infections that commonly involve the respiratory system.
- Bacterial: Pneumonias, tuberculosis, and enteric fever
- Fungal: Aspergillosis and other fungal pneumonias
- Viral: Hanta virus, dengue, and influenza
- Parasitic: Protozoal—malarial parasites, *Entamoeba histolytica*, *Leishmania donovani*, *Toxoplasma gondii*, *Babesia*
- Helminthic: *Echinococcus granulosus*, Filariasis, Schistosomiasis, *Ascaris lumbricoides*

> **BOX 97.2:** Important pulmonary complications of malaria.
>
> - Pulmonary edema—noncardiogenic
>   - Fluid overload—Iatrogenic
>   - Acute respiratory distress syndrome
> - Cardiac pulmonary edema (following malarial myocarditis)
> - Pneumonias:
>   - Malarial
>   - Postconvulsive aspiration
>   - Nosocomial
> - Acute asthma-like presentation

Acute Respiratory Distress Syndrome

Pulmonary edema is common in patients with hyperparasitemia, renal failure, and pregnancy, commonly associated with hypoglycemia and metabolic acidosis. It may develop suddenly after delivery, due to fluid overload. Pulmonary edema is the terminal event in many cases of fatal falciparum infection. Cerebral edema is commonly present in these cases. Pulmonary edema has been rarely described in patients with *P. ovale* and *P. vivax* infections. *P. vivax* is emerging as an important cause of severe malarial complication, including acute respiratory distress syndrome (ARDS) in children. The first indications of impending pulmonary edema include tachypnea and dyspnea, followed by hypoxemia and respiratory failure requiring intubation.

It can also develop in patients with normal capillary wedge pressures. Such cases may happen due to the increased permeability of pulmonary capillaries. It is generally produced by a disturbance in pulmonary microcirculation. Sequestration of red cells, hypoalbuminemia, clogging of pulmonary microcirculation, and disseminated intravascular coagulation with immune complex disease may also play their role in pathogenesis. A central mechanism with hypothalamic dysfunction due to disturbed oxidative metabolism leading to pulmonary venular spasm has also been suggested.

The most severe form is acute pulmonary edema, which manifests with acute respiratory distress, is rapidly progressive and occurs in the absence of cardiac decompensation or fluid overload. It has been proposed that *P. vivax*-infected erythrocytes may sequester within the pulmonary microvasculature and cause greater inflammatory response to a given parasite burden than with *P. falciparum*.

Refractory to the usual treatment of cardiogenic pulmonary edema, it has a high mortality with up to 50% of the patients succumbing to the complication. The mechanism of pulmonary edema is not clearly understood. It has a close resemblance to adult respiratory distress syndrome. Multiple mechanisms have been hypothesized. Overhydration has been proposed as the cause in some cases of pulmonary edema. This, compounded by venous and lymphatic obstruction, leads to elevated capillary wedge pressure.

Other Manifestations

Acute asthma-like picture has been also described. Clinical features may develop rapidly, even after initial response to antimalarial treatment and clearance of parasitemia. The various pulmonary symptoms of malaria include cough (80%), dyspnea (40%), expectoration (32%), chest pain (18%), and hemoptysis (4%). The common signs are tachypnea, tachycardia, and hypotension. Chest radiographic abnormalities range from confluent nodules to basilar and/or diffuse bilateral pulmonary infiltrates. Benign forms have rarely been described in the literature. These cause minimal or no respiratory difficulty, and can present as pleural effusions, interstitial edema, and lobar consolidation. They often go undiagnosed and unrecognized as part of the clinical and radiologic spectrum of acute malaria, and are probably more common than reported.

Management

Fluid overload should be avoided at all costs, especially in pregnant women. The central venous pressure should be maintained between 0 cm of H_2O and 5 cm of H_2O by regulating fluid intake and nursing the patient propped up at 45°. All intravenous fluids should be stopped immediately and diuretics may have to be administered. Initial management of pulmonary edema includes treatment with oxygen, backrest, and diuretics if there is evidence of fluid overload. Injectable furosemide (40 mg intravenously) increased to 200 mg in the absence of a desired response is generally used. Fluid volume can be further reduced by venesection and letting of 250 mL of blood initially. This blood or its packed cells can be retransfused once the problem settles down. The procedure can be repeated carefully if needed. If the patient deteriorates with conservative treatment, mechanical ventilation is indicated.

Antimalarial treatment in addition to the respiratory support is an important component of overall management. Antibiotics, bronchodilators, and other symptomatic treatments are required depending upon the presence of complications. Antimalaria drugs like mefloquine are occasionally associated with pulmonary complications, such as pneumonitis.

TYPHOID

Typhoid is a systemic febrile illness caused by *Salmonella typhi*. It develops due to the consumption of contaminated food and water or contact with chronic infected carrier.

The involvement of lung in typhoid fever is not an uncommon entity (Box 97.3). The exact pathogenesis is not known. Because of hematogenous spread of the organism, it has been long tried to isolate the organism from the lungs. The endotoxin released from organism is considered responsible for the signs and symptoms of pulmonary disease. Predisposing factors for lung involvement include, but are not limited to immunocompromised host, alcoholism, sickle cell disease or preexisting pulmonary disease. Fever, toxemia, and abdominal pain are the most common manifestations of typhoid

> **BOX 97.3:** Pulmonary complications of important tropical infections.
>
> - *Enteric fever:*
>   - Typhoid bronchitis
>   - Pneumonia and sepsis
>   - Acute respiratory distress syndrome
>   - Salmonella lung abscess—rarely
> - *Leptospirosis:*
>   - Pulmonary hemorrhages
>   - Acute respiratory distress
>   - Leptospiral pneumonia
> - *Dengue fever:*
>   - Hemoptysis
>   - Severe pulmonary hemorrhage
> - *Amebiasis:*
>   - Pulmonary amebiasis (pneumonia and empyema)
>   - Hepatobronchial/hepatobronchopleural fistula

fever, while 10–15% of the patients with illness lasting more than 2 weeks develop systemic complications.

The incidence of pulmonary manifestations ranges from 1% to 7%. Pneumonia is uncommon (1%) but can occur in 50% of patients with empyema, bronchopleural fistula, lung abscess or effusion. Bronchopneumonia is more common, although lobar pneumonia may also be seen rarely in these patients. In advanced disease, secondary bacterial pneumonia may occur due to aspiration or other organism. ARDS in most patients manifests in the early phase, i.e. first 2 weeks of illness.

Nonspecific radiographic infiltrates are seen in one-fourth of the patients with pulmonary symptoms. It is rare to isolate *Salmonella* from the sputum though blood culture may be positive in majority, which is the best test to diagnose salmonellosis. Occasionally, lung abscess caused by *S. typhi*, sometimes in a preexisting hydatid cyst, has been reported. The treatment of typhoid involves the appropriate and timely use of antibiotics along with supportive respiratory care. Steroid use decreases the mortality from typhoid fever. Outcome of ARDS is frequently fatal. Ventilatory and other supportive care are crucial to management.

LEPTOSPIROSIS

Leptospirosis caused by *Leptospira interrogans*, is a reemerging zoonosis occurring as large outbreaks throughout the world. This is especially so in Asian countries with an enormous load of diseases due to tropical pathogens. The natural reservoirs are the mammals (rodents, cattle, dogs, horses, and sheep) with humans getting incidentally infected after contact with contaminated animal urine. Risk factors include outdoor activities like walking barefoot, gardening, and forest activities. Wet soil, refuse around the home, pets at home, and skin wounds may also help in promoting the spread of disease.

Leptospirosis can manifest with variable clinical picture ranging from mild subclinical illness to multiorgan failure (Box 97.3). Pulmonary involvement is often mild with symptoms of cough, dyspnea, and hemoptysis. Severe forms include the presence of intra-alveolar hemorrhage which can occasionally present with a fatal outcome. Severer course is particularly described in the elderly patients.

The pathophysiology of pulmonary hemorrhages is unclear and probably related to vascular injury and focal hemorrhages. The incidence of pulmonary hemorrhage seems to increase in the recent reports. The etiology of pulmonary hemorrhages is probably multifactorial. It could possibly be sepsis related with disturbed platelet function. Linear deposition of immunoglobulin and complement on the alveolar surfaces may play a role in causing hemorrhages. Two mechanisms related to damage have been proposed: one, toxin-mediated capillary vasculitis and second, the immune-mediated damage by host.

A possibility of primary noninflammatory vascular damage has also been considered. *Leptospira* are found in a lesser number than in the liver suggesting that the toxins generated by the liver circulate in the body and cause damage at a distant site. Respiratory symptoms could occur during both the anicteric and the icteric phases, include hemoptysis, chest pain, cough, and dyspnea. ARDS is a serious complication with high rates of mortality. Severe pulmonary form of leptospirosis appears in 4–6 days of illness, is the most serious form with deaths (30–60%) occurring within 72 hours. Chest radiographs may show small nodular densities (57%), confluent consolidation (16%) or a ground glass appearance (27%). High-resolution computed tomography chest delineates the picture better. It may show ground glass opacities, pleural effusion or consolidation.

Sometimes, chest manifestations occur preterminally and suddenly. It is therefore important to keep a strict vigil for the problems in patients with severe leptospirosis.

It often goes unnoticed because of the lack of clinical suspicion, varying clinical presentation, and lack of adequate molecular diagnostic facilities. Diagnostic tests like Dot test or enzyme-linked immunosorbent assay (ELISA) for *Leptospira* immunoglobulin M (IgM) antibody and polymerase chain reaction (PCR) for 16s rRNA on blood and urine samples are used for confirmation. Pulmonary involvement and hemoptysis is shown as a strong predictor of mortality in patients with severe leptospirosis.

The treatment of leptospirosis should be initiated early based on epidemiological and clinical features to shorten the illness, and because respiratory involvement needs urgent care. Besides the supportive care, plasma exchange with immunosuppression is shown to improve survival in the presence of pulmonary hemorrhage. Activated protein C was shown to be helpful in sepsis attributed to dual infection with *P. falciparum* and leptospirosis. Assisted ventilation should be started at the first sign of clinical suspicion of respiratory failure.

DENGUE

Dengue fever is a common tropical illness with high morbidity. It was identified as the most common cause of systemic febrile illness among travelers to the developing countries. Dengue is now considered a threat to about half of the world's population. It is an endemic illness especially in the countries of Africa, Southeast Asia, and the Eastern Mediterranean. It presents with a wide range of manifestations ranging from mild illness to a severe shock-like state.

Dengue is caused by dengue virus, which is a *Flavivirus*, spread by the bite of *Aedes* mosquito. There are four serotypes of dengue virus (DENV-1 to 4). Infection with one serotype leads to classic dengue fever with lifelong immunity to that serotype. Infection with second serotype leads to dengue hemorrhagic fever with severe manifestations. Complications like massive gastrointestinal bleeding, pneumonia, and shock syndrome are important causes of death. There are only a few case reports of respiratory involvement in dengue hemorrhagic fever (DHF). It may manifest with cough, sore throat or nasal congestion. Pneumonitis or pleural effusion may develop as reactive phenomena. Hemoptysis has been reported to develop in 1.4% and pulmonary hemorrhages occur in a small number of cases. Pulmonary hemorrhages may present with mild hemoptysis and bilateral areas of consolidation on chest roentgenogram. Sometimes, the hemorrhages are rather fatal. Occasionally, dengue can also present with ARDS-like picture.

The development of clinical manifestations is related to pulmonary capillary leak. Dengue virus causes endothelial cell dysfunction. The virus attaches to the endothelial surface may serve as target for antibody binding and complement activation. Cytokines like tumor necrosis factor-alpha (TNF-α), interleukin (IL-8), interferon (IFN)-γ, and free vascular endothelial growth factor (VEGF) have been observed in patients with DHF. Besides this, abnormalities in the coagulation cascade, thrombocytopenia, platelet dysfunction, disseminated intravascular coagulation, and vascular defects all play a role in the development of DHF.

Radiologically, pulmonary hemorrhages are seen as ground glass opacities. There may be pleural effusion, associated consolidation, and diffuse infiltrates in the lung fields. Hemagglutination inhibition (HI) assay remains the gold standard serologic test for dengue virus-specific antibodies. Immunoglobulin M assay for dengue virus is less sensitive and specific than HI assay and becomes positive only after 10–14 days of acute phase. The dengue viral nonstructural protein 1 (NS1) can be detected in plasma, especially during the first 5–6 days of illness, high levels early in infection were associated with DHF. Treatment of DHF with pulmonary manifestations is primarily supportive to maintain vital function. There is no specific therapy for DHF. Careful early intervention with appropriate intensive care can decrease the mortality to less than 1%.

AMEBIASIS

Amebiasis caused by a protozoan *Entamoeba histolytica* is relatively rare these days. It is still endemic in some of the developing countries, responsible for high morbidity and mortality. Transmission occurs by consumption of contaminated food and water or oroanal contact. The infectious form is the cyst which after being ingested, excysts in the lumen of intestine, converts to trophozoite, attach to the wall of the intestine causing symptoms. As is well known, it causes gastrointestinal manifestations ranging from diarrhea to severe colitis with bloody diarrhea.

Extraintestinal manifestations occur mainly in the liver as abscess formation, which can spread to lung tissue. It can manifest as reactionary pleural effusion or the abscess may rupture into the lung parenchyma causing respiratory distress, empyema, and lung abscess development. Hematogenous spread may also occur to the lung. There may be sputum production ranging from mild to copious. Rarely, superior vena cava syndrome due to pulmonary amebiasis is reported. If hepatobronchial fistula develops, sputum may be purulent with an anchovy sauce appearance. There is no eosinophilia. Jaundice is uncommonly seen in hepatic amebiasis.

Diagnosis of amebiasis rests on detection of trophozoites or cysts in the stool. It is not a very sensitive or specific test for extraintestinal manifestations. Antigen detection in the stool or pus is more reliable for *E. histolytica*. Most patients develop antibodies against *E. histolytica*, which can be detected in the serum. Immunoglobulin M antibody detection is a useful test for acute infection. Immunoglobulin G antibodies may be detected years after active infection; its presence does not indicate active disease.

Metronidazole or tinidazole are highly effective for intestinal or extraintestinal manifestations. To prevent recurrence, luminal agents like iodoquinol are effective. Mild pleural effusion does not require treatment. Drainage along with antiamebic antibiotics is necessary to manage a lung abscess or empyema to prevent complications.

Pulmonary involvement can occur in several other tropical infections either in isolation or along with other system manifestations. Several such syndromic manifestations are region specific described in different parts of the world. Readers are advised to refer to different chapters of this book or other specific texts for details on conditions of interest.

CHAPTER
98

Pulmonary Diseases in Pregnancy

Lakhbir K Dhaliwal, Preeti Verma, Umesh Jindal

A number of pulmonary disorders are encountered during pregnancy. Moreover, a number of hormonal changes in pregnancy cause significant alterations in pulmonary physiology, which are important to understand for the appropriate interpretation of diseased state. There may be hyperemia, mucosal edema, hypersecretion, and increased mucosal friability of the upper respiratory tract structures. The diaphragm is pushed upward by as much as 4 cm by the enlarged uterus although the function of the diaphragm remains normal. There are significant changes in the lung volumes and lung capacities (Box 98.1).

The lung compliance is not altered but the chest wall and the total respiratory compliance are reduced at term. Increases in basal oxygen consumption and physiological hyperventilation are responsible for increased kidney bicarbonate excretion. Therefore, serum bicarbonate levels fall to about 15-20 mEq/L, causing mild alkalosis.

BOX 98.1: Lung function changes during pregnancy.
- Increase in vital capacity and inspiratory capacity
- Decreased expiratory reserve volume
- Increase in tidal volume but constant respiratory rate
- Increased minute ventilation—increases by about 30–40%
- Increase in arterial pressure of O_2 from 100 mm Hg to 105 mm Hg
- Carbon dioxide production increases but pressure of CO_2 decreases from 40 mm Hg to 32 mm Hg due to increase in the diffusion capacity and alveolar hyperventilation
- Residual volume decreases.

DYSPNEA DURING PREGNANCY

Mild dyspnea which does not impair routine daily activities is seen in almost 60% of women in early pregnancy. Possibly this is attributable to the increased progesterone level which causes hyperventilation. Breathlessness caused by diseases complicating pregnancy should be distinguished from the physiologic dyspnea with the help of clinical features and other relevant investigations.

ASTHMA IN PREGNANCY

Asthma is reported amongst 3-12% of pregnant women worldwide. Pregnancy outcomes are adversely affected by asthma, especially when it is poorly controlled. The clinical picture of asthma may vary from mild wheezing and bronchospasm to severe bronchoconstriction and respiratory failure.

Effect of Pregnancy on Asthma

Asthma during pregnancy is variably affected—about a quarter of patients may improve, while 30% may become worse during pregnancy. Intrapartum exacerbation may be present in 20% of patients. Worsening of asthma is usually seen between 24 weeks and 36 weeks of gestation. Symptoms are less troublesome in the peripartum period. Asthma severity returns to the prepregnant state within about 3 months of delivery in most cases; it may be worse in rare cases.

Effect of Asthma on Pregnancy

In the recent years, pregnancy outcome in asthmatic women has improved. Clinical features are the same as in the nonpregnant state. Severe disease may affect the pregnancy outcome. There is increased risk of preeclampsia, preterm labor, placental abruption, preterm rupture of membranes, low-birth-weight infants, and perinatal mortality. Asthma medication and poor asthma control leading to hypoxia have been hypothesized to explain these observations.

The risks of obstetrical complications are not higher in asthmatic pregnant women than in nonasthmatics except for depression, miscarriage, and cesarean delivery. Complications during pregnancy are related to the disease severity. In a severe case, complications such as pneumothorax, pneumomediastinum, acute cor pulmonale, and cardiac arrhythmias can often prove to be life-threatening.

The fetus is threatened by poorly controlled asthma or severe asthma exacerbations because of increased maternal hypoxemia and diminished uterine artery blood flow, secondary to hypocapnic vasoconstriction. The leftward shift of oxyhemoglobin dissociation curve due to alkalotic state is responsible for fetal hypoxia. Perinatal outcomes are good with reasonable control of asthma. The possible teratogenic and adverse effects of drugs in asthma are important concerns. However, there is enough evidence that the commonly used drugs cause no harm to the fetus.

> **BOX 98.2:** Components of asthma management during pregnancy.
>
> - Patient education
> - Avoidance or control of environmental precipitating factors
> - Objective assessment of pulmonary function and fetal well-being
> - Pharmacological therapy to provide baseline control and treat exacerbations.

Management of Chronic Asthma

Aggressive management of asthma is required during pregnancy not only to alleviate symptoms, but also to restore and maintain normal lung function. A multipronged approach to management is recommended by the Working Group on Asthma and Pregnancy (Box 98.2).

Asthma pharmacotherapy: The primary asthma therapy is aimed at relief from bronchospasm and to resolve the inflammation in the airways to improve pulmonary function and reduce airway hyperresponsiveness. Asthma therapy during pregnancy is somewhat affected due to differences in maternal physiology and pharmacokinetics which alter the absorption, distribution, metabolism, and clearance of drugs. There is possibly some tissue refractoriness to cortisol and changes in cellular immunity during pregnancy. Although the drugs are considered safe to use but firm data on the issue is hard to obtain since the pregnant women are usually excluded from clinical trials. The standard pharmacotherapy with inhaled corticosteroids (ICSs) and long-acting beta-2 agonists is recommended. These drugs are not reported to cause any adverse pregnancy outcome.

- Inhaled β_2-agonists: Salbutamol (albuterol) or terbutaline are used for mild occasional asthma attacks. For continued maintenance treatment, long-acting agents like salmeterol and formoterol are used in combination with ICSs. Formoterol has the advantage of a rapid onset of effect for the relief of acute bronchospasm. Side effects of selective β_2-agonists are few but may include tremors, tachycardia, and palpitations.
- Inhaled corticosteroids: These constitute the cornerstone of management of asthma. ICSs produce clinically important improvements in symptoms as well as bronchial hyperresponsiveness. There is no reported evidence of any increase in neonatal malformations or other adverse perinatal outcomes. There is little difference between different ICS but budesonide is generally a preferred medication, unless a woman is well-controlled by a different ICS before pregnancy.

Theophylline: It is used as an additional treatment when β_2-agonists and inhaled anti-inflammatory agents do not adequately control symptoms. It is not effective for the treatment of acute exacerbations during pregnancy.

Leukotriene moderators: Both zafirlukast and montelukast, the leukotriene receptor antagonists, are considered to be safe (pregnancy category β drugs) but there are minimal data regarding the efficacy or safety of these agents.

Oral (systemic) corticosteroids: Use of oral corticosteroids during the first trimester of pregnancy is associated with a threefold increase of risk for isolated cleft lip with or without cleft palate. Their use is occasionally indicated for an acute, life-threatening exacerbation of asthma.

Antenatal Management

Adverse outcomes of pregnancy are more in case the asthma severity and exacerbations are underestimated and inadequately managed. Detailed medical history and appropriate attention to medical conditions should happen at the very first prenatal visit. The patient should be asked about the presence and severity of symptoms, episodes of nocturnal episodes, the number of the days of work missed due to asthma exacerbations, history of acute asthma emergency care visits, and the smoking history. Asthma medications should be inquired and recorded in details.

Scheduling of prenatal visits for pregnant mothers with moderate or severe asthma should be based on clinical judgment. Pulmonary function [forced expiratory volume in one second or peak expiratory flow (FEV_1 or PEF)] should be done in addition to routine care and asthma evaluations. Antenatal fetal surveillance with regular ultrasonography is important in patients with moderate and severe asthma. It is necessary to establish true pregnancy dating since asthma is a frequent cause of intrauterine growth restriction and preterm birth. Ultrasonography is also helpful to evaluate fetal viability, anatomy, amniotic fluid volume, placental location, and interval fetal growth. The intensity and frequency of antenatal fetal surveillance should be based upon the severity of asthma.

Management of Acute Asthma

The treatment of acute asthma is generally the same as in nonpregnant state. Hypoxia must be prevented with aggressive management. Continuous fetal monitoring must be assured if gestation has advanced to the point of potential fetal viability. Besides oxygen administration, nebulization with short-acting β-agonists, such as terbutaline or salbutamol (2.5–5 mg every 20 minutes for three doses, then 2.5–10 mg every 1–4 hours as needed, or 10–15 mg/hr continuously), should be delivered. In severe cases, systemic administration of corticosteroids is necessary. Both nebulized and intravenous magnesium sulfate are shown to be safe to control acute exacerbation. Monitoring should be done for oxygenation through pulse oximeter or arterial blood gases, the general level of activity, color, pulse rate, use of accessory muscles, and airflow obstruction. Treatment is assessed as good, incomplete or poor depending upon various monitoring parameters (Box 98.3).

Acute Severe Asthma and Respiratory Failure

Severe asthma of any kind not responding after 30–60 minutes of intensive therapy was previously known as status asthmaticus. Early intubation and

> **BOX 98.3:** Assessment of response to initial treatment of acute asthma.
>
> *Good response:*
> - FEV_1 or PEF >70%
> - Response sustained 60 minutes after last treatment
> - No distress
> - Physical examination: Normal
> - Reassuring fetal status
> - Discharge home
>
> *Incomplete response:*
> - FEV_1 or PEF 50% but <70%
> - Mild or moderate symptoms
> - Continue fetal assessment until the patient stabilized
> - Monitor FEV_1 or PEF, O_2 saturation, pulse
> - Continue inhaled salbutamol and oxygen
> - Inhaled ipratropium bromide
> - Systemic (oral or intravenous) corticosteroid
> - Individualize decision for hospitalization
>
> *Poor response:*
> - FEV_1 or PEF <50%
> - PCO_2 >42 mm Hg
> - Physical examination: Severe symptoms, drowsiness, and confusion
> - Admit to hospital intensive care
> - Continue fetal assessment.
>
> (FEV_1: forced expiratory volume in one second; PEF: peak expiratory flow)

mechanical ventilation may be needed. Management in intensive care has resulted in good outcome.

Labor and Delivery Management

Asthma management should continue during labor and delivery. Adequate hydration and analgesia should be assured in order to decrease the risk of bronchospasm and other complications. Intravenous corticosteroids (hydrocortisone 100 mg q 8 hours) should be administered during labor and for the 24-hour period following delivery to prevent adrenal crisis, especially if systemic corticosteroids had been used in the previous 4 weeks.

Cesarean delivery is rarely necessary for an acute asthma exacerbation. Aggressive medical management is usually successful to control maternal and fetal compromise. Labor induction may be done with oxytocin and prostaglandin (PG) E_2 or E_1. Oxytocin and prostaglandin E2 may be needed for postpartum hemorrhage. Carboprost (15-methyl PGF_2-alpha) and methylergonovine are contraindicated since they are known to cause bronchospasm. Magnesium sulfate is a safe choice for treating preterm labor. Indomethacin can induce bronchospasm in the aspirin-sensitive patient. There are no reports of the use of calcium channel blockers for tocolysis among women with asthma.

It is better to use lumbar epidural anesthesia to reduce oxygen consumption and minute ventilation during labor. Fentanyl is a better analgesic than meperidine. Meperidine which causes histamine release is occasionally associated with the onset of bronchospasm during labor. Conduction analgesia is preferred since tracheal intubation can trigger bronchospasm.

Breastfeeding

Antiasthma drugs are safe for the infant even though they are shown to present in the breast milk in very small amounts. There is no contraindication for breastfeeding in case the mother is on any of these drugs such as prednisone, theophylline, antihistamines, beclomethasone, β_2-agonists, and cromolyn. Theophylline may occasionally cause toxic effects in the neonate, including vomiting, feeding difficulties, jitteriness, and cardiac arrhythmias.

PNEUMONIA IN PREGNANCY

There is no increase in the incidence of pneumonia in the pregnant than the nonpregnant women. But because of the physiologic alterations of pregnancy, pneumonia during pregnancy carries greater morbidity and mortality. There are decreases in pulmonary functional residual capacity and cell-mediated immunity. Therefore, a higher level of surveillance is important during pregnancy.

Currently, pneumonia has been classified into several types: (1) community-acquired pneumonia (CAP)—commonly seen in young and pregnant women; (2) hospital-acquired pneumonia; (3) healthcare-associated pneumonia (HCAP); and (4) ventilator-associated pneumonia. The fetus poorly tolerates hypoxemia and acidosis due to severe pneumonia, which may frequently stimulate preterm labor. Chest radiography should be done in any pregnant woman suspected to have pneumonia.

Bacterial Pneumonia

Incidence and causes: Bacterial pneumonias during pregnancy are commonly caused by the same organisms that are responsible in general population, i.e. *Streptococcus pneumoniae, Haemophilus influenzae, Chlamydia pneumoniae, Mycoplasma pneumoniae,* and *Legionella pneumophila*. But the causative organisms may not be identified in 50% or more of cases even with extensive diagnostic testing. The common risk factors for pneumonia include asthma and other chronic respiratory diseases, human immunodeficiency virus or acquired immunodeficiency syndrome (HIV or AIDS), smoking, and drug use.

Diagnosis: Signs and symptoms of bacterial pneumonia in pregnancy are the same as in nonpregnant individuals. Cough, sputum production, dyspnea, and pleuritic chest pain are the more common symptoms. Chest radiograph should be done in all patients in whom pneumonia is suspected such as those who have the findings of fever, crackles, and abnormal breath sounds. The chest radiograph is important to confirm pneumonia or rule out other diagnoses. It also helps to suggest a possible bacterial or other etiology and aid

> **BOX 98.4:** Criteria for severe community-acquired pneumonia.
>
> - Respiratory rate ≥30/min
> - PaO_2/FiO_2 ≤250
> - Multilobular infiltrates
> - Confusion or disorientation
> - Uremia
> - Leukopenia—WBC <4,000/µL
> - Thrombocytopenia—platelets <1,00,000/µL
> - Hypothermia—temperature <36°C
> - Hypotension requiring aggressive fluid resuscitation
>
> (PaO_2, partial pressure of arterial oxygen; FiO_2, fraction of inspired oxygen; WBC, white blood cell)

in determining the severity of illness. Multilobar involvement is a more severe form of pneumonia than single lobar involvement (Box 98.4).

Management: Pregnant women with pneumonia are generally hospitalized for observation and initial therapy. Investigations should include a complete blood count, serum electrolytes, and assessment of oxygenation; blood cultures have been found to be positive only 7–15% of the times. Intravenous antibiotic therapy should be empirically started. Erythromycin, azithromycin or a β-lactam, such as ceftriaxone or ampicillin are recommended as initial choice for mild CAP. For severe disease, the American Thoracic Society recommends: (1) fluoroquinolone—levofloxacin or moxifloxacin; (2) a β-lactam plus a macrolide. Clinical response in most patients is seen within 3 days. Treatment should not change in the first 72 hours unless there is significant clinical deterioration. X-ray resolution takes longer up to 6 weeks. Pleural effusion may be seen in up to 20% of patients. Treatment is given for a minimum period of 5 days.

Pregnancy outcome with pneumonia: Depending upon the severity and response to treatment, several complications of bacterial pneumonia may occur, such as meningitis, arthritis, endocarditis, empyema, and pericarditis. Severe pneumonia can be complicated by serious problems such as sepsis, heart failure, renal failure, and acute respiratory distress syndrome (ARDS). Aggressive and/or intensive care treatment may be required in such cases. ARDS in pregnancy can result from other obstetric causes such as pre-eclampsia, amniotic fluid embolism, and retained products of conception.

Obstetric complications of pneumonia include fetal distress secondary to poor oxygenation and preterm birth. Women, who have pneumonia, are significantly more likely to deliver before 34 weeks. Preterm birth has been reported to be more common when the woman who has pneumonia, has some underlying comorbid condition. Anemia has also been reported in several studies of pneumonia during pregnancy. Birth weights of infants born to women having antepartum pneumonia have been found to be significantly less than the controls.

Prevention: Pneumococcal vaccine is 60–70% protective. The vaccine is not recommended for otherwise healthy pregnant women. It is recommended for immunocompromised patients like those with HIV infection, diabetes, cardiac or renal disease, and asplenia such as sickle cell disease.

Influenza

Historically, influenza in pregnant women is reported to be associated with high morbidity and mortality.

Pregnant women constitute an important high-risk group; the risk is even more if there is an underlying medical condition, or advanced age. In one study, women in the third trimester had 3–4 times as much risk for hospitalization for an acute cardiopulmonary illness during influenza season as in postpartum women.

Clinical presentation: The influenza virus spreads via aerosolized droplets. Pregnancy does not alter the clinical presentation of influenza. Influenza virus has an incubation period of 1–4 days, with an average of 2 days. Patients are generally infectious a day before the onset of symptoms and for 5 days thereafter. Virus shedding may last for much longer periods of time in young children and immunocompromised adults.

Cough, fever, malaise, rhinitis, myalgias, headache, chills, and sore throat are most commonly present. Less common symptoms include nausea and vomiting, otitis, and conjunctival burning. Physical findings include the presence of fever, tachycardia, facial flushing, clear nasal discharge, and cervical adenopathy. Fever in adults may generally last for 3 days while resolution of other symptoms may take about a week. Cough and malaise may sometimes persist for longer than 2 weeks.

Diagnosis: Influenza is usually diagnosed by the clinical features during the influenza season. Culture is important for definitive diagnosis. Nasal samples provide a higher level of sensitivity than do throat samples. Immunofluorescence or immunoassay has the advantage of providing rapid diagnosis but do not have the same sensitivity as that of culture. Culture is essential for patients with a highly suggestive clinical picture but with a negative rapid test. Viral culture is also helpful to subtype influenza, as well as for drug sensitivities.

Management: Uncomplicated cases generally respond to supportive and symptomatic treatment with antipyretics and bedrest. The antiviral agents, amantadine and rimantadine, are active against influenza A only. They are 70–90% effective for chemoprophylaxis to prevent influenza. Given within the first 48 hours of symptoms, they also help to reduce the symptom duration.

Prevention or vaccination: Vaccination is the primary method of influenza prevention. All women with likelihood of pregnancy during the influenza season shall receive the vaccine. Vaccination can be safely given in any trimester. Breastfeeding also is not a contraindication to vaccination. The inactivated vaccine is used for pregnant women, as well as for all other high-risk groups.

Effects on pregnancy: Pneumonia, either viral or superimposed bacterial, typically occurs 2-14 days after the symptoms of influenza have resolved. Postinfluenza pneumonia during pregnancy should be managed more aggressively on the same lines as stated earlier. Other important complications of influenza include myopathy, rhabdomyolysis and myoglobinuria, carditis, and encephalopathy.

Fetal effects: There are no significant differences in the incidence of congenital malformations in babies born to women who had serum-confirmed influenza and those born to women without influenza. According to some studies, influenza may sometimes be associated with limb reduction and neural tube defects, including anencephaly. No association was found between influenza and anencephaly by other investigators. Increased incidence of cleft lip has also been reported.

Varicella Pneumonia

Varicella virus infection occurs in 0.7 per 1,000 pregnancies and pneumonia is the most common complication. Smoking and the presence of 100 or more skin lesions are the important risk factors for varicella pneumonia. Pulmonary symptoms (cough, hemoptysis, dyspnea, tachypnea, and pleuritic chest pain) usually occur 2-5 days after the onset of rash and fever. Treatment is given with intravenous acyclovir, although its value is not proven.

Congenital varicella syndrome characterized by limb hypoplasia, chorioretinitis, cutaneous scars, and cortical atrophy occurs in 1-2% of cases of maternal varicella, depending on gestational age. Varicella pneumonia has also been associated with preterm labor. The infection in susceptible individuals can be prevented or at least attenuated with varicella-zoster immunoglobulin given within 96 hours of exposure to varicella. Varicella-zoster immunoglobulin is not contraindicated in pregnancy but the varicella vaccine, a live-attenuated vaccine, is not recommended.

Severe Acute Respiratory Syndrome

Severe acute respiratory syndrome (SARS) occurs due to a novel coronavirus. SARS pneumonia can also be complicated by respiratory failure, superimposed bacterial infections, and disseminated intravascular coagulation (DIC). There are high rates of morbidity and mortality with the case fatality rate of 25%. During pregnancy, a large number of cases are complicated by first-trimester spontaneous abortions, preterm births, and intrauterine growth restriction. There are no reported cases of vertical transmission. Treatment consists of broad-spectrum antibiotics to cover superimposed bacterial infections, high-dose steroids, and possibly ribavirin. Ribavirin has been shown to have teratogenic effects in animals; its use in pregnancy has not been established.

Fungal Pneumonia

Fungal pneumonias with *Aspergillus, Candida,* and *Cryptococcus* are seen in those women who are immunocompromised or hospitalized. Management of these opportunistic fungal infections during pregnancy is same as in nonpregnant women. These are generally serious, life-threatening conditions. With the physiologic suppression of cell-mediated immunity in pregnancy, endemic fungal pneumonias can be seen in otherwise healthy women. There have only been a handful of cases of pneumonia secondary to histoplasmosis. With the increasing number of pregnant women infected with HIV, *Pneumocystis jiroveci* pneumonia (PJP), previously known as *Pneumocystis carinii,* is a common complication. Symptoms include dry cough, dyspnea, and tachypnea. A diffuse infiltrate is seen on chest radiograph.

Treatment is given with trimethoprim-sulfamethoxazole or pentamidine. HIV-infected patients who have a CD4+ T-lymphocyte count of less than 200/mL, a history of oropharyngeal candidiasis, or an AIDS-defining illness should receive prophylaxis. The preferred regimen is trimethoprim-sulfamethoxazole, one double-strength tablet per day. Prophylaxis is 90–95% effective.

TUBERCULOSIS AND PREGNANCY

The diagnosis and management of tuberculosis in pregnancy is of utmost importance, especially since the untreated disease poses much greater risk to both the mother and the fetus.

Clinical Presentation

About half to two-thirds of pregnant women with tuberculosis may remain asymptomatic. The clinical presentation of tuberculosis in the pregnant women is similar to that in the nonpregnant patients (Table 98.1). Nonspecific symptoms like lethargy, alteration in bowel habit, or failure to gain weight are commonly interpreted as usual symptoms of pregnancy, hence the cause of delay in the diagnosis.

During pregnancy, pulmonary tuberculosis is more common than extrapulmonary tuberculosis. Only 5–10% of pregnant women have extrapulmonary disease most commonly of lymph nodes, pleura, genitourinary tract, bones, joints, meninges, and peritoneum.

Effect of Pregnancy on Tuberculosis

Tuberculosis gets flared up by the stress of pregnancy, especially if associated with poor nutritional and immunodeficient states, or coexistent diseases.

TABLE 98.1: Symptoms of tuberculosis in pregnancy.

Common	Less common
Cough, sputum	Lethargy, malaise
Weakness, weight loss	Abdominal distension
Fever, sweating	Irritability, headache
Hemoptysis	Skin lesions, lymph nodes
Fatigue, tiredness	Alteration in bowel habit

> **BOX 98.5:** Effects of tuberculosis on pregnancy.
>
> - Spontaneous abortions
> - Intrauterine death
> - Premature labor
> - Small for gestational age neonates
> - Low birth weight
> - Increased perinatal mortality

Effect of Tuberculosis on Pregnancy (Box 98.5)

The pulmonary and extrapulmonary forms of tuberculosis affect pregnancy in several ways. With the advent of chemotherapy, several studies have demonstrated that tuberculosis does not increase complications of pregnancy and labor.

Diagnosis

It is important to identify pregnant women with tuberculosis since an early diagnosis and treatment will result in better maternal and neonatal outcomes. History of exposure to tuberculosis and the similarities of symptoms between tuberculosis and pregnancy should be kept in mind.

Chest radiograph: In the past, chest X-ray was advocated to detect tuberculosis. In view of the risk of radiation exposure, the routine use of chest radiograph is not justified. If tuberculin skin test is greater than 10 mm of induration, a chest radiograph should be obtained in asymptomatic patient with proper abdominal shielding preferably after first trimester.

Tuberculin skin test: In India, the routine use of the tuberculin test for diagnosis of tuberculosis remains questionable since about half of the population is tuberculin positive. Positive tuberculin test is an indication of present or past mycobacterial infection or exposure. Tuberculin test is considered as a safe and useful method for screening tuberculosis infection in pregnancy. But it does not imply the presence of active disease. HIV-positive women may have diminished or negative tuberculin reaction, an area of 5 mm or greater induration in an HIV-positive patient is considered positive.

Microbiological methods: Essential laboratory methods for diagnosis of tuberculosis include microscopy, culture, nucleic acid amplification assays, and drug susceptibility testing. Bronchoscopy may be required to obtain bronchial secretions if the patient is unable to produce sputum.

Treatment of Tuberculosis in Pregnant Women

Antituberculosis treatment (ATT) should be initiated without delay when tuberculosis is diagnosed in pregnant women. The decision to treat tuberculosis in pregnancy must keep into account the potential benefits and risks to mother and fetus. It is widely considered that the benefits of treating tuberculosis in pregnancy outweigh any risk of treatment. The indications for treatment of active tuberculosis in pregnant women are the same as for nonpregnant women. None of the first-line ATT, i.e. two months of intensive phase with isoniazid (INH), rifampicin, pyrazinamide, and ethambutol followed by four months of maintenance phase with isoniazid (INH), rifampicin and ethambutol, was found to be teratogenic, except streptomycin which can cause ototoxicity in fetus. Most of the second-line drugs including the fluoroquinolones are contraindicated during pregnancy. It is therefore advisable to terminate pregnancy in a patient on those drugs.

The same regimens are recommended for use in pregnancy as for the nonpregnant state with the exception of streptomycin. As per the WHO recommendation, pyrazinamide should also be used for treatment.

Treatment of Tuberculosis in Lactating Women

Treatment for tuberculosis is not a contraindication to breastfeeding women even though small concentrations of antituberculosis drugs are excreted in breast milk. Breastfeeding of neonates is recommended regardless of the mother's tuberculosis status.

Care of newborn: The infant needs evaluation for active tuberculosis with chest radiograph and/or examination of gastric aspirate or sputum for acid-fast bacilli (AFB) if the mother is sputum-positive or on ATT. The newborn should receive vitamin K at birth to avoid the risk of postnatal hemorrhage in case the mother has received rifampicin during pregnancy.

Isoniazid prophylaxis is given to the infant born to a mother with tuberculosis if there is no evidence of active tuberculosis. Prophylaxis is either provided for 3 months or until after the mother's sputum becomes negative and the baby is tuberculin negative. Bacillus Calmette–Guérin (BCG) vaccination may be postponed or done with INH-resistant BCG vaccine in this situation. The INH prophylaxis is extended to a total period of 6 months if the infant is tuberculin positive but active tuberculosis is ruled out. INH prophylaxis has no role if the mother is suffering from multidrug-resistant tubercle bacilli (MDR-TB). In such cases, the infant should receive BCG vaccination, which has been shown to have a protective effect. BCG is contraindicated in HIV-positive children.

The prognosis for both the mother and the child is good if tuberculosis is diagnosed and treated appropriately and early. It is highly desirable that TB care is integrated with prenatal care to improve the management of tuberculosis during pregnancy.

Contraception: Rifampicin accelerates the metabolism of oral contraceptives and other drugs resulting in subtherapeutic serum levels. So, the reliability of oral contraceptive is decreased in women taking ATT. All other contraceptive measures can be considered in postpartum women taking ATT.

PULMONARY THROMBOEMBOLISM

Venous thromboembolism (VTE) during antenatal period (from conception to delivery) is about 7–10 times higher than the incidence in age-matched controls. On an average, 5-12 events of VTE are reported per 10,000 pregnancies with similar risk in all three trimesters. Pulmonary embolism (PE) occurs in 10-15% cases of VTE. There are no specific signs and symptoms of PE—tachypnea, dyspnea, chest pain (pleuritic), apprehension, and crackles are present in at least 50% of patients as are seen in nonpregnant patients. Chest radiographic abnormalities seen in 80% or more of patients and electrocardiogram findings seen in about 70% of patients with PE are not diagnostic. Arterial oxygen tension is low in most of the patients.

Both VTE and PE require objective diagnostic testing to confidently confirm or exclude the diagnosis. This is particularly important during pregnancy to determine duration of therapy, requirement for prophylaxis during future pregnancies, and recommendation regarding avoidance of oral contraceptive pills.

Compression ultrasonography is the first objective test for VTE. Pulmonary perfusion scanning is done initially while the ventilation scan is added when perfusion defects are noted. CT pulmonary angiography is mostly diagnostic of PE. Pulmonary angiography, the gold standard test for PE diagnosis, is done if lung scan findings are of low probability or are indeterminate and the clinical suspicion remains high.

Intravenous unfractionated heparin is administered immediately in patients in whom PE is strongly suspected unless there is a high risk or contraindication for the use of any anticoagulant. Heparin does not cross the placenta and is therefore the safest anticoagulant to use during pregnancy. The initial loading dose of 5,000-10,000 units is followed with an infusion of 18 U/kg. Activated partial thromboplastin time should be monitored and kept in the therapeutic range of 1.5-2 times the baseline value.

Low-molecular-weight heparin (LMWH) is the treatment of choice for PE in pregnant (and nonpregnant) patients. LMWH is at least as effective and safe as unfractioned heparin (UFH) in nonpregnant women for the treatment of acute VTE. Although only a relatively modest amount of data has been gathered, LMWH, which does not cross the placenta, can be given once a day and does not require monitoring. LMWH has not been shown to increase the risk of bleeding with surgical procedures, including with the cesarean delivery.

Warfarin should be avoided throughout the pregnancy. It can result in embryopathy characterized by mental retardation, optic atrophy, cleft lip, cleft palate, and cataracts in addition to hemorrhage. The teratogenic effects are particularly common during the first trimester. Warfarin crosses the placenta; it can cause fetal and neonatal hemorrhage and placental abruption.

Anticoagulation therapy with heparin is essential throughout the pregnancy for patients with antepartum VTE or PE. Warfarin should be started after delivery and heparin discontinued once an adequate international normalized ratio (INR) is achieved. Warfarin is continued for at least 6 weeks postpartum or after at least 3 months of anticoagulant therapy.

Use of unfractionated heparin for more than 6 months is reported to cause osteopenia and osteoporosis while the problem is less likely with LMWH. There are no definite beneficial effects of concomitant multivitamins, calcium or vitamin D supplementation, though providing optimum supplementation is reasonable for all patients receiving long-term heparin administration during pregnancy.

The recurrence rate of VTE in a subsequent pregnancy is more (4–15%) in women with previous history of VTE during pregnancy. The risk of VTE during pregnancy is also increased in women with a known hypercoagulable state. All these high risk groups should receive prophylaxis with either unfractionated heparin or LMWH. Unfractionated heparin is administered twice daily with an average daily dose of 16,400 IU/day or 225 IU/kg of body weight per 24 hours. The amount of heparin required for adequate prophylaxis is likely to increase through the second and third trimester. LMWH is preferable for prophylaxis in view of its single daily dose, no requirement for laboratory monitoring, and a lower risk of osteoporosis and bleeding.

PREGNANCY-SPECIFIC PROBLEMS

Besides the lung diseases, which complicate pregnancy, there are several pregnancy-specific problems (Box 98.6), which may frequently pose problems of diagnosis and treatment.

Amniotic Fluid Embolism

Amniotic fluid embolism is a rare complication which usually occurs during labor and delivery. This can be occasionally associated with uterine manipulation, uterine trauma, and the early postpartum period. The condition is frequently fatal with a mortality rate of 10–80%. The embolic material consists of amniotic fluid containing particulate cellular elements which enters the circulation through endocervical veins or uterine tears. The emboli in the lungs obstruct the pulmonary vessels causing vascular spasms and pulmonary hypertension. Occasionally, the episode may also cause acute left ventricular failure.

Usually, the patient will complain of a sudden onset of severe dyspnea, hypoxemia, and cardiovascular collapse. Other, relatively less common presentations may include hemorrhage caused by disseminated intravascular coagulation and fetal distress. The diagnosis of amniotic fluid embolism is usually made from the characteristic history and clinical picture. Presence of fetal squamous cells in a wedged pulmonary capillary aspirate may support the diagnosis, but not specific. Other conditions in the differential diagnoses include septic shock, pulmonary thromboembolism, ruptured placentae, tension pneumothorax, and myocardial ischemia.

BOX 98.6: Some important pregnancy-specific pulmonary problems.
- Amniotic fluid embolism
- Tocolytic pulmonary edema
- Preeclampsia and pulmonary edema
- Peripartum cardiomyopathy
- Gestational trophoblastic disease

Treatment consists of routine resuscitative and supportive measures. Urgent attention should be given to adequate oxygenation, ventilation, and inotropic support. There is no specific therapy for this condition. Use of corticosteroids remains debatable. Disseminated intravascular coagulation, ARDS, or both may develop in the survivors.

Tocolytic Pulmonary Edema

Pulmonary edema during pregnancy has been reported to develop in 0.3–9% of women for whom there is use of β-adrenergic agonists (particularly salbutamol, ritodrine, and terbutaline) for inhibition of uterine contractions and preterm labor. Several mechanisms have been proposed for this complication such as the prolonged exposure to catecholamines (which causes myocardial dysfunction), increased capillary permeability, and a large volume of intravenous fluids administered in response to maternal tachycardia. Glucocorticoids administration in cases of preterm labor may also contribute to fluid retention. The clinical presentation consists of acute respiratory distress and pulmonary edema. Tocolytic pulmonary edema should be distinguished from cardiogenic pulmonary edema, amniotic fluid embolism, and aspiration pneumonia. Pulmonary edema usually resolves rapidly after discontinuation of β-agonist therapy and supportive diuresis.

Preeclampsia and Pulmonary Edema

Patients with preeclampsia, who are usually volume depleted, may sometimes receive aggressive fluid replacement which may result in pulmonary edema in about 3% of cases. Most commonly this occurs in the early postpartum period. Pulmonary edema in such situations is further contributed by reduced albumin concentration and myocardial dysfunction. The standard treatment consists of restriction of fluids, supplemental oxygen, and diuresis. Invasive monitoring might be useful if inotropic vasodilator therapy becomes necessary.

Peripartum Cardiomyopathy

Cardiogenic pulmonary edema is an important problem in the differential diagnosis of acute respiratory distress during pregnancy. Preexisting heart disease may or may not be present. Hypertensive disease of pregnancy and peripartum cardiomyopathy usually during the last month of pregnancy or during the postpartum period are important causes of pulmonary edema in women with no known cardiac illness. Peripartum cardiomyopathy is of idiopathic origin and is associated with significant mortality. Tachycardia and increased cardiac output during labor and early postpartum can precipitate pulmonary edema.

Gestational Trophoblastic Disease

Benign hydatidiform or molar pregnancy may be complicated by pulmonary hypertension and pulmonary edema due to trophoblastic PE. This may commonly occur while the uterus is evacuated. The incidence of pulmonary complications is higher in later gestations. Molar pregnancy can lead to the development of choriocarcinoma, which is often characterized by the presence of multiple discrete pulmonary metastases and occasional pleural effusions.

In summary, there are several pulmonary problems seen among pregnant women. While some of these problems are specific to the state of pregnancy, the others are general medical or surgical conditions which may be either preexisting or occur during pregnancy. In either state, one needs to be careful while managing these conditions since both the investigations and the management involve special issues of additional risks to the fetus in utero. Ideally, the decision should be made after mutual consultation between the gynecologists and pulmonary physicians.

CHAPTER
99

Rare Lung Diseases

Sanjeev Mehta, PS Shankar

Rare lung diseases, sometimes referred to as orphan lung diseases, are rare in incidence but important from clinical presentation and management points of view.

PULMONARY ALVEOLAR PHOSPHOLIPOPROTEINOSIS

Pulmonary alveolar proteinosis (PAP) is characterized by the presence of a large amount of surfactant within the alveolar spaces. Abnormal alveolar surfactant accumulation can occur due to various conditions associated with functional impairment or reduced numbers of alveolar macrophages when PAP is called as secondary PAP. On the other hand, there is no identifiable cause in case of idiopathic or primary PAP.

Etiology and Pathophysiology

Pulmonary alveolar proteinosis is likely a common phenotypic response to a number of biochemical or molecular abnormalities, resulting in altered surfactant homeostasis, i.e. excessive production and/or reduced clearance of surfactant, by defective function of the alveolar macrophage and the growth factor necessary for its maturation, the granulocyte-macrophage colony-stimulating factor (GM-CSF). More likely, these are due to mutations in the genes encoding surfactant protein B or C or the C chain of the receptor for GM-CSF. Exact etiology is unknown but most patients are smokers. Secondary PAP which develops in association with various conditions is now being increasingly recognized (Box 99.1).

> **BOX 99.1:** Causes of secondary pulmonary alveolar proteinosis.
>
> - Subjects exposed to volcanic ash, aluminum dust, titanium, chlorambucil, and busulfan
> - Conditions, where alveolar macrophage function may be altered or suppressed:
>   - Immunodeficiency states
>   - Hematological malignancies, e.g. myeloid leukemias, neutropenia, and lymphomas
>   - Fanconi anemia
>   - Immunoglobulin G monoclonal gammopathy
>   - Silico-proteinosis (in sandblasters)
>   - Atypical mycobacterioses
>   - *Pneumocystis carinii* pneumonia
>   - Mycoses
> - Pulmonary diseases associated with or aggravated by smoking:
>   - Chronic obstructive pulmonary disease
>   - Interstitial pulmonary fibrosis
>   - Bronchogenic carcinoma
>   - Calcification of pleural plaques in asbestosis
>   - Pulmonary eosinophilic granuloma
>   - Alveolar hemorrhage in Goodpasture syndrome.

Pathology

On light microscopy with periodic acid-Schiff (PAS) stain, there is presence of eosinophilic, granular lipoproteinaceous material in the alveoli and terminal bronchioles. This fluid is rich in phospholipids and surfactant proteins A, B, C and D, tubular myelin, and membranous vesicles. On electron microscopy, one can also identify lamellar bodies which consist of phospholipids that are identical to inclusions found in normal type II pneumocytes. Bronchoalveolar lavage (BAL) fluid will show predominance of enlarged, foamy macrophages, which contain numerous complex phospholipoprotein inclusions. In secondary PAP, septal thickening, edema, and lymphocytic and neutrophilic infiltration can be seen.

Symptoms and Signs

Pulmonary alveolar proteinosis has been noted in young and middle aged individuals. Males are often more affected than females. The disease involves only the lungs. Clinically, nearly one-third are asymptomatic or minimally symptomatic. Most patients with acquired PAP complain of insidious onset of progressive exertional dyspnea and cough. Less frequently, there may be fever, chest pain or hemoptysis, especially if there is any secondary infection.

In some patients, PAP may begin with an initial febrile episode, followed later by progressive dyspnea, productive cough, low-grade fever, chest pain, and loss of weight. Cough is minimally productive with gelatinous white "chunky" expectoration. Hemoptysis is rare.

Physical examination may be unremarkable, but crackles are present in about 50%, cyanosis in 25%, and clubbing in a smaller number of patients.

Radiology

The extent of radiographic abnormalities is often disproportionate to the severity of the symptoms and physical findings. The chest X-ray (Fig. 99.1) usually reveals bilateral air space infiltrates with an ill-defined acinar nodules, ground glass opacification or confluent pattern, greater in the lower two-thirds of the lungs. It may be asymmetric in 20%. The "classic" perihilar "bat wing" or "reverse pulmonary edema" pattern is seen in about 50% cases. Air bronchograms are not a predominant feature of this disease. As the disease progresses, the alveolar infiltrates become denser. High-resolution computed tomography (HRCT) scan of the chest shows ground glass opacities which reflect alveolar filling or patchy airspace consolidation. Thickened interlobular septae, which are predominantly perihilar with relative sparing of the peripheral lung, are also seen. Presence of the proteinaceous material in the septal interstitium causes accentuation of the interlobular septae. An appearance of "crazy paving", i.e. sharp transition between the normal and the abnormal lung, is a characteristic feature on HRCT. However, "crazy paving" is not seen only in PAP. Interstitial infiltration may be seen in chronic cases.

Laboratory Tests

Routine laboratory tests are generally unremarkable. There may be mild leukocytosis. Elevated serum lactate dehydrogenase (LDH) may be a useful marker. Pulmonary function tests usually reveal a restrictive ventilatory defect, with reduced lung volumes and a disproportionate reduction in diffusing capacity of carbon monoxide. Hypoxemia caused by ventilation–perfusion

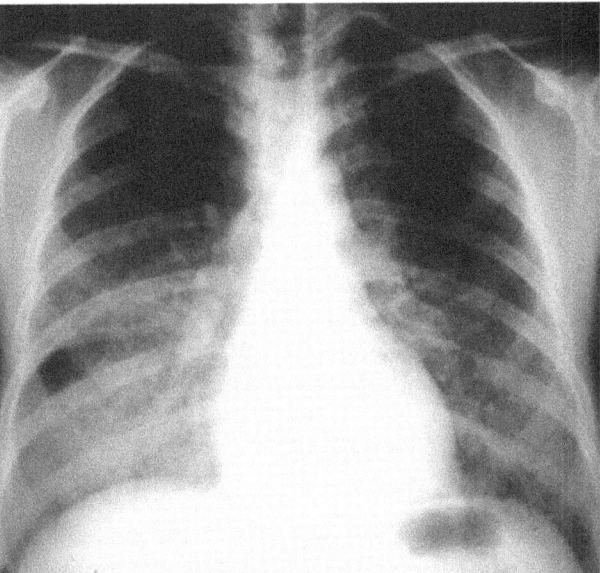

Fig. 99.1: Chest roentgenograph of pulmonary alveolar proteinosis—bilateral air space infiltrates, acinar nodules, and ground-glass opacification.

inequality and intrapulmonary shunting is common, resulting in a widened alveolar–arteriolar diffusion gradient. Open lung biopsy has been the gold standard for diagnosis, but bronchoscopic lung biopsy may suffice. BAL is also helpful. Aspiration of opaque milky or sandy or light-brown fluid from an affected segment is characteristic. Differentiation of the phospholipoprotein aggregates from mucins can be made on different staining characteristics of BAL fluid which stains pink with PAS, but negative with alcian blue. Surfactant protein-A (SP-A) concentrations are 400 times higher in patients with PAP than in controls on assay using monoclonal antibodies to SP-1. This can be a useful test for diagnosis of PAP, especially when lung biopsy is contraindicated. Serum LDH may be elevated but not specific to PAP.

Treatment

Therapy is essentially supportive. About 30% patients may improve spontaneously, especially those with a partial pressure of arterial oxygen (PaO_2) more than or equal to 70 mm Hg or pulmonary alveolar-arterial (A-a) O_2 less than or equal to 40 mm Hg. Steroids have not shown to be beneficial. Treatment of the underlying cause should be undertaken, wherever possible. Aggressive attempts should be made at cessation of smoking.

Whole lung lavage, using normal saline, one lung at a time is the mainstay of therapy. The usual reported benefit is for 15 months. Patients with severe and/or recurrent disease require repeated lavages at intervals of several weeks to months. When whole lung lavage cannot be performed, segmental or lobar lavage, using flexible bronchoscope, can be attempted. Whole lung lavage is not having any effect on the pathogenetic mechanisms and is often associated with many complications. Subcutaneous and inhaled administration of GM–CSF has been reported to be effective, but this strategy, while promising, remains experimental. Aerosolized trypsin has been used to treat PAP, but the results are not consistent. Treatment of infection and supportive care, such as the use of oxygen, should be administered as appropriate. Lung transplantation is rarely indicated for an advanced disease.

Progress and Complications

Progressive respiratory failure occurs from disease persistence. Interstitial fibrosis develops in chronic cases. Infection with unusual organisms, such as *Nocardia* species, *Aspergillus* species, *Mycobacteria*, *Pneumocystis*, *Cryptococcus neoformans* and other organisms, is known to occur.

PULMONARY CALCIFICATION AND OSSIFICATION SYNDROMES

Pulmonary calcification commonly seen on chest X-ray is usually an incidental finding. It may be metastatic, benign or malignant or dystrophic in origin. The list of causes is rather exhaustive. Frequency-wise, the dystrophic causes of infectious etiology are more common (Box 99.2). The condition is possibly

BOX 99.2: Causes of pulmonary calcification.

- Dystrophic calcification:
  - Tuberculosis
  - Sarcoidosis
  - Histoplasmosis and other fungal infections
  - Postvaricella pneumonia
  - Smallpox handler's lung
  - Parasitic infections: Paragonimiasis
  - Amyloidosis
  - Silicosis
  - Coal worker's pneumoconiosis
  - Pulmonary vascular calcification
  - Idiopathic: Pulmonary alveolar microlithiasis
- Metastatic:
  - Chronic renal insufficiency on hemodialysis
  - Primary hyperparathyroidism
  - Hypervitaminosis D
  - Excess exogenous administration of calcium and vitamin D (milk-alkali syndrome)
  - Osteopetrosis
  - Osteitis deformans (Paget's disease)
  - Malignant causes: Parathyroid carcinoma, multiple myeloma, lymphoma/leukemia, and choriocarcinoma

due to abnormalities in serum calcium and phosphate concentration, alkaline phosphatase activity, and local pH and other physicochemical conditions.

Pathophysiology

Metastatic calcification commonly occurs due to elevated calcium-phosphate product of 70 mg^2/dL^2 (normal <40). Calcification at normal or low serum calcium can be seen in azotemia (previous or current), high parathyroid hormone levels, and/or exogenous vitamin D administration. In the presence of other risk factors, ectopic calcification results from hypercalcemia and alkalosis which act synergistically to predispose.

Dystrophic calcification may occur with normal serum calcium levels in the injured or the abnormal tissues as is often seen in granulomas and in lymphadenopathy associated with tuberculosis, fungal diseases, and sarcoidosis. It is sometimes seen in other conditions such as amyloidosis, coal workers pneumoconiosis.

Sarcoidosis-related calcification could be dystrophic or metastatic, secondary to hypercalcemia or both. It may sometimes mimic pulmonary alveolar microlithiasis (PAM) with a calcified micronodular pattern. Pulmonary vascular calcification is a dystrophic condition due to shear stress. PAM is an autosomal recessive disorder of unknown etiology characterized by formation of calcium phosphate microliths in the alveoli. The distinct histologic and radiographic features seen in PAM are not seen in metastatic or dystrophic calcification.

> **BOX 99.3:** Causes of pulmonary ossification.
>
> - Preexisting pulmonary disorders:
>   - Tuberculosis
>   - Sarcoidosis
>   - Pulmonary amyloidosis
>   - Idiopathic pulmonary fibrosis
>   - Metastatic breast cancer
>   - Histoplasmosis
>   - Chronic busulfan therapy
>   - Pulmonary metastases of osteogenic sarcoma
>   - Metastatic melanoma
> - Other systemic causes:
>   - Primary and secondary hyperparathyroidism
>   - Hypervitaminosis D
>   - Mitral stenosis
>   - Chronic left ventricular failure
>   - Pyloric stenosis with alkalosis
>   - Idiopathic hypertrophic subaortic stenosis
> - Idiopathic pulmonary ossification

Pulmonary ossification is another idiopathic condition attributable to complex mechanisms, such as angiogenesis, chronic venous congestion, lung fibrosis, and/or the influence of various growth factors. It can also result from a variety of underlying pulmonary, cardiac, or extracardiopulmonary disorders (Box 99.3). Rarely, malignant pulmonary metastases can become calcified or ossified.

PULMONARY ALVEOLAR MICROLITHIASIS

Pulmonary alveolar microlithiasis is a rare and idiopathic disorder, characterized by the intra-alveolar deposition of a large number of minute calcific concretions, throughout both the lungs.

Etiopathology

The etiology is undetermined. A local alteration in the cells of alveolar septa appears to predispose to the occurrence of calcification. There is no abnormality of calcium metabolism. Nucleotide mutations in exon 6 have been occasionally reported. The cases have been reported in age group 30–50 years. Females are affected more than males. There is a familial incidence with a tendency to appear in siblings.

Clinical Features

Although the condition presents with abnormal chest radiograph in an asymptomatic patient, the advanced cases can present with cough, dyspnea, and respiratory failure. Hemoptysis may occasionally occur and very rarely calcified bodies may be coughed. There can be occurrence of recurrent pneumothoraces. Physical examination of the chest often does not reveal any abnormality, even in the presence of markedly abnormal chest radiograph. In advanced stages, the disease may show the presence of inspiratory crackles and ultimately, the signs of cor pulmonale.

Investigations

The chest radiograph gives widespread snowstorm appearance from minute calcified mottled shadows. They may be so profuse, as to make the lung diffusely white, especially in mid and lower lung zones obscuring the cardiac borders. Pleural calcification gives pencil-thin sharp dense white lines along the costal surfaces and over the hemidiaphragm. Presence of bullae may be considered to be a feature of advanced stage of disease. The radiological appearance of stenosis, talc granulomatosis, and calcified military histoplasmosis may simulate microlithiasis, but the lesions in those conditions are larger and have different distribution.

The lungs appear like sack of sand containing innumerable homogeneous intra-alveolar deposit of calcium-containing bodies. The lungs are solid containing sand-like grains (calcospherite) that are distributed diffusely, more so at the bases, a saw may be required to cut the lung. Under microscope, they appear as "onion-skin" bodies in the alveoli and are densely calcified. There can be emphysematous blebs at the apices or along anterior margins of the lungs. Pulmonary interstitium is not involved. Such calcification is not encountered in other organs. Lung biopsy reveals alveolar spaces containing animated calcific microliths, with fibrosis and thickening of the alveolar walls.

Extensive microcalcific deposits may be seen on computed tomography in the posterior and inferior subpleural spaces and along bronchovascular bundles. In addition, there may be findings suggestive of interstitial fibrosis and bronchiectasis. Calcified nodules larger than 1 mm (up to 5 mm) are visible on HRCT scans. Scintigraphy shows intense uptake of radiotracer technetium-99m by calcified spherules.

Pulmonary function studies do not show any abnormality despite extensive radiographic changes. In the later stages of disease, there is a restrictive pattern of lung volumes due to alveolar filling and a reduction in diffusing capacity.

Treatment

There is no specific treatment. The disease is variable in its course. It remains static in some cases while it is slowly progressive in others leading to the development of chronic cor pulmonale, respiratory or cardiac failure. Nasal continuous positive airway pressure ventilation has been tried to improve oxygenation in patients with respiratory failure. Bilateral sequential lung transplantation may be the other alternative.

CHAPTER 100

Ethics in Respiratory Care

Basil Varkey

INTRODUCTION

In all physician–patient interactions there is a moral component; some interactions [e.g. withdrawal of ventilator in an intensive care unit (ICU)] pose an obvious and dramatic ethical consideration while others (e.g. decisions on aggressive treatments in end-stage diseases in office settings) are less obvious. Patient care decisions involve more than selecting a treatment or intervention on a scientific basis; the physician's ethical obligation to benefit the patient and to avoid or minimize harm and the values and preferences of the patient and family members are all very much in play. Competence in ethics has been shown to improve the quality of care in certain areas and is a requisite to provide competent patient care.

ETHICS EDUCATION

The goals of ethics education are: (i) to appreciate the ethical dimensions of patient care; (ii) to understand ethical principles (principlism) of medical profession; (iii) to have competence in "core ethical behavioral skills"; (iv) to know the commonly encountered ethical issues in general and in one's specialty; (v) to have competence in analyzing and resolving ethical problems; (vi) to appreciate cultural diversity and how it impacts ethics; and (vii) to share one's knowledge in ethics with colleagues, trainees, and students. Core behavioral skills in ethics include obtaining informed consent, assessing decision-making capacity, discussing resuscitation status and use of life-sustaining treatments, advanced care planning, breaking bad news, and effective communication. Ethics education has been shown to improve learner awareness, attitudes, confidence, knowledge, and in moral reasoning.

Ethics and Morality

Ethics is a generic term covering different ways of examining the moral life. Some moral norms about right conduct are common to human kind—transcends cultures, regions, religions, and other group identities—and constitute *common morality*; examples of which include—not to kill or harm or cause suffering to others, not to steal, not to punish the innocent, to be truthful, to obey law, to nurture the young and dependent to help the suffering, and rescue those in danger. *Particular morality* norms bind groups special because of their culture, religion, profession, etc. and include responsibilities, ideals, professional standards, etc. and the explication or adjudication in some cases may need experts or religious authorities.

Professional moralities that include moral codes and standards of practice are one form of *particular morality*. Physicians have specialized knowledge and training and a commitment to provide services to patients. The standards and rules of their organizations attempt to keep them competent and trustworthy so that they can fulfill their obligations to their patients. These obligations are based on the accepted role of a physician then form in a basic level, the ethics of the profession. Physicians' organizations have also codified their standards to reduce the vagueness of professional morality based on "the accepted role of a physician". Codes, although well intentioned, may simplify moral requirements and may lead physicians to mistakenly consider that they are fulfilling the moral norms by complying with the codes.

The Four-principles Approach to Medical Ethics (Principlism)

Common morality is the base from which the four principles of biomedical ethics evolved. They are (i) respect for autonomy, (ii) nonmaleficence, (iii) beneficence, and (iv) distributive justice. The principles of respect for autonomy and justice evolved later than the other two.

Respect for Autonomy

The philosophical underpinning for autonomy is that all persons have intrinsic worth and therefore should have the power to make rational decisions and moral choices and each should be allowed to exercise his or her capacity for self-determination.

Autonomy, as is true for all four principles, needs to be weighed against competing moral principles and in some instances may be overridden; an obvious example would be if the liberty for autonomous action causes harm to another person or persons. The principle of autonomy does not extend to persons who lack the capacity (competence) to act autonomously; examples include infants and children and incompetence due to developmental, mental or physical disorder. A rigid distinction between incapacity (assessed by health professionals) and incompetence (determined by court of law) is not of practical use as a clinician's determination of a patient's lack of decision-making capacity has the same practical consequences as a legal determination of incompetence.

These views, on careful consideration, do not negate the principle of patient autonomy if one appreciates that autonomous choice is a right of a patient and the patient may choose a family member or members to make decisions for him or her. Physicians have a professional obligation to ensure that their patients have the right to choose, and inherently the right to accept or decline information.

Respecting the principle of autonomy also obliges the physician to disclose medical information and treatment options that are necessary for the patient to exercise self-determination. The proper understanding of the principle of autonomy supports other moral rules, such as informed consent, truth-telling, and confidentiality.

Informed consent: In order for a consent for a medical or surgical procedure or intervention or for research to meet the requirements of an informed consent, the patient or subject (i) must be competent to understand and decide, (ii) receives a full disclosure, (iii) comprehends the disclosure, (iv) acts voluntarily, and (v) consents to the proposed action.

Since competence is the first of the requirements for informed consent, one should know how to detect incompetence. Standards (used singly or in combination) that are generally accepted for determining incompetence are based on the patient's inability to state a preference or choice, inability to understand one's situation and its consequences, and inability to reason through a consequential life decision.

Incompetent (nonautonomous) patients and previously competent (autonomous) but presently incompetent patients would need a surrogate decision-maker. In a nonautonomous patient either a substituted judgment standard (what would the patient wish in this circumstance not what the surrogate's wish) or a best interests standard (highest net benefit to the patient by weighing risks and benefits) can be used by the surrogate. In a previously autonomous, but presently incompetent patient, the previously expressed preferences (prior autonomous judgments) should be respected even in the absence of a written formal advance directive.

A pattern that is not uncommonly followed, in nonwestern countries, is to disclose the information to the family and not to the patient. This violates patient autonomy unless the patient chooses this option and authorizes the physician to do so. The likely reasons for resistance of physicians to convey bad news are concern that it may cause anxiety and loss of hope, uncertainty of about the outcome, belief that the patient would not be able to understand the information and may not want to know. An autonomous patient has a right to choose not to know, but the physician must know about this choice. Providing full information, with tact and sensitivity, to patients who want to know should be the standard. The sad consequences of not telling the truth regarding a cancer include depriving the patient of an opportunity for completion of important life-tasks: writing a history for one's children, putting financial affairs in order, reconciling with estranged family members, attaining spiritual order by reflection, prayer, and religious sacraments.

Confidentiality: Physicians are obligated not to disclose confidential information given by the patient to another party without the patients' authorization. An obvious exception (with implied patient authorization) is the sharing necessary of medical information for the care of the patient from the primary physician to consultants and other healthcare teams. In the present day, modern hospitals with multiple points of tests and consultants and the use of electronic medical records there has been an erosion of confidentiality. However, individual physicians must exercise discipline in not discussing patient specifics with their family members or in social gatherings.

There are some noteworthy exceptions to patient confidentiality. These are legally required reporting of gunshot wounds and venereal diseases and exceptional situations that may cause major harm to another; examples are partner notification in HIV disease and relative notification of certain genetic risks.

Nonmaleficence

Nonmaleficence is the obligation of a physician not to harm the patient. This simply stated principle supports several moral rules—do not kill, do not cause pain or suffering, do not incapacitate, do not cause offense, and do not deprive others of the goods of life. The practical application of nonmaleficence is to have the physician is weigh the burdens against benefits of all treatments, to eschew those that are inappropriately burdensome, and to choose the best course of action for the patient. This is particularly important and pertinent in difficult end-of-life (EOL) care decisions on withholding and withdrawing life-sustaining treatment, medically administered nutrition and hydration, and in the doctrine of double effect in pain and other symptom control.

Beneficence

The principle of beneficence is the obligation of physician to act for the benefit of the patient and supports a number of moral rules—to protect and defend the right of others, prevent harm, remove conditions that will cause harm, help persons with disabilities, and rescue persons in danger. Note in distinction to nonmaleficence the language is one of positive requirements. The principle calls for not just avoiding harm but to benefit patients and to promote their welfare. Rather than the idealized view of physicians' beneficence as based on altruism and philanthropy, an argument can be made that it is based on reciprocity for the debt to society (education, in some instances subsidized by state governments, and privileges) and to their patients (for learning from them in practice and research).

Distributive Justice

Distributive justice is by one definition fair, equitable and appropriate distribution determined by justified norms that structure the terms of social cooperation. Several markedly different principles of distributive justice to each person have been proposed: an equal share, according to need, according to effort, according to contribution, according to merit, and according to free-market exchanges. It is easy to see the difficulty in choosing, balancing, and refining these principles to form a coherent and workable solution to distribute medical resources. This large healthcare policy discussion is beyond the scope of this chapter.

However, issues of justice are encountered daily in hospital practice and office practice. A few examples: allotting scarce equipment (e.g. ventilator), giving expensive drugs when the budget is tight, dealing with uninsured patients, providing a benefit not covered by insurance and even in allotting time for outpatient visits (on what basis: equal time for every patient or based on need or complexity or based on social status). Difficult as it may be, and in spite of the many constraining forces, physicians must accept the requirement of fairness contained in this principle. Fairness to the patent assumes a role of primary importance when there are conflicts of interests. A flagrant example of violation of this principle would be when a particular option of treatment is chosen over other(s) because it financially benefits the physician.

Conflicts between Principles

Each one of the principles is to be taken as a *prima facie* obligation that must be fulfilled unless it conflicts, in a specific instance, with another principle. When faced with such a conflict, the physician has to determine the actual obligation to the patient by examining the respective weights of the competing *prima facie* obligations based on the content and context. Consider an example of a conflict that has an easy resolution: a patient in shock treated with urgent fluid-resuscitation and placement of an indwelling intravenous catheter caused pain and swelling. Here the principle of beneficence overrides that of nonmaleficence. Many of the conflicts that physicians face, however, are much more complex and difficult. Consider a competent patient's refusal of a potentially lifesaving intervention (mechanical ventilation) or request for a potentially life-ending action (withdrawing mechanical ventilation).

Beneficence has enjoyed a historical role in the traditional practice of medicine. However, giving it primacy over patient autonomy is *paternalism** that makes a physician–patient relationship analogous to that of a father to a child. A father may refuse a child's wishes, may influence a child by a variety of ways—nondisclosure, manipulation, deception, coercion, etc., consistent with his thinking of what is best for the child. Paternalism can be further divided into soft and hard.

In soft paternalism the physician acts on grounds of beneficence (and at times nonmaleficence) when the patient is nonautonomous or substantially nonautonomous (examples are cognitive dysfunction due to severe illness, depression, drug addiction). Soft paternalism is complicated because of the difficulty in determining whether the patient was nonautonomous at the

---

*Although paternalism is a term well entrenched in bioethics literature a more appropriate term for modern times would be the gender-inclusive term *parentalism*.

time of decision-making, but is ethically defensible as long as the action is in concordance with what the physician believes to be the patient's values. Hard paternalism is an action by a physician, intended to benefit a patient, but contrary to the voluntary decision of an autonomous patient who is fully informed and competent. In contrast to soft paternalism, hard paternalism is ethically indefensible with very rare exceptions.

On the other end of the scale is consumerism, a rare and extreme form of patient autonomy, which holds the view that the physician's role is limited to providing all the medical information and the available choices for interventions and treatments while the fully informed autonomous patient selects from the available choices. In this model, because of the limited role a physician cannot use his or her knowledge and skills to benefit the patient and therefore partaking in this model of care is a form of patient abandonment.

Faced with the contrasting paradigms of beneficence and respect for autonomy and the need to reconcile these to find a common ground, beneficence can be inclusive of patient autonomy as "the best interests of the patients are intimately linked with their preferences" from which "are derived our primary duties to them".

Several models to analyze and resolve ethical problems have been proposed. One model uses a systematic four points approach as follows: (i) medical (identifying medical problems, treatment options, goals of care); (ii) patient (finding and clarifying patient preferences on treatment options and goals of care); (iii) quality-of-life (QOL) (effects of medical problems, interventions, and treatments on patient's QOL with awareness of individual biases on what constitutes an acceptable QOL); and (iv) context (many factors that include family, cultural, spiritual, religious, economic, and legal). Using this model the physician can identify the principles that are in conflict, ascertain by weighing and balancing what should prevail and when in doubt turn to ethics literature and expert opinion. The foregoing theoretical discussion on principles of ethics has practical application in clinical practice in all settings (Table 100.1).

ETHICS IN END-OF-LIFE CARE

Having laid the ground work on ethical principles as they apply to clinical practice in the preceding discussions, this segment will focus on ethics in EOL care of particular importance to pulmonary and critical care physicians. A substantial number of patients die with unrelieved symptoms that are poorly recognized and poorly treated, physicians are often unaware of patients' wishes regarding EOL care and interventions are often done that are not consistent with patients' preferences while a significant number of patients end their lives in the hospital, hooked up to machines, and surrounded by strangers and not by their family.

Besides cognitive skills the physician needs to have affective skills to provide emotional support to the patient while respecting the patient's values, skills to communicate with patient and family, and ability to coordinate and communicate with the care team. Dealing with EOL issues, more than any other

TABLE 100.1: Application of principles of ethics in patient care.

Beneficence	Clinical assessment
Nonmalfeasance:	Nature of illness (acute, chronic, reversible, terminal)?
	Goals of treatment?
	Treatment options and probability of success for each option?
	Adverse effects of treatment and does benefit outweigh harm?
	Effects of no medical or surgical treatment?
	If treated, plans for limiting treatment? Stopping treatment?
Respect for autonomy:	Patient rights and preferences:
	Information given to patient on benefits and risks of treatment? Patient understood the information and gave consent?
	Patent mentally competent? If competent, what are his or her preferences?
	If patient mentally incompetent, are patient's prior preferences known?
	If preferences unknown who is the appropriate surrogate?
Beneficence	Quality-of-Life (QOL)
Nonmalfeasance:	Expected QOL with and without treatment?
Respect for autonomy:	Deficits—physical, mental, social—may have after treatment?
	Judging QOL of patient who cannot express himself or herself? Who is the judge?
	Recognition of possible physician bias in judging QOL?
	Rationale to forgo life-sustaining treatment(s)?
Distributive justice:	External forces and context:
	Conflicts of interests—does physician benefit financially, professionally by ordering tests, prescribing medications, seeking consultations?
	Research or educational considerations that affect clinical decisions, physician orders?
	Conflicts of interests based on religious beliefs? Legal issues?
	Conflicts of interests between organizations (clinics, hospitals), third party payers?
	Public health and safety issues?
	Problems in allocation of scarce resources?

patient or family and physician, interactions, has the potential to compromise decision-making that is influenced by the physician's personal and cultural values and religious and spiritual beliefs.

Pulmonary and critical care physicians provide care in various milieus (outpatient, inpatient hospital, and ICU) for patients with cancer and chronic life-limiting diseases, such as chronic obstructive pulmonary disease (COPD) and pulmonary fibrotic diseases. In the latter group, prognostication is difficult and therefore it is hard to decide when to initiate advanced care planning and EOL care. The quality of EOL care in chronic lung disease is poor, and patients with COPD are more likely to die in the ICU than patients with cancer, while on mechanical ventilation and with dyspnea. In the United States approximately 20% of all deaths occur in the ICU and a substantial number of them involve a decision to withhold or withdraw life-supporting therapy (see Chapter 101).

A CONCEPTUAL MODEL FOR PATIENT CARE

Drawing upon a life-time experience as a physician and teacher to physicians, I present a conceptual model of patient care in Flowchart 100.1. This model requires a physician to be both competent and virtuous and integrates elements in the text. Morality, both common and particular, and ethical principles have already received due attention in this chapter. The focal virtues expected of a physician (also applicable to other healthcare professionals) are depicted in the Flowchart 100.1.

Compassion, a prelude to caring, combines an active regard for another person's welfare with an imaginative awareness and emotional response of sympathy, tenderness, and discomfort at that person's misfortune or suffering. Compassion presupposes sympathy and is expressed in acts of beneficence as in relieving pain and suffering.

Discernment is the ability to make fitting judgments and reach decisions without being unduly influenced by extraneous conditions and while keeping personal emotions in check. A discerning physician will thus recognize even in the face of conflicting options when comfort is paramount and provide the right type of consolation and care to the patient. Discernment is a particularly valuable virtue in situations where principles of ethics collide.

Trustworthiness leads to a good climate of trust between people, when trust is taken to be acceptance of being to some degree and some respects, in another person's power. Trustworthiness is an essential virtue as patients, at a time when they are most vulnerable and needy, place themselves in the hands of their physicians.

Integrity involves the coherent integration of one's emotions, knowledge, and aspirations while being faithful to one's moral values and defending them when necessary. A person is deficient in integrity if he or she lacks firmly held moral convictions or fails to act on the one's convictions. Physicians will need to practice with both professional integrity and personal integrity. In the former, adherence to not only professional standards that are codified but also adherence to moral and ethical principles that may not be codified

Flowchart 100.1: A conceptual model of patient care by a physician that integrates morality, ethical principles, virtues, and competencies.

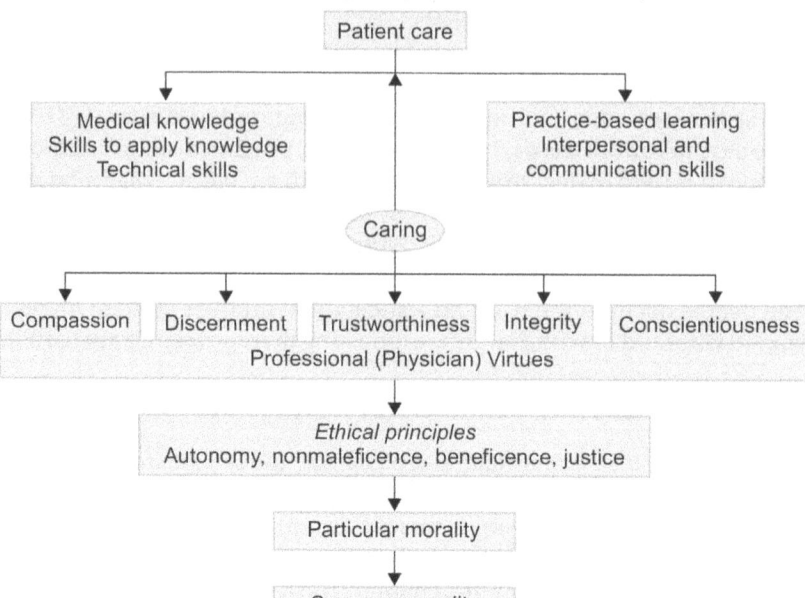

(examples are prescribing drugs that are not effective, placing monetary gain over patient's welfare, inappropriate relationships with patient, treatments without informed consent) are called for.

A physician's personal integrity based on religious and moral convictions may face a challenge in some clinical situations (examples are abortions, removal of life-sustaining treatments); in such situations the physician, in defense of one's moral convictions, can refuse to participate in action that compromises his or her integrity. However, these situations can be avoided or at least reduced by anticipating these problems; if facing such a situation is unavoidable, any adverse impact on the patient must be prevented by using institutional resources (policies, consultation, ethics committee) and delegation of care to another physician.

Conscientiousness is the virtue that motivates a person to do what is right, after diligently determining what is right. Conscience is not a special moral faculty and does not confer a self-justifying moral authority; rather it is an internal checking mechanism requiring critical reflection on good vs. bad, right vs. wrong, and obligatory acts vs. prohibited acts.

The virtues of compassion, discernment, trustworthiness, integrity, and conscientiousness are the necessary building blocks for the fundamental virtue of caring. Caring is the defining virtue for all healthcare professionals and there is no greater duty for a physician than patient care.

CHAPTER 101

End-of-life Care

Jeba S Jenifer, SK Jindal

INTRODUCTION

End-of-life (EOL) care is an interdisciplinary clinical domain, which most physicians find stressful and challenging. The World Health Organization (WHO) defines palliative care as *"an approach that improves the quality of life (QOL) of patients and their families facing the problems associated with life-threatening illness, through the prevention and relief of suffering by means of early identification and impeccable assessment and treatment of pain and other problems, physical, psychosocial and spiritual".* QOL is represented by the difference, or the gap, between the hopes and expectations of the individual and that individual's present experiences at a given time. EOL care is not synonymous with palliative care. Many principles and aspects of palliative care are applicable earlier in the course of an illness, in conjunction with disease modifying therapy and supportive care. It is also important that palliative care continues on to provide bereavement support. Provision of EOL care can be influenced by cultural, social and religious beliefs and practices.

Patients with chronic lung diseases at the EOL have physical and psychosocial needs at least as severe as patients with lung cancer. Breathlessness, fatigue and anxiety are more common in chronic obstructive pulmonary disease (COPD) than in advanced cancer, heart disease or renal disease, but they are less likely to receive medication for symptom control, as compared with lung cancer patients. This occurs despite the fact that most COPD patients prefer treatment focused on symptom control rather than on prolonging life and COPD patients are equally as likely as lung cancer patients to prefer not to receive cardiopulmonary resuscitation. Although the reasons for this discrepancy are not entirely clear, it could be due to poor or infrequent patient-physician communication about EOL care and treatment preferences. Even when recovery/prognosis is uncertain it is better to discuss the uncertainty rather than give false hope.

COMPONENTS

The recognition that a patient is deteriorating, calls for a shift in focus from disease management to patient's priorities, symptoms and comfort. It becomes crucial to assess the current physical, psychosocial and spiritual needs of the patient and family and identify strategies to meet them. Assessment of unconscious patients will require paying close attention to physical signs like facial expression, grimacing, groaning, movements and breathing, along with discussion with family and the entire medical team. Ten key elements of care of the dying have been mentioned in Box 101.1.

There is depth of evidence, mostly from cancer patients, that inclusion of palliative care is associated with reduction in pain and other symptoms, improvement in QOL with enhanced family and patient satisfaction and longer survival. Home palliative care services increase the chance of dying at home and reduce symptom burden particularly in cancer patients. Unrelieved symptoms and unmet needs can result in bitter memories and would be difficult to forget for relatives. It is important to focus and provide good psychosocial and spiritual care.

COMMON SYMPTOMS

One of the essential components in EOL care is achieving maximal symptom control. The most common physical symptoms at the EOL include pain, breathlessness, agitation, nausea and vomiting, and constipation.

Pain

Comprehensive pain evaluation, routine assessment, appropriate analgesic prescription and titration until adequate pain relief are requisites for optimal pain management. The WHO analgesic ladder can be used for the treatment of pain in advanced chronic lung diseases.

BOX 101.1: Care of the dying—key elements.

- Diagnosing dying
- Good communication with patient and family
- Spiritual care
- Anticipatory prescribing
- Interventions focused on patient's best interests
- Decision on hydration—to commence or stop
- Decision on nutrition—to commence or stop
- Discussion of care plan with patient and family
- Regular assessment
- Care after death

The principles to consider in the use of WHO analgesic ladder include use of analgesics at the right dose, at the right time (round the clock), at the right frequency, by the right route (oral), with analgesics given appropriately for breakthrough pain. Oral route should be preferred as it is convenient, noninvasive and cost-effective. The choice of analgesia should be based on the pain severity in a step-wise fashion and not on the stage of disease. To prevent side effects of opioids, prophylactic antiemetics and laxatives should be prescribed. This would enhance patient compliance. Opioids should be used at a reduced dose in the elderly and at a reduced frequency in those with renal/hepatic failure.

Adjuvants are drugs which are not primarily analgesics but produce analgesic effect in some painful conditions (e.g. corticosteroids, tricyclic antidepressants, anticonvulsants, and bisphosphonates). These can be combined with any of the steps, especially in neuropathic pain, spinal cord compression, and bone metastasis. Palliative radiotherapy can also provide pain relief in painful bone metastasis. In difficult pain appropriate referral for expert opinion should be obtained.

Dyspnea

Dyspnea is a distressing and frightening symptom to both the patient and the carers. It significantly affects the physical, emotional and social well-being and results in poor QOL. As a refractory symptom, it is associated with a five-time increased probability of sedation at EOL.

The three treatment categories in a patient with dyspnea include the correction of the correctable, use of nonpharmacological interventions and use of drugs to palliate dyspnea.

Dyspnea could be related to the disease, treatment or other comorbidities. In advanced cancer patients, the cause of dyspnea is often multifactorial. It is important to identify and treat the common reversible conditions in malignant and nonmalignant respiratory diseases. Symptomatic treatment is indicated when there is no clear underlying correctable cause, the disease specific treatment is ineffective, difficult to tolerate or not consistent with patient preference. A few nonpharmacological measures that can be effective are listed in Box 101.2.

In advanced respiratory disease due to interstitial lung disease or COPD, palliative drugs are indicated when standard treatments including pulmonary

> **BOX 101.2:** Nonpharmacological treatment for palliation of dyspnea.
> - *Explanation*: Acknowledge symptom and address anxiety.
> - *Education*: Handling sudden episode of dyspnea/panic, activity pacing.
> - *General measures*: Keep window open, use fan, loose clothing around neck.
> - Breathing techniques
> - Chest physiotherapy
> - Relaxation therapy
> - Pulmonary rehabilitation

rehabilitation, bronchodilators, antibiotics, corticosteroids, long-term oxygen therapy (LTOT) or noninvasive ventilation have failed to relieve dyspnea or are not feasible on a long-term basis. Though the exact mechanism is unknown, opioids at much lower doses, than used for pain, have been shown to improve the sensation of breathlessness. Opioid titration reduces the respiratory rate without producing significant changes in PaO_2 and $PaCO_2$. The side effects of morphine need to be addressed prophylactically. Morphine when used judiciously, with careful titration does not produce respiratory depression (i.e. does not increase CO_2 retention).

Anxiety often coexists with and significantly affects the intensity of dyspnea, resulting in a vicious cycle. Benzodiazepines are considered useful where there is significant anxiety or panic attacks that worsen dyspnea. Combination of benzodiazepine with opioid is often found better than using either of them alone. Benzodiazepines probably help through anxiolytic and sedative effect and possibly muscle relaxation. Care should be taken with diazepam, as it can accumulate due to its long half-life. Lorazepam (1–2 mg) is shorter acting and when given sublingually, provides immediate relief, hence especially useful during panic attacks.

Cough

Cough is a normal but complex physiological mechanism that protects the airways and lungs by removing mucus and foreign matter from the larynx, trachea and bronchi; it has both voluntary and involuntary control. Cough can be classified as productive, with or without the patient being able to cough effectively and nonproductive. Several causes of cough may coexist in one patient.

The first step should be to address and reverse the cause of cough, whenever possible. Nonpharmacological measures like physiotherapy, teaching the patient to cough effectively and steam inhalation may be helpful. Simultaneously appropriate drugs to produce symptom relief should be prescribed. Protussives include nebulized saline, compound benzoin tincture, menthol, guaifenesin, and carbocisteine. Antitussives include simple linctus (demulcent) and opioids (codeine/morphine) and opioid derivatives like dextromethorphan.

Hemoptysis

Massive hemoptysis in advanced lung cancer and chronic lung disease is rare, but can be very frightening and visually traumatic. The cause of hemoptysis in malignant or nonmalignant situations is not always established. Management depends on the cause and prognosis. If this occurs in a patient who is otherwise terminally ill, with palliative goals, the treatment aims to reduce awareness and fear. Use dark towels (green or red) to cover blood. Being physically present with the patient continually is very supportive. Benzodiazepines (diazepam or midazolam) can be given parenterally to reduce panic and awareness, intravenous route is preferred if there is peripheral vascular shutdown.

Stridor

Stridor is a harsh inspiratory wheezing sound heard due to the obstruction of the larynx or of major airways. Corticosteroids can be beneficial in the initial stages. Dexamethasone can be given in high doses (8-24 mg/day). However, the symptom will progress and worsen if the primary cause is not reversible. Explanation to the patient and the carers is crucial. In the terminal phase, palliative sedation can be used after discussion with the relatives to reduce the distress.

Respiratory Secretions

During the terminal phase, many patients develop audible respiratory secretions, called death rattle; caused by patient's inability to clear the throat and the secretions in the hypopharynx oscillating with every inspiration and expiration are responsible for the rattling noise. This symptom causes more distress to the carers and hence it is important to explain to the family/carers that the patient is unaware and not distressed. Positioning the patient semiprone will help in drainage of secretions. Antimuscarinics reduce production of secretions and are hence helpful, if started early on. These drugs can cause dry mouth, and extra attention should be paid to mouth care. Oropharyngeal suction should not be routinely used and should be reserved for unconscious patients.

Nausea and Vomiting

Nausea and vomiting are common in many advanced diseases. The etiology can be multifactorial at EOL (bowel obstruction, constipation, hypercalcemia, uremia, brain metastasis, drugs, etc.). The appropriate antiemetic should be chosen based on the understanding of the likely cause. Antiemetics can be combined and when necessary specialist palliative care advice should be obtained.

Constipation

Most patients can be constipated at EOL, because of immobility, poor diet, dehydration and drugs such as opioids. It is important to assess constipation. Treatment should consist of a combination of stimulant laxative (bisacodyl) and stool softener (cremaffin, senna, docusate sodium). If patients are unable to take orally, use of rectal suppositories can be considered.

DIAGNOSING DYING AND PROVIDING TERMINAL CARE

Diagnosing dying is an important clinical skill. The last few weeks of life may be characterized by progressive physical decline, frailty, lethargy, worsening mobility, loss of interest in food and drink, difficulty in swallowing and little or no response to medical interventions. This phase although usually anticipated can sometimes be rapid and sudden. Fluctuant consciousness, confusion and restlessness are not uncommon toward EOL. Such physical restlessness and delirium when severe is called terminal agitation. Prior to making a diagnosis of terminal agitation, all reversible causes of delirium should be excluded. Antipsychotics (e.g. haloperidol 2.5-5 mg) or benzodiazepines (midazolam 2.5-5 mg) can be used.

There are three key principles in prescribing at the EOL: (i) stop nonessential drugs; (ii) convert essential drugs to subcutaneous (SC) route; and (iii) use anticipatory prescribing. Only the essential drugs that would help in symptom control or patient comfort should be continued. Previously "essential" drugs like vitamin and iron supplements, antihypertensives, hypoglycemics, statins, etc. may not be needed anymore. Analgesics, antiemetics, and sedatives may form the new "essential" list. The route of administration should be decided based on patient's ability to take orally. Drugs may need to be given parenterally, preferably by SC route. A microdrip set or syringe driver can be used to give the drugs as SC infusions depending on its availability. Irrespective of the current symptoms all dying patient should have "as needed" prescriptions for an analgesic, anxiolytic, antiemetic and drugs to reduce bronchial secretions.

END-OF-LIFE CARE IN THE INTENSIVE CARE UNIT

Most patients who die in the ICU die as life-supporting measures are withheld or withdrawn. Decisions surrounding life-sustaining treatments can be difficult, because they often involve complex ethical decision-making. Refusal of life-prolonging therapy may result in conflict of interests among medical professionals or between the medical professional and patient/family. Physicians may agree to the family's inappropriate demands for aggressive life prolonging therapy because they may be worried that angry families will sue if therapy is withheld (although this fear does not have any legal justification) or may not want to put the family through tough decisions or may not be fully convinced themselves. In India, EOL decisions have additional challenges.

Discussion about patient's preferences on treatment during EOL or the use of advanced directives is not common. In such an instance it is the family members who decide the EOL issues for the patient. Often, family members are not well-informed or do not want to take any decision themselves. A vast majority is poor and many families end up selling all their property or take loans just to spend on their relative in ICU, often losing their assets and their loved one at the end. A common cause of conflict with families is poor communication. Most conflicts can be avoided by facilitating communication through a formal family conference. Family meetings are an opportunity to foreshadow EOL discussions and allow family members to psychologically prepare themselves. It is crucial to make the family feel that they are cared for and not abandoned at any stage. Nonabandonment (or fidelity) is also a central moral obligation of a physician. It is also important to ensure that decisions to forgo a particular treatment due to futility are not seen as withdrawing care.

Communication

Good communication forms the foundation for good EOL care. Physician-patient communication about EOL decisions and treatment preferences is crucial. There is evidence that patients with chronic lung disease receive suboptimal palliative care largely due to insufficient communication with their physicians. As accurate prognostication in an individual will remain difficult due to the variability inherent with chronic lung diseases, educating patients and families about the uncertainty in prognosis of lung diseases must be an essential feature of EOL care and decision-making.

There are many patients and physician-related factors that are barriers to effective communication and understanding them would be the first-step toward better communication. It is good to communicate with patients and their carers about prognosis and establish goals of care as early as possible. Discussion with a colleague/team in dealing with the situation will be helpful. Discussing EOL care or giving bad news can never make a clinician feel good. The most important principle is to do it in a sensitive manner and at the individual's pace. Most patients/caregivers want some discussion at the time of diagnosis of an advanced, progressive, life-limiting illness or shortly after.

Index

Page numbers followed by *b* refer to box, *f* refer to figure, *fc* refer to flow chart, and *t* refer to table

A

Abdomen and rib cage, expansion of 700
Abductor palsy, bilateral 257
Abortions 752
    spontaneous 731
Acanthosis nigricans 400, 402
Acetaminophen 539
Acid maltase deficiency 699
Acid-base
    abnormality 32, 34*t*, 36, 39
    disorders 34, 36, 37
    disorders, types of 34
    pathophysiology, overview of 33
Acidemia 243
Acid-fast bacilli 56, 80, 97, 331, 644
Acidosis 37, 527
    adverse effects of 37
    metabolic 34, 37, 197
    primary metabolic 35
    respiratory 34, 38, 173
    severe 37
        metabolic 528
Acinar nodules 739*f*
Acinetobacter 124, 139
Aclidinium 231
Acquired immunodeficiency syndrome 41, 102, 283, 640, 670, 726
Acute asthma 715
    attack 175*t*
    exacerbations 171, 172*b*, 725
        management 173
    initial treatment of 725*b*
    management of 724
    severe 500
    treatment of 724
Acute hypoxemia, severe 242
Acute interstitial pneumonia 267, 275, 282
    diagnosis 282
    prognosis 282
    signs 282
    symptoms 282
    treatment 282
Acute kidney injury 528
    clinical presentation 528
    management 528
    prevention 529
Acute lung injury 500, 577
    transfusion-related 508, 527
Acute pancreatitis 508, 525, 707
    pulmonary complications of 707*b*
    severe 525
Acute respiratory distress syndrome 115, 296, 370, 455, 458, 500, 507, 508*b*, 511, 555, 577, 609, 669, 707, 708, 715, 727
    cause of 507
    clinical picture 508
    etiology 507
    management 509
    pathophysiology 508
    postoperative 374
    prognosis 513
Acute respiratory syndrome, severe 729
Acute withdrawal syndrome, symptoms of 619
Adenocarcinoma 378, 385, 387, 392, 400
    invasive 387
Adenopathy, mediastinal 692
Adenosine deaminase 642
    enzyme activity 642
    levels 642*b*
    role of 75
Adenosine triphosphate 419
    depletion of 37
Adenosquamous carcinoma 388
    small group of 385
Adenovirus 151, 313

Adenyl cyclase activity, modulate 196
Adjunctive therapy 111
Adrenal insufficiency, acute 530
Adrenal metastases 395
Adult respiratory distress syndrome 568, 688, 691
Advanced mediastinal disease, treatment of 414
Adverse drug reactions 87, 417
Aerosolized trypsin 740
Afatinib 416
African-American populations 75
Air embolism 631
    treatment of 631
Air flow obstruction, degree of 225
Air pollutants 172
Airborne droplet 44
Airflow limitation, chronic 164
Airflow obstruction 168
    chronic 164
    severe 567
Airway 120, 536, 598
    artificial 144, 602
    bypass stents 238
    disease 164, 368
        chronic obstructive 475
        obstructive 563
        types of 164
    epithelial cells 155
    epithelium 154
    function, measurement of 156
    hyperresponsiveness 30
    inflammation 153, 167, 168
        noninvasive markers of 160
    injury 601
    management 602, 605
    muscle mass 153
    obstruction 190, 681, 683
        extrathoracic 706
        major 392
        mechanical 163
        proximal 661
    pressure
        release ventilation 510, 565
        generate 243
    remodeling 164
    resistance 30
    responsiveness, measurement of 160
    sensitization 151
    smooth muscles 156
    viral infection 240

Albumin 36, 188
Alcohol 538, 650
Aldehydes 367
Alkalemia 536
Alkaline phosphatase 405
Alkalosis 38, 742
    metabolic 34, 38, 39, 527
    primary metabolic 35
Alkalotic pleural fluid 652
Allen's maneuver 580
Allergen 151, 178
    desensitization 177
        indications 178
        pregnancy 182
        side effects and risks 181
    environmental 172
    immunotherapy 169, 177, 180, 182
        duration of 180
        mechanisms of 177
Allergic alveolitis 113
Allergic asthma 153, 178
Allergic bronchopulmonary aspergillosis 113, 148, 149, 200, 295, 303
    clinical features 202
    diagnosis of 205*b*
    diagnostic criteria 205
    management 205
    pathogenesis 201
    pathology 201
Allergic bronchopulmonary mycosis 200, 207
Allergic diseases 150
Allergic rhinitis 150, 153, 154, 178, 180, 215, 298
Allergic status 158
    measures of 161
Allergy 190
Allopurinol 243
Alpha-1 antitrypsin deficiency 253
Alternative airway techniques 607
Aluminum 291, 344, 345
Alveolar damage, diffuse 282, 464, 465
Alveolar proteinosis, secondary pulmonary 738*b*
Alveolitis, acute 287
Amebiasis 717, 719
Amenorrhea 82
American Thoracic Society 209, 246, 386
Amikacin 60, 86
Aminoglycosides 92, 135
Aminophylline 174, 231

Amiodarone 302, 313, 455, 463, 508
Ammonia 367, 524
Amniotic fluid embolism 734
Amoxicillin 88, 236, 543
Amphotericin B
  colloidal dispersion 116
  lipid
    complex 116
    formulations of 116
Ampicillin 124
Amyl nitrite 539
Amyloidosis 54, 305, 429, 741
  diffuse pulmonary 687
  laryngeal 306
  nodular pulmonary 306
  pulmonary 305, 742
Anaerobic bacteria, aspiration of 126
Anaerobic infections 127, 142, 650
  pathognomonic of 144
Analgesia 610b
  management of 612
  protocols 617
Anaphylaxis 190, 198
Anaplastic lymphoma kinase 415, 418
  inhibitors 418
  translocations 383
Ancylostoma 295
Anderson-Fabry disease 307
Anemia 392, 414, 526, 712
Anesthesia 587
  effect of 554
Aneurysm 486
Angina, unstable 178
Angioedema 190, 198
  atopic dermatitis 178
  hereditary 260
Angiography, pulmonary 478
Angiotensin
  converting enzyme inhibitors 163
  renin axis 543
Anidulafungin 117
Animal products 355
Anion gap 36
Anionic proteins 36
Ankylosing spondylitis 492, 684, 692
  pulmonary manifestations of 692b
Ankylosing spondylosis 447, 450
Anorexia 84, 400, 402
Antiasthma drugs 187, 726

Antibiotics 146, 169, 175, 236, 242, 243, 375
  agents 375t
  and infection source control 518
  factors 109
  prophylaxis, role of 485
  therapy 111, 121, 129
  treatment 652
Antibody
  monoclonal 191
  therapy 376
Anticholinergics 231, 236, 538, 539
  agents 167, 174, 198
  clinical use 231
  drugs 232
  short-acting 174
  side effects 232
Anticholinesterases 539
Anticoagulant therapy 479
Anticoagulation 471
  therapy, duration of 480
Antifibrotic agents 272
Antiglomerular basement membrane
    disease 463
Anti-immunoglobulin E monoclonal
    antibodies 191
Anti-inflammatory
  agents 187
  drugs 376
  effect 233
  therapy 168, 272
Antileukotrienes 168
Antimethicillin-resistant *Staphylococcus
    aureus* 124
Antimicrobial 119, 375
  peptides 47
Antineutrophil cytoplasmic antibody 310
Antinuclear
  antibody 374
  cytotoxic antibodies 298
  factor 271, 310
Antioxidant 237, 272
  response element 221
Antiphospholipid antibody syndrome,
    primary 455
Anti-*Pseudomonas* 123
  agent 123, 124
Antiretroviral drugs 99
Antiretroviral therapy 72
  active 99
  combination of 100

Anti-snake venom 542
Antitubercular
   drugs 63, 64, 87, 93, 94
   therapy 75, 100
   treatment 89, 94, 731
Antituberculosis
   drugs, grading of activities of 65t
   duration of 89
Anti-tumor necrosis factor 376
Antitussives 237
Antivenin 544
Anxiety 240
   symptoms of 245
Anxiousness 190
Aorta, coarctation of 453
Aortic arch 436
Apical bullous disease 681, 684
Apnea 494
   hypopnea index 495
Apoptosis 221
Arrhenius 33
Arrhythmia 30, 37, 226, 502, 601
Arsenic 368
Arterial blood 501
   gas 32, 315, 574, 579, 724
      analysis 108, 502, 585
      interpretation of 32
Arterial dissection, pulmonary 306
Arterial hypoxemia 19
   subclinical 708
Arterial oxygen
   alveolar 501
   partial pressure of 628
   saturation 241, 588
Arteriovenous malformation 429
   pulmonary 482, 483b
Arthralgia 190, 456
Arthritis 604
   tuberculous 78
Asbestos 348, 368
   fiber 350
      inhalation, health risks of 348
   pneumoconiosis 348
Asbestosis 290, 348, 349, 349b
Ascaris 295
Ascitic fluid 525
Aspergilloma 17, 200
   formation 114
Aspergillosis 113, 291, 429
   chronic pulmonary 203
   invasive 114
   pulmonary 113

Aspergillus 114, 126, 200$_p$ 204$_p$ 205, 255, 671, 729, 740
   antigen 113, 205
   fumigatus 133, 139, 200
      antigens 202
   hypersensitivity 200
   sensitized asthma 200
   skin test 202
Asphyxiation 632
Aspiration 141, 508
   bronchiolitis, diffuse 313-315
   endocavitary 256
   pneumonia 703, 705, 706
   pneumonitis 686
   simple 669
Aspirin 302
Assist-controlled mode, pressure tracing of 562f
Asteroid bodies 287
Asthma 18, 147, 148, 148b, 149, 150, 153, 154, 156, 157, 161, 164, 165, 169, 180, 184, 187, 189, 209, 215, 224, 255, 258, 261, 295, 299, 354, 368, 392, 456, 488, 491, 492, 555, 671
   acute severe 175b, 724
   aspirin exacerbated 148
   care, essential components of 166
   chronic severe 188
   coexisting 234
   control 165, 186
   development of 181
   diagnosis of 17, 158, 163, 164
      difficult 156
   education
      contents of 186
      primary aim of 184
      programs 185
      strategy of 185
   episode of 171
   exacerbation 171
      moderate-to-severe 198
   exercise induced 148
   immunological occupational 355
   in pregnancy 722
      effect of 722
   irritant-induced 369
      workplace 148
   knowledge of 185
   management 165, 170, 229, 725
      cornerstone of 187
      during pregnancy, complications of 723b
      objectives of 165

methods and settings 185
mild 156
monitoring 167
nocturnal 151, 491
    symptoms of 491
nonimmunological occupational 355
persistent 167
pharmacotherapy 167, 723
presence of 158
prevalence of 149, 150
problems 186
risk factors of 149
severe 153, 200, 724
severity 185
symptoms 169
treatment 169, 192
    global initiative for 147, 184
    goals of 165
triggers 166
    control of 165
uncontrolled 168
unstable 178
work-exacerbated 354
Asthmatic airway 156
Ataxia-telangiectasia 313
Atelectasis 25, 429, 556, 656, 707
Atomic mass unit 5
Atoms, types of 4
Atresia, bronchial 429
Atropine 538, 539
Attack, acute 171
Augmentin 236
Autoimmune
    diseases 686
    disorders 182, 338
Autonomic nervous system, tumors of 446
Aviation and space travel 322
Azathioprine 292, 302, 689
Azithromycin 105
Aztreonam 135
Azulfidine 375
Azygos vein 436

B

Bacillus Calmette-Guérin vaccination 70, 101, 286
Bacteria 59, 649
Bacterial infections, recurrent 131
Bacterial pneumonia 267, 650, 726
    causes 726
    diagnosis 726

    incidence 726
    management 727
    prevention 728
Bacterial translocation 525
Bacteriology 650
Bacteroides fragilis 146
Bambuterol 195, 231
Barbiturate 189, 538
Barium 345
Barotrauma 243
Basal metabolic
    profile 531
    rate 592
Basophils 154
B-cell 301
    deficient 49
Beclomethasone 302
Bedsore prevention 599
Bee sting allergy 180
Behçet disease 21, 462
Behçet syndrome 455, 461, 486
Benzodiazepines 534, 539, 614, 615, 756
Bernoulli's principle 10
Berylliosis 290, 340, 341
    acute 340
    types of 341
Beryllium 291, 340, 344, 345
    disease 340, 341
    exposure 341t
    hypersensitivity 341
    lymphocyte proliferation test 342
    sensitization 341
Best supportive care 411
Beta agonists, short-acting 167, 187
Beta-2-agonists 232
    and theophylline 236
    side effects 232
Beta-human chorionic gonadotropin 443
Bevacizumab 678
Bicarbonate 32, 34
Bileveled positive airway
    pressure 565
    therapy 496
Bilirubin 422
Biogas 230
Biologic therapies 169
Biological drugs 191
Biomass fuel exposure 368
Birth weight, low 731
Bispectral index 612
Bladder transitional cell carcinoma 302
Blastomyces 126

Blastomycosis 291
Bleeding, intracranial 513
Bleomycin 302, 313, 374, 662, 677
Blood
    brain barrier 80, 524
    counts, complete 422
    flow
        bronchial 696
        hepatic 37
        pulmonary 2
    gas
        abnormalities 579
        analysis 581
        monitoring 579, 581
    pressure 18, 29
        elevated 193
        elevation, substantial 30
        increases 637
        noninvasive 30
    stream 142
    sugar 422
    vessels 681
Bloody gastric lavage 523
Body mass index 225, 451
Bone
    fractures 475
    marrow 313
        transplantation 455
    tuberculosis 76
        treatment of 79
Bordetella pertussis 132
Borrelia burgdorferi 286
Bovine cough 393
Bowel disease, inflammatory 708
Bowel sounds, role of 597
Boyle's law 8, 322
Bradycardia 502, 519
Bradypnea 18
Brain
    activity 612
    function 612
    injury, hypoxic 601
    metastases 395
    natriuretic peptide 477, 550
Brass chills 371
Brazier's disease 371
Breast cancer 655
    metastatic 742
Breastfeeding 726, 732

Breath
    cycling of 556
    shortness of 163
    triggering of 556
Breathing 1, 536, 598
    altered control of 622
    awareness of 16
    pattern 18
    trials, spontaneous 625
Breathlessness 51, 163, 164, 263, 392, 656
    severity of 241
British Thoracic Society Rules 109
Bromide 538
Bronchi, conducting 603
Bronchial asthma 200, 205, 320, 576, 706
    epidemiology 147
    pharmacotherapy of 187
Bronchiectasis 17, 103, 131, 254, 429, 681,
        684-686, 706
    central 205
    complications 136
    cystic 131
    diagnosis 133
    etiology 132, 132*b*
    long-term management of stable
        disease 135
    microbiology 134
    pathology 131
    physiology 132
    prognosis 136
    proximal 201
    signs 132
    symptoms 132
    treatment 134
Bronchiolar disorders 314*t*
    diagnosis of 315
    general features of 312
Bronchiolar luminal impaction 314
Bronchiolar wall thickening 314
Bronchiole, respiratory 218, 312
Bronchiolectasis 314
Bronchiolitis 190, 312, 315*fc*, 368, 681
    clinical classification of 313*b*
    constrictive 312, 315
    drug induced 313
    eosinophilic 313
    infectious 313, 314
    lymphocytic 313
    obliterans 281, 295, 312, 315, 370, 375
        organizing 681
    obliterative 683
    respiratory 275, 313, 315

Bronchitis 327, 344, 368, 706
Bronchoalveolar lavage 56, 127, 270, 275, 276, 290, 337, 342, 364, 377, 420, 457, 738
  bronchoscopic 122
  development of 330
  fluid 685
Bronchodilators 105, 192, 231t, 242
  inhaled 242
  short-acting 174
Bronchoprovocation tests 158
Bronchopulmonary sequestration 482, 486
Bronchoscopic techniques 262
Bronchoscopy 128, 259, 457, 583
  electromagnetic navigational 435
Bronchospasm, acute severe 197
Brucella 291
Brucellosis 295, 642
Bullae 27
  causes of 253b
Bullous disease, idiopathic 253
Bullous lung diseases 252
  clinical presentation 254
  complications 255
  etiology 253
  natural history 255
  pathogenesis 252
  radiologic features 254
  treatment 255
Bungarus caeruleus 541
Burkholderia cepacia 671
  complex 138, 139
Busulfan 313, 374
  therapy, chronic 742

C

Cachexia 400, 402, 414
Cadmium 344, 368
Caffeine 197
Calcification 432, 681
  metastatic 741
Calcinosis 269
Calcium 36, 422, 593
  channel blocker 539
  chloride 539
  metabolism, abnormalities of 289
  oxalate crystals 287
Calcospherite 743
Calorie requirements 595

Cancer 178
  chemotherapy 374, 374t
    agents 373
    therapeutic strategy for 374f
  esophageal 264
  treatment of 632
Candida 729
  infection, high risk of 115
  pneumonia, diagnosis of 115
Candidal bronchopneumonia, primary 115
Capillaritis, pulmonary 455
Capillary membrane, alveolar 509
Caplan's syndrome 329, 338, 339, 681-683
Capnography, cutaneous 585
Capreomycin 60, 86, 88
Carbamazepine 189, 302, 536
Carbapenems 123
Carbohydrate antigens 659
Carbon dioxide 34, 492
  arterial 698
    partial pressure of 32
  monitoring 588
  partial pressure of 501, 555, 585
Carbon monoxide 27, 538, 632, 704
  inhalation 372
  poisoning 631, 632
Carcinoid syndrome 402
Carcinoid tumor, atypical 388
Carcinoma 429
  bronchogenic 400, 486
  in situ 385
  sarcomatoid 385
Cardiac arrest 631
Cardiac arrhythmias 233, 529, 631, 632
  risk of 233
Cardiac catheterization 583
Cardiac cycle 485
Cardiac disease 461
Cardiac failure 226, 502, 743
  congestive 475, 656
Cardiomyopathy
  congenital 467
  peripartum 734, 735
Cardiopulmonary exercise testing 28, 29, 589
Cardiopulmonary resuscitation 547, 672
  basic 547
Cardiovascular diseases 695
Cardiovascular drugs 374
Carmustine 313

Caspofungin 117
Castleman disease 426
Catamenial pneumothorax 666, 671
Cathelicidin 47
Catheter embolectomy 481
Cathode 581
Cavitation 432
Cavity formation 114
Cefaclor 236
Ceftazidime 135
Ceftriaxone 124
Cell
    carcinoma, alveolar 685
    mediated immunity, antigen-specific 345
Central airways obstruction 257
Central nervous system 196
    infection 534
    tuberculosis 74, 79
Central sleep apnea 488, 493, 494, 497, 697
    syndrome 497
Central venous pressure 550, 551
Centriacinar emphysema 218
Centrilobular nodules 314, 315
Cephalosporin 236
Cerebellar hematoma 533
Cerebral
    abscess, chances of 485
    activity 612
    air embolism 631
    edema 243
    metabolic activity 545
    state index 612
Cerebrovascular
    accidents 484, 532
    disease 490
Cervical
    disk abnormalities 604
    lymphangiomas 445
    ribs 452
Cervix, squamous cell carcinomas of 302
Charcot-Leyden crystal protein 294
Charcot-Marie-Tooth syndrome 492
Charles' law 8
Chemokines 48, 592
Chemotherapy 63, 409-412, 660, 677
    adjuvant 411
    combination adjuvant 677
    complications of 414
    duration of 63
    first-line 410, 412
    induction 678
    maintenance 410, 412
    neoadjuvant 411
    second-line 411, 412, 678
Chest
    and upper extremities 484
    computed tomography test 438
    contrast-enhanced computed tomography of 432f
    discomfort 262
    drain 662
    examination of 19
    imaging 456, 459
    pain 16, 190, 392, 656, 667, 689, 713, 733
    nonpleuritic 676
    physiotherapy 139
    radiograph 128, 349, 430, 482, 731
        conventional 437
        lateral 316
    radiographic abnormalities 716
    radiography 116, 158, 270, 468
    radiology 55
    skiagram, examination of 21
    tightness 163
    ultrasonogram of 651f
    wall 2, 447, 697
        diseases of 447
        disorders of 16
        hernias 453
        nonmuscular diseases of 447b
        tumors of 453
    X-ray 276, 313, 315, 700
Cheyne-Stokes breathing 490
Chills 728
Chinese hamster ovary cells 191
Chlamydia 151
    pneumoniae 169, 286, 642, 726
Chlorambucil 374
Chlorhexidine 119
Chloride, concentrations of 36
Cholesterol
    crystals 681
    pneumonia 309
Chondroma 78, 429
Chromium 344
Chronic asthma 216
    management of 723
Chronic beryllium
    disease 291, 340, 341, 344
    exposure 341

Chronic eosinophilic pneumonia,
    idiopathic 297, 303
Chronic obstructive pulmonary disease
    17, 23, 103, 107, 114, 156, 159, 208,
    209, 211, 213, 215, 216, 218, 220,
    221, 223, 230f, 231t, 239, 245, 255,
    258, 273, 320, 322, 368, 369, 414,
    466, 467, 488, 491, 499, 500, 555,
    568, 573, 575, 624, 671, 753
  acute exacerbation of 239, 500
  anticholinergics 231
  bronchodilators 230
  burden of 208
  causes of 240
  economic burden of 211
  environmental risk factors 229
  exacerbation 239
  management of 240, 242
  pathogenesis 223
  pharmacotherapy 230
  prevalence of 209
  prevention 229
  primary care 240
  risk factors 229
  symptoms of 240
  systemic manifestations of 224, 225b
  treatment of 229
  wasting and weight loss 225
Churg-Strauss syndrome 148, 168, 190,
    192, 271, 295, 298
Ciliary dyskinesia, primary 103
Cilomilast 196
Ciprofloxacin 94, 243
Circulation 598
Cirrhosis 290
Cisapride 597
Cisplatin 677
Clarithromycin 105, 243
Clavulanic acid 236
Clenbuterol 195
Clinical Pulmonary Infection Score 121
Clofazimine 88
Clofibrate 302
Clubbing 402
Coagulation disorders 455, 465
Coal dust 368
  exposure, clinical features of 327
  lung disease 327
Coal workers pneumoconiosis 327, 741
  pathology of 329
Co-amoxiclav 139

Cobalt 344, 345
  asthma 345
Cobb's angle 448, 448f
Cocaine 302, 313, 538
Coccidioidomycosis 291, 295, 429, 642
Codeine 756
Coinfection 240
Colchicine 686
Cold abscess 75
Coliforms 134
Colistin 135, 375
Collagen vascular diseases 313, 468, 680
Coma 537, 555
  cocktail 537
Comet tail sign 431
Community-acquired pneumonia 106,
    144
  diagnostic testing 108
  prognosis 109
  severe 727b
  treatment 110
Complex airways diseases, management
    of 601
Compliance, rate, oxygenation, pressure
    index 624
Compression ultrasonography 477
Computed tomography 405, 422, 431,
    433, 437
  contrast-enhanced 422
  pulmonary arteriography 477
  scan 297
Computer-aided diagnosis techniques
    434
Confusion 727
Conjunctivitis 459
Connective tissue 436
  diseases 267, 295, 313, 315, 338, 467,
    486, 666, 680
  disorders 267
  related lung diseases, treatment of
    694b
Consciousness, levels of 241
Constipation 757
Constrictive pericarditis, effusive 84
Continuous positive airway pressure 261,
    321, 496, 504, 563, 564f, 570, 595,
    624, 626, 702
Contraceptive pills, oral 475
Copper 344, 345
  sulphate 345

Cor pulmonale 330
   chronic 226, 338, 341, 743
   signs of 449
Coronary artery disease, severe 178
Corticosteroids 174, 187, 233, 242, 520, 694
   inhaled 167, 206, 226, 723
   oral 169, 206, 724
   role of 646
   side effects 234
   therapy 227
Costochondritis 452
Cotton dust 368
Cough 15, 51, 237, 262, 341, 363, 392, 630, 667, 713, 728, 730, 756
   chronic 706
      nonproductive 689
   drug-induced 163
   hygiene 69
   nonproductive 275
   variant asthma 162
Crack cocaine inhalation 455
Creatinine 422
Crest syndrome 685
Cricothyroidotomy 608
Critical care, nonpulmonary 522
Critical flow rate 12
Crusty rhinitis 456
Cryoglobulinemia 455
Cryoglobulinemic vasculitis 462
Cryptococcosis 291, 429
   pulmonary 115
Cryptococcus 729
   neoformans 740
Cryptogenic organizing pneumonia 267, 272, 275, 282, 313, 688, 690
   diagnosis 281
   etiology 281
   prognosis 281
   signs 281
   symptoms 281
   treatment 281
Cryptosporidium 56
Crystalline silica 334, 368
Cuff pressure 120
Cushing's syndrome 396, 402
Cutis laca 253
Cyanide 538, 539
Cyanosis 19
Cyclophosphamide 374, 459
   infusion 311
   oral 459

Cycloserine 88, 99
   crosses placenta 91
Cysts
   bronchogenic 429, 444
   enterogenous 445
   infected 254
   large clusters of 131
   mediastinal 444
   neuroenteric 445
   pericardial 445
Cystic adenomatoid malformation, congenital 486
Cystic fibrosis, atypical 137
Cytokine 48, 161, 592
   levels 592
   mediators, number of 224
   storm 515
Cytomegalovirus 670
Cytotoxic drug 292
   therapy 455

D

Dacomitinib 416
Dalton's law 7
Danders 166
Dantrolene 302
Dapsone 302, 536
Daytime sleepiness, excessive 489
Decompression sickness 629, 630
Deep coma 538
Deep venous thrombosis 414, 473
   formation of 474fc
   prophylaxis 599
   testing 477
Defensin 3, 47
Delirium
   management of 620
   prevention of 620
   treatment of 620
Dendritic cells 44, 48
Dengue 464, 718
   fever 717, 718
   hemorrhagic fever 719
   viral nonstructural protein-1 719
   virus 719
Deoxyribonucleic acid 373
Depression 190, 240, 414
   symptoms of 245
Dermatitis
   atrial 150
   exfoliative 400, 402

Dermatomyositis 267, 313, 400, 680, 691, 691*b*
Desquamative interstitial pneumonia 267, 269, 272, 275
   diagnosis 280
   etiology 279
   signs 279
   symptoms 279
   treatment 280
Dexmedetomidine 613, 616, 617
Dextrose 539
Diabetes 113, 114
   and lung function 704
   and tuberculosis 704
   mellitus 290, 599, 604, 650, 703, 712
      pulmonary complications of 703*b*
   type 1 704
   type 2 704
Diabetic foot 631
Diabetic ketoacidosis 531
   management 531
Diaphragm dysfunction, severe 702
Diaphragm imaging 701
Diaphragm paralysis
   bilateral 700*t*
   unilateral 700*t*, 701
Diaphragmatic paralysis 492, 699
   etiology of 699*t*
Diarrhea 97, 234, 418, 598
Diazepam 613, 756
Diet 169
Diethylenetriaminepentaacetic acid 271
Diffuse alveolar hemorrhage 310, 454, 455, 463, 464
   causes of 455*b*
   syndromes 454
Diffusion 2, 13, 14
Digital clubbing 399
Digoxin 471, 539
   specific antibodies 539
Dimorphic fungi 115
Diphenhydramine 538
Diphenylhydantoin 455
Diprophylline 197
Direct puncture technique 580
Directly observed treatment 89
Disability adjusted life years 211
Discoid lesions 21
Disease modifying antisarcoid drugs 292
Disorientation 727
Disseminated intravascular coagulation 676

Diuresis 233
Diuretics 471
Dizziness 193
Dobutamine 519, 552
Domiciliary oxygen 235
Dopamine 552
Doripenem 123
Dorsalis pedis 579
Doxofylline 233
Doxycycline 236, 677
D-penicillamine 313
Drowning 547
Drug 295
   interactions 194
   reactions 291
   regimen 123
   resistance, prevention of 63
   resistant tuberculosis 86, 87
      surgical management of 89
   therapies 236
Dry cough 281, 604, 683
Dry mouth 190
Dry pericarditis 83
Dying, care of 754*b*
Dyspnea 16, 37, 133, 225, 248, 349, 363, 449, 484, 630, 667, 679, 683, 686, 689, 700, 713, 722, 733, 755
   mechanisms of 696*b*
   palliation of 755*b*
   progressive 262, 275
   psychogenic 16
   treatment of 237
Dysrhythmias 543
Dystrophic calcification 741

E

Eaton-Lambert syndrome 398, 492
Echinococcosis 295
Echocardiogram 469
Echocardiography 550
Eczema 190
Edema 19
   cardiac pulmonary 715
   laryngeal 500
   neurogenic pulmonary 508
   peripheral 498
   pulmonary 543, 712, 715, 734, 735
Egg shell calcification 337
Ehlers-Danlos syndrome 253
Elastic recoil, balance of 635
Electrocardiogram 422, 468

Electrocardiography 476
Electromagnetic navigation systems 434
Embolectomy, surgical 481
Embolotherapy 485
Empey's index 258
Emphysema 27, 221, 253, 555, 692
　diffuse nonbullous 254
　severe 238
　subcutaneous 665
Empyema 143, 642, 646, 648, 650, 681
　diagnostic of 651
　formation of 143
　necessitans 647
Encephalomyelitis 398, 402
End-expiratory pressure, auto-positive 622
Endobronchial ultrasound 290
　guided transbronchial needle aspiration 441
Endocarditis, subacute bacterial 455
Endocrine
　diseases 703
　disorder 226, 402, 703
　syndromes 396
End-of-life care 753, 758
Endometriosis 429
Endoscopy 583
Endosonographic procedures 404
Endotracheal intubation 3, 505
　confirmation of 606
Endotracheal tube 119, 606
　cuff pressure 120
End-stage diseases 744
End-tidal carbon dioxide
　monitoring 586
　　advantages 586
　　limitation 587
　　tension 585
Endurance shuttle walk test 247
Energy
　conservation 249
　requirements, estimation of 596
Entamoeba histolytica 719, 720
Enteral nutrition 594, 598
Enteric fever 717
Enterobacter 124, 134
Envenomation 535
Environmental tobacco smoke 210, 214, 368, 380
Enzyme 189, 356
　acid sphingomyelinase 308

group of 196
linked immunosorbent assay 718
Eosinophil 154, 294
　cationic protein 294
　derived neurotoxin 294
Eosinophilia 294
　peripheral 204
　primary pulmonary 295
　secondary pulmonary 295
Eosinophilic pneumonia, acute 295, 296, 303
Epidermal growth factor receptor 383, 415, 416*t*
　gene mutations 383
Epiglottitis 260, 555
Epilepsy 243
Epinephrine 192, 519
Episcleritis 456, 459
Epistaxis 484
Epithelial cells 140, 155
　alveolar 44
Epithelial injury 369
Epithelial tumors 386
Epstein-Barr virus 426
Epworth sleepiness scale 491
Erlotinib 416, 678
Eryptogenic organizing pneumonia 272
Erythema 192, 456
　gyratum repens 400, 402
　multiforme 400, 402
　nodosum 21, 78
Erythrocyte sedimentation rate 422, 682
Erythroderma 402
Erythromycin 597
Escherichia coli 126
Esophageal dysfunction 141, 269
Esophagitis, eosinophilic 190
Esophagomediastinal fistula 76
Esophagus 16, 26, 436
　involvement of 394
Essential initial test 108
Ethambutol 65, 75, 88, 92, 99, 645
Ethanol 230, 538, 539
Ethionamide 88, 94, 99
Ethylene glycol 538, 539
European Respiratory Society 209, 246, 386
Exacerbation 250
　acute severe 172*b*
　management of 173
Excretion 34

Exercise 172, 249
   testing 28, 583
      basic modalities 28
Extracellular matrix deposition 153
Extracorporeal membrane oxygenation 506, 513
Extrapulmonary tuberculosis 55, 57, 64, 74, 75
   diagnosis 74
Extrapyramidal syndrome 620
Extravascular lung water 696
Exudative effusion, diagnosis of 642b
Eyes 289, 680

F

Fabry's disease 253
Facemask 606
Facial
   flushing 728
   palsy 289
   wrinkling 216
Fatal pulmonary hemorrhage 462
Fatigue 341, 449, 730
Fatty acid metabolism 43
Feeding
   position of 597
   tube 597
Fenoterol 195
Fentanyl 613, 614
Fetal
   nephrotoxicity 91
   ototoxicity 91
Fever 281, 364, 400, 402, 456, 728, 730
   inhalation 368
Fiberoptic bronchoscopy 56, 434, 578
   role of 56
Fibrinolytics, intrapleural 653
Fibrinopurulent stage 649
Fibrosis 314, 685
   apical 692
   cystic 3, 103, 131, 136-138, 190, 200, 667, 671
   diffuse pulmonary 682
   interstitial 681
   post-tubercular 253
   pulmonary 341, 368
Fick's law 13
Fine-needle aspiration
   biopsy, endoscopic ultrasound-guided 441
   cytology 76, 434

Finger clubbing 349
Fish proteins 356
Fistula, bronchopleural 647
Five factor score 299
Fixed airway obstruction 257
Flail chest 447, 452
   treatment 452
Flattened thoracic cage 283
Flexible bronchoscopy 589, 607
Flock worker's lung 313
Flucloxacillin 139
Fluconazole 117
Fluid
   management 512
      strategy of 512
   overload 554
   status 550
Flumazenil 539
Fluorodeoxyglucose positron emission tomography 433f
Fluoroquinolone 92, 124, 146
   resistant tuberculosis 110
Fluoroscopic sniff test 701
Fluoroscopy 700
Fluxes 357
Follicular bronchiolitis 314
Food
   allergens 166
   allergy 178
Forced vital capacity 278, 337, 700
Formaldehyde 538
Formoterol 195, 231
Foundry fever 371
Fracture, traumatic 78
Free silica 338
Fresh frozen plasma 523
Full cardiopulmonary exercise tests 247
Functional residual capacity 635, 685, 696
Fungal
   ball 113
      formation of 200
   infections 291, 295, 429, 703
   pneumonia 729
   proteases 201
   respiratory tract infection 113b
   rhinosinusitis 113
      allergic 113
      eosinophil-related 113
      invasive 114
   sensitization 200
Fungi 514

Fungus ball 692
Funnel chest 450
Fusarium infections 115, 117
Fusidic acid 139
Fusobacterium necrophorum 143

G

Gallium scanning 290
Gamma-aminobutyric acid 614
Gamma-glutamyl transpeptidase 405
Gangrene, pulmonary 129
Gases
    absorption 665
    exchange 2, 563, 698
        abnormalities 513, 712, 713
    flow of 11
    gangrene 631
    laws 8
    molecules 6
    physical properties of 5
    pressure 7
    properties of 4
    solution and tension 10
    volumes, expression of 11
Gastric acid 196
Gastric retention 614
Gastroesophageal reflux 151, 233, 650
    disease 163, 277, 706, 706*b*
Gastrointestinal
    bleeding 509, 522, 523
    decontamination 536
    disease 522, 706
    tract 169, 188
        manifestations 299
        tuberculosis of 81
    tuberculosis 62
Gaucher's disease 290, 307, 308, 467
Gauge pressure 7
Gay-Lussac's law 9
Gefitinib 416, 678
Gemifloxacin 146
Genetic defects 3
Genitourinary
    cancers 655
    tuberculosis 62, 74, 82
Genome-wide association studies 285
Gentamicin 135, 375
Germ cell tumors 442
    mediastinal 442
Gestational trophoblastic disease 734, 735

Giant cell
    arteritis 461
    granuloma 345
    multinucleated 201
Glasgow coma score 518
Glaucoma 289
Globotriaosylceramide 307
Globulin 188
Glomerulonephritis 400
    idiopathic 455
    signs of 456
Glucagon 539, 592
Glucocorticoid receptor complex 168
Gluconeogenesis 592
Glucose control 520
Glutethimide 538
Glycogen storage disease 467
Glycolysis, anaerobic 37, 38
Glycopyrronium 231
Goiter, mediastinal 443
Gold salts 302
Goldenhar syndrome 604
Gonadal hormones 245
Good's syndrome 148
Goodpasture's syndrome 271, 455, 459
Graft-versus-host disease 190
Graham's law 9, 13
Grain dusts 313
Gram's staining 80, 121
Gram-negative bacilli 146
Granular immune complex 459
Granulocytosis 399
Granuloma
    eosinophilic 267
    formation 640
Granulomatosis 457
    eosinophilic 298, 460
    lymphomatoid 425
    treatment of 459
Granulomatous
    diseases 368
    inflammation 286-288, 290
    vasculitis, antineutrophil cytoplasmic
        antibody-associated 455
Great vessels 16, 436
Ground-glass
    attenuation 431
    opacity 277
Growth
    hormones 592
    stimulatory pathways 383

Guillain-Barré syndrome 500, 699
Gut dialysis 536
Gynecomastia 402

H

H1N1 464
Haemophilus influenzae 124, 132-134, 138, 139, 236, 260, 650, 652, 726
Halo sign 116, 431
Haloperidol 620
Hamartoma 429
Hamazaki-Wesenberg bodies 287
Hand hygiene 119
Hard metal 345
    lung disease 344
Headache 233, 234, 728
Headcheese sign 314
Healthcare-associated pneumonia 118, 726
Heart 16, 394, 436, 680
    disease 38, 467, 753
        congenital 467, 475
        coronary 194
        ischemic 712
    failure 392, 455, 498, 695, 695*b*, 697, 727
        chronic 500
        congestive 163, 529
        diffusion abnormalities 696
        sleep abnormalities 697
        ventilatory abnormalities 696
    involvement 458
    rate 29, 550, 552
    rhythm 550
Heat stroke 546
Heavy metals 539
Heliox 13
    therapy 175
Helium 4, 13
Hemagglutination inhibition 719
Hematochezia 523
Hematological disorders 467
Hematological syndromes 399
Hematology 633
Hematoma 429
Hemiazygos vein 436
Hemodialysis 93, 536
Hemoglobin 245
Hemolytic anemia
    chronic 467
    Coombs-positive 676

Hemoptysis 16, 51, 391, 730, 756
    massive 756
    mechanisms of 51
Hemorrhage
    alveolar 454, 458, 463, 688
    bland pulmonary 455
    diffuse pulmonary 306
    gastrointestinal 484
    idiopathic pulmonary 455
    intracerebral 532
    pulmonary 306, 666, 690
    subarachnoid 532
Hemorrhagic telangiectasias, hereditary 483
Hemosiderosis, idiopathic pulmonary 310, 465
Henderson-Hasselbalch equation 33, 34, 34*t*
Henoch-Schönlein purpura 455
Henry's law 9, 10
Heophylline 196
Heparin therapy, regimens of 479*t*
Hepatic disease 616
Hepatic disorders 709
Hepatic tuberculosis 84, 85
    clinical diagnosis of 84
Hepatitis
    acute 290
    B surface antigen 422
    C virus 422
    drug induced 94
Hepatopulmonary syndrome 710, 710*b*, 711*t*
    clinical features 710
    diagnosis 710
    treatment 711
Hepatotoxicity 93
    drug induced 93
Herd immunity effects 111
Hermansky-Pudlak syndrome 308
Heroin exposure 302
Herpes zoster infection 97
High cuff pressure 264
High flow nasal cannula 504
High molecular weight compounds 355
High positive end expiratory pressures 439
High resolution computed tomography 276, 277, 364, 376
    findings 314
    imaging 290
    scan 314, 349, 370

High-attenuation mucoid impaction 204f
High-resolution computed tomography
    277t, 314t, 456, 682
  abnormalities 692b
Hilar lymph nodes 336
Hip replacement 475
Histiocytosis, pulmonary 467
Histoplasma 126
  capsulatum 303
Histoplasmosis 291, 295, 429, 642, 742
Hodgkin's disease 301
Hodgkin's lymphoma 420, 423, 444
  nodular sclerosing type of 444
Hormone
  adrenocorticotropic 591
  replacement therapy 475
Horner's syndrome 19, 394, 667
Hospital-acquired pneumonia 118, 726
  prevention of 119
Host's genome 140
Host's immune response 95, 594
Household air pollution 214, 381
Human disease 103
  clinical features 103
  diagnosis 104
  treatment 105
Human immunodeficiency virus 41, 53, 74,
    95, 96, 98, 125, 422, 467, 640, 726
  disease, risk of 100
  infection 6b, 95-97, 117, 253, 338, 382,
    645
  treatment of 99
Human plasma 36
Humidity 10
Humoral immunity 49
Hydatidiform, benign 735
Hydralazine 302
Hydrochloric acid 39, 367
Hydrocortisone 188
Hydrogen 4
  ions 33
  peroxide 161
  potential of 32, 34t, 241
Hydromorphone 613, 614
Hydrostatic equilibrium model 637
Hydrothorax, hepatic 709
Hydroxychloroquine 292
Hydroxyurea 374
Hyperbaric oxygen 629, 630, 633
  beneficial effects of 629
  complications 634

contraindications 633
indications 630
mechanism of action of 629
rationale of 628
therapy 628, 629, 634
Hypercalcemia 396, 538, 676
  nonmetastatic 402
Hypercalcitonemia 402
Hypercapnia 19, 173, 227, 243
  arterial 498
  nocturnal 702
Hypercapnic respiratory failure 502,
    575, 602
Hypercarbia 242, 700
Hypereosinophilic syndrome 296, 300,
    303
  idiopathic 295
Hypergammaglobulinemia 271
Hyperglycemia 197
Hyperkalemia 527, 528, 538
Hypermagnesemia 538
Hypernatremia 536
Hyperosmolar hyperglycemic state 531
Hyperparathyroidism
  primary 742
  secondary 742
Hyperplasia
  atypical adenomatous 385
  neuroendocrine 388
Hyperresponsiveness 168
  bronchial 149, 164, 696
Hypersensitivity 243
  disorders 362t
  pneumonia 291, 295
  pneumonitis 200, 267, 315, 361, 364b,
    366, 368
    clinical presentation 363
    diagnosis 364
    etiology 361
    management and prevention 365
    pathogenesis 362
    pathology 363
    prognosis 366
  skin tests 161
Hypertension 194, 495, 601, 712
  chronic thromboembolic 467, 469
  portal 467
  portopulmonary 711, 711t
  progressive pulmonary 694
  pulmonary venous 466, 553
  severe 243

Hyperthermia 546
   management 547
Hyperthyroidism 243, 402, 699
Hypertrichosis lanuginose, acquired 402
Hypertrophic subaortic stenosis, idiopathic 742
Hyperventilation 37
Hypervitaminosis D 742
Hypoalbuminemia, prevalence of 36
Hypoglycemia 38, 402, 527, 676
Hypokalemia 38, 197, 536
Hypomagnesemia 38, 197, 527
Hypopharyngeal misplacements 586
Hypophosphatemia 38
Hypopnea 490, 494
   syndrome 493, 494
Hypotension 503, 543, 614, 716
   arterial 515
   sepsis induced 514, 519
Hypothermia 544, 727
   epidemiology 545
   pathophysiological changes 545
   treatment 545
Hypothyroidism 699, 705
   treatment of 705
Hypouricemia 400
Hypoventilation 490, 491, 498
   diagnosis of 491
   disorders, alveolar 467
   nocturnal 488
Hypoxemia 227, 235, 331, 482, 484, 488, 492, 502, 506, 689, 700, 707, 713
   acute reversible 688, 690
   arterial 707, 713
   syndromes 491
   syndromes, diagnosis of 491
Hypoxemic failure 502
Hypoxemic respiratory failure 500, 576
   primary mechanism of 501f
Hypoxia 18, 549, 554, 669, 697
   mild 502
   presence of 224
Hypoxic respiratory failure 602

I

Idiopathic nonspecific interstitial pneumonia 267, 275, 278
   diagnosis 279
   etiology 278
   prognosis 279
   signs 279
   symptoms 279
   treatment 279
Idiopathic pleuroparenchymal fibroelastosis 267, 275, 283
   diagnosis 283
   treatment 283
Idiopathic pulmonary fibrosis 253, 267, 268, 275, 276, 295, 328, 375, 382, 455, 500, 706, 742
   acute exacerbation of 273
   diagnosis 277
   epidemiology 276
   etiology 276
   prognosis 278
   signs 277
   symptoms 277
   treatment 278
Idiopathic pulmonary ossification 742
Imatinib 678
Imipenem 123
Imipramine 302
Immune cells 155
   activation of 155
Immune deficiency 133
Immune reconstitution inflammatory syndrome 76, 100
Immune system 44
Immunity
   adaptive 48
   cell mediated 45, 48
   innate 47, 48
Immunoglobulin
   A nephropathy 313
   E antibodies 153
Immunotherapy 409, 413
   allergen specific 169, 177
   contraindications of 178b
   indications of 178b
   subcutaneous 182
   sublingual 182
Incremental shuttle walk test 247
Indacaterol 231
Indoor air pollutants 150
Indwelling central vein catheter 475
Indwelling pleural catheter 677
Infarction, pulmonary 429, 666, 707
Infections 151, 260, 267, 303, 464, 608, 691
   bacterial 139, 240
   chronic 649
   prevention of 111

severity of 108
tuberculous 81
Inflammation 314
  chronic 154
  effector cells of 154
Inflammatory cells 196, 201, 509, 649
Inflammatory disease 153
Influenza 151, 728
  A 464
  clinical presentation of 728
  diagnosis 728
  effects on pregnancy 729
  fetal effects 729
  management 728
  prevention 728
  vaccination 111, 728
  vaccine 237
  virus 728
Inhalational bronchiolitis obliterans 370
Inhalational injury 313
  clinical presentation of 368
  determinants of 367
Inhalational therapy 187
Inhaled steroids, high doses of 188
Injuries
  environmental 535, 544
  inhalation 508
Innate lymphoid cells 156
Innominate veins 436
Insomnia 193, 489
Inspiratory positive airway pressure 572
Inspired oxygen, fraction of 175f
Intensive care unit 526, 542b, 548, 550, 552, 553, 578, 591, 758
  costs of 621
  management in 176
Intercellular-cellular adhesion molecule-1 219
Intercostal tube drainage 662
Interferon 678
  gamma release assays 98
Interleukins 678
International Association for Study of Lung Cancer 386
International Classification of Radiographs 336
International Classification of Sleep Disorders 488
International Labour Organization 336
Interstitial lung disease 266, 275, 295, 312, 315, 321, 418, 467, 468, 500, 666, 682, 684, 691-693

acute exacerbation of 273
causes of 267b
classification 266
diffuse 266
epidemiology 268
etiology 266
idiopathic group of 275
pathogenesis 268
pathology 268
primary 266
secondary 266
Interstitial pneumonia
  chronic 291
  major idiopathic 267
  nonspecific 267, 278, 685
Interstitial pneumonitis, lymphocytic 687
Intestinal pseudo-obstruction 402
Intracellular leukocyte killing 631
Intrauterine death 731
Intravenous drug abuse 650
Iodopovidone 662
Ipratropium 174, 231
  bromide 198
Iridocyclitis 456
Iron
  deficiency anemia 484
  overload 113
Ischemia 30
Isocyanate exposure 455
Isoniazid 42, 63-65, 75, 93, 94, 99, 105, 302, 645
  high dose 88
  prophylaxis 732
Isoprostanes 161

J

Joint tuberculosis 74, 76
  treatment of 79
Jugular venous pressure 553

K

Kanamycin 60, 88, 96, 99
Kaposi's sarcoma 21, 670
Keratitis 459
Keratoconjunctivitis sicca 686
Ketone production 592
Kidney 517
  failure 113
Klebsiella 124, 134
  pneumoniae 126

Knee replacement 475
Kussmaul respiration 37
Kyphoscoliosis 447, 448, 468, 492

L

Lactate dehydrogenase 422, 681, 739
    levels of 530
    low 649
Lactation 91
Lactic acidosis 173, 400
Lactoferrin 3
Lambda sign 290
Lambert-Beer law 582
Lambert-Eaton myasthenic syndrome 397, 402
Lane-Hamilton syndrome 311
Langerhans cell
    granulomatosis 301
    histiocytosis 253, 295
        pulmonary 270
Large-cell carcinoma 385, 387, 392
Laryngeal edema, acute 260
Laryngeal nerve palsy, recurrent 393
Laryngitis 368
Laryngoscopy 605
    direct 605
Larynx 19
Latest National Cancer Registry Programme 378
Legionella 108
    pneumonia 703
    pneumophila 726
Lemierre's syndrome 143
Leprosy 290
Leptospira 718
    interrogans 717
Leptospirosis 464, 717
Leukemia, eosinophilic 300, 301
Leukopenia 190, 727
Leukotriene 189
    antagonists 175
    moderators 723
    pathway modifiers 168
    receptor antagonists 189
Levofloxacin 86, 124
Lieomyoma 429
Limb-girdle muscular dystrophy 699
Linear atelectasis 688
Linezolid 88
Lipid soluble drugs 188
Lipoid pneumonia 309, 368

Liposomal amphotericin B 116
Lipoteichoic acid 107
Lipoxygenase inhibitor 189
Liquefied petroleum gas 230
Lithium intoxication, acute 538
Liver
    biopsy 672
    cirrhosis of 113
    disease 93
        alcoholic 93
        chronic 18, 114
        preexisting 94
    dysfunction 418
    failure, acute 524
    function parameters 615
Living donor lobar lung transplantation 273
Löffler's endocarditis 300
Löffler's syndrome 295, 296
Löfgren's syndrome 288, 290
Long-acting beta agonists 167, 232
Long-term oxygen therapy 241, 323, 756
    assessment of 589
Lorazepam 613, 615
Low molecular weight
    compounds 356
    heparin 478, 479
Lower respiratory tract infections 215, 240
L-tryptophan 302
Ludwig's angina 143, 260
Lung 16, 302, 655, 680, 697, 704
    abscess 125, 128, 129, 142, 144, 146, 429, 706
        classification 125
        clinical features 127
        complications 128
        computed tomography 128
        epidemiology 125
        etiology 126
        hematological 127
        laboratory diagnosis 127
        metastatic 127
        microbiological diagnosis 127
        pathogenesis 126
        pathology 126
        percutaneous drainage 130
        prognosis 130
        signs 127
        surgical care 129
        symptoms 127
        treatment 129
        ultrasound examination 128

anaerobic bacterial infections of 141
biopsy 271
bullae 253
cancer 215, 344, 348, 353, 368, 378, 380*b*, 384, 391, 402*b*, 655, 684-686
   classification of 386
   clinical manifestations 391
   diagnosis of 401
   epidemiology of 378
   etiopathogenesis of 378
   local manifestations 391
   major histological types of 378
   management of 407
   metastatic 411
   molecular biology of 383
   risk factors 379
   staging of 401
   treatment of 407, 416*t*
carcinoma 21
collapse 25
diffusing capacity of 27
diseases 22, 55, 294, 295, 320, 327, 633, 665, 737
   ankylosing spondylitis-related 692*b*
   chronic obstructive 18
   eosinophilic 301, 302*b*, 304
   fibrosing 382
   four types of 691*b*
   laboratory tests 739
   obstructive 666
   progress and complications 740
   radiology 739
   restrictive 18
   signs 738
   structural 382
   symptoms 738
   treatment 740
disorders 295
entrapment 657, 663
fibrosis 26
function 167, 229, 686
   aspects of 22
   bedside measurement of 21
   low 160
   measurement of 159
   tests 135, 162
gangrene 125
hematolymphoid neoplasm of 420
infections 138, 144, 392, 692
   anaerobic 141, 142, 146

infiltrates, noncavitating 143
injury
   causes of 513
   ventilator induced 510
involvement 458
lymphoid neoplasm of 420
masses 428
mechanics 563
neuroendocrine lesions of 388
nodules, presence of 484
parenchyma 2, 106, 218, 252, 656
reexpansion 508
resection 25
sliding 667
stretch receptors, stimulation of 696
toxicity, chemotherapy-induced 392
transplantation 140, 278
   advantages of 140
tumors
   pathology of 385
   staging of 389
volume 698
   reduction surgery 238, 256
Lupus pernio 288
Lupus pneumonitis
   acute 688, 689
   chronic 688, 689
Lymph node 436
   biopsy 422
   disease 75
   intrapulmonary 429
   malignant 657
   metastases 395
   peripheral 290
   tuberculosis 75
Lymphadenitis, tuberculous mediastinal 83
Lymphadenopathy 19
   mediastinal 76, 306
Lymphangioleiomyomatosis 267, 270, 467
Lymphangiomas 445
Lymphangitis carcinomatosis 500
Lymphoblastic lymphoma 444
Lymphoid disorders 426
Lymphoid interstitial pneumonia 272, 275, 282
   diagnosis 283
   etiology 282
   signs 283
   symptoms 283
   treatment 283

Lymphoma 78, 291, 293, 420, 421, 429, 655
  Ann Arbor staging of 421b
  mediastinal 444
  pulmonary 424, 687
  workup of 422b
Lysosomal storage disorders 307
Lysozyme 3

M

Macklin effect 665
Macrolide antibiotics 111
Macrophages 220
  alveolar 330
Maculopapular eruptions 288
Magnesium 36
  sulfate 175, 725
Magnetic resonance imaging 404, 405, 433, 437
Major histocompatibility complex 285
Malaise 728
Malaria 464, 714
  important pulmonary complications of 715b
  management 716
  pulmonary symptoms of 716
Malignant pleural effusions 393, 655
  and pleurodesis 655
  diagnosis 657
  etiology of 655
  management 659
Malignant solitary pulmonary nodules 430t
Malnutrition 591, 592
  in critical illness 591
    epidemiology 591
    prevalence 591
Mantoux test 85
Marfan syndrome 253, 450, 486
Marijuana smoking 253
Massive fibrosis, progressive 327, 335
Mast cell 154
  stabilizers 191
Mastocytosis 190
Mastoiditis 457
Maximal expiratory pressure 31
Maximal inspiratory pressures 31
Maximal transdiaphragmatic pressure 700
Mean pulmonary artery pressure 548, 550
Measles 313

Mechanical ventilation 69, 263, 569t, 619, 621
  assist-controlled 560f
  basic aspects of 556
  complications of 568
  controlled 558, 558f
  discontinuation of 621
  general principles 555
  indications of 555
  initiating 567
  invasive 509
  modern 557
  modes of 555, 557
  newer modes of 565
Mediastinal
  abscess 707
  compartments, contents of 436t
  large cell lymphoma, primary 425
  masses, anterior 442
  staging 404
Mediastinitis 439
  acute 440
  chronic 440
  fibrosing 467
Mediastinoscopy 404
Mediastinum
  cysts of 441
  diseases of 438
  imaging of 437
  tumors of 441
Mediterranean fever 642
Melanoma, metastatic 742
Melena 523
Melphalan 302, 374
Memory T cells, role of 49
Meningitis, tuberculous 62, 74, 80
Menorrhagia 82
Mepolizumab 192
Meropenem 123, 135
Mesothelial cells 636, 641, 658, 666, 675
Mesothelioma 642, 674
  malignant 352, 657, 676
  pleural 674
Metabolic disorders 467
Metabolic syndrome 495
Metabolism 189
Metal-fume fever 344, 371
  treatment of 347
Metal-induced asthma 344
  diagnosis of 346
Metal-induced lung disease 344, 345

approach 346
clinical presentation 345
epidemiology 344
pathogenesis 345
treatment 347
types 344, 345, 346, 347
Metallic stents 265
Metastasis 78, 429
component 390
extrathoracic 394
hepatic 395
pathogenesis of 656
staging 405
Metastatic
brain lesion, signs of 21
disease, treatment of 414
malignancy, clinical pointers of 405t
stage, sign of 655
Metered-dose inhaler 231
use of 120
Methacholine challenge 160
Methanol 538
Methicillin resistant *Staphylococcus aureus* 134
Methotrexate 292, 302, 374
Methylphenidate 302
Methylprednisolone 188
Methylxanthines 196, 243
Metoclopramide 597
Metronidazole 543, 720
Micafungin 117
Microalbuminuria 704
Midazolam 613, 615, 756
infusions 615
Middle mediastinum, tumors of 444
Miliary tuberculosis 52
Milrinone 552
Mineral dusts 313
Mineralocorticoid activity 188
Minimal persistent inflammation 156
Minimally invasive adenocarcinoma 387
Minocycline 302, 313, 375
Miscarriages 92
Mites 166
Mitogen-activated protein 675
Mitomycin-C 374
Mitral stenosis 455, 742
Mixed connective tissue
disease 269, 693, 699
disorder 455
Monday morning fever 371

Monitor carbon dioxide 587
Monocyte chemotactic factors 636
Monod's sign 114
Mononeuritis 456
multiplex 402
Mononuclear cell infiltrate 682
Mononucleosis, infectious 642
Montelukast 189, 190
Moraxella catarrhalis 134, 236
Morning dry mouth 489
Morning headache 449, 489, 498
Morphine 613, 756
Mosquito coil smoke 215
Motor neuron disease 500
Moxifloxacin 86, 88, 124, 146
Mucin stains 387
Mucolytics 236
Mucormycosis 114
Mucosa-associated lymphatic tissue 314, 420
lymphoma 424, 424f
Mucosal disease, stress-related 599
Mucosal ulceration, stress-related 599
Mucous glands, bronchial 153
Mucus, production of 3
Multidetector computed tomography 482, 523
Multidrug resistant 67, 123
gram-negative bacilli 124
pathogens 123
Multidrug resistant tuberculosis 73, 86, 97, 645
adverse drug reactions 89
diagnosis 87
diagnostic modalities 87
management 87
new drug delivery system 88
pretreatment evaluation 87
treatment 87
Multilobular infiltrates 727
Multineuritis 456
Multiparameter nutritional indices 593
Multiple organ dysfunction 518
score 516
Multisystem organ failure 516
Muscle
cramps 193
intercostal 2
load indices 624
paralysis 543
weakness 681

Musculoskeletal symptoms 456
Mustard gas 368
Myalgia 456, 728
Myasthenia gravis 455, 492, 500
Mycobacteria 40, 50, 53, 97, 100, 102, 132, 740
   atypical 41, 291
   environmental 102
   nontuberculous 41, 102
   pathogenic 42
   species identification of 59
Mycobacterial cultures 56
Mycobacterial disease 105
   nontuberculous 102
Mycobacterial drug resistance 43
Mycobacterial identification 42
Mycobacterial infection 47, 286
Mycobacterium 41, 286
   abscessus 41
      complex 42
   africanum 41
   avium 41, 42, 102, 104
      complex 41, 103, 105
      intracellulare 139
   bolletii 41
   bovis 41
   chelonae 41, 102, 105
   fortuitum 41, 102
   gordonae 103
   infections, nontuberculous 104
   intracellulare 41, 102, 104
   kansasii 41, 102, 103, 105, 139
   leprae 41
   marinum 41, 103
   massiliense 41
   scrofulaceum 41, 102
   smegmatis 102
   terrae complex 41
   tuberculosis 40-44, 52, 54, 55, 58, 59, 70, 95, 96, 102, 110, 335, 641
      complex 41
      infection 44, 46, 48, 49, 96
   ulcerans 103
   xenopi 41, 103
Mycophenolate 689
Mycoplasma 151, 291
   pneumoniae 169, 236, 313, 642, 726
Mycotic infection 78
Myelofibrosis 311
Myeloid leukemia, chronic 309
Myeloma, multiple 78, 455
Myeloperoxidase 155
Myeloproliferative disorders 467
Myocardial dysfunction 735
Myocardial infarction 475, 547
Myoclonus 399
Myopathic disorders 492, 699
Myxedema coma 530
   clinical and diagnostic features 530
   management 530

N

N-acetylcysteine 272, 539
Naja naja 541
Naloxone 539
Naproxen 302
Narcotic 535, 555
Narcotrend index 612
Nasal
   cannula 606
   cavity 19
   lesion, discharging 19
   polyposis 150, 298
   septum, perforation of 368
   sinuses 19
   symptoms 172, 456
Nasogastric tube 119
Nasojejunal feeding 597
Nasopharynx 19, 302
Nasotracheal intubation 606
Natural killer cells 47
Natural ventilation 69
Nausea 193, 233, 234, 630, 757
Near-drowning 547
Neck swelling 143
Necrobiotic nodules 682
   intrapulmonary 682
Necrotizing fasciitis 631
Necrotizing infections 631
Necrotizing myelopathy 402
Nedocromil sodium 191
Neodymium: yttrium-aluminum garnet laser 422
Neomycin 375
Neonatal intensive care unit 588
Neoplasia 78
Neoplasm 486
Neoplastic disorders 295, 301
Nephrotic syndrome 400

Nerves
  intercostal 436
  peripheral 680
  sheath tumors 445
Nervous system 458, 517
Neuraminidase, inhibitors of 237
Neuroendocrine cell hyperplasia, diffuse idiopathic 385
Neurofibromatosis 253, 311
Neurological disorders 531, 555, 699
Neurological syndromes 397, 402
Neuromuscular diseases 697, 702
Neuromuscular disorders 492, 500, 698
Neuropathy, peripheral 414
Neuropsychiatric derangements 227
Neurosarcoidosis 289
Neurotoxins 524
Neutrophil 155, 219, 640
  role of 219
Nickel 344
Nicotinic acetylcholine receptor 382
Niemann-Pick disease 308
Nimesulide 302
Nitric oxide 161
  exhaled 161
  inhaled 512
Nitrofurantoin 302, 313, 375, 455
Nitrosoaminoketone, nicotine-derived 379
Nitrosourea 374
Nocardia 56
Nocturia 489
Nodular opacities 370
Nodule
  location of 431
  metastatic 21
  necrotizing 338
  subcutaneous 288, 456
Non-*Aspergillus fumigatus* fungi 207
Non-bullous lung 252
Noncaseating granulomatous inflammation 201
Nonchromogens 41
Non-Hodgkin's disease 301
Non-Hodgkin's lymphoma 420, 423, 446
  high-grade 425
Noninvasive methods 404
Noninvasive positive pressure ventilation 243, 571–573, 573b, 574, 575, 577
  application 578
  location of 573
  volume targeted 572

Noninvasive ventilation 175, 504, 505, 505b, 507, 511, 570, 577, 588, 626
  application of 626
  indications of 449b
  role of 626
  technical aspect of 570
  types of 570
  use of 511
Nonmetabolizable ions 37
Nonmetastatic disease, treatment of 414
Non-small cell
  carcinoma 386
    combined 389
  lung cancer 379, 391, 408fc, 415
  staging of 403
Nonspecific bronchial
  hyperresponsiveness 354
  inhalation challenge 358
Nonsteroidal anti-inflammatory drugs 260, 292, 302, 522, 681
Norepinephrine 552
Nosocomial pneumonia 118, 119
  diagnosis 121
  pathogenesis 119
  response to therapy 122
  treatment 123
Nucleic acid
  amplification 58
    cartridge-based 87
    tests 61
    use of 58
  extraction of 61
Nucleotide excision repair gene 382
Nutrition 34, 245, 654
  support
    quantity of 595
    volume of 595
    timing of initiation of 594
Nystagmus 630

O

Obesity 447, 451, 492, 498, 556
  hypoventilation syndrome 451, 494, 498, 500
  morbid 451
  simple 451
Obstructive sleep apnea 488, 493, 494, 697
  diagnosis 495
  pathophysiology 494
  symptoms 494
  treatment 495

Index

Occupational asthma 164, 354, 355
   diagnosis of 164, 357
   management 359
   pathogenetic mechanisms of 357
   prognosis 360
   sensitizer-induced 354
Occupational exposure 333, 336, 381
Ocular disease 459
Odorless poisonous gas 631
Off-target sedation, consequences of 610*b*
Ofloxacin 86, 88, 99, 105
Omalizumab 191
Opiates 508
Opioids 539, 540
   analgesics 613
   mechanism of action of 613
   side effects of 614
Opportunistic infections 98
Opsoclonus 399
Optic neuritis 459
Optical plethysmography 582
Optimal tuberculosis test 62
Oral anticoagulants
   monitoring of 480
   newer 480
Oral azathioprine 459
Oral azoles 206
Oral beta agonists 195, 233
Oral cavity 484
Orciprenaline 194
Organ restricted eosinophilic syndromes 296
Organic dust 313
   toxic syndrome 365, 371
Organophosphate 538
Oropharynx 19, 126
Orotracheal intubation 606
Orthodeoxia 484
Orthopedics trauma 632
Orthopnea 700
Oseltamivir 237
Osler-Weber-Rendu disease 21
Osmosis 14
Ossification syndromes 740
Osteoarthropathy, hypertrophic 399, 402
Osteogenic sarcoma, pulmonary
   metastases of 742
Osteomyelitis 631
Osteonecrosis, bisphosphonates-associated 633
Osteoporosis 227

Otitis
   chronic 457
   subacute 457
Otorhinolaryngology 633
Outdoor air pollutants 150, 215, 381
Out-of-center sleep testing 488, 490
Overlap syndrome 164, 227, 491
   management of 491
Oxidative stress 221, 524
   role of 220
Oximetry 582
Oxitropium 231
Oxygen 4, 250, 506
   administration 174
   analysis 580
   arterial partial pressure of 241, 288
   carrying capacity 550
   delivery, types of 504
   mixture of 13
   partial pressure of 555, 581, 665
   saturation 504
   therapy 243, 249, 471, 496, 504
   toxicity 634
Oxygenation
   abnormalities 32
   assessment of 108
Oxytocin 725

P

Packed red blood cell 526
Pain 754
   assessment 610, 611
      methods 611
   neuropathic 679
   risk profile 611
   substernal 630
Palisading epithelioid cells 682
Palliative therapy 678
Palpitations 489
Panbronchiolitis, diffuse 313-315
Pancoast's syndrome 393, 394
Pancoast's tumor 394
Pandemic influenza infections 106
Panton-valentine leukocidin 464
Papillary dermatosis 400
Para-aminosalicylic acid 88, 92, 302
Paradoxical embolism 482
Paragonimiasis 295, 642
Paragonimus 126
Parainfluenza 151, 313
   virus 260

Paralysis, bilateral diaphragmatic 702
Paralytic ileus 198
Paraneoplastic
   cerebellar degeneration 398
   syndromes 396, 401, 402*b*
Paraplegia 77
Parapneumonic effusion 648
Parasitic
   abscesses 126
   infections 741
   infestations 295
Parathyroid glands, substernal extensions of 436
Parenchyma 263
   necrobiotic nodules 681
   peribronchial 201
Parenchymal lung diseases, diffuse 25, 268, 344
Parietal pleura 635, 637
   fibrosis of 351
   histology of 636
Partial pressure arterial oxygen 175*f*
Patient state index 612
Peak airway pressure 558
Peak expiratory flow 25, 159
Peak inspiratory negative pressure 570
Pectus carinatum 447, 450
Pectus excavatum 447, 450
Pediatric tracheomalacia 261
Pelvic surgery 475
Penicillamine 302, 376, 455
Penicillin 302
   allergy 260
Percutaneous catheter drainage 146
Peribronchiolar alveolar sacs 312
Pericardial fat 436
Pericardiocentesis 84
Pericarditis
   constrictive 83
   effusive 83
Pericardium 394, 436, 674
Periodic acid-Schiff stain 738
Peripheral blood
   eosinophilia 205
   inflammatory 224
Peripheral capillary oxygen saturation 175*f*
Peripheral neuropathy, risk of 93
Peritoneal cavities 636, 674
Peritonitis, spontaneous bacterial 525
Persistent air leak 669

Phagocytic cells 40, 47
Pharyngitis, triad of 143
Phencyclidine 538
Phenothiazine 538
Phenylbutazone 302
Phenylephrine 552
Phenytoin 189, 243, 302, 313, 536, 538
Phosphate, inorganic 36
Phosphodiesterase 552
   inhibitors 234
Phosphorus 422, 593
Photodynamic laser therapy 422
Phrenic nerve 436
   paralysis 392, 393
   stimulation 701
Phthisis 40
Physostigmine 539
Picture archiving and communication systems 434
Pierre Robin syndrome 604
Piperacillin 124, 146
Pirbuterol 194
Piroxicam 302
Pituitary function 226
Plain chest radiography 468
Plant proteins 356
Plasma
   cell dyscrasias 426
   proteins 188
Plasmodium
   falciparum 714, 715
   vivax 715
Platelet-activating factor, effects of 191
Plethora 498
Pleura 16, 635, 680
   anaerobic bacterial infections of 141
   anatomy of 635
   effusion 681
   histology of 636
   physiology 635
Pleural biopsy 644, 658
Pleural canals 636
Pleural cavity 635, 636
Pleural cytology 658
Pleural disease 254, 306, 492, 686, 688, 712
Pleural effusion 53, 76, 348, 648, 655, 685, 688, 692, 693, 705, 707, 708, 713
   chronic persistent 646
Pleural empyema 142

Pleural fluid
    analysis 641, 652, 657
    aspiration 651
    culture and smear 644
    lactate dehydrogenase 641
    levels 659
    nonpurulent 648
    normal 637
    normal volume and cellular contents 636
    pressure of 635
    small amount of 636
    turnover
        pathophysiology of 637
        physiology of 637
Pleural glucose level 658
Pleural inflammation, chronic 641
Pleural involvement 640, 680
Pleural membranes, development of 636
Pleural mesothelioma 348
    malignant 674
Pleural metastases 656
Pleural physiology 638
Pleural plaques 348, 351
Pleural porosity 666
Pleural pressures 701
Pleural space 350
    infections of 649
Pleural thickening 646, 681, 685
Pleural ultrasound 639
Pleuritic chest pain 689
Pleurodesis 256, 660, 662, 669, 677
Pleuroscopy 659
Pneumococcal disease, invasive 111
Pneumococcal infections 109
Pneumococcus 106–108
Pneumoconiosis 267, 291
    environmental 334
Pneumocystis 291, 740
    carinii 116
    jirovecii 270, 286, 671, 692
        infection 112
        pneumonia 730
    respiratory tract infection 116
Pneumolysin, detection of 108
Pneumomediastinum 438, 439
    spontaneous 438
Pneumonia 25, 97, 109, 111, 114, 242, 243, 429, 500, 506, 508, 576, 656, 715, 726, 727
    acute anaerobic 142
    atypical 267
    chronic eosinophilic 267, 295, 313
    interstitial 682
    necrotizing 125, 142, 146
    organizing 281, 295, 315, 375, 429, 683
    pneumococcal 111
    postobstructive 392
    postvaricella 741
    risk of 109
Pneumonitis 142, 681, 707
    acute anaerobic 144
    chemical 341
    chronic
        anaerobic 143, 145
        hypersensitivity 268
    drug induced 691
Pneumothorax 20, 240, 283, 321, 500, 556, 608, 638, 664, 665, 667, 670, 681, 685, 692, 693
    etiology 665
    iatrogenic 671
    open 664
    pathophysiology 665
    primary spontaneous 664, 667, 668, 668*b*
    recurrence rates 668
    recurrent 664
    resolution of 665
    secondary 665
        spontaneous 666*t*, 670
    spontaneous 254, 671
    traumatic 664, 672
    treatment 668
Poisoning 535
Poliomyelitis 699
Pollen grains 166
Polyangiitis 298, 457, 459, 460
    microscopic 339, 455, 456, 460
Polyarteritis nodosa 460-462
Polychondritis 262
    relapsing 262
Polycyclic aromatic hydrocarbons 379
Polycythemia 484
    vera 311
Polyglandular autoimmune syndrome 455
Polymer fume fever 371
Polymerase chain reaction 59, 104, 644
Polymorphisms, genetic 95
Polymyalgia rheumatica 461
Polymyositis 267, 313, 400, 455, 680, 691
    syndrome 691*b*

Polymyxin 124, 375
Polysomnography 495
   nocturnal 490
Polyvalent pneumococcal vaccine 237
Polyvalent polysaccharide vaccine 111
Poncet's disease 78
Portable oxygen 236
Positive airway pressure 493
   expiratory 572
   therapy 495, 496
Positive beryllium lymphocyte
   transformation test 341
Positive end-expiratory pressure 175, 507,
   510, 549, 559, 562, 562*f*, 570
   advantages 562
   complications 563
   indications 563, 564
Positive pressure ventilation 554, 569, 571
Positron emission tomography 271, 291,
   404, 405, 422, 433, 437
Posterior mediastinum, tumors of 445
Postextubation respiratory failure 577
Postintubation tracheal stenosis 257
Postlung transplant 295, 508
Post-polio syndrome 492
Post-tracheostomy tracheal stenosis 263
Post-transplant lymphoproliferative
   disorders 426
Potassium 36, 593
Potato nodes 287
Pott's disease 76, 77
Pott's paraplegia 77
Precursor T-cell
   leukemia 425
   lymphoma 425
Prednisone 188
Predominate 498
Preeclampsia 734, 735
Pregnancy 91
   on tuberculosis, effect of 730, 731
   specific pulmonary problems 734*b*
   termination of 92
Preinvasive lesions 385
Pressure 11
   controlled ventilation 559
      advantages 559
      disadvantage 559
   cycled ventilation 557
   set ventilation 558
   support ventilation 562, 624, 625
   targeted noninvasive positive pressure
      ventilation 572
   volume relationship curve 511*f*
Prevotella intermedia 144
Prima facie obligation 748
Primary lung involvement, overview of
   421
Primidone 189
Procarbazine 374
Propionibacterium 286
Propofol 613, 616
   infusion syndrome 616
Propylthiouracil 455
Prostaglandin 725
Protease inhibitors 99
Protein
   major basic 294
   requirements 596
Proteinosis, alveolar 338, 368
Proteolysis 592
Prothrombin complex concentrate 523
Proton pump inhibitors 120, 599
   role of 120
Protozoa 514
Pruritus 400, 402
Pseudallescheria boydii 114, 115
Pseudoaneurysm 486
Pseudomonas 124, 136
   aeruginosa 110, 124, 132, 134-139, 671
   infection 110
Psittacosis 642
Pulmonary adenocarcinoma, diagnosis
   of 387
Pulmonary airway malformation,
   congenital 482, 486
Pulmonary alveolar microlithiasis 742
   clinical features 742
   etiopathology 742
   investigations 743
   treatment 743
Pulmonary alveolar
   phospholipoproteinosis 737
   etiology 737
   pathology 738
   pathophysiology 737
Pulmonary alveolar proteinosis 309,
   666, 737
   chest roentgenograph of 739*f*

Index

Pulmonary arterial hypertension 467, 468, 470, 548, 551, 553, 554, 685
   management of 552
   preexisting 551
Pulmonary artery 550
   aneurysm 429, 486
      congenital 482
   catheterization 551
   congenital 486
   enlarged 686, 689
   hypertension 18
   pressure 466
   pseudoaneurysm 482
   sling 485
   stenosis 485
      congenital 482
   wedge pressure 466
Pulmonary aspergillosis, chronic necrotizing 17, 114
Pulmonary calcification 712, 740
   causes of 741b
Pulmonary diffusing capacity, measurement of 27
Pulmonary disease 21, 97, 103, 467, 492, 721
   general 488
Pulmonary disorders 721
   preexisting 742
Pulmonary edema
   acute 500
   cardiogenic 576, 735
   photographic negative of 297
Pulmonary embolism 163, 243, 392, 473, 475, 475t, 508, 555, 656
   acute 549
   massive 478
   pathophysiology of 474fc
Pulmonary eosinophilia 294
   toxin induced 303
Pulmonary eosinophilic disorders 294, 295b, 296, 303fc
Pulmonary fibrosis, massive 338
Pulmonary function tests 22, 28, 158, 204, 254, 270, 276, 280, 301, 313, 315, 358, 365, 376, 451, 470, 503, 686, 698, 700
   basic purpose of 24
Pulmonary fungal infections 112
   types of 112

Pulmonary hypertension 226, 254, 306, 320, 338, 466, 467, 486, 548-550, 552-554, 681, 684, 685, 688, 694, 697
   development of 272
   evaluation of 469fc
Pulmonary infections 112
   diagnosis of 116
Pulmonary mycoses 112
   diagnosis of 116
   therapy of 116
   treatment of 117
Pulmonary neuroendocrine cells, primary diffuse hyperplasia of 313
Pulmonary nodules, peripheral 434
Pulmonary ossification, causes of 742b
Pulmonary parenchyma, loss of 485
Pulmonary rehabilitation 245
   program 250
      core components of 248
      role and definition of 245
Pulmonary stenosis, congenital 486
Pulmonary thromboembolic disorders 320
Pulmonary thromboembolism 414, 473, 476, 478, 732
   diagnosis 476
   management 478
   pathophysiology 473
Pulmonary tuberculosis 46, 50, 51, 76, 81, 132, 216
   physical examination 53
   signs 51
   symptoms 51
Pulmonary vascular endothelial activation 527
Pulmonary vascular malformations 482, 482b, 485
   clinical features 484
   diagnosis of 482
   investigations 484
   management 485
   pathogenesis 483
Pulmonary veno-occlusive disease 690
Pulsations, abnormal 18
Pulse oximeters 503, 582
Pupil size 538
Pupillary alterations 538t
Pure red cell aplasia 442
Purified protein derivative 54
Pyloric stenosis 742

Pyogenic osteomyelitis 78
Pyrazinamide 63-65, 75, 88, 92-94, 99, 105
Pyridoxine 91, 93
Pyrimethamine 302

Q

Quantitative sputum cell 160
Quiet eye 289

R

Racemic salbutamol 174
Radial probe endobronchial ultrasound 434
Radiation 295, 374, 381, 392, 660
   pneumonitis 313
   therapy 455
Radioisotope ventilation-perfusion scan 477
Radionuclide imaging 437
Radiotherapy 409, 410
Radon 381
   progeny 368
Rapid eye movement 702
Rapid shallow breathing index 624
Rash 190, 198
Raynaud's phenomenon 269
Reactive airways dysfunction syndrome 355, 369, 369b
Red blood cell 27
   transfusion 526
Refeeding syndrome 593
Regulatory T cells, role of 49
Rehabilitation 245
   team 250
Remifentanil 613, 614
Renal disease 290, 528, 616, 712, 753
Renal failure 37, 456, 712, 727
   chronic 93, 467
   pulmonary complications of 712b
Renal insufficiency 92
Renal replacement therapy 528
Rendu-Osler-Weber syndrome 483
Reperfusion injury 508
Respiration 34
   disorders of 488
Respiratory acidosis, superadded 35
Respiratory alkalosis, 34, 38, 39
   primary 36
Respiratory allergic syndrome, chronic 153

Respiratory bronchiolitis-associated interstitial lung disease 267, 280
   diagnosis 280
   signs 280
   symptoms 280
   treatment 280
Respiratory defenses 3
Respiratory depression 614
Respiratory disease 18, 184, 209, 491
   advanced 755
   chronic 209, 726
   drug induced 373, 376
   infectious 69
   primary 246
Respiratory distress 143
Respiratory disturbances 705
Respiratory dysfunction 709
Respiratory failure 262, 330, 499, 537, 577, 707, 724
   acute 499, 501fc, 505b, 621
   causes of 500t
   chest radiograph 503
   chronic 338, 499
   classification 499
   clinical manifestations 502
   diagnosis 502
   management of 504
   mechanisms 500
   postoperative 577
   symptoms of 51
   treatment 503
Respiratory function 256
Respiratory infections 115, 133, 338
   anaerobic 142
Respiratory muscle 2
   distribution of 702
   dysfunction 622
   function 31
      assessment of 698
      integrated function of 698
      strength assessment 699
   weakness 622, 691-693, 696
Respiratory quotient 592
Respiratory rate 18, 558
Respiratory regulatory system 2
Respiratory secretions 757
Respiratory sleep disorders 488, 493
   classification 493, 494b
Respiratory stimulants 243
Respiratory symptoms, risk of 215
Respiratory syncytial virus 151, 313

Respiratory system 2, 35, 491, 714*b*
   amyloidosis 306
   function of 2, 697
Respiratory tract 2, 3
   infections 172
Restlessness 193, 233
Restrictive pulmonary function tests 349
Reticulonodular opacities 370
Retinal
   perivasculitis 289
   scarring 289
   vasculitis 456
Retinoic acid toxicity 455
Retinopathy, cancer associated 398, 402
Retrognathia 494
Retrograde intubation 607
Retro-orbital pseudotumor 459
Revised National Tuberculosis Control Program 88, 99
Rhabdomyolysis 197
Rheumatoid
   arthritis 21, 114, 267, 268, 313, 455, 642, 680
      pulmonary complications of 681*b*
   factor test, positive 683
   interstitial lung disease 682
   lung nodules, types of 682
   nodule 429, 682
   pneumoconiosis 683
Rhinitis 190, 368, 728
Rhinorrhea 368
Rib 2
   notching 453
Rickettsia helvetica 286
Rifabutin 105
Rifampicin 64, 65, 67, 75, 92-94, 99, 105, 189, 645
   regimen 65
   resistance determining region 60
Rifampin 63, 64
   drug-resistant isolates 42
Rosenberg-Patterson criteria 205
Rubella 313
Rubeola 313
Runyon classification 41
Ruptured emphysematous bulla 670

S

Saccharomyces boulardii 598
Salbutamol 193, 231, 724
Salicylates 508, 538
Saliva 166
Salivary gland tumors 385
Salmeterol 195, 231
Salmonella typhi 716, 717
Samter's triad 148
Saprophytic aspergillosis 114
Saprophytic fungal growth 114
Sarcoid
   galaxy sign, appearance of 287
   granulomatosis, necrotizing 291
Sarcoidosis 21, 78, 253, 263, 267, 285-287, 289, 295, 429, 467, 500, 741, 742
   chest radiographic staging of 288*t*
   clinical features 287
   clustering of 285
   diagnosis of 289, 291*b*
   etiology and risk factors 285
   pathogenesis and immunology 286
   pathology 286
   prognosis of 293
   treatment 291
Saturation point 11
Sauropus androgynus 370
Scar carcinoma 338
Scedosporium
   apiospermum 115
   infections 115, 117
Schaumann bodies 287
Schistosomiasis 295, 467
Schnitzler syndrome 148
Scleritis 459
Sclerodactyly 269
Scleroderma 400, 455, 604, 686
   interstitial lung disease 382
   lung disease 686
Sclerosant, choice of 661
Sclerosis 256
   amyotrophic lateral 492, 699
   multiple 699
   tuberous 267, 666
Scorpion
   bite 544
      treatment 544
   envenomation 543
   sting 543
   venom 543
Secondhand smoke 380
Sedation
   daily interruption of 617, 618
   protocols, analgesia based 618

Sedative drugs 614
Seminoma, mediastinal 443
Semisynthetic penicillins 146
Sensitive molecular tests 61
Sensory neuropathy 398
    subacute 402
Sepsis 243, 508, 506, 514, 518*t*
    clinical features and evaluation 515
    goals of care 520
    management 517
    pathogenesis 514
    prognosis 516
    severe 517*t*
    special considerations 521
Septal
    amyloidosis, diffuse alveolar 306
    erosions 456
    thickening 738
Septic
    embolic abscesses 127
    embolus 429
    shock 111, 517*t*, 521
Serous otitis 457
Serum angiotensin-converting enzyme 271, 290
Serum glutamate pyruvate transaminase 422
Serum glutamic oxaloacetic transaminase 422
Severe exacerbations, course of 173
Sézary syndrome 301
Shock 508
    hemodynamic 632
    hemorrhagic 526
Short-course chemotherapy 63
Sickle cell anemia 311
Silica, substantial amount of 336
Silicomycosis 338
Silicosis 290, 333, 334, 338*b*, 741
    accelerated 335, 338
    acute 335, 336, 338
    chronic 334, 338
    classic 334
    forms of 334
    simple chronic 335
Silicotic nodule 336
Silicotuberculosis 338
Simple weaning 621
Simplified acute physiology score 518
Single-agent adjuvant chemotherapy 677
Sinusitis 150, 298, 456
Six-minute walk test 247, 278, 470, 685

Sjögren's syndrome 267, 313, 680, 686
    primary 687
    pulmonary complications of 687*b*
Skeletal
    disorders 402
    metastases 395
    muscle 222
        dysfunction 225
        function 245
    tuberculosis 62
Skin 288, 302, 680
    biopsy of 290
    changes 456
    decontamination of 536
    manifestations 458
    prick test 179
    rashes 341, 418
    test and serology 358
    tuberculosis 83
Sleep
    abnormalities 702
    apnea 705, 706, 712
        complex 497
        severity of 488
        syndrome 692, 693
    disorder 493
        breathing 190, 467
    history 488
    hygiene, components of 496*b*
    laboratory 589
    questionnaires 491
Small cell
    carcinoma 385-387, 389
    large cell carcinoma, combined 389
    lung cancer 378, 391, 409*fc*, 412
    staging of 405
Small for gestational age neonates 731
Smallpox handler's lung 741
Smelter shakes 371
Smoke inhalation lung injury 372
Smoking, prevalence of 213
Smooth muscle contraction, bronchial 196
Snake envenomation 541
    clinical features 541
    treatment 542
Snake venom 541
Snakebite 542*b*
    treatment 542*b*
Sneezing, excessive 172
Sniff nasal inspiratory pressure 31

Sodium 36
   nitrite 539
   thiosulfate 539
Solid organ tumors 295
Solitary pulmonary nodule 428, 432*f*
   benign 430*t*
   clinical evaluation 430
   etiological causes of 429*b*
   etiology 429
   imaging studies 430
   management 435
   terminology 428
Space travel 325
Specific *Aspergillus* antigens, role of 204
Specific inhalation challenge testing 359
Spherocytosis, hereditary 311
Spinal cord
   compression 395
   injury 492
   transection 699
Spinal tuberculosis 76, 78
Spirometry 22, 25, 159, 258
   contraindications 22
   indications 22
Splenectomy 467
Spores 166
Sputum 15, 730
   cell counts 160
   collection area 70
   microscopy 55
Squamous cell carcinoma 378, 385, 386, 658
Squamous dysplasia 385
St. George's Respiratory Questionnaire 133, 248
Stable asthma
   control of 165
   management of 165
   treatment of 167
Staphylococcus aureus 126, 127, 134, 138, 139, 464, 650
   infection 260
Staphylococcus haemolyticus 650
Starling's forces and lymphatic drainage 636
Static lung volumes 26
Status epilepticus 534
Stenotrophomonas maltophilia 139
Sterile water-filled syringe 673
Steroids 189, 513
   fixed dose combinations of 189
Sting allergy 178

Stinging 192
Streptococcus 143
   milleri 652, 653
   pneumoniae 106, 110, 124, 126, 133, 134, 236, 650, 652, 726
Streptomycin 63-65, 91, 92, 302, 375
Stridor 262, 757
Stroke 555
   acute ischemic 531
   thrombotic 531
Strongyloides 295
Strongyloidiasis, disseminated 295
Subepithelial fibrosis 153
Subglottic secretions, aspiration of 120
Subpleural, basal predominance 277
Sudden extrathoracic obstruction 163
Sulbactam 124
Sulfasalazine 313
Sulfate 36
Sulfonamides 302, 375
Sulfonylureas 302
Sulfur dioxide 367, 368
Superficial venous thrombosis 475
Superior vena cava 18, 436
   syndrome 393, 440, 444, 446
   symptoms of 393
Supraglottic airway
   device 607
   ventilation 601
Surfactant protein-A 740
Surfactant therapy 512
Surgery, abdominal 475
Surviving sepsis campaign 521
Sweating 730
Sweet's syndrome 400
Synchronized intermittent mandatory ventilation 560, 561*f*, 626
Syndrome of inappropriate antidiuretic hormone 397, 402
Synovitis 456
Syphilis 78
Systemetic vascular resistance 552
Systemic corticosteroids 174, 242
   therapy 188
Systemic disease 295, 313, 463
   part of 21
Systemic disorders 467
Systemic eosinophilia 190
Systemic febrile illness 716
Systemic glucocorticoid 311
   therapy 206
Systemic hematopoietic disorders 426

Systemic immunosuppression 41
Systemic inflammation 227, 515
   disease of 221
   response syndrome 514, 529
Systemic lupus erythematosus 264, 267, 313, 335, 400, 455, 456, 463, 680, 687, 699
   pulmonary manifestations of 688b
Systemic perfusion 550
Systemic sclerosis 267, 335, 680, 684
   pulmonary complications of 685b
Systemic steroid 188
   sparing effect 189
Systemic syndromes 402
Systemic vasculitides 267
Systemic vasculitis 339

T

T-lymphocytes 155
   role of 219
Tabin asthma education programs 185t
Tachyarrhythmias
   atrial 552
   low-risk of 519
Tachycardia 193, 194, 198, 546, 601, 716, 728, 735
Tachypnea 18, 476, 716, 733
Takayasu's arteritis 461
Talc granulomatosis 743
Tap sign 543
Tazobactam 124, 135
T-cell
   leukemia 301
   lymphoma 425
Telangiectasia 21, 269
Temperature alteration 537
Tension pneumothorax 500, 664, 672
Teratoma 429, 442
Terbutaline 195, 231, 724
Tetracycline 236, 302, 677
Thalassemia 311
Thalidomide 678
Theophylline 168, 174, 196, 197, 231, 233, 243, 723
   side effects 233
Therapeutic
   drug monitoring 197
   pleural puncture 664
   thoracentesis 660
Thermal lung injuries 367

Thermoneutral water immersion 325
Thiacetazone 65
Thiazides 302
Thoracic
   cage
      involvement 684
      tuberculosis of 453
   cavity 2
   duct 436
   gas volume 26
   muscle cage dyspnea 681
   ultrasound 667
Thoracoplasty 447, 449
   history of 492
Thoracoscopic bullapasty 256
Thoracoscopy 644, 670
   medical 659
Thoracotomy, open 670
Thrombocytopenia 100, 527, 727
   heparin-induced 479
Thrombocytosis 399, 676
Thromboembolism 399
Thrombolytic therapy 480
Thrombophlebitis, migratory 676
Thrombotic disorders 475
Thymoma 442
Thymus gland 436
Thyroid
   disorders 467
   dysfunction, pulmonary complications of 705b
   function 226
   glands, substernal extensions of 436
   stimulating hormone 529
   storm 529
      management 529
Thyroiditis, chronic 313
Ticarcillin 146
Tidal volume 510
Tietze syndrome 452
Tinidazole 720
Tinnitus 630
Tiotropium 231
   bromide 199
Tiredness 730
Tissue
   injury 153
   resident 295
   sampling techniques 434
Titanium 291, 344, 345
T-lymphocyte functions 52

Tobacco
    consumption 213
    smoking 213, 214, 227, 253
Tobramycin 135
Tocolytic 508
    pulmonary edema 734, 735
Tofimilast 196
Total lung capacity 255, 283, 685, 696
Total oxygen-carrying capacity 628
Toxic fumes 313
Toxic ingestion 535
Toxic inhalations 367
Toxicity 197
Toxicology screening 539
Toxin 295
    ingestion 37
Trachea 436, 603
Tracheal ring fracture 608
Tracheal stenosis 259*f*, 263
Tracheal tumors, primary 264
Tracheobronchial amyloidosis 262, 305
Tracheobronchial aspergillosis 114
Tracheobronchial secretions 393
Tracheobronchitis, acute 341
Tracheobronchomalacia 261
Tracheomalacia 259, 261
Tracheopathia osteochondroplastica 262
Tracheostomy 3, 261, 608
    percutaneous 608
    role of 627
Traction bronchiectasis 277
Transbronchial lung
    biopsy 56, 271, 276, 315
    cryo-biopsy 275
Transbronchial needle aspiration 56, 290, 441
Transcutaneous carbon dioxide 590
Transcutaneous oxygen
    measurement 584
    tension 583
Transdiaphragmatic pressure 31
Transthoracic needle aspiration 403
Transtracheal jet ventilation 607
Trauma 492, 508
Treacher Collins syndrome 604
T-regulatory cells 48
Tremor 190
Trench mouth 144
Trichinella 295
Trigger asthma symptoms 163
Trimellitic anhydride 455

Tropical pulmonary eosinophilia 295, 302
Trousseau's syndrome 399
Tube
    placement, confirmation of 606
    thoracostomy 669, 677
Tubercle bacilli 40, 44, 77, 79, 83, 102
Tubercular disease, site of 64
Tubercular pleural effusion 640
    clinical features 641
    complication of 646
    diagnosis 641
    management 645
    medical management 645
    pathology and pathogenesis 640
Tuberculin skin
    reaction 101
    test 54, 71, 75, 98, 290, 644, 731
        positive 290
Tuberculoma 55
Tuberculosis 40, 46, 50-53, 58, 74, 86, 95, 96*b*, 263, 291, 295, 429, 640, 642, 670, 703, 730, 730*t*, 741, 742
    abdominal 81
    characteristics of 338*b*
    congenital 92
    diagnosis of 54, 58
    effects of 731*b*
    endobronchial 263
    irregular treatment of 17
    management of 63
    miliary 267
    molecular diagnosis of 58
    osteomyelitis 79
    pathogenesis of 45
    pericardial 83
    pleural fluid 641
    postprimary pulmonary 50
    prevention of 68
    primary prevention 68
    secondary prevention 70
    tertiary prevention 73
    treatment of 63, 91-93, 339, 731, 732
Tuberculous lymphadenitis 62
    diagnosis of 76
Tumor
    angiogenesis 383
    architecture 387
    benign 163
    carcinoid 385, 429
    diameter, measurement of 389
    malignant 163

multinodularity of 389
multiple primary 390
necrosis factor 509, 719
neurogenic 445
oncogenes 383
size 389
staging, primary 403
Tungsten carbide 345
Tunica vaginalis 674
Tylosis 402
Typhoid 716
Typical carcinoid tumor 388
Tyrosine kinase inhibitors 415, 416*t*

U

Ulceration 368
Ulcerative colitis 313, 455
Ultrasonography, endobronchial 437
Ultrathin bronchoscopy 435
Upper airway 368, 489, 603
 disease 683
 obstruction 257, 683
  acute 259, 508
  chronic 261
Upper gastrointestinal bleeding 522
Upper lobe
 cavities 692
 fibrosis 692
Upper respiratory syndromes 143
Upper respiratory tract 19
 colonization 115
 diseases 368
 history of 17
 symptoms 17
Urea 422
Ureagenesis 592
Uremia 727
Uremic complications 528
Uric acid 422
Urinary nitrogen losses 592
Urticaria 190, 198, 400, 402
 chronic idiopathic 178
Usual interstitial pneumonia 275
 pattern 277*t*
Uveitis 289
 nongranulomatous 288

V

Vaccines 237
Vagus nerves 436

Validated scales and tools, use of 611
Valproic acid 534
Valvular disease 467
Vanishing lung syndrome 255, 688, 689
Vapor pressure 10
Variceal hemorrhage, acute 524
Varicella pneumonia 729
Varicella syndrome, congenital 729
Various sedation scales 612*b*
Vascular endothelial growth factor
 expression of 154
 inhibitors 419, 719
 overexpression of 399
Vasculitis 463, 486, 681
 drug associated 463
Vasodilator therapy 472
Vasopressin 552, 592
Veins, fullness of 18
Veno-occlusive disease 688
Venous thromboembolism 475, 732
Ventilation 2, 587
 adaptive support 496
 assist-control mode of 559
 biologically variable 566
 failure, chronic 578
 high frequency 511, 565
 invasive 505
 mode of 510, 572
 perfusion 501
  mismatch 696
  relationships 2
  scan 469
 proportional assist, 565
 pulmonary 2
 volume controlled 558
Ventilator associated pneumonia 118, 119, 144, 577, 726
 management 123*fc*
 treatment of 124
Ventilatory disorders 321
Ventilatory pump failure 556
Ventilatory support 519
 withdrawal of 621
Ventricular dysfunction 226
Vertigo 190
Video-assisted thoracic surgery 654
Video-assisted thoracoscopic surgery 434
 technique 434
Videolaryngostroboscopy testing 163
Vincent's angina 144
Virchow's triad 473
Visceral larva migrans 295

Visceral pleura 637
    fibrosis of 350
    movement of 667
Vital capacity 288
Vitamin
    A 599
    C 599
    D
        administration, exogenous 741
        deficiency 227
        levels of 169
    E 599
    K 92
        antagonists 480
Vocal cord 257
    dysfunction 163, 261, 706
    palsy, bilateral 264
Voice, hoarseness of 630
Volatile anesthetic sedation 617
Vomiting 233, 234, 630, 757
von Recklinghausen's disease 311, 666
Voriconazole 117

W

Weaning
    index, simplified 623
    outcome of 623
    pathophysiology of 622
    techniques of 624

Wegener's granulomatosis 19, 271, 291, 313, 425, 429, 456, 457, 666
Weight loss 341, 456
Welder's ague 371
Wheeze 163, 261, 263
White blood cells 527
Whole body plethysmography 26
Whooping cough 132
Wood dusts 356
World trade center lung 313
Worsening peripheral edema 241
Wounds, nonhealing 633

X

Xanthines 196, 198
Xerostomia 686

Z

Zafirlukast 168
Zanamivir 237
Ziehl-Neelsen staining 40
Zileuton 189, 190
Zinc chills 371
Zirconium 345
Zygomycetes 114

EU GSPR Authorised Reprsentative
Logos Europe, 9 rue Nicolas Poussin
1700, La Rochelle, France
Phone: +33 (0) 6 67 93 73 78
E-mail: contact@logoseurope.eu

www.ingramcontent.com/pod-product-compliance
Ingram Content Group UK Ltd.
Pitfield, Milton Keynes, MK11 3LW, UK
UKHW050455150426
5217IPUK00025B/1701